Diabetes: Comorbidities, Therapeutics and Insights

Diabetes: Comorbidities, Therapeutics and Insights

Guest Editor

Tomislav Bulum

MDPI

Basel • Beijing • Wuhan • Barcelona • Belgrade • Novi Sad • Cluj • Manchester

Guest Editor
Tomislav Bulum
Vuk Vrhovac University Clinic
for Diabetes, Endocrinology
and Metabolic Diseases
Merkur University Hospital
Zagreb
Croatia

Editorial Office
MDPI AG
Grosspeteranlage 5
4052 Basel, Switzerland

This is a reprint of the Special Issue, published open access by the journal *Biomedicines* (ISSN 2227-9059), freely accessible at: https://www.mdpi.com/journal/biomedicines/special_issues/527D74BU6Q.

For citation purposes, cite each article independently as indicated on the article page online and as indicated below:

Lastname, A.A.; Lastname, B.B. Article Title. *Journal Name* **Year**, *Volume Number*, Page Range.

ISBN 978-3-7258-5557-5 (Hbk)
ISBN 978-3-7258-5558-2 (PDF)
https://doi.org/10.3390/books978-3-7258-5558-2

Contents

About the Editor

Tomislav Bulum

Tomislav Bulum is employed at the Vuk Vrhovac University Clinic for Diabetes, University Hospital Merkur, Croatia's Referral Center for Diabetes, where he currently serves as a Specialist in internal medicine and a Subspecialist in endocrinology and diabetology. He received his PhD in 2010 from the Faculty of Science, University of Zagreb. Since 2020, he has been an Assistant Professor and Scientific Adviser at the Medical School, University of Zagreb. He lectures undergraduate courses as well as Postgraduate specialist and PhD studies in biomedicine and health sciences at the Medical School, University of Zagreb.

He has authored over 100 scientific papers published in Web of Science, Scopus, and Index Medicus-indexed journals, as well as over 90 scientific and professional abstracts, with his work cited over 1000 times. He has served as Guest Editor for 10 Special Issues in MDPI journals, including *Biomedicines, Journal of Clinical Medicine, Diagnostics,* and *Biology.* In 2023, he received the annual award from the Croatian Medical Chamber for scientific advancement in medicine and professional excellence. He is a member of the Croatian Academy of Medical Sciences.

biomedicines

MDPI

Article

Circulating Isthmin-1 Levels and Their Relationship with Diabetes and Metabolic Diseases in Kuwaiti Adults

Eman Alshawaf [1,†], Sulaiman K. Marafie [1,†], Mohamed Abu-Farha [1,2], Ahmed N. Albatineh [3], Tahani Alramah [1], Aldana Albuhairi [1], Yafa Al Qassar [1], Reem Zinoun [1], Rawan Shalabi [1], Sarah Behbehani [1], Dalal Mohammed [1], Fahad Alajmi [2], Mohammed A. Abdalla [2], Ebaa Al-Ozairi [4], Mohammad Shehab [5], Muhammad Abdul-Ghani [2,6], Fahd Al-Mulla [2,*] and Jehad Abubaker [1,*]

1 Department of Biochemistry and Molecular Biology, Dasman Diabetes Institute, Dasman 15462, Kuwait; eman.alshawaf@dasmaninstitute.org (E.A.); sulaiman.marafie@dasmaninstitute.org (S.K.M.); mohamed.abufarha@dasmaninstitute.org (M.A.-F.); tahani.alramah@dasmaninstitute.org (T.A.); aldanalbuhairi@gmail.com (A.A.); yafa.qassar@gmail.com (Y.A.Q.); reemadnan694@gmail.com (R.Z.); rawan-shalabi@hotmail.com (R.S.); sarah.behbehani@ucdconnect.ie (S.B.); dalalomaralk85@gmail.com (D.M.)

2 Department of Translational Research, Dasman Diabetes Institute, Dasman 15462, Kuwait; fahad.alajmi@dasmaninstitute.org (F.A.); mohammed.ahmed@dasmaninstitute.org (M.A.A.); abdulghani@uthscsa.edu (M.A.-G.)

3 Department of Community and Population Health, College of Health, Lehigh University, Bethlehem, PA 18015, USA; aha424@lehigh.edu

4 Clinical Research Unit, Dasman Diabetes Institute, Dasman 15462, Kuwait; ebaa.alozairi@dasmaninstitute.org

5 Division of Gastroenterology, Department of Internal Medicine, Mubarak Alkabeer University Hospital, Kuwait University, Kuwait City 31470, Kuwait; mohammad.shehab@dasmaninstitute.org

6 Division of Diabetes, University of Texas Health Science Center, San Antonio, TX 78229, USA

* Correspondence: fahd.almulla@dasmaninstitute.org (F.A.-M.); jehad.abubakr@dasmaninstitute.org (J.A.)

† These authors contributed equally to this work.

Abstract: Background/Objectives: Obesity and type 2 diabetes (T2D) are associated with significant alterations in various metabolic biomarkers. Isthmin-1 (Ism1) has recently emerged as a potential marker of metabolic health and was shown in animal studies to associate with metabolic-associated fatty liver disease (MAFLD). In this study, we aimed to investigate the circulatory levels of Ism1 in individuals with obesity compared to non-obese individuals and evaluate their association with insulin resistance, MAFLD, and T2D. The primary outcomes of this study are obesity, insulin resistance, MAFLD, and T2D, while the secondary outcome is hypertension; Methods: This is a cross-sectional study involving 450 participants, who were divided based on their obesity status into people with obesity (n = 182) and those without obesity (n = 265). Circulating Ism1 levels were measured by ELISA and were compared between the groups. Insulin resistance was assessed using the homeostasis model assessment of insulin resistance (HOMA-IR), and fatty liver was evaluated using Fibroscan; Results: Our results showed a significant reduction in circulating Ism1 levels in individuals with obesity (p-value = 0.002). Ism1 levels were negatively associated with the odds of T2D, possibly suggesting a protective role. Additionally, individuals with higher CAP scores demonstrated significantly lower Ism1 levels, and the Spearman's rank correlation revealed a negative association between Ism1 and both CAP scores (r = −0.109, p-value = 0.025) and insulin resistance (r = −0.141, p-value = 0.004). Logistic regression analysis further supported Ism1 as an independent significant protective factor against obesity-related metabolic dysfunction. This significance persisted after adjusting for several confounders. Furthermore, our ROC results indicate that circulatory Ism1 levels possess significant diagnostic capability for identifying individuals with obesity-related metabolic imbalances with an area under the curve of 0.764 (95% CI = 0.718, 0.811). Finally, the adjusted multinomial analysis suggested that higher levels of Ism1 may play a protective role against pre-diabetes (AOR

= 0.88, 95% CI = 0.838, 0.925) and T2D (AOR = 0.87, 95% CI = 0.814, 0.934); Conclusions: This study suggests that reduced Ism1 levels are linked to increased insulin resistance, MAFLD, and T2D in obese individuals. Our findings further corroborate the protective role of Ism1 and highlight its potential utility as a biomarker for monitoring obesity-related metabolic diseases.

Keywords: obesity; pre-diabetes; diabetes; MAFLD; metabolic diseases; Isthmin-1; adipokines

1. Introduction

Metabolic diseases refer to a broad range of diseases by which the process where the body turns food into energy is disrupted [1]. Obesity is categorized as a chronic illness where individuals have a body mass index (BMI) of over 30 kg/m^2 with excess adiposity. According to the World Health Organization (WHO), in 2022, one in eight people around the world were obese, a figure which has more than doubled since 1990 [2]. Kuwait ranks among the highest countries in the world for obesity, with a substantial proportion of the adult population classified as overweight or obese. Different organs are impacted by obesity, raising the chance of developing other comorbidities, including type 2 diabetes (T2D), insulin resistance, cardiovascular diseases, and cancer. Additionally, obesity can be influenced by a combination of genetic susceptibility, metabolic pathways, and environmental factors [3].

Insulin resistance is associated with obesity, driven by reduced glucose uptake in fat tissue and muscle and altered hepatic insulin action [4]. Consequently, the combination of increased BMI and distributions of abdominal fat has been shown to enhance the likelihood of developing T2D [5]. T2D is characterized by chronic hyperglycemia emanating from deficiencies in insulin production, insulin action, or both. Management of T2D requires a combination of lifestyle modifications and pharmacological interventions [6]. Obesity, insulin resistance, and T2D are closely linked to the accumulation of excess fat in the liver, leading to the development of fatty liver disease (FDL) [7]. FLD progresses through several stages, starting from simple fatty liver (steatosis) and advancing to metabolic dysfunction-associated fatty liver disease (MAFLD). In MAFLD, fat makes up 5–10% of the liver's weight, which could potentially further progress to metabolic-associated steatohepatitis (MASH). MASH is characterized by severe inflammation that contributes to fibrosis and liver damage [8,9]. It has also been reported that MASH could further evolve to develop cirrhosis, leading to liver failure or even hepatocellular carcinoma (HCC) [10]. Taken together, the various developmental stages of fatty liver highlight the crucial link between metabolic risk factors, such as obesity, insulin resistance, and T2D, and the progression of FLD itself.

One of the key signaling pathways involved in T2D regulation is the AMP-activated protein kinase (AMPK) pathway [11]. AMPK also plays a regulatory role in glycogen metabolism, promoting its production. Other key players involved in insulin signaling are the phosphoinositide 3-kinase (PI3K) and protein kinase B (Akt) signaling pathways implicated in enhancing insulin sensitivity [12]. Additionally, insulin receptor substrate 1 (IRS-1) and phosphoinositide-dependent protein kinase 1 (PDK1) are essential for the overall regulation of insulin sensitivity and hyperglycemia management in T2D [13,14]. The mammalian target of rapamycin (mTOR) is another crucial regulator of insulin signaling that lies both upstream and downstream of Akt. Once activated, it regulates various cellular functions, including protein biogenesis and cell growth [15]. Taken together, the

PI3K/Akt/mTOR pathway is a significant player and therapeutic target for the prevention and treatment of metabolic diseases [16]. Recent studies have demonstrated that Ism1 plays a role in regulating glucose uptake via the PI3K/Akt/mTOR signaling pathway [17–19]. Ism1 is an adipokine that has also been implicated in different signaling pathways, including cancer suppression and apoptosis regulation [20–22]. Recently, Jiang et al. revealed a dual role of Ism1, where it caused increased adipocyte glucose uptake while suppressing hepatic lipid synthesis in a PI3K/Akt/mTOR-dependent manner [23]. This led to improved hyperglycemia and reduced lipid accumulation in mice. This finding suggests a potential therapeutic role for Ism1 to simultaneously treat T2D and FLD, a promising avenue for future research and clinical applications. Other studies have reported reduced Ism1 levels in obese individuals with T2D compared to their non-diabetic counterparts, indicating a potential link between Ism1 deficiency and the development of T2D [24].

Obesity and T2D are highly prevalent in Kuwait and the Arabian Gulf region [25,26]. This study aimed to estimate the correlation between Ism1 levels and several anthropometric and blood biomarkers in the Kuwait population and investigate its potential association with metabolic disease risk factors such as obesity, insulin resistance, MAFLD, and T2D.

2. Materials and Methods

2.1. Study Population

The Kuwait Adult Diabetes Epidemiological Multidisciplinary (KADEM) program is a study conducted at the Dasman Diabetes Institute, which was approved by the DDI ethical committee (Study Number RA-2019-030) and registered on clinical trials.gov (NCT06115876, accessed on 23 May 2022). This study was conducted in accordance with the ethical framework of the Helsinki Declaration. All participants signed a consent form before participating in this study. A total of 450 participants who were either non-diabetic or diagnosed with type II diabetes were enrolled in the KADEM. People with type 1 diabetes were excluded from participation. Anthropometric measures were recorded, including age, gender, and BMI, as well as clinical lab tests evaluating lipid profiles, liver function tests, and glucose. BMI was calculated by dividing the weight in kilograms by the square of height in meters, an electronic weighing scale determined weight, and portable inflexible measuring bars were used to measure height (BMI = kg/m^2), where individuals were classified as non-obese (BMI < 30 kg/m^2) and obese (BMI $\geq$ 30 kg/m^2). Blood pressure and heart rate readings were obtained as the average of three measurements, taken using an Omron HEM-907XL digital sphygmomanometer, with a 5 to 10 min rest interval between each measurement. Participants with malignancies, autoimmune diseases, active infections, endocrine disorders other than diabetes, chronic kidney disease, or those who were pregnant or lactating were excluded.

MAFLD was assessed by a trained specialist using vibration-controlled transient elastography (VCTE) Fibroscan elasticity techniques. To assess clinical variables, participants were asked to fast for at least 10 h overnight for blood samples to be collected for measuring lipid and glycemic profiles, including triglycerides (TG), hemoglobin A1c (HbA1c), fasting plasma glucose (FPG), total cholesterol (TC), high-density lipoprotein (HDL), and low-density lipoprotein (LDL). A Siemens Dimension RXL chemistry analyzer was used for glucose and lipid profiles, while HbA1c levels were determined by the VARIANT™ II Hemoglobin Testing System.

2.2. Blood Processing

Blood samples were collected in EDTA tubes and centrifuged at 400× g for 10 min at room temperature to separate the plasma. The plasma was centrifuged at 800× g for 10 min to obtain a clear supernatant, which was aliquoted into fresh tubes. Plasma samples were stored at −80 °C for future tests. For the ELISA assay, the required plasma samples were thawed at room temperature and centrifuged at 10,000× *g* for 5 min to remove any particles or precipitates. Samples were aliquoted into the appropriate plate layout.

2.3. Measurement of Circulating Levels of Isthmin-1 by ELISA

Levels of human Ism1 in plasma were determined using the Isthmin-1 ELISA Kit (Human) (Cat. No. AG-45B-0032-KI01) from Adipogen Life Sciences, Liestal, Switzerland. Plasma samples were diluted 1:4 with 1X sample diluent from the kit, and an ELISA assay was performed following the manufacturer's protocol. The ELISA plate was read at 450 nm using a plate reader within 30 min of stopping the reaction. Color intensity is directly proportional to Ism1 levels in the samples. The concentration of Ism1 in the samples was extrapolated from the Ism1 standard curve. The intra-assay and inter-assay coefficients of variation (CV%) were less than 10%.

2.4. Statistical Analysis

All analyses were performed using SPSS V.29.0 software (IBM Corp., Chicago, IL, USA). Data were coded and checked for any abnormalities. Categorical variables were presented as counts and percentages, while continuous variables were presented as the median (IQR) to represent the center due to skewness. To test for an association between categorical variables, the Pearson chi-square test of independence was implemented if the expected cell counts for 80% of the cells were more than 5; otherwise, the Fisher exact test was implemented. The Mann–Whitney U test was implemented to compare the median of the groups due to the non-normality of the variables. To measure the strength of the linear relationship between two continuous variables and due to the presence of outliers, the Spearman's rank correlation was implemented. Finally, to model the association between the binary outcome and a set of covariates, multiple logistic regression modeling was implemented, and the receiver operating characteristic (ROC) curve was produced to shed light on the model's predictive ability. Furthermore, the multiple logistic regression model was checked for significance using the omnibus test and for fitting the data well using the Hosmer and Lemeshow test. All tests were two-tailed, and a significant level was set at 5%.

3. Results

3.1. Study Population Characteristics

The investigated sample involved 450 participants, and a comprehensive descriptive analysis of the comparison of an array of variables stratified by the primary outcome of obesity is presented in Table 1. The sample was divided based on BMI and included a total of 265 non-obese (BMI < 30 kg/m^2) and 182 obese participants (BMI $\geq$ 30 kg/m^2). The results showed a significant difference in the medians for weight, BMI, waist circumference, hip circumference, waist-to-hip ratio, wrist circumference, systolic blood pressure (SBP), diastolic blood pressure (DBP), FBG, albumin, TG, HDL, homeostasis model assessment of insulin resistance (HOMA-IR), Ism1, controlled attenuation parameter (CAP) score, aspartate aminotransferase (ALT), alanine aminotransferase (ALT), ALT/AST ratio, Fibrosis-4 (FIB-4), platelet, and aspartate aminotransferase-to-platelet ratio index (APRI) (AST/platelet) between individuals with obesity compared to those from the non-obese group (p-value < 0.05). Additionally, participants with obesity presented significantly increased insulin resistance reflected by a higher HOMA-IR median and a significant increase in the median of CAP scores, while showing significantly lower Ism1 median levels compared to the non-obese group. Furthermore, obese participants showed significantly higher medians for ALT, ALT/AST ratio, and platelets but significantly lower medians for the FIB-4 index and APRI (AST/platelet), as shown in Table 1.

Table 1. Descriptive analysis of biochemical parameters comparing non-obese with obese participants.

	All Participants n [c] = 450 (100%)	Non-Obese (BMI < 30) n = 265 (59.3%)	Obese (BMI ≥ 30) n = 182 (40.7%)	*p*-Value
Gender				
Male	234	145 (62.5)	87 (37.5)	0.151 [a]
Female	216	120 (55.8)	95 (44.2)	
Age (years)	49 (15.3)	48 (16)	49.5 (14.3)	0.099 [b]
Height (cm)	167 (15)	168 (15)	165 (15.6)	0.151 [b]
Weight (kg)	81.7 (25.0)	72 (18)	97 (19.8)	**<0.001**
BMI (kg/m^2)	28.7 (7.7)	25.9 (4.38)	33.8 (5.15)	<0.001
Waist Circumference (cm)	98 (20.5)	89 (15)	109 (13)	**<0.001**
Hip Circumference (cm)	107 (16)	101 (10)	117 (12.5)	**<0.001**
Waist/Hip Ratio	0.905 (0.11)	0.891 (0.12)	0.931 (0.12)	**<0.001**
Wrist Circumference	17 (1.9)	16.4 (1.85)	17 (1.55)	**<0.001** [b]
SBP (mmHg)	126 (19)	125 (20)	129 (16)	**<0.001** [b]
DBP (mmHg)	79 (14)	78 (14)	80 (11)	**0.047** [b]
Heart Rate	76 (14)	74.5 (14)	78 (13)	0.053 [b]
FBG (mmol/L)	5.2 (1.1)	5.2 (1.1)	5.3 (0.97)	**0.032** [b]
Albumin (g/L)	40 (4)	41 (5)	39 (4)	**<0.001** [b]
Total Chol (mmol/L)	5.15 (1.4)	5.1 (1.5)	5.2 (1.3)	0.402 [b]
TG (mmol/L)	0.98 (0.71)	0.83 (0.68)	1.14 (0.77)	**<0.001** [b]
HDL Cholesterol (mmol/L)	1.43 (0.47)	1.46 (0.5)	1.38 (0.41)	**0.026** [b]
LDL Cholesterol (mmol/L)	3.2 (1.3)	3.2 (1.3)	3.2 (1.3)	0.369 [b]
HbA1c (%)	5.6 (0.8)	5.5 (0.8)	5.6 (0.9)	0.066 [b]
HOMA-IR	2.87 (3.2)	2.19 (2.71)	3.83 (3.98)	**<0.001** [b]
Ism1 (ng/mL)	4.11 (7.45)	5.17 (8.28)	3.15 (5.79)	**0.002** [b]
CAP Score	247 (74)	232.0 (62)	275.0 (77)	**0.002** [b]
ALT	28.0 (16)	27 (15)	30 (16)	**0.036** [b]
AST	20.0 (8)	20 (8)	20 (7)	0.192 [b]
ALT/AST Ratio	1.44 (0.61)	1.375 (0.61)	1.556 (0.62)	**<0.001** [b]
Platelet	266 (83)	260 (84)	273.5 (93)	**0.012** [b]
FIB-4 Index	0.65 (0.43)	0.760 (0.35)	0.570 (0.32)	**0.034** [b]
APRI (AST/platelet)	0.075 (0.04)	0.078 (0.05)	0.071 (0.04)	**0.005** [b]

[a] *p*-value calculated using Pearson chi-square test of independence, [b] *p*-value calculated using Mann–Whitney U test due to non-normality of at least one of the groups. [c] The numbers do not add up to N due to missing values. Bold values in the table indicate statistically significant findings ($p < 0.05$).

3.2. Levels of Ism1 Correlate with Various Clinical Parameters

To better understand the nature of the relationship between Ism1 and clinical covariates, we applied the Spearman's rank correlation. Our data revealed a significant negative correlation between Ism1 levels and various parameters, including age, BMI, hip circumference, SBP, FBG, HbA1c, HOMA-IR, and CAP score (Table 2). To further explore the relationship between obesity and various variables including Ism1, we employed univariate analysis (Table 3). Our analysis indicated that Ism1, SBP, TG, HDL cholesterol, HOMA-IR, and CAP scores are significantly and independently associated with obesity.

Additionally, adjusted analysis demonstrated that increased Ism1 and HDL levels have a protective effect against obesity. Specifically, a one-unit increase in the Ism1 level was associated with a 5.6% decrease in the odds of being obese (AOR = 0.944; 95% CI: 0.904–0.987, *p*-value = 0.010). Similarly, a one-unit increase in HDL is associated with a 47.6% reduction in the odds of being obese (AOR = 0.524; 95% CI: 0.314–0.875, *p*-value = 0.014). It is worth noting that the multiple logistic regression model presented in Table 3 produced an area under the ROC curve of 0.764 (95% CI: 0.718, 0.811) (Figure 1), indicating a good predictive ability for Ism1 to discriminate between obese and non-obese participants. According to the omnibus test, the multiple logistic regression model was significant (chi-square = 92.15, *p*-value < 0.001) and fits the data (chi-square =11.92, *p*-value = 0.155) according to the Hosmer and Lemeshow test.

Table 2. Spearman's rank correlation between Ism1 and various parameters in the study participants (n = 450).

Variables	[a] Correlation	*p*-Value
Age (years)	−0.153	**0.002**
Height (cm)	0.045	0.354
Weight (kg)	−0.093	0.055
Body Mass Index (kg/m^2)	−0.143	**0.003**
Waist Circumference (cm)	−0.091	0.117
Hip Circumference (cm)	−0.123	**0.011**
Waist/Hip Ratio	0.001	0.999
Wrist Circumference	−0.009	0.850
SBP (mmHg)	−0.138	**0.004**
DBP (mmHg)	−0.023	0.644
Heart Rate	−0.015	0.753
Fasting Glucose (mmol/L)	−0.140	**0.004**
Albumin (g/L)	−0.013	0.785
Total Cholesterol (mmol/L)	0.039	0.426
TG (mmol/L)	−0.080	0.100
HDL Cholesterol (mmol/L)	0.092	0.060
LDL Cholesterol (mmol/L)	0.034	0.493
HbA1c (%)	−0.247	**<0.001**
HOMA-IR	−0.141	**0.004**
CAP Score	−0.109	**0.025**
ALT	0.006	0.900
AST	0.070	0.152
ALT/AST Ratio	−0.057	0.247
FIB-4 Index	−0.155	0.241
Platelet	−0.018	0.713
APRI (AST/platelet)	0.076	0.117

[a] Due to the skewness of most covariates, the Spearman's correlation coefficient was implemented to down-weight the effect of outliers. Bold values in the table indicate statistically significant findings ($p < 0.05$).

Table 3. Multiple logistic regression modeling showing the association between obesity and Ism1 (n = 450).

Covariate	Univariate Analysis OR (95% CI)	*p*-Value	Adjusted Analysis AOR (95% CI)	*p*-Value
Ism1 (ng/mL)	0.937 (0.902, 0.974)	**<0.001**	0.944 (0.904, 0.987)	**0.010**
SBP (mmHg)	1.020 (1.007, 1.033)	**0.002**	1.008 (0.992, 1.025)	0.308
FBG (mmol/L)	1.032 (0.925, 1.152)	0.574	0.788 (0.611, 1.018)	0.068
Total Chol (mmol/L)	1.043 (0.961, 1.131)	0.317	1.026 (0.904, 1.164)	0.696
TG (mmol/L)	1.439 (1.113, 1.860)	**0.006**	1.132 (0.770, 1.663)	0.528
HDL Chol (mmol/L)	0.524 (0.314, 0.875)	**0.014**	0.685 (0.338, 1.386)	0.293
LDL Chol (mmol/L)	1.144 (0.926, 1.413)	0.213	1.015 (0.758, 1.360)	0.920
HbA1c (%)	1.046 (0.932, 1.174)	0.442	0.986 (0.727, 1.338)	0.929
HOMA-IR	1.131 (1.069, 1.197)	**<0.001**	1.076 (1.001, 1.158)	**0.048**
CAP Score	1.017 (1.013, 1.022)	**<0.001**	1.015 (1.010, 1.021)	**<0.001**

Estimates in the adjusted analysis are adjusted for age and gender. OR: odds ratio, AOR: adjusted odds ratio. Bold values in the table indicate statistically significant findings ($p < 0.05$).

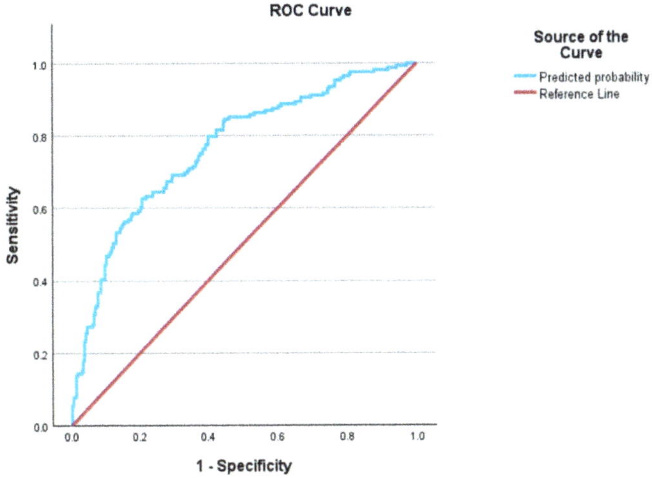

Figure 1. Area under the receiver operating characteristic curve for the model presented in Table 3.

To investigate the significance of Ism1 further, we examined the relationship between T2D and Ism1 with other variables (Table 4). Our analysis indicated that Ism1 and TG are significantly and independently associated with pre-diabetes and T2D. Adjusted analysis showed that increased Ism1 levels have a protective role against T2D. Compared to people with no diabetes (reference group), a one-unit increase in Ism1 resulted in a 12% decrease in the pre-diabetes odds after adjusting for all other covariates included in the model. Additionally, compared to the reference group, people with no diabetes showed that a one-unit increase in Ism1 resulted in a 12.8% decrease in the odds of having T2D after adjusting for all other covariates included in the model. Our analysis implies that higher levels of Ism1 could potentially provide a protective effect against pre-diabetes or T2D compared to people without diabetes.

Table 4. Multinomial logistic regression modeling showing the association between diabetes status and Ism1.

Covariate	Pre-Diabetes * AOR (95% CI)	*p*-Value	T2D * AOR (95% CI)	*p*-Value
Ism1 (ng/mL)	0.880 (0.838, 0.925)	**<0.001**	0.872 (0.814, 0.934)	**<0.001**
SBP (mmHg)	1.011 (0.993, 1.029)	0.249	1.014 (0.991, 1.036)	0.229
Total Cholesterol (mmol/L)	1.180 (0.607, 2.295)	0.625	0.987 (0.352, 2.771)	0.980
TG (mmol/L)	1.958 (1.113, 3.444)	**0.020**	2.934 (1.437, 5.992)	**0.003**
HDL Cholesterol (mmol/L)	0.398 (0.145, 1.094)	0.074	0.378 (0.090, 1.588)	0.184
LDL Cholesterol (mmol/L)	0.787 (0.377, 1.642)	0.523	0.648 (0.215, 1.955)	0.441

* Estimates in the adjusted analysis are adjusted for age and gender. AOR: adjusted odds ratio, the outcome reference group is the non-diabetic one. Bold values in the table indicate statistically significant findings ($p < 0.05$).

4. Discussion

Ism1 is a newly studied adipokine with potential roles in obesity and T2D, in particular [23,24]. However, a comprehensive understanding of its distribution, function, and association with various phenotypic parameters remains elusive. Previous studies reported a link between higher levels of Ism1 and improved glucose tolerance with lower T2D risk [23,24], while others linked the severity of albuminuria to a substantial increase in serum Ism1 in people with T2D [24,27]. The primary cause of such differences and ambiguous correlations might have resulted from differences related to sample size, study design, and population characteristics, in particular an incomplete adjustment for potential confounders. In this study, we investigated the circulating Ism1 as a potential biomarker for conditions of metabolic diseases in a well-phenotyped population of individuals with obesity compared to those without obesity. Our data showed a significant reduction in Ism1 levels in people with obesity, in addition to increases in insulin resistance and MAFLD indicated by increased HOMA-IR and CAP scores, respectively. Our analysis also revealed a negative association between Ism1 and odds of T2D, suggesting a protective role for Ism1 against T2D. Similarly, individuals with high CAP scores showed significantly reduced Ism1 levels, and a negative correlation with Ism1 according to Spearman's rank correlation. As a result, our logistic regression analysis suggests Ism1 as an independent protective factor to monitor obesity progression.

People with obesity, in particular abdominal obesity, are at increased risk of developing T2D and MAFLD [28–30]. Several studies reported that in over 50% of patients, T2D was accompanied by MAFLD [31,32]. Many studies have shown that metabolic comorbidities, including obesity, T2D, dyslipidemia, and hypertension, significantly influenced the prevalence and incidence of MAFLD [33]. In line with other studies, our study sample demonstrated that obese individuals, with a median BMI of 33.8 kg/m^2 and waist size of 109 cm depicting abdominal obesity, were more likely to have increased CAP scores, which is reflective of MAFLD and increased insulin resistance. This group of participants was presented with significantly reduced levels of circulating Ism1 (3.15 ng/mL) compared to those without obesity (5.17 ng/mL). These findings were consistent with those of a recent study by Wang et al., where they reported low levels of Ism1 as an independent risk factor for the development of T2D [24]. However, they did not find a clear link between changes in Ism1 levels and the development of MAFLD in people with T2D [24].

Considering the strong association between Ism1 and obesity, we evaluated the diagnostic potential of circulating Ism1 for obesity using ROC analysis. Our ROC results indicate that serum Ism1 levels possess significant diagnostic capability for identifying individuals with obesity. The area under the ROC curve was 0.764, indicating good predictive ability in distinguishing the outcome. These findings suggest that Ism1 may serve as a promising novel biomarker for assessing obesity-related metabolic disorders and predicting the risk of developing obesity-related comorbidities.

Additionally, our findings indicate that low levels of Ism1 are significantly associated with an increased risk of developing pre-diabetes and T2D. Specifically, compared to people with normal glucose, the adjusted odds ratios suggest that for each unit increase in Ism1, the odds of pre-diabetes decrease by 12% (AOR = 0.88, 95% CI = 0.838, 0.925, $p < 0.001$) and the odds of T2D decreases by 13% (AOR = 0.87, 95% CI = 0.814, 0.934, $p < 0.001$). These results underscore the protective role of Ism1 against the development of diabetes. The significant association implies that maintaining higher levels of Ism1 may be beneficial in reducing the risk of transitioning from normal glucose regulation to pre-diabetes and subsequently to T2D. Given that pre-diabetes is a critical stage where intervention can prevent the progression to T2D, Ism1 could potentially serve as a valuable biomarker for the early identification of individuals at risk. This highlights the importance of further research into Ism1's mechanisms and its potential as a target for therapeutic strategies aimed at preventing diabetes onset.

Some of this study's strengths are the large sample size and the rigorous data analysis and biostatistical modeling techniques implemented. Additionally, the covariates used in the analysis were measured in the laboratory, so there was no recall bias. However, some limitations include the fact that, due to the cross-sectional design, the results can be used only to establish associations but not causations or temporality. Also, the sampling conducted was a non-probability sampling technique.

5. Conclusions

In conclusion, our findings demonstrated an association between T2D and increased insulin resistance with reduced Ism1 levels. Furthermore, we observed reduced levels of circulating Ism1 in people with obesity and MAFLD. Collectively, our findings suggested a potential protective role for Ism1 against obesity and its complications, indicating it as a potential biomarker or diagnostic tool for early detection of metabolic diseases, warranting further investigation into its therapeutic potential.

Author Contributions: F.A.-M., M.A.-F. and J.A. designed this study, helped in writing, reviewed the manuscript, and supervised the experiments. E.A. and S.K.M.—writing, directing the laboratory investigation, and revising the manuscript. A.N.A.—data analysis, management, and statistical analysis. T.A., F.A., M.A.A., E.A., M.S., E.A.-O. and M.A.-G. critically reviewed and revised the manuscript. A.A., Y.A.Q., R.Z., R.S., S.B. and D.M. performed the ELISA assays and analyzed the data. E.A. and S.K.M. contributed equally to this work. All authors have read and agreed to the published version of the manuscript.

Funding: This work was supported by the Kuwait Foundation for the Advancement of Sciences (KFAS) under project RA-2019-030 and registered on clinical trials.gov (NTC06115876).

Institutional Review Board Statement: This study was conducted in accordance with the Declaration of Helsinki and approved by the Ethical Review Board of the Dasman Diabetes Institute (protocol code RA-2019-30 and approval date 3 March 2020).

Informed Consent Statement: Informed consent was obtained from all subjects involved in this study.

Data Availability Statement: The original contributions presented in the study are included in the article, further inquiries can be directed to the corresponding author.

Acknowledgments: We are grateful to the Clinical Laboratory and Special Services Facility at the DDI for their contribution in handling the samples. The corresponding authors had full access to all the data in this study and had final responsibility for the decision to submit for publication. The authors would like to thank the staff at the Tissue Bank and Clinical Laboratory for their assistance throughout this study.

Conflicts of Interest: The authors declare no conflicts of interest.

References

1. Agus, A.; Clément, K.; Sokol, H. Gut microbiota-derived metabolites as central regulators in metabolic disorders. *Gut* **2021**, *70*, 1174–1182. [CrossRef]
2. WHO. Obesity and Overweight. 1 March 2024. Available online: https://www.who.int/news-room/fact-sheets/detail/obesity-and-overweight (accessed on 23 May 2022).
3. Busebee, B.; Ghusn, W.; Cifuentes, L.; Acosta, A. Obesity: A Review of Pathophysiology and Classification. *Mayo Clin. Proc.* **2023**, *98*, 1842–1857. [CrossRef] [PubMed]
4. Wondmkun, Y.T. Obesity, Insulin Resistance, and Type 2 Diabetes: Associations and Therapeutic Implications. *Diabetes Metab. Syndr. Obes.* **2020**, *13*, 3611–3616. [CrossRef] [PubMed]
5. Klein, S.; Gastaldelli, A.; Yki-Järvinen, H.; Scherer, P.E. Why does obesity cause diabetes? *Cell Metab.* **2022**, *34*, 11–20. [CrossRef]
6. Sugandh, F.; Chandio, M.; Raveena, F.; Kumar, L.; Karishma, F.; Khuwaja, S.; Memon, U.A.; Bai, K.; Kashif, M.; Varrassi, G.; et al. Advances in the Management of Diabetes Mellitus: A Focus on Personalized Medicine. *Cureus* **2023**, *15*, e43697. [CrossRef] [PubMed]
7. Forlano, R.; Sigon, G.; Mullish, B.H.; Yee, M.; Manousou, P. Screening for NAFLD-Current Knowledge and Challenges. *Metabolites* **2023**, *13*, 536. [CrossRef] [PubMed]
8. Dam-Larsen, S.; Franzmann, M.; Andersen, I.B.; Christoffersen, P.; Jensen, L.B.; I A Sørensen, T.; Becker, U.; Bendtsen, F. Long term prognosis of fatty liver: Risk of chronic liver disease and death. *Gut* **2004**, *53*, 750–755. [CrossRef]
9. Ekstedt, M.; Franzén, L.E.; Mathiesen, U.L.; Thorelius, L.; Holmqvist, M.; Bodemar, G.; Kechagias, S. Long-term follow-up of patients with NAFLD and elevated liver enzymes. *Hepatology* **2006**, *44*, 865–873. [CrossRef]
10. Loomba, R.; Friedman, S.L.; Shulman, G.I. Mechanisms and disease consequences of nonalcoholic fatty liver disease. *Cell* **2021**, *184*, 2537–2564. [CrossRef]
11. Zheng, T.; Yang, X.; Wu, D.; Xing, S.; Bian, F.; Li, W.; Chi, J.; Bai, X.; Wu, G.; Chen, X.; et al. Salidroside ameliorates insulin resistance through activation of a mitochondria-associated AMPK/PI3K/Akt/GSK3β pathway. *Br. J. Pharmacol.* **2015**, *172*, 3284–3301. [CrossRef]
12. Yan, J.; Wang, C.; Jin, Y.; Meng, Q.; Liu, Q.; Liu, Z.; Liu, K.; Sun, H. Catalpol ameliorates hepatic insulin resistance in type 2 diabetes through acting on AMPK/NOX4/PI3K/AKT pathway. *Pharmacol. Res.* **2018**, *130*, 466–480. [CrossRef]
13. Aierken, A.; Li, B.; Liu, P.; Cheng, X.; Kou, Z.; Tan, N.; Zhang, M.; Yu, S.; Shen, Q.; Du, X.; et al. Melatonin treatment improves human umbilical cord mesenchymal stem cell therapy in a mouse model of type II diabetes mellitus via the PI3K/AKT signaling pathway. *Stem Cell Res. Ther.* **2022**, *13*, 164. [CrossRef]
14. Xiao, F.; Huang, Z.; Li, H.; Yu, J.; Wang, C.; Chen, S.; Meng, Q.; Cheng, Y.; Gao, X.; Li, J.; et al. Leucine deprivation increases hepatic insulin sensitivity via GCN2/mTOR/S6K1 and AMPK pathways. *Diabetes* **2011**, *60*, 746–756. [CrossRef] [PubMed]
15. Le Bacquer, O.; Queniat, G.; Gmyr, V.; Kerr-Conte, J.; Lefebvre, B.; Pattou, F. mTORC1 and mTORC2 regulate insulin secretion through Akt in INS-1 cells. *J. Endocrinol.* **2013**, *216*, 21–29. [CrossRef] [PubMed]
16. Zhang, Y.; Wang, Y.; Luo, M.; Xu, F.; Lu, Y.; Zhou, X.; Cui, W.; Miao, L. Elabela protects against podocyte injury in mice with streptozocin-induced diabetes by associating with the PI3K/Akt/mTOR pathway. *Peptides* **2019**, *114*, 29–37. [CrossRef]
17. Humphrey, S.J.; Yang, G.; Yang, P.; Fazakerley, D.J.; Stöckli, J.; Yang, J.Y.; James, D.E. Dynamic adipocyte phosphoproteome reveals that Akt directly regulates mTORC2. *Cell Metab.* **2013**, *17*, 1009–1020. [CrossRef] [PubMed]
18. Luo, J.; Manning, B.D.; Cantley, L.C. Targeting the PI3K-Akt pathway in human cancer: Rationale and promise. *Cancer Cell* **2003**, *4*, 257–262. [CrossRef]
19. Zhao, M.; Jung, Y.; Jiang, Z.; Svensson, K.J. Regulation of Energy Metabolism by Receptor Tyrosine Kinase Ligands. *Front. Physiol.* **2020**, *11*, 354. [CrossRef]
20. Xiang, W.; Ke, Z.; Zhang, Y.; Cheng, G.H.-Y.; Irwan, I.D.; Sulochana, K.N.; Potturi, P.; Wang, Z.; Yang, H.; Wang, J.; et al. Isthmin is a novel secreted angiogenesis inhibitor that inhibits tumour growth in mice. *J. Cell. Mol. Med.* **2011**, *15*, 359–374. [CrossRef] [PubMed]
21. Wu, Y.; Liang, X.; Ni, J.; Zhao, R.; Shao, S.; Lu, S.; Han, W.; Yu, L. Effect of ISM1 on the Immune Microenvironment and Epithelial-Mesenchymal Transition in Colorectal Cancer. *Front. Cell Dev. Biol.* **2021**, *9*, 681240. [CrossRef]
22. Chen, M.; Zhang, Y.; Yu, V.C.; Chong, Y.-S.; Yoshioka, T.; Ge, R. Isthmin targets cell-surface GRP78 and triggers apoptosis via induction of mitochondrial dysfunction. *Cell Death Differ.* **2014**, *21*, 797–810. [CrossRef]

23. Jiang, Z.; Zhao, M.; Voilquin, L.; Jung, Y.; Aikio, M.A.; Sahai, T.; Dou, F.Y.; Roche, A.M.; Carcamo-Orive, I.; Knowles, J.W.; et al. Isthmin-1 is an adipokine that promotes glucose uptake and improves glucose tolerance and hepatic steatosis. *Cell Metab.* **2021**, *33*, 1836–1852.e11. [CrossRef] [PubMed]
24. Wang, C.; Xu, M.; Feng, R.; Zhang, L.; Yin, X.; Feng, R.; Liang, K.; Liu, J. Serum isthmin-1 levels are positively and independently correlated with albuminuria in patients with type 2 diabetes mellitus. *BMJ Open Diabetes Res. Care* **2022**, *10*, e002972. [CrossRef] [PubMed]
25. Weiderpass, E.; Botteri, E.; Longenecker, J.C.; Alkandari, A.; Al-Wotayan, R.; Al Duwairi, Q.; Tuomilehto, J. The Prevalence of Overweight and Obesity in an Adult Kuwaiti Population in 2014. *Front. Endocrinol.* **2019**, *10*, 449. [CrossRef] [PubMed]
26. Alkandari, A.; Alarouj, M.; Elkum, N.; Sharma, P.; Devarajan, S.; Abu-Farha, M.; Al-Mulla, F.; Tuomilehto, J.; Bennakhi, A. Adult Diabetes and Prediabetes Prevalence in Kuwait: Data from the Cross-Sectional Kuwait Diabetes Epidemiology Program. *J. Clin. Med.* **2020**, *9*, 3420. [CrossRef]
27. Liao, J.; Li, Y.; Gui, X.; Zhang, Y.; Hu, X.; Cheng, L.; Hu, W.; Bai, F. Serum Isthmin-1 Was Increased in Type 2 Diabetic Patients but Not in Diabetic Sensorimotor Peripheral Neuropathy. *Diabetes Metab. Syndr. Obes.* **2023**, *16*, 2013–2024. [CrossRef] [PubMed]
28. Ruze, R.; Liu, T.; Zou, X.; Song, J.; Chen, Y.; Xu, R.; Yin, X.; Xu, Q. Obesity and type 2 diabetes mellitus: Connections in epidemiology, pathogenesis, and treatments. *Front. Endocrinol.* **2023**, *14*, 1161521. [CrossRef] [PubMed]
29. Godoy-Matos, A.F.; Júnior, W.S.S.; Valerio, C.M. NAFLD as a continuum: From obesity to metabolic syndrome and diabetes. *Diabetol. Metab. Syndr.* **2020**, *12*, 60. [CrossRef] [PubMed]
30. Chen, X.; Shi, F.; Xiao, J.; Huang, F.; Cheng, F.; Wang, L.; Ju, Y.; Zhou, Y.; Jia, H. Associations Between Abdominal Obesity Indices and Nonalcoholic Fatty Liver Disease: Chinese Visceral Adiposity Index. *Front. Endocrinol.* **2022**, *13*, 831960. [CrossRef] [PubMed]
31. Alexopoulos, A.S.; Duffy, R.; A Kobe, E.; German, J.; A Moylan, C.; Soliman, D.; Jeffreys, A.S.; Coffman, C.J.; Crowley, M.J. Underrecognition of Nonalcoholic Fatty Liver Disease in Poorly Controlled Diabetes: A Call to Action in Diabetes Care. *J. Endocr. Soc.* **2021**, *5*, bvab155. [CrossRef] [PubMed]
32. Qi, Y.; Fan, L.; Ran, D.; Xu, J.; Wang, Y.; Wu, J.; Zhang, Z. Main Risk Factors of Type 2 Diabetes Mellitus with Nonalcoholic Fatty Liver Disease and Hepatocellular Carcinoma. *J. Oncol.* **2021**, *2021*, 7764817. [CrossRef]
33. Cariou, B.; Byrne, C.D.; Loomba, R.; Sanyal, A.J. Nonalcoholic fatty liver disease as a metabolic disease in humans: A literature review. *Diabetes Obes. Metab.* **2021**, *23*, 1069–1083. [CrossRef] [PubMed]

biomedicines

MDPI

Article

Material Technologies for Improved Diabetic Foot Ulcer (DFU) Treatment: A Questionnaire Study of Healthcare Professionals' Needs

Marian Gabriela Vargas Guerrero [1,2], Lieve Vonken [3], Erwin Peters [1], Jimmy Lucchesi [4] and Jacobus J. C. Arts [1,2,5,*]

1 Department of Orthopaedic Surgery, Maastricht University Medical Centre (MUMC+), 6229 HX Maastricht, The Netherlands; marian.vargasguerrero@maastrichtuniversity.nl (M.G.V.G.)
2 Laboratory for Experimental Orthopaedics, Faculty of Health, Medicine & Life Sciences, Maastricht University, 6229 ER Maastricht, The Netherlands
3 Department of Health Promotion, Faculty of Health, Medicine & Life Sciences, Maastricht University, 6229 HA Maastricht, The Netherlands
4 Bonalive Biomaterials, 20750 Turku, Finland
5 Department of Orthopaedic Biomechanics, Faculty of Biomedical Engineering, Eindhoven University of Technology, 5600 MB Eindhoven, The Netherlands
* Correspondence: j.arts@mumc.nl

Abstract: Background/Objectives: Diabetic foot ulcers (DFUs) are a common and severe complication of diabetic patients, with significant global prevalence and associated health burdens, including high recurrence rates, lower-limb amputations, and substantial associated economic costs. This study aimed to understand the user needs of healthcare professionals treating diabetic foot ulcers for newly developed material technologies. **Methods:** An open-ended questionnaire was used to identify user needs, identify the limitations of current treatments, and determine the specific requirements for ideal treatment. This information was used to develop a list of key considerations for creating innovative material technologies to improve diabetic wound treatment results. **Results:** Most respondents indicated that they followed published treatment guidelines for DFUs but noted that treatment often required a case-specific approach. Antibiotics and surgical debridement were commonly used for infection control. The participants showed a strong preference for wound dressings with lasting antibacterial properties. Respondents identified ideal properties for new products, including ease of use, enhanced antibacterial properties, affordability, and targeted biological activity. The respondents also highlighted the importance of a holistic approach to DFU management, integrating product development with comprehensive care strategies and patient education. **Conclusions:** This study highlights the complexity of DFU care, emphasizing that no single product can address all treatment needs. Future materials could focus on combination therapies and specific use cases. Additionally, understanding global variations in treatment practices and educating users on the proper application of newly developed material technologies is crucial for improving the management of DFUs and patient outcomes.

Keywords: diabetic foot ulcers; osteomyelitis; wound care; wound dressings; material technologies; user needs

1. Introduction

Diabetic foot ulcers represent a significant health burden, characterized by high incidences, recurrence rates, and substantial associated economic costs. Diabetic foot ulcers have an annual incidence rate of 2% in the general diabetic population [1]. However, individuals with established neuropathy are at an even higher risk, experiencing ulceration rates between 5.0% and 7.5% [2]. Throughout their lifetime, diabetic patients face a 19 to 34% risk of developing a foot ulcer. This translates into 9.1 million to 26.1 million diabetic patients with foot ulcers per year [2]. Following the initial ulceration, morbidity remains high. Recurrence rates reach 65% within 3–5 years, and patients experience a 20% lifetime risk of lower-limb amputation alongside a 50–70% mortality rate within 5 years [3–6]. The consequences of DFUs extend beyond patient well-being, imposing a significant economic burden on healthcare systems. In Europe, for instance, annual costs per DFU patient range from EUR 7000 to EUR 13,500, with substantial variations attributable to healthcare systems, treatment approaches, and study methodologies [7]. However, these costs pale compared to the lifetime costs associated with amputation, estimated at USD 350,465–USD 509,2645 per patient [5,8]. DFUs present a global prevalence of 6.3% [9] and are caused by a combination of neuropathy (nerve damage), trauma, peripheral artery disease (PAD), excessive pressure on the foot [10], and chronic kidney disease [11]. DFUs are susceptible to infection [12,13], with over 50% of ulcerations developing an infection [14]. This high rate of infection is attributed to compromised immune function [15], poor circulation [16], edema, neuropathy, and prolonged inflammation, all of which may be present in diabetic patients [17].

The specific classification of a DFU is crucial for providing appropriate wound care and therapeutic interventions [10]. DFUs can be classified as neuropathic [18], ischemic [19], or neuroischemic [20]. Neuropathic ulcers develop due to nerve damage, leading to sensory loss, callus formation, and increased pressure on the foot, often resulting in deep, painless ulcers on the plantar surface [18]. Ischemic ulcers arise from reduced blood flow caused by peripheral artery disease (PAD), presenting as painful, pale wounds with poor healing potential [19]. Neuroischemic ulcers, the most prevalent type of DFUs, combine features of both neuropathic and ischemic ulcers, occurring in individuals with both nerve damage and reduced blood flow [20,21]. A study performed in Catalonian primary care centers shows that the prevalence of neuroischemic ulcers among DFUs was 44.1% while 20.3% were neuropathic, and 20.3% were ischemic [21].

The International Working Group on the Diabetic Foot (IWGDF) Guidelines recommends that DFU treatment should involve a multidisciplinary team to provide individualized care tailored to the complex needs of each patient [22]. This guideline recommends that treatment consists of extensive surgical debridement, antibiotic therapy [23], topical dressings, wound decompression, vascular assessment, and glycemic control [24,25]. Dressings play a fundamental role in the quality and speed of wound healing [26]; however, dressings suitable for chronic wounds, such as diabetic foot ulcers are not currently available [27]. DFUs remain a complex therapeutic challenge despite recent advances in diabetes treatment and wound dressings [16,28,29]. Hyperglycemia in diabetes leads to inflammation, hypoxia, and immune dysfunction, increasing infection risk due to delayed leukocyte migration [30]. Fibroblasts exhibit impaired differentiation and cytokine release, hindering adaptive wound healing [31]. Epithelial cells such as keratinocytes have their migration and proliferation inhibited, delaying re-epithelialization and prolonging wound closure [32]. Diabetes also impairs the signaling of vascular endothelial growth factor (VEGF), which is key in promoting angiogenesis; this affects the growth and function of endothelial cells which are essential for new blood vessel formation [33]. If the wound becomes infected, the healing process is further challenged [34]. The prolonged inflammation in DFUs delays wound healing; additionally, bacteria produce enzymes that break down newly formed tissue and extracellular matrix components [17,35]. These factors underscore the complexity of DFUs and the need for specialized treatment.

Traditional and modern dressings are readily available, although all of them present limitations in wound management [36]. Traditional dressings require frequent replacement due to inadequate exudate absorption, leading to potential tissue damage and increased patient discomfort [37]. Moreover, they tend to create a dry wound environment [38], hindering granulation tissue formation and delaying wound healing [36,37]. Modern wound dressings offer significant advancements in wound healing, including enhanced granulation tissue formation, reduced inflammation, and antibacterial properties [39,40]. However, while offering numerous benefits, they also present limitations. For instance, the moist environment they create can lead to maceration of surrounding skin if not managed properly [41]. Dressings such as foams do not allow us to visualize the wound without removal, and this makes clinical monitoring difficult [41]. Modern wound dressings are also more expensive than traditional dressings [27] and may require a secondary dressing to ensure adhesion to the wound bed. Many new materials used in advanced dressings require complex manufacturing techniques that limit widespread production and availability [42]. Storage can also be an issue, as some advanced dressings may have specific storage requirements or are more difficult to handle than traditional dressings [27]. Given the advantages and limitations of current wound dressings, we decided to explore the user needs of healthcare professionals who use advanced dressings to treat diabetic foot ulcers (DFUs). The poor clinical outcomes of diabetic ulcers in comparison to non-diabetic ulcers [2,43] made it clear that this investigation was necessary. This led us to create a user needs questionnaire to investigate what an ideal product for treating DFUs would resemble from the perspective of healthcare professionals directly involved in such treatments.

This exploratory study uses a questionnaire to ascertain what healthcare professionals and material scientists experienced in DFUs consider relevant when developing therapeutic material technologies and products.

1. First, we inquired about the current challenges, limitations, and unmet needs.
2. Secondly, we inquired about what healthcare professionals consider an ideal treatment.
3. Third, we created an overview of what user needs should be considered when developing innovative therapeutic material technologies to treat DFUs.

2. Methods

2.1. Research Design

The open-ended questionnaire was distributed from January 2023 to September 2023 to purposively sample healthcare professionals and material experts with experience in DFU treatment.

Questionnaire development

The first draft of the user needs questionnaire was developed (MV) based on a systematic literature review of emerging materials for DFU treatment, published by our group [44], and an existing user needs questionnaire by a product manager specializing in biomaterials. Subsequentially, material experts (n = 3) and clinicians (n = 2) were consulted to review and formulate the final version of the questionnaire.

The final questionnaire (Appendix A) included three sections and sixteen questions.

- Section 1 (7 questions): addressed objective 1, which involved identifying current treatment options and shortcomings.
- Section 2 (7 questions): focused on objective 2, exploring the desired user needs of a treatment product for DFUs.
- Section 3 (2 questions): provided respondents with the opportunity to offer additional insights and clarify any points in the questionnaire.

2.2. Data Collection

The questionnaire was distributed by a QR code with a link to a Google Forms questionnaire, through the European Wound Management Association (EWMA), the 14th Pisa International Diabetic Foot Course in Pisa, the Oxford Bone Infection Conference (OBIC), and the Annual Meeting of the European Bone & Joint Infection Society (EBJIS). These channels ensured respondents had experience in the clinical wound treatment field. Respondents could complete the questionnaire on paper or online through a Google Form. Questionnaires filled out on paper were transcribed to the Google Form (MV).

2.3. Data Analysis

The questionnaire data were extracted to Microsoft Excel, and all answers were read by MV and JA to familiarize themselves with the data. Then, MV coded sections of the respondents' answers using the hybrid approach to thematic analysis as described by Feredey and Muir-Cochrane [45]; answers were coded inductively as well as deductively. Qualitative content analysis was applied to further analyze reoccurring themes. The frequency of occurrence of these themes was reported. The quantitative data were supplemented with quotes from respondents. The codes used can be found in Appendix B.

3. Results

3.1. Sample Characteristics

The questionnaire received 29 responses. All respondents had experience in the treatment of DFUs or the development of DFU material technologies. Respondents most often worked in Europe (n = 24; Australia [n = 2], the United States [n = 2], or the Philippines [n = 1]). Most respondents worked in a hospital (n = 19), which was most often a university hospital (n = 12). The other respondents (n = 10) worked in peripheral clinics, as wound consultants, or were self-employed. Respondents worked in plastic surgery, orthopedics, dermatology, internal medicine, or the development of medical devices. Most professionals mentioned they were experts in wound healing (n = 15), and this includes physicians and nurses.

The results presented correspond to the analysis of the information from the user needs questionnaire, which was divided into three sections.

3.2. Section 1: Participant Background—Profiles of Commonly Treated Patients and Wounds Managed

3.2.1. Medical and Demographic Characteristics of Patients Treated for Diabetic Wounds

The characteristics of patients treated by the healthcare professionals (respondents) are as follows:

Age: Sixteen respondents indicated that they generally treat patients above 60 years of age. Ten respondents did not specify an age or just mentioned that all age groups were difficult to treat for different reasons. Three respondents said that young people were more difficult to treat as they wanted to be more physically active.

Medical Status: Many patients treated by the respondents have additional health issues such as cardiovascular disease, obesity, neuropathy, and immune system impairments. These comorbidities significantly affect wound healing and treatment approaches. Out of the 29 respondents, 25 answered this question. In total, 32% of the respondents (n = 8) mentioned that patients treated presented several comorbidities. For the several comorbidities category, obesity was mentioned in combination with cardiovascular disease (twice) and hepatic disease (once). The remaining respondents in this category (n = 5) indicated that patients generally have various comorbidities but did not specify. Cardiovascular diseases were reported by 28% (n = 7) of respondents as common among their patients, followed by obesity at 24% (n = 6), and hepatic diseases at 16% (n = 4).

The respondents noted that medical treatment is often hindered by patients' non-compliance, low levels of education, and low socioeconomic status, which also limits access to available treatment options.

3.2.2. Distribution of Encountered DFU Types

The healthcare professionals who answered the questionnaire indicated that they handle various types of wounds, including neuropathic, ischemic, or neuroischemic wounds located at different pressure points on the foot. Each wound varies in depth, size, and infection status. Ten respondents said they often encounter wounds on patients' toes. Eight respondents did not specify a location, seven found more on the plantar area of the foot, and four found them on the heels.

3.2.3. Diabetic Foot Guidelines

Most of the respondents (59%, n = 17) reported following a published treatment guideline, while 31% (n = 9) indicated they did not follow any guidelines because of the heterogeneity of the patient population. The guidelines referenced by respondents include IWGDF, M.O.I.S.T. (moisture balance, oxygen balance, infection control supporting strategies, and tissue management) [46], T.I.M.E. (Tissue management, Infection and inflammation control, Moisture balance, and Edge of the wound) [47], the Diagnostic Therapeutic Care Path, ESVS Guidelines, the MD Approach, Best Practice Guidelines, and the DF Protocol, as well as various national and international guidelines.

3.2.4. Infected DFUs

Most respondents (69%, n = 20) stated that they commonly encounter infected wounds, 17% (n = 5) said that the wounds they treat are usually not infected, 7% indicated that it is variable (n = 2), and 7% (n = 2) did not answer.

Fifteen distinct treatment options for infection were mentioned, and as respondents could answer more than once, a total of 45 answers were registered. Antibiotics were the most frequently mentioned intervention (31.1%, n = 14), followed by surgical debridement (26.7%, n = 12). Silver-based products (13.3%, n = 6) and antimicrobial dressings (6.7%, n = 3) were also reported. The remaining interventions (22.2%, n = 10) included a variety of approaches such as skin grafts, betadine, negative pressure wound therapy, honey, Granudacyn solution, topical oxygen therapy, and iodine.

3.2.5. Wound Healing Time

Respondents mentioned that wound healing time depends on multiple factors as illustrated by the following quote:

> *"Healing time is often related to the type of ulcer (...). The factors that most contribute to the delay in healing are infection, ischemia, compliance, and I would add the process of management."* [P21, wound care specialist]

Some respondents provided an estimated healing time for the wounds they usually encounter; these values were divided into categories by the authors. In total, 31.0% (n = 9) of the respondents did not give an approximate healing time; they mentioned that it varies greatly from case to case. A total of 27.5% (n = 8) of respondents indicated that wounds took between 1 and 3 months to heal, and an additional 27.5% (n = 8) mentioned that wounds took more than 3 months to heal; most wounds taking more than 3 months to heal were specified to be neuroischemic. At the same time, 14.0% (n = 4) stated that the wounds they treat heal between 1 and 4 weeks.

3.2.6. Current Treatment Techniques and Limitations

There is a considerable variation in the products used by medical professionals for the treatment of DFUs, with respondents mentioning a total of twenty-eight different products. Forty-eight answers were recorded, as respondents could provide more than one answer. Silver-based materials were the most mentioned by the respondents (28%, n = 8) in the treatment of infected wounds. Honey-based products were also commonly mentioned (17%, n = 5) for treating wounds with extensive necrotic tissue, as honey provides a wound healing environment.

To achieve non-load bearing on the wounds, respondents often used casting, noting that in such cases, additional wound care products need to be long-lasting (7 to 14 days) to minimize the frequency of cast removal. Respondents also pointed out that the high moisture levels commonly found in DFUs can make it challenging for patches like Urgotul to manage exudates effectively, requiring supplementary bandages. Limitations cited included the availability and affordability of specialized wound care products, as well as the fact that these specialized dressings are not always covered by insurance. Additionally, the need for tailored treatments and dressings at different stages of wound healing was seen as a drawback of current treatment options.

3.3. *Section 2: Material Development*

3.3.1. Medical Professionals' Perspectives on Ideal Treatment Features

According to the respondents, ideal features in material technologies for DFU treatment include the following:

- **Product application**: Medical professionals emphasize the importance of products that are easy to apply and manage, with some suggesting features like color change to indicate loss of functionality.
- **Treatment outcome**: Antibacterial activity is desired, with many respondents indicating a preference for materials that provide antibacterial effects.
- **Health economics**: Treatments should be affordable and ideally reimbursed by health insurance to ensure broader accessibility and adherence.
- **Healing time**: Products that expedite the healing process of DFUs are highly desired.
- **Additional properties**: Other desired properties include moisture control, non-adherence to the wound, breathability, and the ability to determine bacterial types present for more targeted treatment.

Figure 1 shows a more detailed overview of the ideal material technology characteristics mentioned by the respondents.

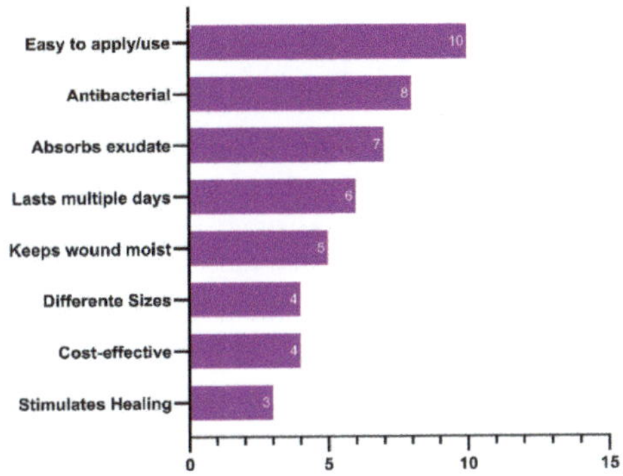

Figure 1. Frequency of desired product characteristics reported by respondents. Data from 29 respondents. Multiple responses were allowed (47 registered responses).

When asked which biological processes should be stimulated, respondents were able to provide more than one answer (see Table 1). They indicated that for effective wound healing, a product should primarily promote processes like angiogenesis (21%, n = 6) and granulation (24%, n = 7), along with re-epithelialization and fibroblast stimulation (14%, n = 4 for both of them). Additionally, 10% (n = 3) of the respondents mentioned that the product should stimulate every process involved in wound healing. Conversely, respondents said that the product should avoid causing adverse effects, particularly inflammation (28%, n = 8) and infection (14%, n = 4), which are critical to prevent. Additional concerns include avoiding the promotion of blood clots and necrosis (with 14% [n = 4] and 7% [n = 2], respectively), as well as minimizing pain and scar tissue formation, and ensuring that the product does not contribute to necrosis (7%, n = 2).

Table 1. Biological processes that are considered essential and detrimental to achieving wound healing according to the respondents.

Essential Product Characteristics	Counts	Detrimental Product Characteristics	Counts
Angiogenesis	6	Inflammation (immune response)	8
Fibroblast stimulation	4	Pain to the patient	1
Granulation	7	Scar tissue	1
Re-epithelialization	4	Blood clots	4
Reduction in inflammation	2	Infection	4
Every process involved in wound healing	3	Necrosis	2

The desired duration of antibacterial properties includes a variety of responses. Most respondents indicated that antibacterial properties should last during the time the material is in direct contact with the wound.

3.3.2. Frequency of Product Exchange

Most respondents (52%, n = 15) expressed they would use a product that required daily exchange if it resulted in faster wound healing. Meanwhile, 24% (n = 7) stated they would not use it, and 10% (n = 3) indicated they would use it depending on the circumstances.

The respondents who answered negatively often mentioned that it is too time-consuming and costly for them to make the change. Respondents who answered "maybe" said they would use the product if the patient could apply it properly and independently. However, they remained concerned about the potential challenges this might pose for patients.

> *"(. . .) we need to consider that patients are usually of advanced age, with poor eyesight and reduced mobility. They will most likely not be able to reach the wound to treat it, they also usually live alone."* [P4, Diabetic foot nurse]

3.3.3. The Most Important Factor in the Wound Healing Process

When asked what they considered the most important factor in the wound healing process, one of the medical professionals said:

> *"It's not just the bandage that heals the patient, it's the diet, physical activity, do they smoke or not? It is a combination of everything."* [P1, Wound consultant]

The need for a holistic approach to wound healing is mentioned by eight of the respondents, as illustrated by the following quote:

> *"The state of the patient, state of the wound, wound pre-treatment, person who treats the wound, material used to cover the wound. Each one of these are key factors in wound healing, together they all contribute to the healing process."* [P22, wound care specialized nurse]

Educating the end users on how to apply the products and their working mechanisms is a recurring topic in the respondents' answers (n = 6):

> *"Education is key, know how to treat the wound and how the product works."* [P1, Wound Consultant]

One of the respondents indicated that current products can be effective when used correctly.

4. Discussion

This study addressed three primary objectives: first, to inquire into the current challenges, limitations, and unmet user needs faced by healthcare professionals and material scientists in treating diabetic foot ulcers (DFUs); second, to inquire into what is considered an ideal treatment for DFUs by these stakeholders; and third, to create an overview of the key considerations for developing innovative therapeutic material technologies for DFU treatment. To achieve these objectives, an open-ended questionnaire was distributed through medical associations and conferences.

Understanding the types of wounds treated by respondents and the context of their patient populations is crucial for developing effective new products. Most respondents treat patients above 60 years of age who have a combination of comorbidities. Respondents also mentioned that these patients usually have lower levels of education, making it difficult for them to follow treatment plans, and they also have a lack of access to treatment options. Consequently, 24% (n = 7) of respondents indicated that patients might not be able to change a product by themselves daily and prefer longer-lasting options that a nurse could manage. Common wound locations mentioned by the respondents were the toes and the plantar area. This information is relevant to determine user and application needs for new material technologies in DFU treatment.

4.1. Product Characteristics

The ideal new product characteristics identified by respondents are consistent with Roger's principles for the diffusion of innovations [48]. Ease of use was the most commonly mentioned feature, aligning with Rogers' concept of minimizing complexity to facilitate adoption [48]. Respondents emphasized that products should be easily adaptable to various wound shapes and sizes, which increases compatibility with the existing practices and needs of healthcare professionals. This adaptability is crucial as it enhances the product's fit within current workflows, thereby increasing the likelihood of clinical adoption.

Cost emerged as another major consideration for the respondents when developing new material technologies, highlighting the importance of relative advantage [48]; new products must be cost-effective to gain acceptance, especially among patients from lower socioeconomic backgrounds who may struggle with expensive treatments. Studies such as the one from Ka et al. (2022) [49] have pointed out that a low socioeconomic level is a barrier to patients' adherence and access to medical treatments. The significance of relative advantage is further underlined by the need for insurance coverage, which can mitigate the financial burden on patients. To achieve this, the newly developed product must show clear evidence of superior efficacy compared to existing alternatives, enhancing its observability by making its benefits more apparent to users [48].

Respondents also pointed out the importance of educational materials accompanying the product, targeted at patients and healthcare professionals. Effective wound treatment options already exist, but improper use due to a lack of education can hinder positive outcomes. By providing these materials, the product enhances its trialability [48], allowing users to learn and experiment with its use in a controlled manner, thereby reducing perceived risk. Education is a well-established behavior change technique [50]; an example of this is an educational intervention carried out by Sikkens et al. (2018) [51]. They performed a study on antibiotic prescribing skills and showed that a targeted e-learning course led to an 11% higher exam pass rate among medical students compared to a control group, demonstrating the long-term effectiveness of educational interventions [51].

In summary, these characteristics—ease of use, adaptability, cost-effectiveness, demonstrable efficacy, and educational support—align with Rogers' innovation characteristics and collectively improve the likelihood of successful product adoption.

4.2. Guidelines for DFU Treatment

There is no single agreed-upon way to treat DFUs, with respondents citing up to 10 available treatment guidelines. Interestingly, 35% (n = 10) of the respondents reported that they did not follow any guidelines and instead tailored treatment to individual patients' needs and comorbidities due to the heterogeneity of patients. In this case, their experience plays a key role in choosing the best treatment.

Implementing DFU treatment guidelines is challenging due to various factors, including resource limitations, disparities in healthcare infrastructure, and the heterogeneity of patient needs. Variability in outcomes, even within the same country, can be attributed to differences in healthcare professionals' training and emphasis on DFU management [45]. In low-resource settings, the limited availability of specialized care and resources further complicates adherence to guidelines [52]. Additionally, DFU treatment often requires a customized approach, depending on factors like ulcer severity, patient comorbidities, and access to offloading devices or surgical options.

Given these challenges, healthcare providers may not strictly adhere to guidelines, opting instead to rely on their clinical experience and judgment. While personalizing care is important, established guidelines based on scientific research [53] advocate for a team-based approach to patient care [54], which can improve outcomes, prevent amputations, and reduce the overall impact of diabetes-related foot disease [25]. This highlights the complex landscape of DFU treatment, where both adherence to guidelines and individual professional experience play crucial roles.

4.3. Infection in DFU

Infections in diabetic foot ulcers (DFUs) are complex [55] and multifaceted. An infected wound in the context of DFUs is generally identified by the presence of clinical symptoms such as redness, warmth, swelling, pain, or discharge [56]. These symptoms can be subtle in diabetic patients due to neuropathy and poor blood circulation [57]. The timing of intervention is particularly challenging, as overtreatment with antibiotics can lead to antimicrobial resistance [58], while delayed treatment of true infections can result in serious complications, including limb loss [59]. Current guidelines recommend initiating treatment when clear signs of infection are present and discontinuing antibiotics when signs of infection have resolved [58], emphasizing the importance of individualized patient assessment.

Reflecting this challenge, 74% (n = 21) of respondents reported that the wounds they treat are often infected and mentioned antibiotics as the most common treatment for infection. Nearly all respondents (93%, n = 27) expressed a desire for products with antibacterial properties, and 33% out of this 93% (n = 9) wanted the antibacterial properties to last as long as the product was in contact with the wound.

Diabetic foot infections (DFIs) affect 50–60% of patients with DFUs [60]. A common pathogen in DFIs is *Staphylococcus aureus*, comprising 20–25% of bacteria isolated from DFIs [61]. *S. aureus* has shown resistance to several antibiotics, including methicillin (MRSA) [62], making it difficult to treat. This suggests a need for wound care products with antibacterial properties that do not rely solely on traditional antibiotics. These products could complement current treatments by having a different mode of action to kill bacteria compared to antibiotics in combating infection.

Debridement, which removes necrotic and avascular tissue [63], was the second most mentioned treatment for infected DFUs. This is a crucial step in treatment since the first stage of a diabetic foot infection by *S. aureus* is the bacteria attaching to surface components of the skin, such as epidermal keratinocytes [64]. Since there are already good methods for debridement, this should not be the main focus in the development of new material technologies for DFUs.

Silver-based products have been used as a complementary treatment for infection in diabetic foot ulcers. This was the third most mentioned treatment by the respondents in our questionnaire. However, the widespread use of silver-containing compounds has led to the emergence of silver-resistant bacteria, including four different *S. aureus* isolates in the study by Hosny et al. (2019) [65]. The potential for resistance development may depend on the specific silver formulation and the exposure conditions. These factors should be taken into consideration during product development.

4.4. Biological Processes in Wound Healing

The respondents indicated specific biological processes that new products should or should not stimulate. Angiogenesis was the most frequently mentioned process that respondents desired the product to stimulate. We understand that angiogenesis is essential for proper wound healing. However, it is important to note that excessive angiogenesis does not necessarily guarantee faster healing and may even have negative consequences [66]. The level of angiogenesis often coincides with the inflammatory response because inflammatory cells produce numerous factors that promote angiogenesis [67]. While inflammation is a necessary part of healing, excessive inflammation can lead to poor healing outcomes and increased scarring [68]. For this reason, it is crucial to carefully tune the material's characteristics. While a few respondents indicated that, ideally, a product should stimulate all processes involved in wound healing, achieving this across all stages of wound healing with a single product is quite challenging. This is one of the reasons why it is important to consider new products and material technologies as pieces of a larger puzzle and to identify other material technologies alongside which they might work well. By identifying complementary products, we can explore the potential benefits of a combination therapy approach.

4.5. Strengths and Limitations

Open-ended questionnaires allow healthcare professionals to freely share their experiences, providing valuable insights into current DFU treatments and their shortcomings. Unlike fixed-choice formats, this approach prevents potential misleading answers and ensures we capture all relevant information. These detailed responses will inform the development of products that align closely with clinicians' needs, are user-friendly, and address existing treatment limitations.

This study acknowledges limitations due to sample size, self-selection bias, and challenges with online surveys. A small sample size and self-selection bias prevent findings from being extrapolated as well as increase the possibility of assuming a false premise as true [69,70]. Finally, the online format makes it difficult to clarify responses, especially for open-ended questions. This can leave unclear or ambiguous data that require extra effort to interpret. While the sample size limits applying the findings to the entire continent, the results still provide valuable insights. They highlight the complex nature of DFU treatment and the importance of a holistic approach.

4.6. Design Recommendations and Future Directions

This paragraph aims to recapitulate the results from our three research objectives, emphasizing the need for material technology innovations in DFU treatment. Recognizing that a single product cannot address all aspects of DFU care, the development of new material technologies should focus on combination therapy and specific use cases. For example, products intended for use alongside offloading therapy should be durable enough to minimize disruptions caused by frequent device removal. The ideal new product for DFU treatment should prioritize features like ease of use, enhanced antibacterial properties for infected wounds, affordability, and targeted biological activity, such as promoting angiogenesis without triggering excessive inflammation. By aligning new materials with these desired characteristics, we can effectively address the limitations of current treatments, leading to improved management of DFUs and, ultimately, better overall patient care. Future research should also explore variations in treatment practices globally, given the differences in healthcare resources [71] and patient demographics.

5. Conclusions

Healthcare professionals pointed out several limitations in current material technologies for the treatment of DFUs, such as the limited availability and high cost of specialized wound care products as well as the need for various treatments and dressings to cover all stages of wound healing. When developing new material technologies, it is crucial to align with the specific needs of users of healthcare professionals. According to healthcare professionals, an ideal product for the treatment of DFUs should feature products that offer long-lasting antibacterial properties, are easy to use, and are cost-effective. Additionally, the education of healthcare professionals and patients emerged as a critical theme, emphasizing the importance of proper technology application and education for optimal treatment results in DFUs.

This study highlights the complex nature of treating diabetic foot ulcers (DFUs). The survey responses suggest that a single, universal treatment solution is unlikely to meet the diverse needs of DFU management. Therefore, when designing new products, developers should not only consider user needs but also how their material technology can work in conjunction with complementary wound healing products.

Author Contributions: Conceptualization, M.G.V.G., J.L. and J.J.C.A.; methodology, M.G.V.G., L.V. and J.J.C.A.; formal analysis, M.G.V.G.; investigation, M.G.V.G., E.P. and J.J.C.A.; data curation, M.G.V.G.; writing—original draft preparation, M.G.V.G.; writing—review and editing, M.G.V.G., L.V., E.P., J.L. and J.J.C.A.; supervision, J.J.C.A.; project administration, M.G.V.G.; funding acquisition, J.J.C.A. All authors have read and agreed to the published version of the manuscript.

Funding: No external funding was received for the execution of this questionnaire.

Institutional Review Board Statement: Not applicable.

Informed Consent Statement: Participants were informed about data usage.

Data Availability Statement: The data retrieved from the user needs questionnaire can be obtained through the following link: https://docs.google.com/spreadsheets/d/1wa4NG0h83wmD5T8WNYUkZb8r5XoVTAI9/edit?usp=sharing&ouid=110983971402187884564&rtpof=true&sd=true (accessed on 22 August 2024).

Acknowledgments: This publication is part of the project DARTBAC (with project number NWA.1292.19.354 of the research program NWA-ORC which is (partly) financed by the Dutch Research Council (NWO)). Grammarly, Inc., was used throughout the writing of this paper as a tool to improve readability.

Conflicts of Interest: The authors declare no conflicts of interest.

Appendix A

User Needs Questionnaire: Diabetic wound treatment

Part 1 (seven questions) focused on gathering background information about the wounds being treated by the respondents and their current treatment methods, part 2 (seven questions) inquired about the desired features of a treatment product for DFUs, and part 3 (two questions) allowed respondents to offer additional insights and address points of the questionnaire that were unclear. Respondents were informed about the study's purpose and the voluntary nature of participation.

Date: ______________________________

Respondent: ______________________________

Field of expertise: ______________________________

Goals:

1. Learn about the different types of diabetic wounds and patients that medical professionals treat, as well as what their ideal treatment for these wounds would be.
2. Obtain input from medical professionals regarding the techniques that they are currently using for the treatment of diabetic wounds and their limitations

Part I. Current Medical Practice

1. What is the type of diabetic wound you usually treat?
    a. Size, position in the body, any other relevant characteristic
        i. If the wound is in the foot, can you specify the area of the foot it is in, as well as the specific characteristics of this location
    b. Are these wounds usually infected, if so:
        i. How do you treat the wound?
        ii. How do you treat the infection?
    c. How do you decide if the wound is infected or not? Do you do a culture? Or do you base your decision in the way the wound looks/smells, other?
        i. Do you need to identify the pathogen in order for the treatment to be effective?
        ii. Do infections cause the wound to be clearly more challenging to treat?
2. What are the demographics of patients that present the previously described wound and the reported comorbidities? Which are the most challenging patient groups to treat?
3. How do you decide the treatment plan? Do you follow a specific guideline?
    a. How do you treat the wound? Can you describe the process? Is there a standard procedure?

b. Which products do you use and why do you use them versus other available products?
c. Which are the limitations you encounter when using these products?
d. How do you keep the product positioned/contained at the wound site?

4. How much time does it usually take the wound to heal? What are risk factors for non-healing wounds?
5. Which type of wounds heal poorly or do not heal?
6. During the wound healing time is the product being exchanged, if so, how often? How often would the ideal exchange time be?
7. If there were a very effective and fast treatment solution that always cleared the infection and healed the wound but required daily exchange, would you use it? Please elaborate on your answer.

Part II. Product Development

1. What would your ideal product be to treat the wounds you usually encounter? Why? How would you like to apply this product?
2. What do you think is the most important factor in the wound healing process? e.g., state of the patient, state of the wound, wound pre-treatment, person who treats the wound, material used to cover the wound...
3. How often should the product be exchanged? If it stays on for 2 weeks, would it be good enough for a wound with a diameter of *2* cm to heal? * wound size previously mentioned*.
4. Should the wound and wound edges remain moist throughout all of the healing process?
5. Which biological processes should the product stimulate (e.g., Clot formation, angiogenesis, fibroblast stimulation, remodeling of granulation tissue, others)?
6. Which biological processes should the product not stimulate?
7. Should the material have antibacterial activity, if so, how long should this activity preferably last?

Part III. Concluding Questions

1. Are there additional properties that were not mentioned previously that you would like to see in your ideal product?
2. Are there any questions regarding this questionnaire?

The data retrieved from the user needs questionnaire can be obtained through the following link: https://docs.google.com/spreadsheets/d/1wa4NG0h83wmD5T8WNYUkZb8r5XoVTAI9/edit?usp=sharing&ouid=110983971402187884564&rtpof=true&sd=true (accessed on 22 August 2024)

Appendix B

Data Analysis: Deductive and Inductive Themes

Deductive Themes: These themes were developed to understand respondents' ideal product characteristics in the context of the patients and wounds they are treating.

Patients' demographics and comorbidities

- Wound characteristics, e.g., healing time, size, and position; this allows us to put answers into context about current product limitations and desired product characteristics
- Presence of infection: to further characterize the wound and assess the need for antibacterial properties in the materials
- Infection treatment: more detail into current medical practices
- Duration of antibacterial activity
- Promotion of angiogenesis
- Promotion of granulation
- Price of the product: important to consider in the design process
- Mode of application of the material: relevant for material design
- Design features, e.g., shape, size, adhesive properties, etc.

Inductive Themes:

- Education of end users on the product's application
- Case-specific approach to DFUs
- Holistic approach to DFU management
- Inflammation control

References

1. Bus, S.A.; Sacco, I.C.N.; Monteiro-Soares, M.; Raspovic, A.; Paton, J.; Rasmussen, A.; Lavery, L.A.; van Netten, J.J. Guidelines on the prevention of foot ulcers in persons with diabetes (IWGDF 2023 update). *Diabetes Metab. Res. Rev.* **2024**, *40*, e3651. [CrossRef] [PubMed]
2. Armstrong, D.G.; Boulton, A.J.M.; Bus, S.A. Diabetic Foot Ulcers and Their Recurrence. *N. Engl. J. Med.* **2017**, *376*, 2367–2375. [CrossRef] [PubMed]
3. McDermott, K.; Fang, M.; Boulton, A.J.M.; Selvin, E.; Hicks, C.W. Etiology, Epidemiology, and Disparities in the Burden of Diabetic Foot Ulcers. *Diabetes Care* **2023**, *46*, 209–221. [CrossRef] [PubMed]
4. Syahrul, S.; Narmawan, N. The risk of diabetic foot complication among type 2 diabetes mellitus patients in Kendari City, Indonesia. *Enfermería Clínica* **2021**, *31*, S713–S717. [CrossRef]
5. Chung, K.C.; Saddawi-Konefka, D.; Haase, S.C.; Kaul, G. A cost-utility analysis of amputation versus salvage for Gustilo type IIIB and IIIC open tibial fractures. *Plast. Reconstr. Surg.* **2009**, *124*, 1965–1973. [CrossRef] [PubMed] [PubMed Central]
6. Yammine, K.; Hayek, F.; Assi, C. A meta-analysis of mortality after minor amputation among patients with diabetes and/or peripheral vascular disease. *J. Vasc. Surg.* **2020**, *72*, 2197–2207. [CrossRef]
7. Waibel, F.W.A.; Uckay, I.; Soldevila-Boixader, L.; Sydler, C.; Gariani, K. Current knowledge of morbidities and direct costs related to diabetic foot disorders: A literature review. *Front. Endocrinol.* **2023**, *14*, 1323315. [CrossRef] [PubMed]
8. MacKenzie, E.J.; Jones, A.S.; Bosse, M.J.; Castillo, R.C.; Pollak, A.N.; Webb, L.X.; Swiontkowski, M.F.; Kellam, J.F.; Smith, D.G.; Sanders, R.W.; et al. Health-care costs associated with amputation or reconstruction of a limb-threatening injury. *J. Bone Jt. Surg. Am.* **2007**, *89*, 1685–1692. [CrossRef]
9. Zhang, P.; Lu, J.; Jing, Y.; Tang, S.; Zhu, D.; Bi, Y. Global epidemiology of diabetic foot ulceration: A systematic review and meta-analysis (dagger). *Ann. Med.* **2017**, *49*, 106–116. [CrossRef]
10. Jais, S. Various Types of Wounds That Diabetic Patients Can Develop: A Narrative Review. *Clin. Pathol.* **2023**, *16*, 2632010X231205366. [CrossRef]
11. Bonnet, J.-B.; Sultan, A. Narrative Review of the Relationship Between CKD and Diabetic Foot Ulcer. *Kidney Int. Rep.* **2022**, *7*, 381–388. [CrossRef] [PubMed]
12. Mazen, S.B. Diabetic Foot Infection. *Am. Fam. Physician* **2008**, *78*, 71–79.
13. Ahmadishooli, A.; Davoodian, P.; Shoja, S.; Ahmadishooli, B.; Dadvand, H.; Hamadiyan, H.; Shahriarirad, R. Frequency and Antimicrobial Susceptibility Patterns of Diabetic Foot Infection of Patients from Bandar Abbas District, Southern Iran. *J. Pathog.* **2020**, *2020*, 1057167. [CrossRef] [PubMed]
14. Hobizal, K.B.; Wukich, D.K. Diabetic foot infections: Current concept review. *Diabet. Foot Ankle* **2012**, *3*, 18409. [CrossRef] [PubMed]
15. Armstrong, D.G.; Lipsky, B.A. Diabetic foot infections: Stepwise medical and surgical management. *Int. Wound J.* **2004**, *1*, 123–132. [CrossRef] [PubMed]
16. Yang, L.; Rong, G.C.; Wu, Q.N. Diabetic foot ulcer: Challenges and future. *World J. Diabetes* **2022**, *13*, 1014–1034. [CrossRef]
17. Baig, M.S.; Banu, A.; Zehravi, M.; Rana, R.; Burle, S.S.; Khan, S.L.; Islam, F.; Siddiqui, F.A.; Massoud, E.E.S.; Rahman, M.H.; et al. An Overview of Diabetic Foot Ulcers and Associated Problems with Special Emphasis on Treatments with Antimicrobials. *Life* **2022**, *12*, 1054. [CrossRef]
18. Ndip, A.; Ebah, L.; Mbako, A. Neuropathic diabetic foot ulcers—Evidence-to-practice. *Int. J. Gen. Med.* **2012**, *5*, 129–134. [CrossRef]
19. Spiliopoulos, S.; Festas, G.; Paraskevopoulos, I.; Mariappan, M.; Brountzos, E. Overcoming ischemia in the diabetic foot: Minimally invasive treatment options. *World J. Diabetes* **2021**, *12*, 2011–2026. [CrossRef]
20. Ndip, A.; Jude, E. Emerging Evidence for Neuroischemic Diabetic Foot Ulcers: Model of Care and How to Adapt Practice. *Int. J. Low Extrem. Wounds* **2009**, *8*, 82–94. [CrossRef]
21. Bundo, M.; Llussa, J.; Serra, M.; la Iglesia, P.P.; Gimbert, R.M.; Real, J.; Vlacho, B.; Mata-Cases, M.; Cos, X.; Franch-Nadal, J.; et al. Incidence and characteristics of diabetic foot ulcers in subjects with type 2 diabetes in Catalonian primary care centres: An observational multicentre study. *Prim. Care Diabetes* **2021**, *15*, 1033–1039. [CrossRef] [PubMed]
22. Swaminathan, N.; Awuah, W.A.; Bharadwaj, H.R.; Roy, S.; Ferreira, T.; Adebusoye, F.T.; Ismail, I.F.N.b.; Azeem, S.; Abdul-Rahman, T.; Papadakis, M. Early intervention and care for Diabetic Foot Ulcers in Low and Middle Income Countries: Addressing challenges and exploring future strategies: A narrative review. *Health Sci. Rep.* **2024**, *7*, e2075. [CrossRef] [PubMed]
23. Khan, T.; Lopez Rowe, V. Diabetic Foot Ulcers Treatment & Management. Available online: https://emedicine.medscape.com/article/460282-treatment?form=fpf (accessed on 20 August 2024).

24. Jiang, P.; Li, Q.; Luo, Y.; Luo, F.; Che, Q.; Lu, Z.; Yang, S.; Yang, Y.; Chen, X.; Cai, Y. Current status and progress in research on dressing management for diabetic foot ulcer. *Front. Endocrinol.* **2023**, *14*, 1221705. [CrossRef]
25. Senneville, E.; Albalawi, Z.; van Asten, S.A.; Abbas, Z.G.; Allison, G.; Aragon-Sanchez, J.; Embil, J.M.; Lavery, L.A.; Alhasan, M.; Oz, O.; et al. IWGDF/IDSA Guidelines on the Diagnosis and Treatment of Diabetes-related Foot Infections (IWGDF/IDSA 2023). *Clin. Infect. Dis.* **2023**, *79*, 286. [CrossRef] [PubMed]
26. Shi, C.; Wang, C.; Liu, H.; Li, Q.; Li, R.; Zhang, Y.; Liu, Y.; Shao, Y.; Wang, J. Selection of Appropriate Wound Dressing for Various Wounds. *Front. Bioeng. Biotechnol.* **2020**, *8*, 182. [CrossRef] [PubMed]
27. Rezvani Ghomi, E.; Khalili, S.; Nouri Khorasani, S.; Esmaeely Neisiany, R.; Ramakrishna, S. Wound dressings: Current advances and future directions. *J. Appl. Polym. Sci.* **2019**, *136*, 47738. [CrossRef]
28. Schmidt, B.M.; Holmes, C.M.; Najarian, K.; Gallagher, K.; Haus, J.M.; Shadiow, J.; Ye, W.; Ang, L.; Burant, A.; Baker, N.; et al. On diabetic foot ulcer knowledge gaps, innovation, evaluation, prediction markers, and clinical needs. *J. Diabetes Complicat.* **2022**, *36*, 108317. [CrossRef]
29. Moura, L.I.; Dias, A.M.; Carvalho, E.; de Sousa, H.C. Recent advances on the development of wound dressings for diabetic foot ulcer treatment—A review. *Acta Biomater.* **2013**, *9*, 7093–7114. [CrossRef]
30. Dasari, N.; Jiang, A.; Skochdopole, A.; Chung, J.; Reece, E.M.; Vorstenbosch, J.; Winocour, S. Updates in Diabetic Wound Healing, Inflammation, and Scarring. *Semin. Plast. Surg.* **2021**, *35*, 153–158. [CrossRef]
31. Xiao, Y.; Qian, J.; Deng, X.; Zhang, H.; Wang, J.; Luo, Z.; Zhu, L. Macrophages regulate healing-associated fibroblasts in diabetic wound. *Mol. Biol. Rep.* **2024**, *51*, 203. [CrossRef]
32. Liu, Y.; Liu, Y.; He, W.; Mu, X.; Wu, X.; Deng, J.; Nie, X. Fibroblasts: Immunomodulatory factors in refractory diabetic wound healing. *Front. Immunol.* **2022**, *13*, 918223. [CrossRef] [PubMed]
33. Kota, S.K.; Meher, L.K.; Jammula, S.; Kota, S.K.; Krishna, S.V.; Modi, K.D. Aberrant angiogenesis: The gateway to diabetic complications. *Indian J. Endocrinol. Metab.* **2012**, *16*, 918–930. [CrossRef] [PubMed]
34. Beyene, R.T.; Derryberry, S.L., Jr.; Barbul, A. The Effect of Comorbidities on Wound Healing. *Surg. Clin. N. Am.* **2020**, *100*, 695–705. [CrossRef]
35. Alfano, M.; Canducci, F.; Nebuloni, M.; Clementi, M.; Montorsi, F.; Salonia, A. The interplay of extracellular matrix and microbiome in urothelial bladder cancer. *Nat. Rev. Urol.* **2016**, *13*, 77–90. [CrossRef]
36. Everett, E.; Mathioudakis, N. Update on management of diabetic foot ulcers. *Ann. N. Y. Acad. Sci.* **2018**, *1411*, 153–165. [CrossRef] [PubMed]
37. Dhivya, S.; Padma, V.V.; Santhini, E. Wound dressings—A review. *Biomedicine* **2015**, *5*, 22. [CrossRef]
38. Pilehvar-Soltanahmadi, Y.; Dadashpour, M.; Mohajeri, A.; Fattahi, A.; Sheervalilou, R.; Zarghami, N. An Overview on Application of Natural Substances Incorporated with Electrospun Nanofibrous Scaffolds to Development of Innovative Wound Dressings. *Mini Rev. Med. Chem.* **2018**, *18*, 414–427. [CrossRef]
39. Mishra, A.; Kushare, A.; Gupta, M.N.; Ambre, P. Advanced Dressings for Chronic Wound Management. *ACS Appl. Bio. Mater.* **2024**, *7*, 2660–2676. [CrossRef]
40. Jones, A.M.; San Miguel, L. Are modern wound dressings a clinical and cost-effective alternative to the use of gauze? *J. Wound Care* **2006**, *15*, 62–65. [CrossRef]
41. Britto, E.J.; Nezwek, T.A.; Popowicz, P.; Robins, M. Wound Dressings. Available online: https://www.ncbi.nlm.nih.gov/books/NBK470199/ (accessed on 22 August 2024).
42. Nguyen, H.M.; Ngoc Le, T.T.; Nguyen, A.T.; Thien Le, H.N.; Pham, T.T. Biomedical materials for wound dressing: Recent advances and applications. *RSC Adv.* **2023**, *13*, 5509–5528. [CrossRef]
43. Jeffcoate, W.J.; Harding, K.G. Diabetic foot ulcers. *Lancet* **2003**, *361*, 1545–1551. [CrossRef]
44. Vargas Guerrero, M.; Aendekerk, F.M.A.; de Boer, C.; Geurts, J.; Lucchesi, J.; Arts, J.J.C. Bioactive-Glass-Based Materials with Possible Application in Diabetic Wound Healing: A Systematic Review. *Int. J. Mol. Sci.* **2024**, *25*, 1152. [CrossRef] [PubMed]
45. Fereday, J.; Muir-Cochrane, E. Demonstrating Rigor Using Thematic Analysis: A Hybrid Approach of Inductive and Deductive Coding and Theme Development. *Int. J. Qual. Methods* **2006**, *5*, 80–83. [CrossRef]
46. Dissemond, J.; Chadwick, P.; Weir, D.; Alves, P.; Isoherranen, K.; Lazaro Martinez, J.L.; Swanson, T.; Gledhill, A.; Malone, M.M.O.I.S.T. Concept for the Local Therapy of Chronic Wounds: An International Update. *Int. J. Low Extrem. Wounds* **2024**, 15347346241245159. [CrossRef]
47. Harries, R.L.; Bosanquet, D.C.; Harding, K.G. Wound bed preparation: TIME for an update. *Int. Wound J.* **2016**, *13* (Suppl. S3), 8–14. [CrossRef] [PubMed]
48. Rogers, E.M. *Diffusion of Innovations*, 5th ed.; Simon and Schuster: New York, NY, USA, 2003.
49. Ka, O.; Sow, D.; Seck, E.M.; Guéye, N.F.N.; Bop, M.C.; Dia, M.E.; Ndiaye, A.A.; Sow, P.G.; Ndour, M.M. Low Socio-Economic Level: A Major Obstacle to Therapeutic Observation (Survey of 125 Diabetic Patients). *Open J. Prev. Med.* **2022**, *12*, 1–9. [CrossRef]
50. Kok, G.; Gottlieb, N.H.; Peters, G.-J.Y.; Mullen, P.D.; Parcel, G.S.; Ruiter, R.A.C.; Fernández, M.E.; Markham, C.; Bartholomew, L.K. A taxonomy of behaviour change methods: An Intervention Mapping approach. *Health Psychol. Rev.* **2015**, *10*, 297–312. [CrossRef]
51. Sikkens, J.J.; Caris, M.G.; Schutte, T.; Kramer, M.H.H.; Tichelaar, J.; van Agtmael, M.A. Improving antibiotic prescribing skills in medical students: The effect of e-learning after 6 months. *J. Antimicrob. Chemother.* **2018**, *73*, 2243–2246. [CrossRef]

52. Van Netten, J.J.; Apelqvist, J.; Bus, S.A.; Fitridge, R.; Game, F.; Monteiro-Soares, M.; Senneville, E.; Schaper, N.C. The International Working Group on the Diabetic Foot: Stories and Numbers Behind Three Decades of Evidence-Based Guidelines for the Management of Diabetes-Related Foot Disease. *Diabetes Ther.* **2024**, *15*, 19–31. [CrossRef]
53. IWGDF. Introduction to the Work of IWGDF Guidelines. Available online: https://iwgdfguidelines.org/introduction (accessed on 3 July 2024).
54. Tchero, H.; Kangambega, P.; Fluieraru, S.; Bekara, F.; Teot, L. Management of infected diabetic wound: A scoping review of guidelines. *F1000Research* **2019**, *8*, 737. [CrossRef]
55. Powlson, A.S.; Coll, A.P. The treatment of diabetic foot infections. *J. Antimicrob. Chemother.* **2010**, *65* (Suppl. S3), iii3–iii9. [CrossRef] [PubMed]
56. Gemechu, F.W.; Seemant, F.; Curley, C.A. Diabetic Foot Infections. *Am. Fam. Physician* **2013**, *88*, 177–184. [PubMed]
57. Gardner, S.E.; Frantz, R.A.; Doebbeling, B.N. The validity of the clinical signs and symptoms used to identify localized chronic wound infection. *Wound Repair Regen.* **2001**, *9*, 178–186. [CrossRef]
58. Lipsky, B.A. Medical Treatment of Diabetic Foot Infections. *Clin. Infect. Dis.* **2004**, *39*, S104–S114. [CrossRef]
59. Mavrogenis, A.F.; Megaloikonomos, P.D.; Antoniadou, T.; Igoumenou, V.G.; Panagopoulos, G.N.; Dimopoulos, L.; Moulakakis, K.G.; Sfyroeras, G.S.; Lazaris, A. Current concepts for the evaluation and management of diabetic foot ulcers. *EFORT Open Rev.* **2018**, *3*, 513–525. [CrossRef]
60. Edmonds, M.; Manu, C.; Vas, P. The current burden of diabetic foot disease. *J. Clin. Orthop. Trauma* **2021**, *17*, 88–93. [CrossRef]
61. Rajab, A.A.H.; Hegazy, W.A.H. What's old is new again: Insights into diabetic foot microbiome. *World J. Diabetes* **2023**, *14*, 680–704. [CrossRef]
62. Rajha, H.; Alsheiks, A.Z.; Mohsen, S.; Zughaier, S.M. Microbiology and Antimicrobial Resistance in Diabetic Foot Infections. In *Diabetic Foot Ulcers—Pathogenesis, Innovative Treatments and AI Applications*; Chowdhury, M.E.H., Zughaier, S.M., Hasan, A., Alfkey, R., Eds.; IntechOpen: London, UK, 2024; pp. 3–6.
63. Salati, S. Debridement: A review of current techniques. *J. Pak. Assoc. Dermatol.* **2021**, *31*, 262–272.
64. Dunyach-Remy, C.; Ngba Essebe, C.; Sotto, A.; Lavigne, J.P. *Staphylococcus aureus* Toxins and Diabetic Foot Ulcers: Role in Pathogenesis and Interest in Diagnosis. *Toxins* **2016**, *8*, 209. [CrossRef]
65. Hosny, A.E.M.; Rasmy, S.A.; Aboul-Magd, D.S.; Kashef, M.T.; El-Bazza, Z.E. The increasing threat of silver-resistance in clinical isolates from wounds and burns. *Infect. Drug Resist.* **2019**, *12*, 1985–2001. [CrossRef]
66. Shi, Z.; Yao, C.; Shui, Y.; Li, S.; Yan, H. Research progress on the mechanism of angiogenesis in wound repair and regeneration. *Front. Physiol.* **2023**, *14*, 1284981. [CrossRef] [PubMed]
67. Jeong, J.H.; Ojha, U.; Lee, Y.M. Pathological angiogenesis and inflammation in tissues. *Arch. Pharm. Res.* **2021**, *44*, 1–15. [CrossRef] [PubMed]
68. DiPietro, L.A. Angiogenesis and wound repair: When enough is enough. *J. Leukoc. Biol.* **2016**, *100*, 979–984. [CrossRef] [PubMed]
69. Faber, J.; Fonseca, L.M. How sample size influences research outcomes. *Dental Press J. Orthod.* **2014**, *19*, 27–29. [CrossRef]
70. Elston, D.M. Participation bias, self-selection bias, and response bias. *J. Am. Acad. Dermatol.* **2021**. [CrossRef]
71. MacKinnon, N.J.; Emery, V.; Waller, J.; Ange, B.; Ambade, P.; Gunja, M.; Watson, E. Mapping Health Disparities in 11 High-Income Nations. *JAMA Netw. Open* **2023**, *6*, e2322310. [CrossRef]

biomedicines

MDPI

Article

Diabetes Control Status and Severity of Depression: Insights from NHANES 2005–2020

Raedeh Basiri [1,2,*], Yatisha Rajanala [3], Megan Kassem [4], Lawrence J. Cheskin [1,2,5], Cara L. Frankenfeld [1,6] and Maryam S. Farvid [1]

1 Department of Nutrition and Food Studies, George Mason University, Fairfax, VA 22030, USA
2 Institute for Biohealth Innovation, George Mason University, Fairfax, VA 22030, USA
3 Department of Health Administration and Policy, George Mason University, Fairfax, VA 22030, USA
4 Department of Global and Community Health, George Mason University, Fairfax, VA 22030, USA
5 Department of Medicine, Johns Hopkins School of Medicine, Baltimore, MD 21205, USA
6 Center for Interdisciplinary & Population Health Research, MaineHealth Institute for Research, Westbrook, ME 04092, USA
* Correspondence: rbasiri@gmu.edu

Abstract: Background/Objectives: Examining the risk of depression among patients with diabetes is crucial for understanding the mental health burden of this chronic condition. This study examined the likelihood of depression severity among participants in the National Health And Nutrition Examination Survey (NHANES) from 2005 to 2020, based on glycemic control status. **Methods:** Depression severity was categorized into three levels using the Patient Health Questionnaire-9 (PHQ-9), and glycemic control status was categorized into five groups based on prior diabetes diagnoses and hemoglobin A1c (HbA1c) levels. Using multinomial logistic regression models, the odds ratio (OR) and 95% confidence intervals (95%CIs) of various severities of depression by glycemic control status were calculated after comprehensive adjustments. **Results:** Out of 76,496 NHANES participants from 2005 to 2020, 37,037 individuals who met our inclusion criteria were analyzed. The likelihood of depression in individuals with prediabetes was not significantly different from those with normoglycemia. In contrast, participants with diabetes had a higher likelihood of having depression versus individuals with normoglycemia even when they kept their HbA1c within the normal range (lower than 5.7%). Among individuals with diabetes, those with HbA1c $< 5.7\%$ had a higher likelihood of mild depression (OR: 1.54, 95%CI: 1.02–2.34), while having HbA1c $\geq 10.0\%$ was significantly associated with a greater likelihood of moderate to severe depression (OR: 1.53, 95%CI: 1.07–2.19) compared to those with HbA1c levels of 5.7–10.0%. **Conclusions:** Our findings highlight the need for a holistic approach to diabetes care that includes mental health considerations, especially for those who are at the extremes of the HbA1c spectrum.

Keywords: diabetes; prediabetes; depression; HbA1c; NHANES; mental health; blood glucose control

1. Introduction

Diabetes and depression pose significant global health challenges, with diabetes (total of type-1 and type-2) affecting 1 in 11 adults worldwide, and depression having a lifetime prevalence of 11–15% [1]. Both conditions contribute to medical and economic burdens, with diabetes accounting for 12% of global health expenditure [2]. Diabetes often coexists with neuropsychiatric comorbidities, particularly depression [3]; however, it remains a neglected condition in patients with diabetes, directly impacting their quality of life. Depression ranks as the fourth leading cause of Disability-Adjusted Life Years (DALYs) in developed countries, while diabetes holds the eighth rank [4].

Depression, a mood disorder defined in the American Psychiatric Association's *Diagnostic and Statistical Manual of Mental Disorders*, Fifth Edition (DSM-5), disrupts emotions, cognition, and behaviors [5,6]. Diagnostic criteria include the core symptom of diminished mood or anhedonia, plus at least four additional symptoms, namely feelings of guilt or worthlessness, fatigue, loss of concentration, suicidal thoughts, at least 5% change in weight, a change in psychomotor activity, or sleep disruptions lasting for at least two weeks [7].

The treatment of depression in patients with diabetes is challenging, often proving ineffective and sometimes refractory [8]. Further complicating matters, some antidepressant medications can adversely affect blood glucose control [9]. On the other hand, the demanding nature of diabetes management for patients, including the complexities of blood glucose control, medication adherence, and lifestyle adjustments, contributes to elevated stress levels. The emotional burden associated with navigating the potential complications of diabetes also significantly heightens a susceptibility to developing or worsening depression [10,11]. Coping with the uncertainty of managing a chronic condition and the potential complications associated with diabetes, such as neuropathy or cardiovascular issues, can further contribute to the development of depression [12].

Studies reveal an increased prevalence of depression in prediabetes and undiagnosed diabetes, with markedly higher rates in individuals with diagnosed diabetes compared to those with a normal glucose metabolism [13]. The interactions between the hypothalamus, pituitary gland, and adrenal glands can cause alterations to cortisol production, which could be an underlying mechanism of an increased depression risk in people with impaired glucose tolerance [14]. Chronic inflammation and fluctuations in blood glucose that could lead to mood swings and impact neurotransmitters could be other potential causes of depression in those with diabetes or prediabetes [15]. Inflammatory markers such as C-reactive protein (CRP) and interleukin-6 (IL-6) are often elevated in individuals with depression, diabetes, and prediabetes. This chronic low-grade inflammation can affect the brain and contribute to the development of depressive symptoms [16,17]. This increased risk is intricately linked to the complex interplay between physical health, lifestyle factors, and the psychological burden associated with managing a chronic condition like diabetes [18,19]. The bidirectional association between diabetes and depression suggests shared biological mechanisms, emphasizing the need for a comprehensive understanding to enhance treatment and outcomes for these interconnected conditions [20]. The early identification and comprehensive management of depression in individuals with diabetes is critical for improving the overall outcomes and enhancing the quality of life of this vulnerable population [21,22]. Thus, recognizing the risk factors of depression among patients with diabetes is essential, and addressing both conditions comprehensively can provide further benefits to overall health.

While the increased risk of depression among individuals with diabetes is widely reported, the association between potential contributing factors—including diabetes control status, anthropometric measures, and demographic variables—and varying degrees of depression severity remains largely underexplored. Thus, it is important to investigate the link between diabetes management and different levels of depression severity, while accounting for potential covariates and stratifying according to influential predictors. This comprehension can assist in identifying vulnerable populations and optimizing patient treatment approaches.

We aimed to assess the likelihood of experiencing varying degrees of depression across different categories of glycemic control status to identify patients with diabetes at the highest risk of depression after a comprehensive adjustment.

2. Materials and Methods

2.1. Source of Data

Data from the National Health And Nutrition Examination Survey (NHANES), a series of cross-sectional, nationally representative health examination surveys, spanning 2005 to 2020 were used [23]. The NHANES, conducted by the Centers for Disease Control and Prevention (CDC), assesses the health and nutritional status of the U.S. population through interviews and physical examinations. Each year, NHANES samples about 5000 individuals using a complex, multistage probability-sampling design to ensure national representativeness. The process begins with geographical stratification, dividing the country into Primary Sampling Units (PSUs) based on factors like region and urbanization. A random sample of PSUs is then selected, followed by smaller geographical segments within each PSU, and then households within these segments. Finally, individuals within these households are randomly chosen, with the oversampling of certain groups such as the elderly, African Americans, Asians, and Hispanics to ensure sufficient data for these populations. The survey is conducted annually, with different participants each year. However, some participants might be re-invited in subsequent survey cycles, although this is not common [24,25]. For this study, the data were obtained from 76,496 participants who had participated in NHANES from 2005 to 2020. Participants were eligible for our analysis if they were aged 18+ years, had available test results for hemoglobin A1c (HbA1c), had answered at least seven questions from Patient Health Questionnaire-9 (PHQ-9) [26], and were non-pregnant/non-lactating. The final analysis included 37,073 participants. Figure 1 details the inclusion and exclusion criteria.

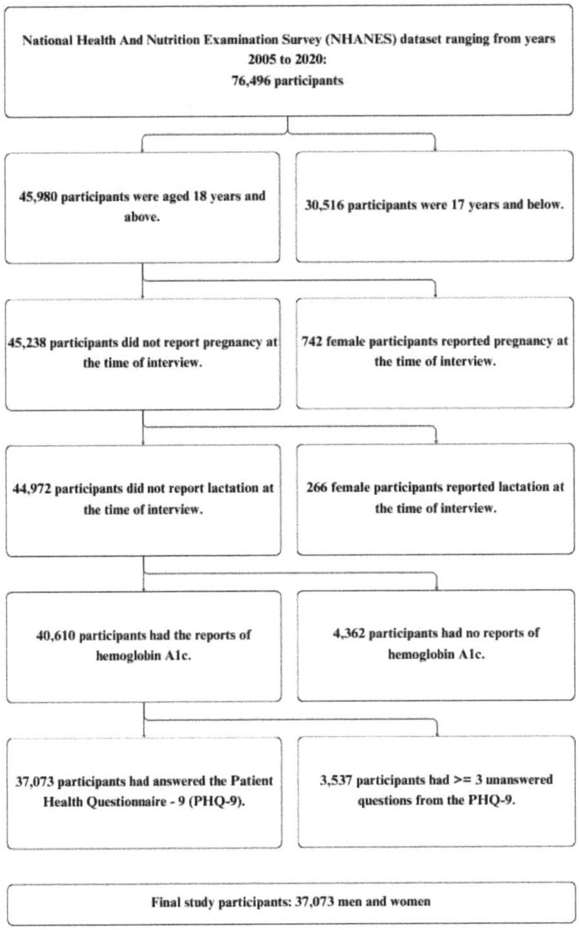

Figure 1. Flowchart of eligible individuals, the National Health And Nutrition Examination Survey (NHANES) 2005–2020.

Based on the participants' responses to the DIQ010 question ("Other than during pregnancy, {have you/has SP}/{have you/has SP} ever been told by a doctor or health professional that {you have/{he/she/SP}has} diabetes or sugar diabetes?") and the availability of data from LBXGH (glycohemoglobin (%)), they were placed in five glycemic control categories as follows: normoglycemia (no prior diagnosis, HbA1c < 5.7%), prediabetes (no prior diagnosis, HbA1c 5.7%– <6.5%), Diabetes (diagnosed for diabetes with HbA1c < 5.7%, Diabetes with 5.7% < HbA1c < 10.0%), and Diabetes with HbA1c ≥ 10.0% [27]. Details about the classification of participants into these categories are outlined in Figure 2.

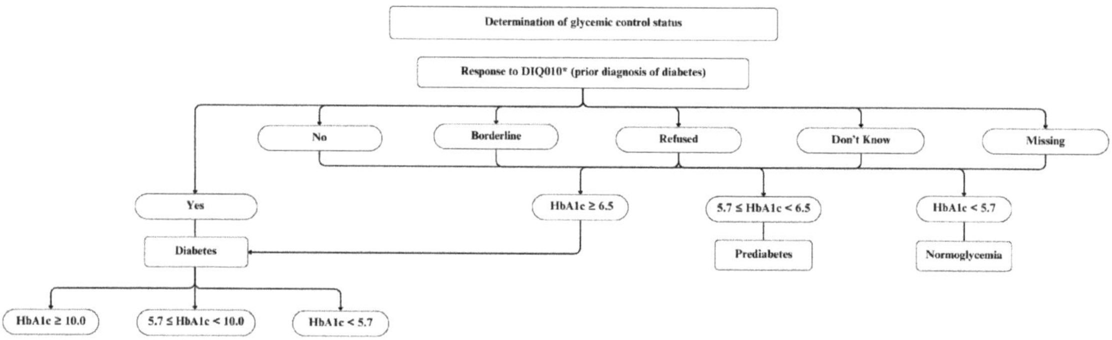

Figure 2. The determination of glycemic control status in the National Health And Nutrition Examination Survey (NHANES) 2005–2020. * DIQ010 question: "Other than during pregnancy, {have you/has SP}/{have you/has SP} ever been told by a doctor or health professional that {you have /{he/she/SP}has} diabetes or sugar diabetes?".

The severity of depression was defined based on the participants' PHQ-9 scores. The PHQ-9 is a screening tool for depression consisting of nine questions about symptoms experienced over the past two weeks. The total scores range from 0 to 27, with higher scores indicating more severe depression. Following NHANES instructions, the total score was determined based on the sum of scores from responses to questions DPQ010 to DPQ090 from the NHANES website [23]. If participants did not respond to more than two questions out of nine, then the data were considered invalid and excluded; however, if one or two questions remained unanswered, then the prorated score calculation method was utilized as suggested in the analytical notes of the PHQ-9 [26]:

Calculating prorated score for determining severity of depression:

$$\text{Partial raw score (PRS)} = \text{sum of available questionnaire scores} \tag{1}$$

$$\text{Total score} = (\text{PRS} \times 9)\ /\ \text{total number of answered questions} \tag{2}$$

The participants were then divided into three categories based on their scores from PHQ-9: no depression (score: 0–4), mild depression (score: 5–9), moderate and severe depression (score: 10–27) [26].

Information about age, sex, and race/ethnicity was obtained from the "Demographic Variables and Sample Weights" data, while the body mass index (BMI) was extracted from the "Body Measures" questionnaires. Participants were categorized into six BMI categories: underweight (<18.5 kg/m^2), normal weight (≥18.5 and <25 kg/m^2), overweight (≥25 and <30 kg/m^2), class I obese (≥30 and <35 kg/m^2), class II obese (≥35 and <40 kg/m^2), and class III obese (≥40 kg/m^2). Participants without information for their BMI were categorized as missing. Physical activity levels were evaluated based on the Metabolic Equivalent of Task (MET) hours per week (MET-hrs./week) using the Global Physical Activity Questionnaire (GPAQ). The physical activity questionnaire used by NHANES differed between the 2005–2006 period and 2007 onward. To ensure consistency in our analysis, we categorized the 2005–2006 population into four distinct groups based on their estimated physical activity intensity and aligned them with the MET categories applied to participants from 2007 onward. Further details on the categorization and alignment of physical activity data from 2005–2006 with the rest of the dataset are provided in the Supplementary Material, Appendix SA. The MET-hrs./week was calculated for data from 2007 to 2020 based on the NHANES guidelines, which assign eight MET points for vigorous work and recreational activities and four MET points for moderate work, recreational activities, and walking/bicycling. The calculation of MET-hrs./week for physical activity involved using these MET scores, alongside the daily duration and frequency of the activities performed each week [28]. Participants with no physical activity (MET-hrs./week = 0) were placed in the lowest category, while the others were divided into four additional categories (quartiles), and a separate category was created for participants with missing data [28].

2.2. Statistical Analysis

The odds ratio (OR) and 95% confidence intervals (CIs) for the association between glycemic control status and severity of depression were evaluated by multinomial logistic regression models. The primary outcome was depression severity. Survey analytic techniques were used in descriptive and regression analyses to incorporate the complex stratified sampling procedure and population weighting [23]. All analyses were conducted using Stata software version 18, with statistical significance set at a two-sided p-value of <0.05.

2.2.1. Examining the Association between Glycemic Control Status and Various Severities of Depression

The odds of various severities of depression in individuals with prediabetes, diabetes with HbA1c < 5.7%), diabetes with HbA1c between 5.7% and 10.0%), and diabetes with HbA1c $\geq$ 10.0%) versus those with normoglycemia were evaluated. Model 1 was adjusted for age, sex, and race/ethnicity, while Model 2 included additional adjustments for BMI, physical activity, and the year of data collection alongside the covariates from Model 1.

2.2.2. Examining the Associations between Diabetes Control Status and Various Severities of Depression

The odds of various severities of depression related to diabetes control status were examined among participants with diabetes. This model was applied to assess the severity of depression in participants with diabetes across different HbA1c categories. Participants with HbA1c levels lower than 5.7%, as well as those with HbA1c $\geq$ 10.0%, were compared to participants whose HbA1c levels were between 5.7% and 10.0%.

2.2.3. Examining the Association between Diabetes Control Status and Various Severities of Depression among Participants with Diabetes, Stratified by BMI and Race/Ethnicity

We investigated whether the relationship between diabetes control status and depression differed by BMI (BMI < 25 kg/m^2 vs. BMI $\geq$ 25 kg/m^2) and race/ethnicity (Non-Hispanic White vs. other races/ethnicities).

3. Results

A total of 37,073 participants were eligible for inclusion in the study. The demographic distribution of the study population is reported in Table 1. In summary, 38.86% of the population with diabetes were 65 years or older. Non-Hispanic Whites were the largest ethnic group in the entire population (67.87%), as well as across all diabetes status subgroups. Among participants with diabetes, 52.19% were males. Overweight and obesity were prevalent among the general population of the study, with 32.50% being overweight and 37.15% in obesity classes I, II, or III.

Table 1. Characteristics of adult participants in the National Health And Nutrition Examination Survey (2005–2020) by glycemic control classification.

Variable (Number of Participants [1])	Total Participants (n = 37,073)	Normoglycemia (n = 22,393)	Prediabetes (n = 8815)	Diabetes (n = 5865)
Depression Categories				
No Depression	76.63%	77.80%	76.91%	69.47%
Mild Depression	15.53%	15.12%	15.01%	18.72%
Moderate to Severe Depression	7.84%	7.07%	8.08%	11.82%
Age Categories				
18–34 Years	28.38%	38.16%	9.86%	4.28%
35–44 Years	17.18%	19.55%	13.56%	9.82%
45–54 Years	19.02%	18.23%	20.88%	20.35%
55–64 Years	16.72%	12.72%	24.23%	26.70%
65+ Years	18.70%	11.34%	31.47%	38.86%
Sex				
Male	49.73%	49.90%	47.70%	52.19%
Female	50.27%	50.10%	52.30%	47.81%
Race/Ethnic Groups				
Non-Hispanic White	67.87%	70.73%	62.69%	60.39%
Non-Hispanic Black	10.68%	8.41%	15.59%	15.20%
Mexican American	8.45%	8.26%	8.29%	9.82%
Non-Mexican Hispanic	5.71%	5.70%	5.55%	6.08%
Other Races—Including Multi-Racial	7.29%	6.91%	7.88%	8.51%
Body Mass Index (BMI) Categories				
Normal Weight	1.60%	2.01%	0.99%	0.31%
Underweight	28.01%	33.96%	18.59%	10.14%
Overweight	32.50%	33.65%	33.08%	24.97%
Class I Obese	20.50%	18.14%	23.51%	28.83%
Class II Obese	9.54%	7.04%	13.17%	17.56%
Class III Obese	7.11%	4.57%	9.97%	16.75%
Missing	0.73%	0.62%	0.70%	1.44%
Physical Activity Categories				
No Activity	18.83%	14.65%	24.00%	33.80%
Quartile 1	19.25%	18.22%	21.56%	21.16%
Quartile 2	24.46%	25.85%	21.28%	21.93%
Quartile 3	18.60%	20.53%	15.95%	12.16%
Quartile 4	18.84%	20.72%	17.18%	10.95%
Missing	0.02%	0.03%	0.02%	0.00%

[1] The participant numbers in the table are based on unweighted data, whereas the percentages are derived from weighted data.

3.1. Glycemic Control Status and Various Severities of Depression

In Model 1, the likelihood of depression in participants with prediabetes was significantly different than those with normoglycemia (OR for moderate to severe depression: 1.25, 95%CI: 1.09–1.45). However, this association didn't remain significant when the data was further adjusted for BMI, year of data collection, and physical activity in Model 2. Additionally, a significantly increased likelihood of different severities of depression was observed in individuals with diabetes withHbA1c < 5.7%, 5.7% ≤ HbA1c < 10.0%, and HbA1c ≥ 10.0% compared to normoglycemia, in both Models 1 and 2. For instance, the odds ratio for moderate to severe depression was 2.00 (CI: 1.40–2.88), 2.14 (CI: 1.81–2.54), and 2.86 (95%CI: 2.07–3.94) for those with HbA1c < 5.7%, 5.7% ≤ HbA1c < 10.0%, and HbA1c ≥ 10.0%, respectively (Table 2, Model 1). This trend remained similar after adding more covariates in Model 2. A greater likelihood of mild depression was also observed in individuals with diabetes compared to the population with normoglycemia.

Table 2. Odds ratio and 95% confidence intervals for the associations between glycemic control status and various severities of depression among participants in the National Health And Nutrition Examination Survey (n = 37,073).

Glycemic Control Status	Number	Depression Categories			
		Mild Depression		Moderate to Severe Depression	
		Odds Ratio	95%CI	Odds Ratio	95%CI
Model 1 *					
Normoglycemia	22,393	1 (reference)		1 (reference)	
Prediabetes	8815	1.07	0.96–1.19	1.25	1.09–1.45
Diabetes (HbA1C < 5.7%)	367	2.11	1.42–3.15	2.00	1.40–2.88
Diabetes (5.7% ≤ HbA1c < 10.0%)	4915	1.48	1.32–1.66	2.14	1.81–2.54
Diabetes (HbA1c ≥ 10.0%)	583	1.71	1.22–2.40	2.86	2.07–3.94
Model 2 **					
Normoglycemia	22,393	1 (reference)		1 (reference)	
Prediabetes	8815	0.97	0.87–1.09	1.10	0.95–1.28
Diabetes (HbA1C < 5.7%)	367	1.90	1.26–2.85	1.70	1.19–2.42
Diabetes (5.7% ≤ HbA1c < 10.0%)	4915	1.24	1.10–1.40	1.63	1.38–1.92
Diabetes (HbA1c ≥ 10.0%)	583	1.49	1.04–2.12	2.31	1.68–3.17

The participant numbers in the table are based on unweighted data. * Model 1 adjusted for sex (men and women), age (18–34, 35–44, 45–54, 55–64, and ≥65 years), race/ethnicity (Non-Hispanic White, Mexican American, Non-Mexican Hispanic, Non-Hispanic Black, and other races—including multi-racial). ** Model 2 adjusted for sex (men and women), age (18–34, 35–44, 45–54, 55–64, and ≥65 years), race/ethnicity (Non-Hispanic White, Mexican American, Non-Mexican Hispanic, Non-Hispanic Black, and other races—including multi-racial), BMI [underweight (<18.5 kg/m^2), normal weight (≥18.5 and <25 kg/m^2), overweight (≥25 and <30 kg/m^2), class I obese (≥30 and <35 kg/m^2), class II obese (≥35 and <40 kg/m^2), class III obese (≥40 kg/m^2), and missing values], year of collecting data (continuous), and physical activity (MET-hrs./week = 0, quartiles, missing).

3.2. Diabetes Control Status and Various Severities of Depression

To examine the effect of diabetes control status on the likelihood of depression, participants with diabetes were compared across different categories of HbA1c levels. Compared to those with an HbA1c between 5.7% and 10.0%, the likelihood of mild depression (OR:

1.54, 95%CI: 1.02–2.34) was significantly higher among individuals with HbA1c < 5.7; while the likelihood of moderate to severe depression (OR: 1.53, 95%CI: 1.07–2.19) was significantly higher in those with HbA1c ≥ 10.0% compared to those with HbA1c levels between 5.7% and 10.0%, as shown in Table 3.

Table 3. Odds ratio and 95% confidence intervals for the associations between diabetes control status and various severities of depression among participants with diabetes in the National Health And Nutrition Examination Survey (n = 5865).

Diabetes Control Status	Number	Depression Categories			
		Mild Depression		Moderate to Severe Depression	
		Odds Ratio	95%CI	Odds Ratio	95%CI
Model 1 *					
Diabetes (HbA1C < 5.7%)	367	1.46	0.99–2.16	0.94	0.65–1.36
Diabetes (5.7% ≤ HbA1c < 10.0%)	4915	1 (reference)		1 (reference)	
Diabetes (HbA1c ≥ 10.0%)	583	1.24	0.87–1.76	1.42	1.01–2.01
Model 2 **					
Diabetes (HbA1C < 5.7%)	367	1.54	1.02–2.34	1.07	0.75–1.54
Diabetes (5.7% ≤ HbA1c < 10.0%)	4915	1 (reference)		1 (reference)	
Diabetes (HbA1c ≥ 10.0%)	583	1.26	0.89–1.79	1.53	1.07–2.19

The participant numbers in the table are based on unweighted data. * Model 1 adjusted for sex (men and women), age (18–34, 35–44, 45–54, 55–64, and ≥65 years), race/ethnicity (Non-Hispanic White, Mexican American, Non-Mexican Hispanic, Non-Hispanic Black, and other races—including multi-racial). ** Model 2 adjusted for sex (men and women), age (18–34, 35–44, 45–54, 55–64, and ≥65 years), race/ethnicity (Non-Hispanic White, Mexican American, Non-Mexican Hispanic, Non-Hispanic Black and other races—including multi-racial), BMI [underweight (<18.5 kg/m^2), normal weight (≥18.5 and <25 kg/m^2), overweight (≥25 and <30 kg/m^2), class I obese (≥30 and <35 kg/m^2), class II obese (≥35 and <40 kg/m^2), class III obese (≥40 kg/m^2), and missing values], year of collecting data (continuous), and physical activity (MET-hrs./week = 0, quartiles, missing).

3.3. Diabetes Control Status and Various Severities of Depression among Participants with Diabetes, Stratified by BMI and Race/Ethnicity

Since BMI and race/ethnicity play an important role in diabetes control and depression [29,30], we also examined the associations between diabetes control status and severity of depression after stratification for these covariates. When stratifying the data by race/ethnicity (Non-Hispanic White vs. other racial/ethnic groups), significant positive associations between HbA1c < 5.7% and all severities of depression were observed only among the other racial/ethnic groups, while the results did not reach statistical significance in the Non-Hispanic White population. When stratified by BMI, significant positive associations were observed between HbA1c < 5.7% and mild depression in participants with a BMI ≥ 25 kg/m^2, and moderate to severe depression in participants with a BMI < 25 kg/m^2 (Table 4).

Table 4. Odds ratio and 95% confidence intervals for the associations between diabetes control status and various severities of depression among participants with diabetes in the National Health And Nutrition Examination Survey (n = 5865), stratified by race/ethnicity and BMI.

Diabetes Control Status	Depression Categories							
	Mild Depression				Moderate to Severe Depression			
	Non-Hispanic Whites		Other Races/Ethnicities		Non-Hispanic Whites		Other Races/Ethnicities	
	Odds Ratio	95%CI	Odds Ratio	95%CI	Odds Ratio	95%CI	Odds Ratio	95%CI
HbA1C < 5.7%	1.53	0.81–2.88	1.66	1.08–2.54	0.74	0.39–1.42	1.81	1.24–2.64
5.7% ≤ HbA1c < 10.0%	1 (reference)		1 (reference)		1 (reference)		1 (reference)	
HbA1c ≥ 10.0%	1.44	0.72–2.85	1.13	0.79–1.63	1.93	0.99–3.74	1.42	0.99–2.04
Diabetes Control Status	Depression Categories							
	Mild Depression				Moderate to Severe Depression			
	BMI < 25 kg/m^2		BMI ≥ 25 kg/m^2		BMI < 25 kg/m^2		BMI ≥ 25 kg/m^2	
	Odds Ratio	95%CI	Odds Ratio	95%CI	Odds Ratio	95%CI	Odds Ratio	95%CI
HbA1C < 5.7%	0.50	0.20–1.29	1.62	1.03–2.55	4.29	1.81–10.17	0.74	0.50–1.10
5.7% ≤ HbA1c < 10.0%	1 (reference)		1 (reference)		1 (reference)		1 (reference)	
HbA1c ≥ 10.0%	1.51	0.53–4.28	1.13	0.79–1.62	2.25	0.84–5.99	1.44	0.98–2.10

The models were adjusted for sex (men and women), age (18–34, 35–44, 45–54, 55–64, and ≥65 years), race/ethnicity (Non-Hispanic White and other ethnicities including Mexican American, Non-Mexican Hispanic, Non-Hispanic Black, and other races—including multi-racial), BMI [underweight (<18.5 kg/m^2), normal weight (≥18.5 and <25 kg/m^2), overweight (≥25 and <30 kg/m^2), class I obese (≥30 and <35 and kg/m^2), class II obese (≥35 and <40 kg/m^2), class III obese (≥40 kg/m^2), and missing values], year of collecting data (continuous), physical activity (MET-hrs./week = 0, quartiles, missing). Note: Race/ethnicity was not included as a covariate in the models when analyses were stratified by race/ethnicity, and similarly, BMI was excluded as a covariate in models stratified by BMI.

4. Discussion

Overall, having diabetes was associated with a higher likelihood of all severities of depression; however, no significant association was found between prediabetes and depression after adjustments for the year of data collection, BMI, and physical activity. In participants with diabetes and HbA1c < 5.7%, the likelihood of mild and moderate to severe depression was 1.90- and 1.70-fold higher than in those with normoglycemia, respectively. Similarly, among participants with HbA1c levels between 5.7% and 10.0%, the likelihood of mild and moderate to severe depression was 24% and 63%, higher, respectively, compared to those with normoglycemia. Additionally, for participants with HbA1c ≥ 10.0%, the likelihood of mild and moderate to severe depression was also notably high—1.49- and 2.31-fold greater than individuals with normoglycemia. Among participants with diabetes, those with HbA1c < 5.7% had a higher likelihood of mild depression (54%), while those with HbA1c ≥ 10.0% had significantly higher chance of moderate to severe depression (53%) than those with HbA1c between 5.7% to 10.0%. These results align with previous studies that reported the risk of depression as being twice as high among individuals with diabetes as among those without diabetes, as well as a higher risk of depression among patients with low and high levels of HbA1c [22,31]. Similarly, in our study population, the odds of depression were higher for individuals with HbA1c < 5.7% and HbA1c ≥ 10.0% compared to those with HbA1c between 5.7% and 10.0%.

We found that individuals with prediabetes had no statistically significant difference in the likelihood of depression compared to individuals with normoglycemia after adjustments for year of data collection, BMI, and physical activity. This differs from other studies, which found an increased risk of depression for the prediabetic population [32,33]. This disparity may be due to comprehensive adjustments in our study, differences in the duration of prediabetes, access to medical services, and other sociodemographic factors [34].

A 54% higher odds of mild depression and a 53% higher odds of moderate to severe depression observed in individuals with diabetes who had HbA1c levels below 5.7% or equal/above 10.0% compared to those with HbA1c levels between 5.7% and 10.0%, suggesting that both tighter glycemic control and higher blood glucose levels may be associated with an increased risk of depression. This may be due to the ongoing psychological stress of managing the condition, biological factors affecting mood regulation, social stigma, a reduced perception of control, and underlying psychological vulnerabilities [17,35]. These findings are aligned with other studies that suggest that the risk of depression in patients with diabetes is not linearly related to HbA1c levels [36,37]. Therefore, integrating mental health support into diabetes care, particularly for those who are at the extremes of the HbA1c spectrum, is crucial for addressing these complex interplays and improving overall well-being.

This data underscores the importance of a comprehensive approach to diabetes management that considers the mental health of patients with this challenging chronic disease in addition to their physical health. While maintaining lower HbA1c levels is recommended and beneficial for reducing the risk of diabetes-related complications, the challenges inherent in adhering to stringent dietary and medical restrictions may also be accompanied by an increased risk of depression and related complications. This aligns with the results of a study by Penckofer et al. [38], as it suggests that managing glycemic variability is not only important for physical health but also for mental well-being and overall quality of life. Healthcare providers should be aware of this potential risk and consider integrating regular mental health screenings and support into the care plan for patients with diabetes, including those who are achieving and maintaining lower HbA1c levels. This is important since it has been shown that depression may be a factor that highly influences the progression of diabetes complications [39].

These findings highlight the need for further research to understand the causal mechanisms behind these associations and to develop targeted interventions to help mitigate the risk of depression in patients with diabetes across the spectrum of glycemic control.

This study has multiple strengths, including the use of a nationally representative sample, the inclusion of 16 consecutive years of data (2005–2020), and comprehensive adjustments for potential confounding factors related to both diabetes and depression. Additionally, analyses were stratified by BMI and race/ethnicity to enhance the robustness of the findings.

The interpretation of the results should consider this study's limitations. The approach we employed, which used cross-sectional data, limits our ability to determine the sequence and timing of events between diabetes and depression, thus restricting our ability to draw causal conclusions. Addressing the timing or two-way relationship between diabetes and depression is a significant gap that is crucial for understanding the underlying causes. Despite these methodological limitations, the present study sheds light on the intricate relationship between diabetes and depression. The findings suggest the need for tailored interventions addressing the varied needs of patient populations, encompassing both physical and mental health aspects. Long-term clinical trials are needed to identify optimal targets for HbA1c, BMI, and physical activity to effectively reduce the depression risk and enhance the overall well-being in this vulnerable group. Additionally, culturally sensitive interventions are essential to accommodate the diverse sociocultural backgrounds and experiences of patients suffering from diabetes, ensuring comprehensive and effective healthcare provision.

5. Conclusions

Our findings highlight the importance of diabetes control status as a risk factor for depression. Patients with HbA1c levels between 5.7% and 10.0% had the lowest odds for depression compared to all the other HbA1c groups. These results underscore the need for a holistic approach to diabetes care that includes mental health, particularly for those who are at the extremes of the HbA1c levels.

Supplementary Materials: The following supporting information can be downloaded at: https://www.mdpi.com/article/10.3390/biomedicines12102276/s1, Appendix SA: calculation of MET Scores for Years 2005–2006 and 2007–2020.

Author Contributions: Conceptualization, R.B.; methodology, R.B. and M.S.F.; software, R.B., Y.R., and M.K.; validation, R.B., M.S.F., and C.L.F.; formal analysis, Y.R. and M.S.F.; resources, R.B.; data curation, R.B., Y.R. and M.K.; writing—original draft preparation, R.B. and Y.R.; writing—review and editing, R.B., Y.R., M.K., M.S.F., L.J.C. and C.L.F.; visualization, R.B. and Y.R.; supervision, R.B.; project administration, R.B. All authors have read and agreed to the published version of the manuscript.

Funding: This research received no external funding.

Institutional Review Board Statement: Ethical review and approval were waived for this study because it utilized publicly available, non-identifiable data, and thus did not involve direct interaction with human subjects or personal data that could identify individuals.

Informed Consent Statement: Not applicable.

Data Availability Statement: Data are publicly available through CDC website; https://wwwn.cdc.gov/nchs/nhanes/ (accessed on 23 September 2024).

Conflicts of Interest: The authors declare no conflicts of interest.

References

1. Lloyd, C.E.; Roy, T.; Nouwen, A.; Chauhan, A.M. Epidemiology of Depression in Diabetes: International and Cross-Cultural Issues. *J. Affect. Disord.* **2012**, *142*, S22–S29. [CrossRef]
2. Roy, T.; Lloyd, C.E. Epidemiology of Depression and Diabetes: A Systematic Review. *J. Affect. Disord.* **2012**, *142*, S8–S21. [CrossRef]
3. Collins, M.M.; Corcoran, P.; Perry, I.J. Anxiety and Depression Symptoms in Patients with Diabetes. *Diabet. Med.* **2009**, *26*, 153–161. [CrossRef]
4. Campayo, A.; de Jonge, P.; Roy, J.F.; Saz, P.; de la Cámara, C.; Quintanilla, M.A.; Marcos, G.; Santabárbara, J.; Lobo, A. Depressive Disorder and Incident Diabetes Mellitus: The Effect of Characteristics of Depression. *Am. J. Psychiatry* **2010**, *167*, 580–588. [CrossRef]
5. Lindekilde, N.; Nefs, G.; Henriksen, J.E.; Lasgaard, M.; Schram, M.; Rubin, K.; Rutters, F.; Kivimaki, M.; Pouwer, F. Psychiatric Disorders as Risk Factors for the Development of Type 2 Diabetes Mellitus: An Umbrella Review Protocol. *BMJ Open* **2019**, *9*, e024981. [CrossRef]
6. Coleman, J. Anxiety and Diabetes. Available online: https://www.thediabetescouncil.com/anxiety-and-diabetes/ (accessed on 12 March 2024).
7. Egede, L.E.; Dismuke, C.E. Serious Psychological Distress and Diabetes: A Review of the Literature. *Curr. Psychiatry Rep.* **2012**, *14*, 15–22. [CrossRef]
8. Markowitz, S.; Gonzalez, J.S.; Wilkinson, J.L.; Safren, S.A. Treating Depression in Diabetes: Emerging Findings. *Psychosomatics* **2011**, *52*, 1–18. [CrossRef]
9. Rubin, R.R.; Peyrot, M. Psychological Issues and Treatments for People with Diabetes. *J. Clin. Psychol.* **2001**, *57*, 457–478. [CrossRef]
10. Pouwer, F. Should We Screen for Emotional Distress in Type 2 Diabetes Mellitus? *Nat. Rev. Endocrinol.* **2009**, *5*, 665–671. [CrossRef]
11. Tabák, A.G.; Akbaraly, T.N.; Batty, G.D.; Kivimäki, M. Depression and Type 2 Diabetes: A Causal Association? *Lancet Diabetes Endocrinol.* **2014**, *2*, 236–245. [CrossRef]
12. Fisher, L.; Hessler, D.M.; Polonsky, W.H.; Mullan, J. When Is Diabetes Distress Clinically Meaningful?: Establishing Cut Points for the Diabetes Distress Scale. *Diabetes Care* **2012**, *35*, 259–264. [CrossRef]
13. Meurs, M.; Roest, A.M.; Wolffenbuttel, B.H.R.; Stolk, R.P.; de Jonge, P.; Rosmalen, J.G.M. Association of Depressive and Anxiety Disorders with Diagnosed versus Undiagnosed Diabetes: An Epidemiological Study of 90,686 Participants. *Psychosom. Med.* **2016**, *78*, 233–241. [CrossRef]
14. Mosili, P.; Mkhize, B.C.; Sibiya, N.H.; Ngubane, P.S.; Khathi, A. Review of the Direct and Indirect Effects of Hyperglycemia on the HPA Axis in T2DM and the Co-Occurrence of Depression. *BMJ Open Diabetes Res. Care* **2024**, *12*, e003218. [CrossRef]
15. Barnard, K.; Peveler, R.C.; Holt, R.I.G. Antidepressant Medication as a Risk Factor for Type 2 Diabetes and Impaired Glucose Regulation: Systematic review. *Diabetes Care* **2013**, *36*, 3337–3345. [CrossRef]
16. Darwish, L.; Beroncal, E.; Sison, M.V.; Swardfager, W. Depression in People with Type 2 Diabetes: Current Perspectives. *Diabetes Metab. Syndr. Obesity Targets Ther.* **2018**, *11*, 333–343. [CrossRef]

17. Basiri, R.; Seidu, B.; Rudich, M. Exploring the Interrelationships between Diabetes, Nutrition, Anxiety, and Depression: Implications for Treatment and Prevention Strategies. *Nutrients* **2023**, *15*, 4226. [CrossRef]
18. Hunter, J.C.; DeVellis, B.M.; Jordan, J.M.; Kirkman, M.S.; Linnan, L.A.; Rini, C.; Fisher, E.B. The Association of Depression and Diabetes across Methods, Measures, and Study Contexts. *Clin. Diabetes Endocrinol.* **2018**, *4*, 1–8. [CrossRef]
19. Svenningsson, I.; Björkelund, C.; Marklund, B.; Gedda, B. Anxiety and Depression in Obese and Normal-Weight Individuals with Diabetes Type 2: A Gender Perspective. *Scand. J. Caring Sci.* **2012**, *26*, 349–354. [CrossRef]
20. Golden, S.H.; Lazo, M.; Carnethon, M.; Bertoni, A.G.; Schreiner, P.J.; Roux, A.V.D.; Lee, H.B.; Lyketsos, C. Examining a Bidirectional Association between Depressive Symptoms and Diabetes. *JAMA* **2008**, *299*, 2751–2759. [CrossRef]
21. Katon, W.J.; Russo, J.E.; Heckbert, S.R.; Lin, E.H.B.; Ciechanowski, P.; Ludman, E.; Young, B.; Von Korff, M. The Relationship between Changes in Depression Symptoms and Changes in Health Risk Behaviors in Patients with Diabetes. *Int. J. Geriatr. Psychiatry* **2010**, *25*, 466–475. [CrossRef]
22. Bădescu, S.V.; Tătaru, C.; Kobylinska, L.; Georgescu, E.L.; Zahiu, D.M.; Zăgrean, A.M.; Zăgrean, L. The Association between Diabetes Mellitus and Depression. *J. Med. Life* **2016**, *9*, 120–125.
23. NHANES. Questionnaires, Datasets, and Related Documentation. Available online: https://wwwn.cdc.gov/nchs/nhanes/continuousnhanes/default.aspx?BeginYear=1999 (accessed on 12 March 2024).
24. National Health and Nutrition Examination Survey (NHANES) | CMS. Available online: https://www.cms.gov/About-CMS/Agency-Information/OMH/resource-center/hcps-and-researchers/data-tools/sgm-clearinghouse/nhanes (accessed on 2 August 2024).
25. NHANES. About the National Health and Nutrition Examination Survey. Available online: https://www.cdc.gov/nchs/nhanes/about_nhanes.htm (accessed on 2 August 2024).
26. Kroenke, K.; Spitzer, R.L.; Williams, J.B.W. The PHQ-9. *J. Gen. Intern. Med.* **2001**, *16*, 606–613. [CrossRef]
27. CDC Diabetes and Mental Health. Available online: https://www.cdc.gov/diabetes/living-with/mental-health.html (accessed on 12 March 2024).
28. Li, C.; Shang, S.; Liang, W. Physical Activity Types, Physical Activity Levels and Risk of Diabetes in General Adults: The NHANES 2007–2018. *Int. J. Environ. Res. Public Health* **2023**, *20*, 1398. [CrossRef]
29. Lim, E.; Davis, J.; Chen, J.J. The Association of Race/Ethnicity, Dietary Intake, and Physical Activity with Depression. *J. Racial Ethn. Health Disparities* **2021**, *8*, 315–331. [CrossRef]
30. Egede, L.E.; Poston, M.E. Racial/Ethnic Differences in Leisure-Time Physical Activity Levels among Individuals with Diabetes. *Diabetes Care* **2004**, *27*, 2493–2494. [CrossRef]
31. Sartorius, N. Depression and Diabetes. *Dialogues Clin. Neurosci.* **2018**, *20*, 47–52. [CrossRef]
32. Engum, A. The Role of Depression and Anxiety in Onset of Diabetes in a Large Population-Based Study. *J. Psychosom. Res.* **2007**, *62*, 31–38. [CrossRef]
33. Wiltink, J.; Beutel, M.E.; Till, Y.; Ojeda, F.M.; Wild, P.S.; Münzel, T.; Blankenberg, S.; Michal, M. Prevalence of Distress, Comorbid Conditions and Well Being in the General Population. *J. Affect. Disord.* **2011**, *130*, 429–437. [CrossRef]
34. Gary-Webb, T.L.; Baptiste-Roberts, K.; Pham, L.; Wesche-Thobaben, J.; Patricio, J.; Pi-Sunyer, F.X.; Brown, A.F.; Jones-Corneille, L.; Brancati, F.L.; Look AHEAD Research Group. Neighborhood Socioeconomic Status, Depression, and Health Status in the Look AHEAD (Action for Health in Diabetes) Study. *BMC Public Health* **2011**, *11*, 349. [CrossRef]
35. Ludman, E.J.; Katon, W.; Russo, J.; Von Korff, M.; Simon, G.; Ciechanowski, P.; Lin, E.; Bush, T.; Walker, E.; Young, B. Depression and Diabetes Symptom Burden. *Gen. Hosp. Psychiatry* **2004**, *26*, 430–436. [CrossRef]
36. Renn, B.N.; Feliciano, L.; Segal, D.L. The Bidirectional Relationship of Depression and Diabetes: A Systematic Review. *Clin. Psychol. Rev.* **2011**, *31*, 1239–1246. [CrossRef] [PubMed]
37. Wium-Andersen, I.K.; Hengeveld, E.M.; Rungby, J.; Jørgensen, M.B.; Osler, M.; Wium-Andersen, M.K. Hemoglobin A1c-Levels and Subsequent Risk of Depression in Individuals with and without Diabetes. *J. Diabetes Its Complicat.* **2021**, *35*, 107946. [CrossRef] [PubMed]
38. Penckofer, S.; Quinn, L.; Byrn, M.; Ferrans, C.; Miller, M.; Strange, P. Does Glycemic Variability Impact Mood and Quality of Life? *Diabetes Technol. Ther.* **2012**, *14*, 303–310. [CrossRef] [PubMed]
39. Lin, E.H.B.; Rutter, C.M.; Katon, W.; Heckbert, S.R.; Ciechanowski, P.; Oliver, M.M.; Ludman, E.J.; Young, B.A.; Williams, L.H.; McCulloch, D.K.; et al. Depression and Advanced Complications of Diabetes: A Prospective Cohort Study. *Diabetes Care* **2009**, *33*, 264–269. [CrossRef]

biomedicines

MDPI

Article

Neonatal Outcomes in Patients with Gestational Diabetes Mellitus Treated with Metformin: A Retrospective Study in Saudi Arabia

Khaled H. Aburisheh [1,*], Mazen M. Barhoush [1], Abdulaziz N. Alahmari [2], Ziyad A. Altasan [3] and Muffarah H. Alharthi [4]

1 University Diabetes Center, King Saud University Medical City, King Saud University, Riyadh 11472, Saudi Arabia; mazen_barhoush@yahoo.com
2 Department of Family Medicine, King Saud University Medical City, Riyadh 11472, Saudi Arabia; abdulaziznh94@gmail.com
3 Ministry of Health, Riyadh 11472, Saudi Arabia; ziyadtasan@gmail.com
4 Department of Family and Community Medicine, College of Medicine, University of Bisha, Bisha 61922, Saudi Arabia; muffarah@hotmail.com
* Correspondence: kaburisheh@ksu.edu.sa; Tel.: +966-542039264; Fax: +966-114671992

Abstract: Background: Gestational diabetes mellitus (GDM) is a common endocrine disease that can occur during pregnancy, increasing the risk of fetal morbidity and mortality. Metformin is a commonly used therapeutic approach for managing GDM. However, there is controversy regarding the effects of metformin on fetal outcomes during pregnancy. This study aimed to evaluate the safety of metformin in relation to neonatal complications, compared to treatment with insulin and/or specialized diets. Method: This was a retrospective study that included pregnant women who were diagnosed with GDM and treated with specialized diets, metformin, or insulin. Data were collected from patients' electronic medical records and analyzed to evaluate the risk of neonatal outcomes in the metformin group compared to the others. Results: The study included 234 women with GDM. There was no difference between the metformin and insulin groups in terms of the rates of neonatal outcomes, while neonatal hypoglycemia, neonatal hyperbilirubinemia, large for gestational age, and respiratory distress were higher in the metformin group when compared to the diet group. Metformin slightly increased the risk of a lower APGAR score compared to diet alone. Conclusions: Metformin was found to be a safe therapy for the fetus when used to manage GDM, compared to insulin therapy. More randomized studies are needed to confirm these findings in the Saudi population.

Keywords: gestational diabetes; neonatal outcomes; metformin; insulin; diet

1. Introduction

Gestational diabetes mellitus (GDM) to refers to any abnormally high glucose value that is diagnosed during pregnancy [1]; however, while this term is typically reserved for women diagnosed in the second or third trimester, it can be diagnosed before that period [2]. The development of GDM is considered the most frequent endocrine disorder in pregnancy, and it is usually associated with adverse outcomes that affect both the mother and the fetus [3]. The overall prevalence of GDM in the Middle East and North Africa has been found to be 13%, and is slightly higher in Arab Gulf countries (14.7%) [4].

Women with GDM have higher incidence of hypertension (HTN), pre-eclampsia, preterm birth, and cesarian section, as well as increased risk of the development of type 2 diabetes mellitus (T2DM) after delivery. Moreover, there is an increased risk of fetal outcomes including higher birth weight, macrosomia, polyhydramnios, birth injury, neonatal hypoglycemia, and neonatal hyperbilirubinemia [5,6].

Early intervention aimed at achieving recommended blood glucose levels may help to delay short-term complications. The primary strategy for managing GDM involves promoting a nutritious diet and advocating for regular physical activity, which could be effective in achieving normal blood glucose levels for approximately 70% of pregnant individuals with GDM [7]. However, in those with uncontrolled levels, the next step is to consider the addition of pharmacological therapy as a means to control hyperglycemia and prevent both maternal and infant complications [8].

Insulin has traditionally been regarded as the standard treatment. This recommendation is consistently supported by the American Diabetes Association (ADA) guidelines [8]. However, it necessitates multiple daily injections and requires patients to undergo training in the technical aspects of treatment. This can result in increased weight gain and higher medical costs. Additionally, approximately 70% of women who use insulin during pregnancy experience episodes of hypoglycemia [9].

Metformin primarily targets the mitochondria, to decrease hepatic gluconeogenesis, regulate hepatic function influenced by glucagon, and improve peripheral insulin sensitivity [10]. Although there is a lack of comprehensive data on the long-term effects of metformin use during pregnancy on offspring as it can cross the placenta [11], it is frequently chosen as the initial treatment option for GDM patients with mild hyperglycemia. Metformin is more cost-effective compared to insulin, has a lower risk of hypoglycemia, and can help to reduce maternal gestational weight gain as well as the occurrence of infants born large for gestational age (LGA) [12]. The use of metformin in pregnancy remains a topic of debate and controversy. While certain studies support its use for glycemic control in pregnant women, others have indicated an elevated risk of adverse events [13,14]. Moreover, to the best of our knowledge, there is no such study considering the Saudi pregnant population diagnosed with GDM.

The present study aimed to assess the neonatal outcomes in Saudi GDM patients treated with metformin compared to diet alone or insulin therapy.

2. Materials and Methods

2.1. Ethical Approval

This study was conducted according to the relevant guidelines and regulations, and the Institutional Review Board of the College of Medicine, King Saud University, Saudi Arabia reviewed and approved the protocol (E-22-6911). As this was a retrospective data collection study, informed consent was waived by the Institutional Review Board of the College of Medicine, King Saud University, Riyadh.

2.2. Study Design

A retrospective observational study was conducted through a review of the medical records of women with GDM who attended gestational diabetes clinics and delivered their child at King Saud University Medical City (KSUMC) in Riyadh, Saudi Arabia, from January 2017 to June 2022.

2.3. Diagnosis and Management of GDM

GDM was diagnosed using a 75 g oral glucose tolerance test (OGTT), with one diagnostic criterion used throughout the study period—either a fasting plasma glucose level of $\geq$5.1 mmol/L, a 1-h plasma glucose level of $\geq$10 mmol/L, or a 2-h plasma glucose level of $\geq$8.5 mmol/L—according to ADA guidelines [15]. After the diagnosis of GDM, patients were referred to diabetes educators and dietitians for dietary advice, including information about a carbohydrate-modified diet. Patients were also advised to monitor their blood glucose levels at least 4 times daily (when fasting and at 2-h post-meals) using a blood glucose meter. Patients were evaluated by an endocrinologist or diabetologist, and management was modified according to the target blood glucose levels (i.e., fasting < 5.3 mmol/L and 2 h post-prandial < 6.7 mmol/L) [8]. Pharmacological therapy was started if the target blood glucose level was not achieved through diet and lifestyle modification alone. The choice of pharmacological therapy between metformin and insulin was dependent on the physician's recommendation and the patient's preference. If metformin was started but was not sufficient to ameliorate hyperglycemia, insulin therapy was initiated.

2.4. Subjects

GDM patients who attended gestational diabetes clinics, delivered their child at KSUMC in Riyadh, and had a complete medical record were collected randomly from the full list covering the study period, consisting of 1607 GDM patients, and were included in the study. We excluded patients with type 1 or type 2 diabetes mellitus, patients with any other disease that could affect blood glucose control (e.g., autoimmune and inflammatory diseases), and those using corticosteroids. Moreover, we excluded those who were treated with a combination of metformin and insulin.

The minimum sample size needed for this study was estimated to be 234 patients based on $\alpha = 0.05$, $\beta = 0.99$, an odds ratio (OR) of 1 to assess neonatal outcomes, and a binomial distribution. The patients were divided into 3 groups according to the means of GDM management (78 patients in the diet-only group, 78 in the insulin-only group, and 78 in the metformin-only group).

2.5. Data Collection

Data were extracted from the patients' electronic medical records, including maternal demographics (i.e., age at pregnancy; body mass index (BMI) in the first trimester; family history ofT2DM; parity; previous history of GDM; previous history of abortions; previous history of macrosomia; gestational age at diagnosis of GDM; gestational age at initiation of pharmacotherapy; OGTT results; glycated hemoglobin (HbA1c) before delivery; the averages of fasting blood sugar (FBS) and 2-h post-prandial glucose (PPG), both calculated from documented home glucose readings before delivery; pre-pregnancy and pregnancy-induced HTN; pre-eclampsia; and gestational age at delivery) and neonatal outcomes (i.e., preterm birth (<37 weeks); neonatal intensive care unit (NICU) admission; neonatal hypoglycemia (<45 mg/dL) and hypocalcemia (<9 mg/dL); congenital anomalies; birth injury; birth weight; perinatal death; five-minute APGAR score at 5 min—this method helps to identify infants requiring respiratory support or other resuscitative measures (with a score of 7–10 considered as reassuring, a score of 4–6 as moderately abnormal, and a score of 0–3 as low); macrosomia, defined as an instance where a fetus is larger than 4000 g; shoulder dystocia; neonatal jaundice or hyperbilirubinemia, where total serum bilirubin is more than 12 mg/dL or is treated with phototherapy; respiratory distress; LGA, defined as birth weight >90th centile for gestational age and gender; and small for gestational age (SGA), defined as birth weight <10th centile for gestational age and gender).

2.6. Statistical Analysis

The analysis was performed using PSPP software (version 1.6.2-g78a33a). Data are presented as the mean and SD or the number and percentage for numerical and categorical variables, respectively. Comparisons were made between all three groups (overall test), and pair-wise comparisons were made between mothers treated with metformin and insulin, as well as between mothers treated with metformin and diet. Differences between groups were compared using Student's independent t-test and one-way analysis of variance (ANOVA) for continuous data, and the chi-squared test for categorical data. To evaluate the independent effect of metformin on neonatal outcomes, multivariate logistic regression was performed to estimate adjusted ORs and CIs. We considered p-values lower than 0.05 to be statistically significant.

3. Results

3.1. Study Population and Demographics

During the study period of January 2017 to June 2022, 234 women with GDM were included in the study. They were categorized equally into three groups, according to their management regimen (i.e., metformin, insulin, or diet). The mean age of all participants was 33.09 ± 5.57 years. Patients who were using metformin were significantly older than those who were treated through diet alone. Most of the patients were obese during the first trimester, with a mean BMI of 33.34 ± 5.47 kg/m^2. There was no significant difference between the metformin and insulin groups; however, the metformin group was significantly heavier than the diet group. Moreover, metformin users were diagnosed with GDM earlier than those who were treated through diet alone, with the mean gestational age of GDM diagnosis for all patients being 27.16 ± 4.51 weeks. The presence of a family history of T2DM, previous macrosomia, and history of abortions was similar in all groups. However, women treated with metformin had more history of previous GDM than those treated through diet, and less history than those treated with insulin. None of the participants had pre-pregnancy HTN, and only a few metformin- or insulin-treated patients developed HTN and pre-eclampsia during pregnancy (3% and 2.1%, respectively), while no patients in the diet group developed these conditions. Furthermore, the mean gestational age of delivery was 38 ± 1.67 weeks and was significantly earlier in the metformin group compared to the diet group (Table 1).

Table 1. Baseline characteristics for women with gestational diabetes mellitus according to treatment group.

Maternal Characteristics	Total (234)	Metformin (78)	Insulin (78)	Diet (78)	Metformin vs. Insulin *p* Value	Metformin vs. Diet Only *p* Value
Maternal age (years ± SD)	33.09 ± 5.57	33.88 ± 5.67	34.59 ± 5.36	30.79 ± 4.97	0.426	0.002 [a]
Maternal BMI (Kg/m^2 ± SD)	33.34 ± 5.47	34.29 ± 5.58	33.16 ± 5.64	32.55 ± 5.12	0.214	0.044 [a]
Parity	2.67 ± 2.05	2.58 ± 1.99	3.09 ± 2.28	2.32 ± 1.8	0.137	0.24
Diagnosis of GDM (weeks ± SD)	27.16 ± 4.51	26.47 ± 4.62	26.84 ± 4.43	28.17 ± 4.36	0.612	0.02 [a]
Previous GDM, *n* (%)	80 (34.2)	27 (34.60)	40 (51.3)	13 (16.70)	0.035 [a]	0.01 [a]
Family history of T2DM, *n* (%)	46 (19.7)	14 (17.90)	22 (28.20)	10 (12.80)	0.128	0.375
Previous macrosomia, *n* (%)	10 (4.3)	3 (3.80)	7 (9.00)	0	0.191	0.08
Previous abortion, *n* (%)	92 (39.3)	32 (41)	28 (35.90)	32 (41)	0.51	1
Pre-pregnancy HTN, *n* (%)	0	0	0	0	NA [b]	NA [b]
Pregnancy-induced HTN, *n* (%)	7 (3)	4 (5.1)	3 (3.8)	0	0.699	0.043 [a]
Pre-eclampsia, *n* (%)	5 (2.1)	3 (3.8)	2 (2.6)	0	0.649	0.08
OGTT 0 h (mmol/L ± SD)	5.34 ± 1.19	5.27 ± 0.85	5.83 ± 1.65	4.94 ± 0.7	0.01 [a]	0.008 [a]
OGTT 1 h (mmol/L ± SD)	10.87 ± 1.85	10.73 ± 1.95	11.39 ± 2.07	10.54 ± 1.54	0.043 [a]	0.489
OGTT 2 h (mmol/L ± SD)	9.16 ± 2.11	9.42 ± 2.13	9.42 ± 2.05	8.67 ± 2.07	0.991	0.027 [a]
Gestational age at initiation of pharmacotherapy (weeks ± SD)	31.46 ± 4.55	30.88 ± 4.65	32.04 ± 4.4	NA	0.114	NA
Total daily dose of metformin reached (mg ± SD)	NA	1166.03 ± 486.61	NA	NA	NA	NA
Total daily dose of insulin reached (units ± SD)	NA	NA	16.88 ± 16.54	NA	NA	NA
Average HbA1c before delivery (%)	6.41 ± 3.7	5.7	6.44 ± 1.12	6.41 ± 4.78	0.525	0.885
Average FBS before delivery (mmol/L ± SD)	5.27 ± 1	5.42 ± 0.73	5.54 ± 1.29	4.69 ± 0.58	0.49	0.000 [a]
Average 2 h PP before delivery (mmol/L ± SD)	7.23 ± 1.53	7.7 ± 1.38	7.53 ± 1.69	6.1 ± 0.74	0.519	0.000 [a]
Gestational age at delivery (weeks ± SD)	38 ± 1.67	37.69 ± 2	37.6 ± 1.24	38.72 ± 1.44	0.737	0.000 [a]

SD: standard deviation, BMI: body mass index, GDM: gestational diabetes mellitus, T2DM: type 2 diabetes mellitus, HTN: hypertension, OGTT: oral glucose tolerance test, HbA1c: glycated hemoglobin, FBS: fasting blood sugar, PP: postprandial, NA: not applicable. [a] $p \leq 0.05$. [b] p value could not be calculated because of zero cell values.

3.2. Glycemic Control

Table 1 presents the OGTT values at diagnosis of GDM, where the mean of fasting and the 1-h and 2-h post-OGTT glucose levels were 5.34 ± 1.19, 10.87 ± 1.85, and 9.16 ± 2.11 mmol/L, respectively. The highest FBS values were observed among the insulin group while the lowest were in the diet group, with significant differences when compared to the metformin group. Furthermore, the metformin group had significantly lower 1-h post-OGTT glucose levels compared to the insulin group (10.73 ± 1.95 vs. 11.39 ± 2.07 mmol/L; p = 0.043) and higher 2-h post-OGTT glucose levels compared to the diet group (9.42 ± 2.13 vs. 8.67 ± 2.07 mmol/L; p = 0.027).

There was no significant difference in HbA1c between the groups before delivery, with a mean HbA1c of 6.41 ± 3.7%; however, the averages of FBS and 2-h PPG were significantly higher in the metformin and insulin groups compared to the diet group.

3.3. Neonatal Outcomes

Table 2 presents the neonatal outcomes for all therapeutic groups. There were no significant differences between the insulin and metformin groups for all neonatal outcome parameters analyzed in this study. Women treated with metformin had a significantly higher rate of neonatal hypoglycemia compared to those treated with diet alone (9 vs. 1.3%; $p = 0.029$). Moreover, neonatal jaundice and hyperbilirubinemia, respiratory distress, and LGA were significantly higher in the metformin group compared to the diet group (26.9 vs. 14.1%, $p = 0.047$; 9 vs. 1.3%, $p = 0.029$; 9 vs. 1.3%, $p = 0.029$, respectively).

Table 2. Neonatal outcomes for women receiving metformin in comparison to those receiving insulin or a specialized diet alone.

Parameter	Metformin	Insulin	Diet	Overall p Value	Metformin vs. Insulin p Value	Metformin vs. Diet Only p Value
Preterm birth (%)	10.30	14.10	5.10	0.168	0.463	0.229
NICU admission (%)	17.90	20.5	9	0.116	0.685	0.101
Neonatal hypocalcemia (%)	2.60	6.40	1.30	0.186	0.246	0.56
Neonatal hypoglycemia (%)	9	10.30	1.30	0.056	0.786	0.029 [a]
Congenital anomaly (%)	10.30	11.50	10.30	0.956	0.797	1
Birth injury (%)	0	0	2.60	0.133	NA [b]	0.155
Birth weight (g ± SD)	3139.27 ± 632.59	3200.58 ± 454.85	3188.26 ± 413.11	0.729	0.488	0.568
Perinatal death (%)	0	2.6	0	0.366	0.316	NA [b]
Five-minute APGAR score ± SD	8.88 ± 0.36	8.84 ± 0.84	8.99 ± 0.3	0.257	0.698	0.055
Macrosomia (%)	2.60	2.60	0	0.362	1	0.155
Shoulder dystocia (%)	0	1.30	1.30	0.604	0.316	0.316
Neonatal jaundice/hyperbilirubinemia (%)	26.9	23.10	14.1	0.134	0.579	0.047 [a]
Respiratory distress (%)	9	12.80	1.3	0.023 [a]	0.441	0.029 [a]
Large for gestational age (>90th percentile) (%)	9	12.80	1.3	0.023 [a]	0.441	0.029 [a]
Small for gestational age (<10th percentile) (%)	3	2.1	2.6	0.835	0.548	0.772

SD: standard deviation, NICU: neonatal intensive care unit, NA: not applicable. [a] $p \leq 0.05$. [b] p value could not be calculated because of zero cell values.

3.4. Multiple Regression Analysis

After multiple regression analyses with the adjustment of multiple factors, metformin did not increase the risk of neonatal outcomes when compared to insulin and diet, except for the five-minute APGAR score, where metformin significantly increased the risk of a lower score compared to diet (standardized beta = −0.18; $p = 0.036$) (Table 3).

Table 3. Multiple regression analysis of the effect of metformin on neonatal outcomes in comparison with insulin or diet alone.

Parameter	Metformin vs. Insulin p Value; Adjusted OR [d] (95%CI)	Metformin vs. Diet Only p Value; Adjusted OR [e] (95%CI)
Preterm birth	0.702; 1.25 (0.39–3.98)	0.304; 2.04 (0.53–7.69)
NICU admission	0.465; 1.42 (0.55–3.66)	0.233; 1.89 (0.66–5.56)
Neonatal hypocalcemia	0.871; 0.85 (0.12–6.21)	0.928; 0.88 (0.05–14.29)
Neonatal hypoglycemia	0.852; 1.13 (0.31–4.19)	0.120; 5.88 (0.63–50)
Congenital anomaly	0.774; 0.85 (0.27–2.61)	0.494; 1.47 (0.48–4.55)
Birth injury	NA	0.511; 0.34 (0.01–8.3)
Birth weight	0.941; 0.01	0.126; −0.13 [c]
Perinatal death	0.177; 3.74 (0.55–25.39)	NA [b]
Five-minute APGAR score	0.641; 0.04	0.036 [a]; −0.18 [c]

Table 3. *Cont.*

Parameter	Metformin vs. Insulin p Value; Adjusted OR [d] (95%CI)	Metformin vs. Diet Only p Value; Adjusted OR [e] (95%CI)
Macrosomia	0.81; 1.3 (0.15–11.1)	0.268; 2.86 (0.44–20)
Shoulder dystocia	NA	0.103; 0.08 (0.004–1.67)
Neonatal jaundice/hyperbilirubinemia	0.280; 1.55 (0.7–3.45)	0.140; 1.92 (0.81–4.55)
Respiratory distress	0.655; 0.77 (0.24–2.45)	0.102; 6.25 (0.69–50)
Large for gestational age (>90th percentile)	0.706; 0.8 (0.24–2.61)	0.152; 5.26 (0.54–50)
Small for gestational age (<10th percentile)	0.874; 1.1 (0.33–3.73)	0.575; 1.43 (0.42–4.76)

NICU: neonatal intensive care unit, NA: not applicable. [a] $p \leq 0.05$. [b] OR could not be calculated because of zero cell values. [c] Adjusted standardized beta. [d] Adjusted for OGTT at 0, OGTT at 1 h, and previous GDM. [e] Adjusted for age at pregnancy, maternal BMI, OGTT at 0, OGTT at 2 h, and previous GDM.

4. Discussion

Our study revealed that there is no significant difference between the effects of metformin and insulin, as therapies for GDM, on neonatal outcomes. Moreover, we found significantly higher rates of neonatal hypoglycemia, neonatal hyperbilirubinemia, respiratory distress, and LGA in the metformin-treated group compared to the diet-only treatment group. However, from the multiple regression analysis, we concluded that metformin has no significant effect on the neonatal outcome, aside from a slightly increased risk of a lower APGAR score when compared to diet alone.

The results of our study indicate that women who were started on metformin were heavier, older, and had earlier diagnoses of GDM than those who received treatment through diet alone. Moreover, OGTT values, average FBS, and PPGlevels were higher in the metformin group. These findings are not surprising, as in people who are obese higher measures of non-esterified fatty acids, glycerol, counterregulatory hormones, and pro-inflammatory cytokines that partake in the advancement of insulin resistance are delivered by adipose tissue [16]. This leads to higher glucose values, and reflects the routine clinical practice of choosing metformin in such patients. Similar data have been reported in many other studies [17–21].

Our study revealed that the metformin-treated group had a higher prevalence of previous GDM when compared to the diet control group, but a lower prevalence compared to the insulin-treated group. This suggests that the need for escalated medication may be associated with insulin resistance. Moreover, the history of previous GDM is considered to be a predictor of insulin initiation in patients with GDM [22].

The outcomes revealed that few patients in the metformin and insulin groups developed gestational HTN and pre-eclampsia. Furthermore, only the difference in the rate of pregnancy-induced HTN was significant when compared to the group treated with diet. Slagjana et al. also observed significantly more cases of pre-eclampsia in those taking metformin and insulin compared to diet [17]. On the other hand, another study concluded that there is no significant difference between all management groups regarding hypertensive complications [23].

Evidence from many studies has demonstrated that treating women with GDM using glycemic-lowering therapy is associated with a slightly earlier gestational age of delivery, as compared with treatment through diet alone [13,20,21,24]. Our data analysis confirmed this evidence. In contrast, this association was not observed in the study by Slagjana et al. when comparing metformin-treated and diet-treated patients [17].

A meta-analysis of five randomized studies comprising 1270 patients with GDM was consistent with our findings, as it concluded that metformin causes similar neonatal complications to insulin [25]. Furthermore, a recent meta-analysis of 24 studies including

4934 participants revealed a reduction in neonatal complications with the use of metformin, especially for macrosomia, LGA, NICU admission, and neonatal hypoglycemia [26].

Slagjana et al. and McGrath et al. both found a significant increase in the rate of incidence of neonatal hypoglycemia in those who used metformin compared to those who were treated through diet only [17,20]. Moreover, another study reported a similar increment in neonatal hypoglycemia; however, the association was not significant [13]. These findings are in agreement with our results. However, other studies did not observe such a difference [13,23,24], with Bashir et al. even concluding that metformin reduces the risk of neonatal hypoglycemia compared to diet alone [19]. The higher rate of newborn hypoglycemia in the metformin group can be explained by the higher average prenatal FBS and PPG in this group compared with the diet group.

Surprisingly, we found that the rates of neonatal hyperbilirubinemia and jaundice were higher when using metformin compared to a specialized diet alone, which contradicts many published studies concluding that metformin therapy has no effect on neonatal jaundice [13,20,27]. However, our results coincide with the findings of D'douza et al. and Callegari et al. [21,28]. This result could be due to the earlier gestational age at delivery and increased severity of the disease in those who were treated with metformin compared to diet alone.

In contrast to the evidence of no increased risk of neonatal respiratory distress with maternal usage of metformin during pregnancy [13,20,21,23], we found a higher rate of this outcome in the metformin group compared to the group treated through diet alone. This finding could also be interpreted according to the advanced disease and earlier delivery in this group.

Notably, SGA and lower birth weight are the most highly reported side effects when metformin is used by pregnant women [29]. Interestingly, our study revealed the opposite finding, as the rate of LGA was significantly higher with metformin treatment compared to diet alone; no difference was observed in the mean birth weight. A study from Qatar shows a comparable result (27 vs. 18%; $p = 0.008$) [28]. The older age, earlier diagnosis of GDM, and higher average blood glucose before delivery in the metformin-treated patients could explain this finding.

It has been shown previously that specific maternal factors are considered to predict several neonatal outcomes inGDM. Maternal metabolic factors such as obesity, high blood pressure, high blood glucose values in the first trimester, and high HbA1c at the diagnosis of GDM have significant associations with increased outcomes. Moreover, previous macrosomia was found to have a strong role in this context. Therefore, risk stratification of the occurrence of neonatal complications based on maternal clinical parameters could guide the strategies of GDM management and the intensification of therapy [30].

After further analysis of our data through multiple regression and adjustment of several risk factors, we determined that those treated with metformin in this study did not have an increased risk of perinatal outcomes when compared to those who underwent insulin and diet treatments. However, there was a slight but significantly increased risk of a lower score for the five-minute APGAR test after metformin treatment compared to diet treatment, which is not clinically significant and is in contrast to what has been reported in the literature [13,17,21,24].

Our study is the first study in Saudi Arabia to evaluate the influence of metformin on neonatal outcomes. Furthermore, we included many different maternal risk factors that could affect the outcomes in our analysis, which serves to strengthen our study. However, the retrospective and observational nature of our study could be one of the limitations, as it could not confirm the causality and the effects of medication on the outcomes. In addition, the lack of randomization in our study may have affected the reliability of our results. Furthermore, we did not match the groups used in the study, and some missing data could affect our results. Moreover, diet compliance by participants was not assessed, which is considered an essential part of GDM management. Finally, the number of women included in the analysis was low.

5. Conclusions

Metformin was found to be a safe therapy for GDM, compared to insulin therapy, when considering the risk of neonatal complications. While the incidences of LGA, neonatal hypoglycemia, neonatal hyperbilirubinemia, and respiratory distress were higher with metformin therapy compared to lifestyle modification, metformin did not increase the risk of these complications after multiple regression analysis. Further prospective randomized studies in the Saudi population with long follow-up periods are required to confirm the safety of metformin with regard to the offspring of women with GDM.

Author Contributions: Conceptualization, K.H.A. and M.M.B.; development and design of methodology, K.H.A., M.M.B., A.N.A., Z.A.A. and M.H.A.; conduction of research and data collection, A.N.A., Z.A.A. and M.H.A.; statistical analysis of study data, K.H.A.; writing of initial draft, M.M.B., A.N.A., Z.A.A. and M.H.A.; critical review and revision of initial draft, K.H.A., M.H.A. and M.M.B.; supervision, K.H.A. All authors have read and agreed to the published version of the manuscript.

Funding: This research received no external funding.

Institutional Review Board Statement: This study was conducted according to the relevant guidelines and regulations, and the Institutional Review Board of the College of Medicine, King Saud University, Saudi Arabia reviewed and approved the protocol (E-22-6911).

Informed Consent Statement: As this was a retrospective data collection study, informed consent was waived by the Institutional Review Board of the College of Medicine, King Saud University, Riyadh.

Data Availability Statement: The data supporting the findings of this study are available from the corresponding author upon reasonable request.

Conflicts of Interest: The authors declare no conflicts of interest.

References

1. McIntyre, H.D.; Catalano, P.; Zhang, C.; Desoye, G.; Mathiesen, E.R.; Damm, P. Gestational diabetes mellitus. *Nat. Rev. Dis. Primers* **2019**, *5*, 47. [CrossRef] [PubMed]
2. Piper, L.K.; Stewart, Z.; Murphy, H.R. Gestational diabetes. *Obstet. Gynaecol. Reprod. Med.* **2017**, *27*, 171–176. [CrossRef]
3. Zhu, Y.; Zhang, C. Prevalence of Gestational Diabetes and Risk of Progression to Type 2 Diabetes: A Global Perspective. *Curr. Diabetes Rep.* **2016**, *16*, 7. [CrossRef]
4. Al-Rifai, R.H.; Abdo, N.M.; Paulo, M.S.; Saha, S.; Ahmed, L.A. Prevalence of Gestational Diabetes Mellitus in the Middle East and North Africa, 2000-2019: A Systematic Review, Meta-Analysis, and Meta-Regression. *Front. Endocrinol.* **2021**, *12*, 668447. [CrossRef]
5. HAPO Study Cooperative Research Group; Metzger, B.E.; Lowe, L.P.; Dyer, A.R.; Trimble, E.R.; Chaovarindr, U.; Coustan, D.R.; Hadden, D.R.; McCance, D.R.; Hod, M.; et al. Hyperglycemia and adverse pregnancy outcomes. *N. Engl. J. Med.* **2008**, *358*, 1991–2002.
6. Lowe, W.L., Jr.; Scholtens, D.M.; Lowe, L.P.; Kuang, A.; Nodzenski, M.; Talbot, O.; Catalano, P.M.; Linder, B.; Brickman, W.J.; Clayton, P.; et al. Association of Gestational Diabetes with Maternal Disorders of Glucose Metabolism and Childhood Adiposity. *JAMA* **2018**, *320*, 1005–1016. [CrossRef]
7. Rasmussen, L.; Poulsen, C.W.; Kampmann, U.; Smedegaard, S.B.; Ovesen, P.G.; Fuglsang, J. Diet and Healthy Lifestyle in the Management of Gestational Diabetes Mellitus. *Nutrients* **2020**, *12*, 3050. [CrossRef]
8. ElSayed, N.A.; Aleppo, G.; Aroda, V.R.; Bannuru, R.R.; Brown, F.M.; Bruemmer, D.; Collins, B.S.; Hilliard, M.E.; Isaacs, D.; Johnson, E.L.; et al. on behalf of the American Diabetes Association. 15. Management of Diabetes in Pregnancy: Standards of Care in Diabetes-2023. *Diabetes Care* **2023**, *46* (Suppl. S1), S254–S266. [CrossRef] [PubMed]
9. Brown, J.; Grzeskowiak, L.; Williamson, K.; Downie, M.R.; Crowther, C.A. Insulin for the treatment of women with gestational diabetes. *Cochrane Database Syst. Rev.* **2017**, *11*, CD012037. [CrossRef]
10. Pernicova, I.; Korbonits, M. Metformin—Mode of action and clinical implications for diabetes and cancer. *Nat. Rev. Endocrinol.* **2014**, *10*, 143–156. [CrossRef]
11. Charles, B.; Norris, R.; Xiao, X.; Hague, W. Population pharmacokinetics of metformin in late pregnancy. *Ther. Drug Monit.* **2006**, *28*, 67–72. [CrossRef] [PubMed]
12. Guo, L.; Ma, J.; Tang, J.; Hu, D.; Zhang, W.; Zhao, X. Comparative Efficacy and Safety of Metformin, Glyburide, and Insulin in Treating Gestational Diabetes Mellitus, A Meta-Analysis. *J. Diabetes Res.* **2019**, *2019*, 9804708. [CrossRef]
13. Tertti, K.; Ekblad, U.; Vahlberg, T.; Rönnemaa, T. Comparison of metformin and insulin in the treatment of gestational diabetes, A retrospective, case-control study. *Rev. Diabet. Stud.* **2008**, *5*, 95–101. [CrossRef] [PubMed]

14. Hellmuth, E.; Damm, P.; Mølsted-Pedersen, L. Oral hypoglycaemic agents in 118 diabetic pregnancies. *Diabet. Med.* **2000**, *17*, 507–511. [CrossRef] [PubMed]
15. ElSayed, N.A.; Aleppo, G.; Aroda, V.R.; Bannuru, R.R.; Brown, F.M.; Bruemmer, D.; Collins, B.S.; Gaglia, J.L.; Hilliard, M.E.; Isaacs, D.; et al. on behalf of the American Diabetes Association. 2. Classification and Diagnosis of Diabetes: Standards of Care in Diabetes-2023. *Diabetes Care* **2023**, *46* (Suppl. S1), S19–S40. [CrossRef]
16. Wondmkun, Y.T. Obesity, Insulin Resistance, and Type 2 Diabetes: Associations and Therapeutic Implications. *Diabetes Metab. Syndr. Obes.* **2020**, *13*, 3611–3616. [CrossRef]
17. Simeonova-Krstevska, S.; Bogoev, M.; Bogoeva, K.; Zisovska, E.; Samardziski, I.; Velkoska-Nakova, V.; Livrinova, V.; Todorovska, I.; Sima, A.; Blazevska-Siljanoska, V. Maternal and Neonatal Outcomes in Pregnant Women with Gestational Diabetes Mellitus Treated with Diet, Metformin or Insulin. *Open Access Maced. J. Med. Sci.* **2018**, *6*, 803–807. [CrossRef]
18. Hughes, R.C.E.; Rowan, J.A. Pregnancy in women with Type 2 diabetes: Who takes metformin and what is the outcome? *Diabet. Med.* **2006**, *23*, 318–322. [CrossRef]
19. Bashir, M.; Aboulfotouh, M.; Dabbous, Z.; Mokhtar, M.; Siddique, M.; Wahba, R.; Ibrahim, A.; Brich, S.A.-H.; Konje, J.C.; Abou-Samra, A.-B. Metformin-treated-GDM has lower risk of macrosomia compared to diet-treated GDM—A retrospective cohort study. *J. Matern.-Fetal Neonatal Med.* **2020**, *33*, 2366–2371. [CrossRef]
20. McGrath, R.T.; Glastras, S.J.; Scott, E.S.; Hocking, S.L.; Fulcher, G.R. Outcomes for Women with Gestational Diabetes Treated with Metformin: A Retrospective, Case-Control Study. *J. Clin. Med.* **2018**, *7*, 50. [CrossRef]
21. Callegari, C.; Algeri, P.; Crippa, I.; Mariani, E.; Mussi, S.; Cameroni, I.; Plevani, C.; Roncaglia, N.; Vergani, P. Is Metformin a Safe and Effective Treatment of Gestational Diabetes Mellitus? *Curr. Res. Diabetes Obes. J.* **2018**, *6*, 29–33. [CrossRef]
22. Priya, G.; Kalra, S. Metformin in the management of diabetes during pregnancy and lactation. *Drugs Context* **2018**, *7*, 212523. [CrossRef]
23. Goh, J.E.L.; Sadler, L.; Rowan, J. Metformin for gestational diabetes in routine clinical practice. *Diabet. Med.* **2011**, *28*, 1082–1087. [CrossRef]
24. Bansal, N.; Chaudhary, P.; Ramola, M.; Saxena, N. Comparison of metformin and insulin in the treatment of gestational diabetes, A retrospective study. *Int. J. Reprod. Contracept. Obstet. Gynecol.* **2016**, *5*, 4356–4360. [CrossRef]
25. Gui, J.; Liu, Q.; Feng, L. Metformin vs insulin in the management of gestational diabetes: A meta-analysis. *PLoS ONE* **2013**, *8*, e64585. [CrossRef]
26. Wu, R.; Zhang, Q.; Li, Z. A meta-analysis of metformin and insulin on maternal outcome and neonatal outcome in patients with gestational diabetes mellitus. *J. Matern.-Fetal Neonatal Med.* **2024**, *37*, 2295809. [CrossRef]
27. Yanachkova, V.E.; Staynova, R.; Stoev, S.; Kamenov, Z. Metformin-associated maternal and neonatal outcomes in women with gestational diabetes–a retrospective cohort study. *Ginekol Pol.* **2024**, *95*, 259–265. [CrossRef]
28. D'Souza, A.; Badri, F.; Abdullahi, H.; Ibrahim, I. FRI632 Metformin Use in Gdm Is Not Associated with Increased Incidence of Preterm Labor and Small for Gestational Age Infants Compared to Diet Control Alone. *J. Endocr. Soc.* **2023**, *7* (Suppl. S1), bvad114-852. [CrossRef]
29. He, K.; Guo, Q.; Ge, J.; Li, J.; Li, C.; Jing, Z. The efficacy and safety of metformin alone or as an add-on therapy to insulin in pregnancy with GDM or T2DM, A systematic review and meta-analysis of 21 randomized controlled trials. *J. Clin. Pharm. Ther.* **2022**, *47*, 168–177. [CrossRef]
30. Pintaudi, B.; Fresa, R.; Dalfrà, M.; Dodesini, A.R.; Vitacolonna, E.; Tumminia, A.; Sciacca, L.; Lencioni, C.; Marcone, T.; Lucisano, G.; et al. The risk stratification of adverse neonatal outcomes in women with gestational diabetes (STRONG) study. *Acta Diabetol.* **2018**, *55*, 1261–1273. [CrossRef]

biomedicines

Article

Study of the Effects of Deuterium-Depleted Water on the Expression of GLUT4 and Insulin Resistance in the Muscle Cell Line C2C12

Masumi Kondo [1], Kaichiro Sawada [2], Yosuke Matsuda [2], Makiko Abe [1], Noriyuki Sanechika [2], Yumi Takanashi [2], Yoshitaka Mori [2], Moritsugu Kimura [2] and Masao Toyoda [2,*]

[1] Division of Nephrology, Endocrinology and Metabolism, Department of Medicine, Tokai University Hachioji Hospital, 1838 Ishikawacho, Hachioji 192-0032, Japan; masumi.k@tokai.ac.jp (M.K.); makiko8031@yahoo.co.jp (M.A.)

[2] Division of Nephrology, Endocrinology and Metabolism, Department of Medicine, Tokai University School of Medicine, 143 Shimokasuya, Isehara 259-1193, Japan; sawada.kaichiro.f@tokai.ac.jp (K.S.); yosuke199260@gmail.com (Y.M.); sanechika.noriyuki.c@tokai.ac.jp (N.S.); takanashi.ym@tokai.ac.jp (Y.T.); mori.yoshitaka.k@tokai.ac.jp (Y.M.); km1689@tokai.ac.jp (M.K.)

* Correspondence: m-toyoda@tokai.ac.jp; Tel.: +81-463-93-1121 (ext. 2490)

Abstract: Deuterium-depleted water (DDW) is used in the treatment of many diseases, including cancer and diabetes. To detect the effect of DDW on gene expression and activation of the insulin-responsive transporter GLUT4 as a mechanism for improving the pathology of diabetes, we investigated the GLUT4 expression and glucose uptake at various concentrations of DDW using the myoblast cell line C2C12 differentiated into myotubes. GLUT4 gene expression significantly increased under deuterium depletion, reaching a maximum value at a deuterium concentration of approximately 50 ppm, which was approximately nine times that of natural water with a deuterium concentration of 150 ppm. GLUT4 protein also showed an increase at similar DDW concentrations. The membrane translocation of GLUT4 by insulin stimulation reached a maximum value at a deuterium concentration of approximately 50–75 ppm, which was approximately 2.2 times that in natural water. Accordingly, glucose uptake also increased by up to 2.2 times at a deuterium concentration of approximately 50 ppm. Drug-induced insulin resistance was attenuated, and the glucose uptake was four times higher in the presence of 10 ng/mL TNF-α and three times higher in the presence of 1 µg/mL resistin at a deuterium concentration of approximately 50 ppm relative to natural water. These results suggest that DDW promotes GLUT4 expression and insulin-stimulated activation in muscle cells and reduces insulin resistance, making it an effective treatment for diabetes.

Keywords: deuterium-depleted water; GLUT4; insulin resistance; diabetes

1. Introduction

Deuterium (D) is a stable isotope of hydrogen (H) with a mass of 2. Natural water contains approximately 150 ppm HDO, and differences in its chemical and physical properties are known to have various effects on living organisms. Its involvement in cancer has attracted attention since the last century. Specifically, it has become clear that high deuterium concentrations promote the growth of cancer cells, whereas low deuterium concentrations inhibit the growth of cancer cells and cause tumor regression [1–3]. As an application for cancer treatment, various animal experiments and clinical studies have reported that drinking deuterium-depleted water (DDW) suppresses the expression of cancer genes and causes tumor regression, indicating the possibility that DDW can be used as a safe anticancer drug [4–7].

It has been proposed that the mechanism of the anticancer effect of DDW involves the function of Na+/H+ transporters and H+-ATPase, as well as the mitochondrial NADPH synthesis pathway, but much remains unknown [8,9].

Studies on cancer treatment with DDW have revealed that in cancer patients with diabetes, DDW improves the condition of diabetes, as well as the effects of cancer treatment. It has been reported to affect glucose metabolism, and recent studies have shown that it affects the activity of glucose transporters (GLUTs), which control glucose uptake [10–12]. GLUT4 is a protein expressed in muscle and fat cells. The uptake of sugar is regulated by insulin. This molecule is directly involved in insulin resistance, which manifests itself as advanced diabetes. In normal cells, GLUT4 translocates to the cell membrane upon insulin stimulation to take up glucose; however, insulin resistance is thought to occur when GLUT4 expression is reduced or membrane translocation is inhibited [13–16].

Recent studies using animal models of diabetes have reported that drinking DDW increases the effect of insulin administration and promotes the membrane translocation of GULT4, indicating the possibility of using DDW as a treatment for diabetes [11,12].

To clarify the mechanism by which DDW improves the pathology of diabetes, we investigated the expression and activation of GLUT4 by DDW in a muscle cell line. Furthermore, we investigated glucose uptake under DDW and measured the effect of DDW on insulin resistance induced in cultured cells, demonstrating the possibility that DDW could significantly improve diabetes and demonstrating the contribution of in vitro systems toward exploring this mechanism.

2. Materials and Methods

Deuterium-depleted water (DDW) was provided by Super Light Water Co., Ltd. (Tokyo, Japan). The deuterium concentration was measured using the δ-D equilibration method with an Isotope Ratio Mass Spectrometer (model DELTA Plus XL, Thermo Fisher Scientific, Waltham, MA, USA) [17]. The deuterium concentration in DDW was 15–20 ppm.

Regarding the cell culture, the mouse myoblast cell line C2C12 was obtained from the JCRB Cell Bank (Osaka, Japan). Cells were cultured in DMEM (high-glucose) (Invitrogen, Carlsbad, CA, USA) supplemented with 10% fetal calf serum, 1× GlutaMAX-1, 50 U/mL penicillin, and 50 mg/mL streptomycin in tissue culture plates in a humidified atmosphere of 95% air/5% CO_2 at 37 °C. After confluence, the medium was replaced with medium supplemented with 2% horse serum to promote myotube differentiation, and the cells were cultured for 10 days or 2 weeks [18–20]. At 48 h before harvest, the medium was replaced with medium adjusted to each deuterium concentration using DDW. To determine the optimal deuterium concentration, media with deuterium concentrations ranging from 25 ppm to 150 ppm were used. Insulin (10 μg/mL) was added 30 min before harvest. Insulin resistance was induced in cells by adding 10 ng/mL tumor necrosis factor-α (TNF-α) or 1 μg/mL resistin in culture medium for 24 h.

For the quantitative real-time polymerase chain reaction (qRT-PCR), complimentary DNAs were prepared from cultured cells using a SuperPrep II Cell Lysis and RT kit for qPCR (Toyobo, Osaka, Japan). The reaction mixture was prepared according to the manufacturer's instructions (TaqMan Gene Expression Assays; Thermo Fisher Scientific) and contained primers and probes for mouse GLUT4 (Assay ID: Mm00436615_m1) and 18S ribosomal RNA endogenous control (Thermo Fisher Scientific). PCR was performed using an ABI StepOne Plus (Thermo Fisher Scientific). Data were analyzed using the comparative Ct method, and GLUT4 mRNA was expressed relative to that of the endogenous control [21].

For Western blotting, cells were lysed using xTractor buffer (Takara Bio, Kusatsu, Japan) with a ProteoGuard protease inhibitor (Takara Bio) and cryonase nuclease (Takara Bio). Sodium dodecyl sulfate–polyacrylamide gel electrophoresis (SDS-PAGE) was performed with NuPAGE 4–12% Bis-Tris gel (Thermo Fisher Scientific), and proteins were transferred to a PVDF membrane with an iBlot2 dry blotting system (Thermo Fisher Scientific). After blocking with 5% BSA in Tris-buffered saline (TBS), the PVDF membrane was treated with a mouse monoclonal antibody against mouse GLUT4 (ab238661; Abcam, Cambridge, UK), washed with TBS containing 0.05% Tween 20, and treated with horseradish peroxidase-conjugated anti-mouse IgG antibody. After washing, the reaction was visualized using

EzWestBlue W solution (ATTO Co., Ltd., Tokyo, Japan) [22]. Image analysis was performed using the ImageJ software (version. 1.54h) [23].

For membrane fraction analysis, membrane fractions were isolated from the cells using a ProteoExtract Transmembrane Protein Extraction Kit (Merck, Darmstadt, Germany) [24]. Membrane proteins from cells cultured in media with various concentrations of DDW were prepared as described in the kit manual, and Western blotting was performed to detect GLUT4, as described above.

For the glucose uptake assay, the glucose uptake in the cells was detected using the Glucose Uptake Assay Kit—Green (DOJINDO LAB. Kumamoto, Japan), according to the manufacturer's instructions [25]. Fluorescence-conjugated glucose was photographed with a fluorescence microscope, and the fluorescence intensity was measured with a fluorescence spectrophotometer SpectraMax i3 (Molecular Devices, San Jose, CA, USA).

Re statistics, R (version. 4.3.2) was used for the statistical calculations [26]. The results are presented as the mean ± standard deviation (SD) of at least three samples. Comparisons between two groups were performed using Student's *t*-test. Statistical significance was set at $p < 0.05$.

3. Results

3.1. Promoting Effect of DDW on the Expression of GLUT4

To investigate the effect of DDW on GLUT4 expression, mouse C2C12 cells were differentiated into myotubes, and the effect of DDW on GLUT4 expression was measured. Fully differentiated myotube C2C12 cells were cultured in media adjusted to various deuterium concentrations for 48 h and harvested after stimulation with insulin for 30 min, and the amount of GLUT4 mRNA was compared. A significant increase in the amount of GLUT4 mRNA was observed in the medium with a lower deuterium concentration than in cells cultured in a medium containing natural water (deuterium concentration of 150 ppm) (Figure 1a). This increase was also detected at a deuterium concentration of 125 ppm but was clear at 100 ppm or less, with a peak at 50 ppm. At this time, the expression was approximately nine times that in the natural water medium. When the deuterium concentration was further reduced, the amount of expression decreased but remained higher than that of natural water.

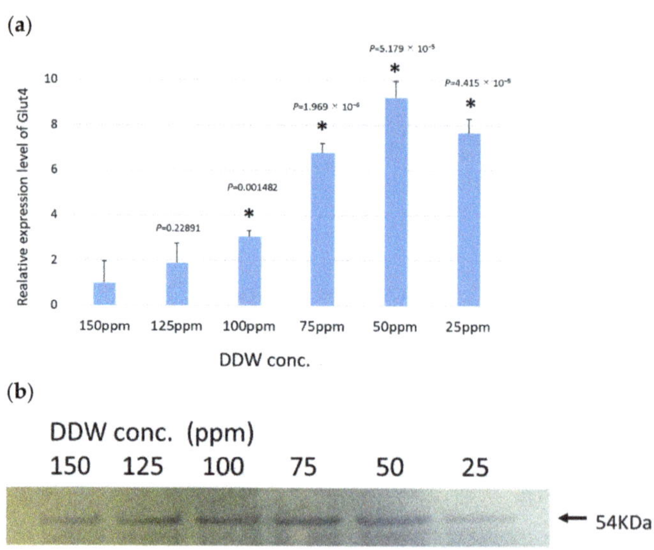

Figure 1. Effect of DDW on the GLUT4 expression in myodifferentiated C2C12 cells. The expression of GLUT4 was examined at the gene and protein levels in the fully differentiated myotubes of C2C12

cells cultured in media adjusted with various concentrations of DDW for 48 h and stimulated with insulin for 30 min before harvest. (**a**) Detection of the expression of GLUT4 by qRT-PCR. The graphs show the relative values compared with those of the natural water medium (150 ppm). Each sample number was ≥3. * Significant difference compared with the natural water medium (150 ppm), $p < 0.05$. (**b**) Diagram of GLUT4 protein expression detected by Western blotting. The arrow indicates the position of the GLUT4 band (54 KDa).

The promoting effect of DDW on the expression of GLUT4 was also confirmed at the protein level (Figure 1b). Western blotting showed that GLUT4 protein, which is difficult to detect in natural water, increased as deuterium concentration decreased, with the maximum amount being at 50–75 ppm deuterium, corresponding to the results at the mRNA level.

These results demonstrated that DDW promoted the expression of GLUT4 in muscle-differentiated C2C12 cells.

3.2. Activation of GLUT4 by DDW

Before insulin stimulation, intracellular GLUT4 accumulates around the nucleus; however, its function is activated by translocation to the cell membrane upon insulin stimulation. To investigate the effect of DDW on GLUT4 activation, fully myotube-differentiated C2C12 cells were cultured for 48 h in media containing various concentrations of DDW, and the GLUT4 in the cell membrane fraction was detected by Western blotting (Figure 2).

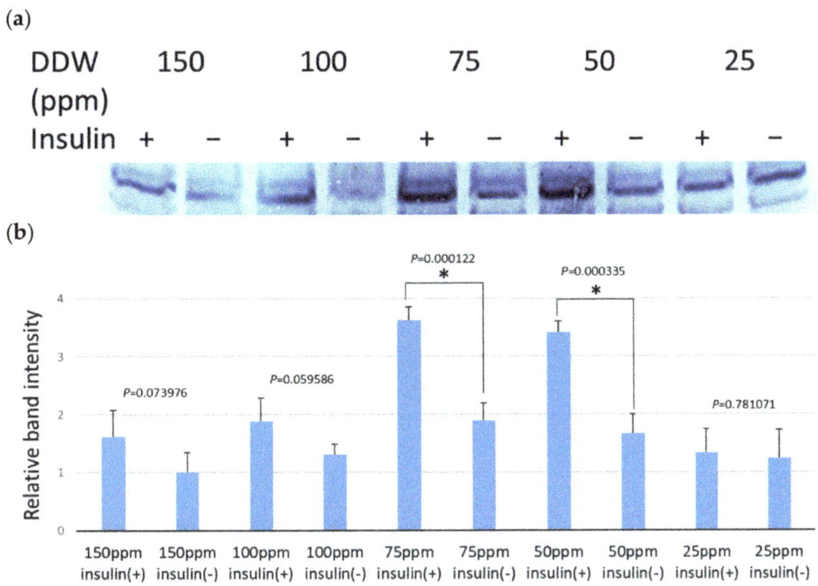

Figure 2. Effect of DDW on the membrane translocation of GLUT4. Fully differentiated C2C12 myotubes were cultured for 48 h in media containing various concentrations of DDW. After insulin stimulation to induce the membrane translocation of GLUT4, the cells were harvested and membrane proteins were extracted. GLUT4 protein was detected and quantified using Western blotting. (**a**) Western blotting of the membrane protein fraction; (**b**) GLUT4 bands were quantified using ImageJ. Values relative to those in cultures without insulin in natural water medium (150 ppm) are shown. The sample size was four. * Significant difference between the presence and absence of insulin in DDW medium at the same concentration ($p < 0.05$).

Even without insulin stimulation, a decrease in deuterium concentration promoted the membrane translocation of GLUT4, reaching a maximum of approximately twice that of natural water at 50–75 ppm. Insulin stimulation in natural water medium induced a 1.6-fold increase in GLUT4 translocation to the membrane relative to the non-stimulated group, while DDW medium further increased GLUT4 translocation. The peak occurred at a deuterium concentration of 50–75 ppm, and approximately 3.5-fold more GLUT4 was translocated to the membrane relative to non-insulin-stimulated natural water medium. This amount was approximately 2.2-fold that of non-insulin-stimulated DDW medium at the same concentration. These results demonstrated that DDW promotes GLUT4 activation through membrane translocation in muscle-differentiated C2C12 cells.

3.3. Effect of DDW on Glucose Uptake and Insulin Resistance

As shown above, DDW promoted the expression and activation of GLUT4; therefore, we observed its effect on the uptake of fluorescence-conjugated glucose into myotube cells.

As a result, in a natural water medium, glucose uptake increased by insulin stimulation by approximately 3.3 times compared with that without insulin stimulation. In DDW medium, even without insulin stimulation, glucose uptake increased with decreasing deuterium concentration, increasing by approximately 2 times at 25–75 ppm. Glucose uptake was significantly increased by insulin stimulation, reaching 7.7 times that of the natural water medium without insulin stimulation at 50 ppm, while it was approximately 3.7 times that of the DDW medium without insulin stimulation at the same concentration. (Figure 3a,d).

Next, to examine the effect of DDW on insulin resistance, myotube-differentiated C2C12 cells were treated with drugs, cultured in medium adjusted with various concentrations of DDW, and then allowed to take up fluorescence-conjugated glucose. To induce insulin resistance, 10 ng/mL TNF-α or 1 μg/mL resistin was added for 24 h. As a result, in a natural water medium, these agents almost completely suppressed the increase in glucose uptake caused by insulin stimulation. In contrast, in DDW medium, these agents had little effect on glucose uptake in the absence of insulin stimulation, and only a slight increase was observed with decreasing DDW concentrations (Figure 3d) before insulin resistance was induced. However, in insulin-stimulated cells, these agents did not sufficiently suppress the uptake of glucose, and at a deuterium concentration of 50 ppm, where the maximum glucose uptake was observed, 45–70% of the glucose uptake before the induction of insulin resistance was confirmed (Figure 3b,c,e,f). These results revealed that DDW attenuated insulin resistance.

(a)

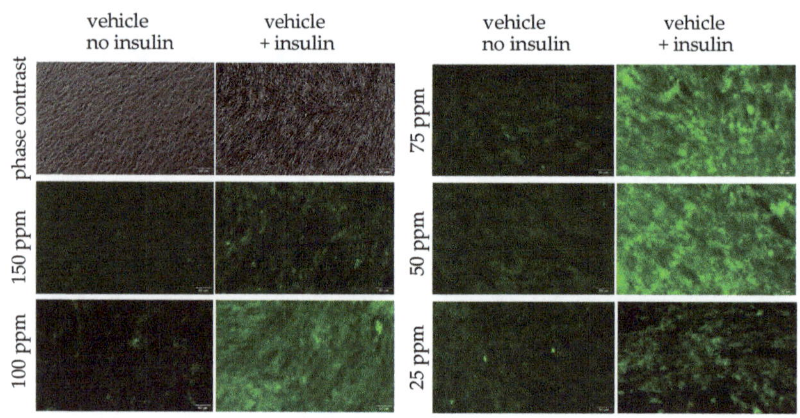

Figure 3. *Cont.*

(**b**)

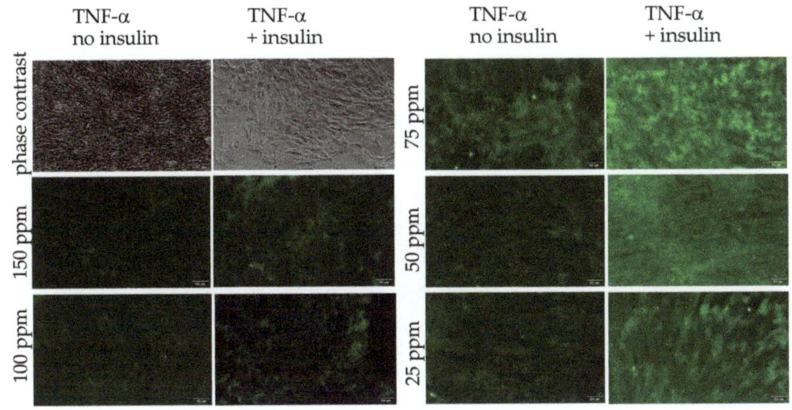

(**c**)

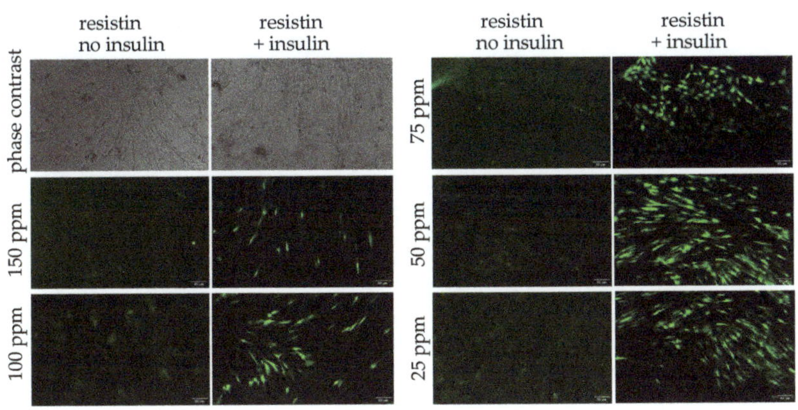

(**d**)

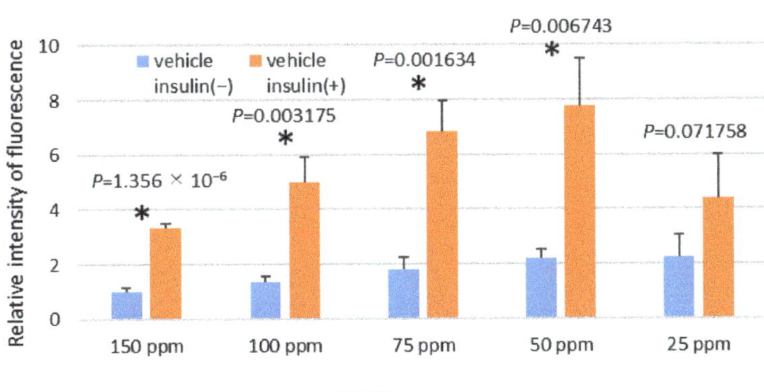

Figure 3. *Cont.*

(e)

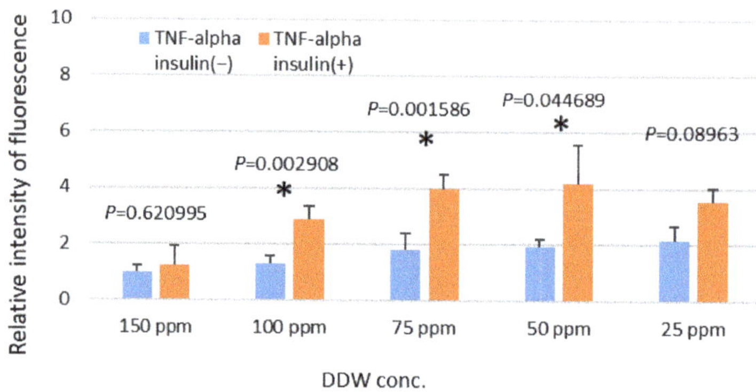

(f)

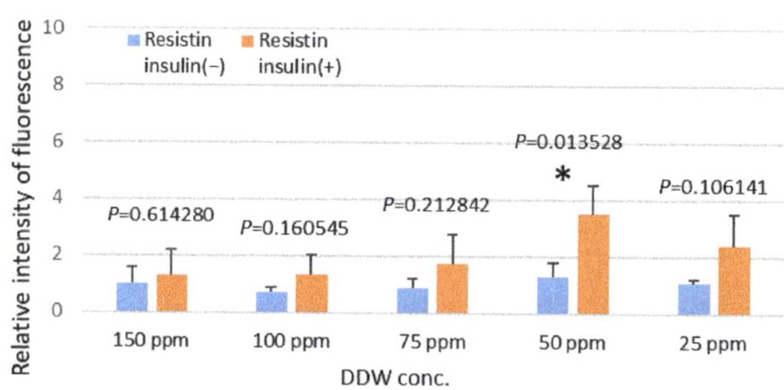

Figure 3. Glucose uptake in myotube-differentiated C2C12 cells. Fully myotube-differentiated C2C12 cells were cultured in a medium containing various concentrations of DDW for 48 h, after which the uptake of fluorescence-conjugated glucose was observed. TNF-α and resistin were added 24 h before harvesting, whereas insulin and fluorescence-conjugated glucose were added 30 min before harvesting. Scale bar: 100 µm. (**a**–**c**) Images of C2C12 glucose uptake. From the left, first and third rows indicate no insulin added; second and fourth rows indicate insulin added. The upper left two images are phase-contrast images of cells cultured in natural water medium (150 ppm) with and without insulin, respectively. The others are fluorescence observations. (**a**) Cells without induction of insulin resistance, (**b**) cells treated with 10 ng/mL TNF-α, and (**c**) cells treated with 10 µg/mL resistin. (**d**–**f**) Fluorescence intensity was measured, and the relative values to culture in natural water medium (150 ppm) without insulin were graphed. The sample size was four. * Significant difference ($p < 0.05$) between the presence (orange bar) and absence (blue bar) of insulin added to DDW medium at each concentration. (**d**) Cells without the induction of insulin resistance, (**e**) cells supplemented with 10 ng/mL TNF-α, and (**f**) cells supplemented with 10 µg/mL resistin.

In addition, although glucose uptake in the presence of TNF-α was observed throughout the myotubes in the absence of an agent, the effect of resistin was different. Glucose uptake was often detected in only a portion of the myotubes, and myotubes were observed to be divided and atrophied (Figure 3c,f).

4. Discussion

Although there have been reports on the effects of DDW on diabetes, the underlying mechanisms remain unclear. Recent studies using diabetic animal models have reported that increased insulin sensitivity due to the activation of GLUT4 promotes disease improvement, but it is unclear whether DDW has a direct effect on diabetes, since the influence of various other effects of DDW on the body cannot be ignored [13].

In this study, we sought to elucidate the mechanism by which GLUT4 is improved in the disease by directly measuring the effect of DDW on muscle cells in vitro while minimizing the impact of the indirect effects that are believed to occur in the body.

The results revealed that the expression and activation (i.e., membrane translocation) of GLUT4 in C2C12 cells were promoted in the medium adjusted with DDW, and the peaks were near a deuterium concentration of 50 ppm. As the peak of glucose uptake was also near 50 ppm, it is speculated that the increase in GLUT4 gene expression owing to the action of DDW is directly reflected in the increase in the amount of GLUT4 protein, membrane translocation, and glucose uptake. Thus, the most important effect of DDW on GLUT4 may be the promotion of GLUT4 transcription.

Two enhancer domains are known in the promoter region of the human GLUT4 gene, and it is known that GLUT4 enhancer factor (GEF) and myocyte enhancer factor 2 (MEF2) bind to them to control transcription. However, in diabetic mice, the binding ability of MEF2 to the enhancer domain is reduced [27,28].

One hypothesis for the mechanism of the anticancer effect of DDW is that deuterium incorporated into proteins and nucleic acids makes these molecules heavier and stickier, inducing abnormalities in intermolecular interactions, while drinking DDW "lightens" proteins and nucleic acids, normalizing intermolecular interactions [8]. DDW may restore the binding ability of the enhancer domain and transcription factors of the GLUT4 gene by "lightening" them.

This hypothesis leads to the conclusion that the lower the deuterium concentration, the better the gene expression. However, our results indicate that there is a peak concentration of 50 ppm for the expression of GLUT4 and activation by DDW. In in vitro experiments using adipogenic 3T3-L1 cells, we also observed that the expression of GLUT4 and activation reached a maximum at 75–100 ppm (unpublished data), suggesting that the effect of deuterium on the expression of GLUT4 and activation has an optimum concentration that may differ depending on the cell type. The details and causes of the effects of deuterium concentrations below the optimal concentration on cells are currently unknown.

Even if DDW has a strong effect on GLUT4 gene expression, the results of this study showed that the increase in gene expression, protein expression, and membrane translocation was not parallel, suggesting the existence of regulation in the process of translation and membrane translocation (exocytosis), and it is quite possible that DDW also affects these processes. The details of how DDW contributes to the mechanisms of transcription, translation, and membrane translocation remain an important topic for future research on the process of GLUT4 activation. Membrane translocation is particularly important for glucose metabolism, and many cutting-edge studies have demonstrated that one of the causes of insulin resistance is the inhibition of this process [29–34].

In this study, two drugs were used to induce insulin resistance in cultured myotubes. Recent studies have reported that adipocytes and related factors secreted by obese enlarged fat cells strongly induce insulin resistance, two of which have been used. TNF-α is an adipocytokine secreted by adipocytes but is also known as an inflammatory cytokine secreted by macrophages [35,36]. Resistin is also an adipocytokine, and excessive secretion of resistin due to obesity is thought to be a cause of diabetes [37]. These agents imparted insulin resistance to myotube-differentiated C2C12 cells and suppressed glucose uptake; however, DDW showed an effect of attenuated insulin resistance. TNF-α is thought to reduce insulin signaling by decreasing the phosphorylation of the insulin receptor substrate-1 (IRS-1) Tyr632 and Akt Ser473, which are downstream effectors of the insulin receptor, thereby resulting in insulin resistance [38–40]. The inactivation of the Akt pathway suppresses the membrane translocation of GLUT4 [41]. In contrast, resistin has been reported to suppress GLUT4 [37]. Since DDW attenuates these effects, it is speculated that DDW acts on both the gene expression and membrane translocation of GLUT4.

In addition, these reagents suppress muscle differentiation and induce muscle degradation, such as atrophy, in differentiated C2C12 cells [42–44]. At the concentrations used in this experiment, only resistin caused myotube disruption (atrophy), but DDW promoted the uptake of glucose, even in atrophied cells, suggesting that myotube maintenance and GLUT4 function are almost independent and that DDW is only involved in glucose metabolism.

Further detailed in vitro and in vivo studies are required to develop novel DDW-based diabetes treatments.

5. Conclusions

A study using cultured muscle cell lines showed that DDW promoted the expression and activation of GLUT4 in muscle cells, with the highest increase occurring at a deuterium concentration of approximately 50 ppm. At the same concentration, the cellular glucose uptake was maximized, and drug-induced insulin resistance was attenuated. These results suggest that DDW is effective in improving diabetes and that an in vitro system is a useful tool for elucidating the detailed underlying mechanisms.

Author Contributions: Conceptualization, M.K. (Masumi Kondo) and M.T.; methodology, Y.T. and Y.M. (Yoshitaka Mori); validation, N.S. and K.S.; formal analysis, M.A. and N.S.; investigation, Y.T., M.K. (Masumi Kondo) and Y.M. (Yosuke Matsuda); data curation, M.K. (Moritsugu Kimura); writing—original draft preparation, M.K. (Masumi Kondo); writing—review and editing, K.S. and Y.M. (Yoshitaka Mori); visualization, M.A. and Y.M. (Yosuke Matsuda); supervision, M.K. (Moritsugu Kimura) and M.T.; project administration, M.T.; funding acquisition, M.T. All authors have read and agreed to the published version of the manuscript.

Funding: This research was conducted with funding provided by TAKAGI Co., Ltd. (Kitakyushyu, Japan, funding number: 23B011000) and Super Light Water Co., Ltd. (Tokyo, Japan, funding number: 19C059003 and 20C056002), based on a Commissioned Research Agreement concluded with the companies regarding the conduct of this research.

Institutional Review Board Statement: Not applicable.

Informed Consent Statement: Not applicable.

Data Availability Statement: The original contributions presented in the study are included in the article, further inquiries can be directed to the corresponding author.

Acknowledgments: We thank the Research Support Center of Tokai University School of Medicine for their valuable technical assistance.

Conflicts of Interest: The authors declare no conflicts of interest. The funders had no role in the study design; the collection, analyses, or interpretation of data; the writing of the manuscript; or the decision to publish the results.

References

1. Gyongyi, Z.; Somlyai, G. Deuterium depletion can decrease the expression of c-myc, Ha-ras and p53 gene in carcinogen-treated mice. *Vivo.* **2000**, *14*, 437–439.
2. Gyongyi, Z.; Budan, F.; Szabo, I.; Ember, I.; Kiss, I.; Krempels, K.; Somlyai, I.; Somlyai, G. Deuterium depleted water effects on survival of lung cancer patients and expression of Kras, Bcl2 and Myc genes in mouse lung. *Nutr. Cancer.* **2013**, *65*, 240–246. [CrossRef] [PubMed]
3. Boros, L.G.; Somlyai, I.; Kovács, B.Z.; Puskás, L.G.; Nagy, L.I.; Dux, L.; Farkas, G.; Somlyai, G. Deutrium Depletion Inhibits Cell Proliferation, RNA and Nuclear Membrane Turnover to Enhance Survival in Pancreatic Cancer. *Cancer Control* **2021**, *28*, 1–12. [CrossRef] [PubMed]
4. Kovács, A.; Guller, I.; Krempels, K.; Somlyai, I.; Jánosi, I.; Gyöngyi, Z.; Szabó, I.; Ember, I.; Somlyai, G. Deuterium depletion may delay the progression of prostate cancer. *J Cancer Ther.* **2011**, *2*, 548–556. [CrossRef]
5. Krempels, K.; Somlyai, I.; Gyongyi, Z.; Ember, I.; Balog, K.; Abonyi, O.; Somlyai, G. A retrospective study of survival in breast cancer patients undergoing deuterium depletion in addition to conventional therapies. *J. Cancer Res. Ther.* **2013**, *1*, 194–200.

6. Cong, F.S.; Zhang, Y.R.; Sheng, H.C.; Ao, Z.-H.; Zhang, S.-Y.; Wang, J.-Y. Deuterium-depleted water inhibits human lung carcinoma cell growth by apoptosis. *Exp. Ther. Med.* **2010**, *1*, 277–283. [CrossRef] [PubMed]
7. Lu, Y.; Chen, H. Deuterium-Depleted Water in Cancer Therapy: A Systematic Review of Clinical and Experimental Trials. *Nutrients* **2024**, *16*, 1397. [CrossRef] [PubMed]
8. Boros, L.G.; Meuillet, E.J.; Somlyai, I.; Jancsó, G.; Jákli, G.; Krempels, K.; Puskás, L.G.; Nagy, I.L.; Molnár, M.; Laderoute, K.R.; et al. Fumarate hydratase and deuterium depletion control oncogenesis via NADPH-dependent reductive synthesis: Mitochondrial matrix water, DNA deuteration and epigenetic events. *Cancer Res.* **2014**, *74*, 1426. [CrossRef]
9. Yaglova, N.V.; Timokhina, E.P.; Obernikhin, S.S.; Yaglov, V.V. Emerging Role of Deuterium/Protium Disbalance in Cell Cycle and Apoptosis. *Int. J. Mol. Sci.* **2023**, *24*, 3107. [CrossRef]
10. Somlyai, G.; Somlyai, I.; Fórizs, I.; Czuppon, G.Y.; Papp, A.; Molnár, M. Effect of systemic subnormal deuterium level on metabolic syndrome related and other blood parameters in humans: A preliminary study. *Molecules* **2020**, *25*, 1376. [CrossRef]
11. Yavari, K.; Gholamali, M.; Yazdian, F. Decreasing of Deuterium Concentration of Water: A Possible Tool in Diabetes Therapy. *Electr. J. Biol.* **2017**, *13*, 314–319.
12. Leney, S.E.; Tavare, J.M. The molecular basis of insulin-stimulated glucose uptake: Signaling, trafficking and potential drug targets. *J. Endocrinol.* **2009**, *203*, 1–18. [CrossRef]
13. Molnar, M.; Horvath, K.; Danko, T.; Somlyai, I.; Kovacs, B.Z.; Somlyai, G. Deuterium-depleted water stimulates GLUT4 translocation in the presence of insulin, which leads to decreased blood glucose concentration. *Mol. Cell. Biol.* **2021**, *476*, 4507–4516. [CrossRef]
14. Stöckli, J.; Fazakerley, D.J.; James, D.E. GLUT4 exocytosis. *J. Cell Sci.* **2011**, *124*, 4147–4159. [CrossRef]
15. Huang, S.; Czech, M.P. The GLUT4 Glucose Transporter. *Cell Metabol.* **2007**, *5*, 237–252. [CrossRef]
16. Gannon, N.P.; Conn, C.A.; Vaughan, R.A. Dietary stimulators of GLUT4 expression and translocation in skeletal muscle: A mini-review. *Mol. Nutr. Food Res.* **2015**, *59*, 48–64. [CrossRef]
17. Martineau, F.; Fourel, F.; Bodergat, A.M.; Lécuyer, C. D/H equilibrium fractionation between H_2O and H_2 as a function of the salinity of aqueous solutions. *Chem. Geol.* **2012**, *291*, 236–240. [CrossRef]
18. Wonga, C.Y.; Al-Salamia, H.; Dass, C.R. C2C12 cell model: Its role in understanding of insulin resistance at the molecular level and pharmaceutical development at the preclinical stage. *J. Pharm. Pharmacol.* **2020**, *72*, 1667–1693. [CrossRef]
19. Terruzzi, I.; Montesano, A.; Senesi, P.; Vacante, F.; Benedini, S.; Luzi, L. Ranolazine promotes muscle diff-erentiation and reduces oxidative stress in C2C12 skeletal muscle cells. *Endocrine* **2017**, *58*, 33–45. [CrossRef]
20. Brown, D.M.; Parr, T.; Brameld, J.M. Myosin heavy chain mRNA isoforms are expressed in two distinct cohorts during C2C12 myogenesis. *J. Muscle Res. Cell Mortil.* **2012**, *32*, 383–390. [CrossRef]
21. Schmittgen, T.; Livak, K.J. Analyzingreal-timePCRdatabythecomparative CTmethod. *Nat. Protoc.* **2008**, *3*, 1101–1108. [CrossRef]
22. Mahmood, T.; Yang, P.-C. Western Blot: Technique, Theory, and Trouble Shooting. *N. Am. J. Med. Sci.* **2012**, *4*, 429–434.
23. Abramoff, M.D.; Magelhaes, P.J.; Ram, S.J. Image Processing with ImageJ. *Biophotonics Int.* **2004**, *11*, 36–42.
24. Waetzig, G.H.; Chalaris, A.; Rosenstiel, P.; Suthaus, J.; Holland, C.; Karl, N.; Uriarte, L.V.; Till, A.; Scheller, J.; Grötzinger, J.; et al. N-linked glycosylation is essential for the stability but not the signaling function of the interleukin-6 signal transducer glycoprotein 130. *J. Biol. Chem.* **2010**, *285*, 1781–1789. [CrossRef]
25. Liu, Y.; Le, Y.; Xu, M.; Wang, W.; Chen, H.; Zhang, Q.; Wang, C. Remodeling on adipocytic physiology of organophosphorus esters in mature adipocytes. *Environ. Pollut.* **2022**, *305*, 119287. [CrossRef]
26. R Development Core Team. *R: A Language and Environment for Statistical Computing*; R Foundation for Statistical Computing: Vienna, Austria, 2016. Available online: http://www.R-project.org/ (accessed on 3 August 2024).
27. Knight, J.B.; Eyster, C.A.; Griesel, B.A.; Olson, A.L. Regulation of the human GLUT4 gene promoter: Interaction between a transcriptional activator and myocyte enhancer factor 2A. *Proc. Natl. Acad. Sci. USA* **2003**, *100*, 14725–14736. [CrossRef]
28. Thai, M.V.; Guruswamy, S.; Cao, K.T.; Pessin, J.E.; Olson, A.L. Myocyte Enhancer Factor 2 (MEF2)-Binding Site Is Required for GLUT4 Gene Expression in Transgenic Mice: Regulation of Mef2 Dna Binding Activity in Insulin-Deficient Diabetes. *J. Biol. Chem.* **1998**, *273*, 14285–14292.
29. Watson, R.T.; Pessin, J.E. GLUT4 translocation: The last 200 nanometers. *Cell Signal.* **2007**, *19*, 2209–2217.
30. Bogan, J.S. Regulation of Glucose Transporter Translocation in Health and Diabetes. *Annu. Rev. Biovhem.* **2012**, *81*, 507–532. [CrossRef]
31. Laurie, S.M.; Cain, C.C.; Lienhardn, G.E.; Castle, J.D. The Glucose Transporter GluT4 and Secretory Carrier Membrane Proteins (SCAMPs) Colocalize in Rat Adipocytes and Partially Segregate during Insulin Stimulation. *J. Biol. Chem.* **1993**, *268*, 19110–19117. [CrossRef]
32. Jaldin-Fincati, J.R.; Pavarotti, M.; Frendo-Cumbo, S.; Bilan, P.J.; Klip, A. Update on GLUT4 Vesicle Traffic: A Cornerstone of Insulin Action. *Trends Endocrinol. Metabol.* **2017**, *28*, 597–611.
33. Tunduguru, R.; Thurmond, D.C. Promoting Glucose Transporter-4 vesicle Trafficking along Cytoskeletal Tracks: PAK-Ing Them Out. *Front. Endocrinol.* **2017**, *8*, 329. [CrossRef]
34. Brewer, P.D.; Habtemichael, E.N.; Romenskaia, I.; Mastick, C.C.; Coster, A.C.F. Insulin-regulated Glut4 Translocation: Membrane protein trafficking with six distinctive steps. *J. Biol. Chem.* **2014**, *289*, 17280–17298. [CrossRef]

35. Jove, M.; Planavila, A.; Sanchez, R.M.; Merlos, M.; Laguna, J.C.; Vazquez-Carrera, M. Palmitate Induces Tumor Necrosis Factor-Expression in C2C12 Skeletal Muscle Cells by a Mechanism Involving Protein Kinase C and Nuclear Factor-B Activation. *Endocrinology* **2006**, *147*, 552–561. [CrossRef]
36. Haghani, K.; Pashaei, S.; Vakili, S.; Taheripak, G.; Bakhtiyari, S. TNF-α knockdown alleviates palmitate-induced insulin resistance in C2C12 skeletal muscle cells. *Biochem. Biophys. Res. Commun.* **2015**, *460*, 977–982. [CrossRef]
37. LI, F.-P.; LI, Z.-Z.; Zhang, M.; Yan, L.; Fu, Z.-Z. Effects of resistin on skeletal glucose metabolism. *Front. Med.* **2010**, *4*, 329–335. [CrossRef]
38. Kanety, H.; Feinstein, R.; Papa, M.Z.; Hemi, R.; Karasik, A. Tumor necrosis factor alpha-induced phosphorylation of insulin receptor substrate-1 (IRS-1). Possible mechanism for suppression of insulin-stimulated tyrosine phosphorylation of IRS-1. *J. Biol. Chem.* **1995**, *270*, 23780–23784.
39. Hotamisligil, G.S.; Peraldi, P.; Budavari, A.; Ellis, R.; White, M.F.; Spiegelman, B.M. IRS-1-mediated inhibition of insulin receptor tyrosine kinase activity in TNFα- and obesity-induced insulin resistance. *Science* **1996**, *271*, 665–668.
40. Storz, P.; Doppler, H.; Wernig, A.; Pfizenmaier, K.; Muller, G. Cross-talk mechanisms in the development of insulin resistance of skeletal muscle cells palmitate rather than tumour necrosis factor inhibits insulin-dependent protein kinase B (PKB)/Akt stimulation and glucose uptake. *Eur. J. Biochem.* **1999**, *266*, 17–25.
41. Ijuin, T.; Takenawa, T. Regulation of insulin signaling and glucose transporter 4 (GLUT4) exocytosis by phosphatidylinositol 3,4,5-trisphosphate (PIP3) phosphatase, skeletal muscle, and kidney enriched inositol polyphosphate phosphatase (SKIP). *J. Biol. Chem.* **2012**, *287*, 6991–6999. [CrossRef]
42. Matsuba, I.; Fujita, R.; Iida, K. Palmitic Acid Inhibits Myogenic Activity and Expression of Myosin Heavy Chain MHC IIb in Muscle Cells through Phosphorylation-Dependent MyoD Inactivation. *Int. J. Mol. Sci.* **2023**, *24*, 5847. [CrossRef]
43. Powrózek, T.; Pigoń-Zajac, D.; Mazurek, M.; Rahnama-Hezavah, M.; Małecka-Massalska, T. TNF-α Induced Myotube Atrophy in C2C12 Cell Line Uncovers Putative Inflammatory-Related lncRNAs Mediating Muscle Wasting. *Int. J. Mol. Sci.* **2023**, *23*, 3878. [CrossRef]
44. Wen, F.; Zhang, H.; Bao, C.; Yang, M.; Wang, N.; Zhang, J.; Hu, Y.; Yang, X.; Geng, J.; Yang, Z. Resistin Increases Ectopic Deposition of Lipids Through miR-696 in C2C12 Cells. *Biochem. Genet.* **2015**, *53*, 63–71. [CrossRef]

biomedicines MDPI

Article

An Assessment of Semaglutide Safety Based on Real World Data: From Popularity to Spontaneous Reporting in EudraVigilance Database

Anca Butuca [1], Carmen Maximiliana Dobrea [1], Anca Maria Arseniu [1], Adina Frum [1], Adriana Aurelia Chis [1], Luca Liviu Rus [1], Steliana Ghibu [2,*], Anca Maria Juncan [1], Andrei Catalin Muntean [1], Antonina Evelina Lazăr [3], Felicia Gabriela Gligor [1], Claudiu Morgovan [1] and Andreea Loredana Vonica-Tincu [1]

[1] Preclinical Department, Faculty of Medicine, "Lucian Blaga" University of Sibiu, 2A Lucian Blaga St., 550169 Sibiu, Romania; anca.butuca@ulbsibiu.ro (A.B.); carmen.dobrea@ulbsibiu.ro (C.M.D.); anca.arseniu@ulbsibiu.ro (A.M.A.); adina.frum@ulbsibiu.ro (A.F.); adriana.chis@ulbsibiu.ro (A.A.C.); liviu.rus@ulbsibiu.ro (L.L.R.); ancamaria.juncan@ulbsibiu.ro (A.M.J.); andreicatalin.muntean@ulbsibiu.ro (A.C.M.); felicia.gligor@ulbsibiu.ro (F.G.G.); claudiu.morgovan@ulbsibiu.ro (C.M.); loredana.vonica@ulbsibiu.ro (A.L.V.-T.)

[2] Department of Pharmacology, Physiology and Pathophysiology, Faculty of Pharmacy, "Iuliu Hatieganu" University of Medicine and Pharmacy, 400012 Cluj-Napoca, Romania

[3] National Institute of Research and Development for Electrochemistry and Condensed Matter, 144 Dr. A. P. Podeanu, 300569 Timisoara, Romania; antonina_pop@yahoo.com

* Correspondence: steliana.ghibu@umfcluj.ro

Abstract: Some glucagon-like peptide-1 receptor agonists (GLP-1 RAs), first used in the treatment of type 2 diabetes mellitus (T2DM), have been approved for the treatment of obesity in patients with or without T2DM (liraglutide—LIR, semaglutide—SEM, and tirzepatide—TIR). Social media had an important influence on the off-label use of GLP-1 RAs for obesity, especially for SEM. We analyzed the Google queries related to SEM to assess people's interest in this drug. We also investigated the occurrence of adverse drug reactions (ADRs) by searching the EudraVigilance database (EV) for Individual Case Safety Reports (ICSRs) that reported SEM as the suspected drug and performed a descriptive and a disproportionality analysis. The data obtained for SEM were compared to other GLP-1 RAs. SEM had the highest proportions of searches on Google associated with the term "weight loss" and presented the lowest number of severe ADRs, but it also had the highest number of ICSRs reported in EV. Even though no unexpected safety issues have been reported for it until now, SEM has a hi3gh tendency for overdose reports. The most frequent off-label use was reported for SEM and TIR. In order to lower the risks of ADRs, the off-label use should be reduced and carefully monitored.

Keywords: semaglutide; obesity; weight loss; overdose; underdose; off-label use; EudraVigilance; GLP-1

1. Introduction

Obesity is considered one of the most common metabolic diseases, often associated with an elevated risk of developing type 2 diabetes mellitus (T2DM), non-alcoholic fatty liver disease, and cardiovascular disorders like hypertension and heart failure with preserved ejection fraction, etc., thus reducing the life expectancy of patients [1–4]. Recent studies show that obesity increases the number of hospitalizations, the need for mechanical ventilation and the incidence of death in patients with SARS-CoV-2 [5]. According to the World Health Organization (WHO), in 2022, 2.5 billion adults were overweight, and of them, 890 million were obese (~12.5%). The same report pointed out that the number of overweight children under the age of five was 37 million. In the 5 to 19 years group, over 390 million children and teenagers were overweight, of which 160 million were obese [6].

Known as one of the biggest challenges of modern society at a global level, the fight against obesity has been declared a real public health emergency [1,5]. On the other hand, diabetes is considered one of the most widespread worldwide medical conditions and T2DM is the most common form [7], with both acute and chronic consequences which decrease the quality of life, reduce life expectancy and increase the mortality rate [8].

One of the global goals of the WHO is to stop the increase in diabetes and obesity by 2025 [6]. Unfortunately, until now, lifestyle changes in terms of daily diet and physical exercise have often proved insufficient in achieving significant weight loss [7,9]. The connection between obesity and diabetes is very close, so a large part of obese people are affected by diabetes or have a very high risk of developing T2DM in a very short period, and many patients with diabetes, especially those with T2DM, start to gain weight, soon becoming overweight or obese [10].

Significant evidence attests that an effective improvement of insulin sensitivity and simultaneous reduction of the risk of diabetes associated with obesity can be achieved through weight loss [10]. Over time, several molecules have been administered for the treatment of obesity, but their limited efficacy and/or adverse reactions led to the limitation of their use or even their withdrawal from the market (e.g., sibutramine, amfepramone, rimonabant, benfluorex, dexfenfluramine etc.) [5,11–13]. In this context, the approval of new drugs with adequate efficiency and safety in obesity treatment has been sought. Thus, the approval of the first glucagon-like peptide-1 (GLP-1) receptors agonist (GLP-1 RAs) in the treatment of T2DM, with structures similar to endogenous hormones, opened a new era in promoting weight loss and improving health outcomes in obese people, including those with comorbidities [14].

GLP-1 and glucose-dependent insulinotropic polypeptide (GIP) are two of the main incretin peptide hormones excreted in the intestinal tract [15], responsible for increasing the secretion of insulin after eating food and also inhibiting the secretion of glucagon [16–19]. GLP-1 reduces gastrointestinal motility, which in turn extends the period when nutrients might be absorbed. It also determines the feeling of satiety, enhances resting metabolic rate, and decreases free fatty acid concentrations in plasma [1]. Because GLP-1 receptors are expressed in extra-pancreatic tissues, GLP-1 presents a lot of extra-pancreatic effects: delayed gastric emptying, appetite suppression, weight loss, glucose uptake in the muscles, decreased glucose production in the liver, cardiovascular protection, neuroprotection, renoprotection etc. [19–22]. These effects determined that the use of GLP-1 RAs has a high potential to reduce body weight and to be considered for the treatment of obesity [15] (Figure 1). GLP-1 RAs have been approved in the treatment of T2DM for improving HbA1c and for reducing the risk of major adverse cardiac events (MACE) in diabetes patients with cardiovascular risk [23,24].

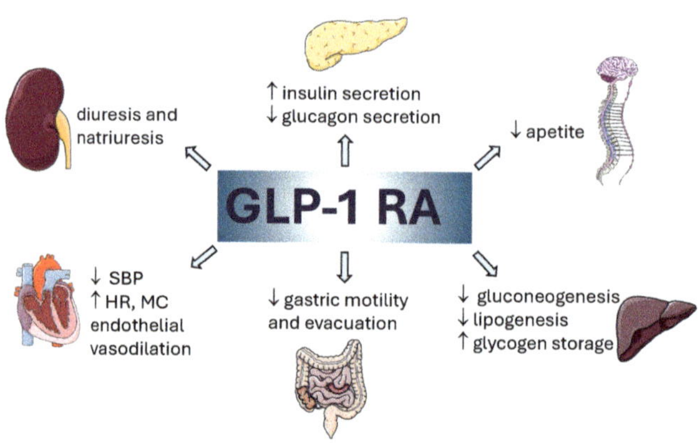

Figure 1. The main biological activities of GLP-1 RAs [25]. SBP—systolic blood pressure; HR—heart rate; MC—myocardial contractility; ↑—increase; ↓—decrease.

Currently, there are several GLP-1 RAs approved worldwide, mainly for the treatment of diabetes. Exenatide (EXE) was the first GLP-1 RA in the world approved by the Food and Drug Administration (FDA), in 2005, for the treatment of T2DM, with two administrations per day before meals [26]. Later, the European Medicines Agency (EMA) (2009) and FDA (2010) approved the second agonist, liraglutide (LIR), as an adjuvant to diet associated with physical exercise in patients with T2DM. Compared to its predecessor, the latter presented a longer half-life with a greater effect on the reduction of HbA1C; at the same time, it showed cardiovascular benefits in addition to its effects of lowering blood sugar. In addition, it can be administered once a day regardless of meals. Moreover, the FDA (December 2014) and EMA (March 2015) approved LIR for the treatment of chronic weight management [26,27]. The manufacturer improved the short-acting time of EXE and a new formulation was approved in 2012 by the FDA. Compared to the old formulation, the prolonged-release suspension of EXE is administered once a week [28]. In 2014, the second GLP-1 RA with weekly administration, albiglutide (ALB), was approved by the FDA for the treatment of T2DM in patients who cannot reach glycemic goals. In 2018, the manufacturer withdrew ALB for commercial reasons [29,30]. Also in 2014, dulaglutide (DUL) was approved by the FDA. It had the advantage of reaching the therapeutic concentration faster than other GLP-1 RAs with weekly administration. Semaglutide (SEM) was launched in 2017 in injectable form, and it had an extended half-life of 7 days. In 2019 the oral form of SEM received approval from the FDA, thus being the first oral GLP-1 RA treatment for adults with T2DM [29,31]. Tirzepatide (TIR), a dual GLP-1 RA and GIP receptor agonist (GIP/RAs), is the latest one launched on the market, approved in 2022. GIP triggers glucose-dependent insulin excretion and is responsible for a larger fraction of the incretin effect than GLP-1. Depending on glycemic status, the glucagon secretion could be increased in normoglycemic or hypoglycemic patients (glucagonotropic effect) or inhibited in hyperglycemic patients (glucagonostatic effect) [22,32,33].

Preclinical studies have shown that GIP can decrease body weight by diminishing food intake and enhancing energy expenditure and, in combination with GLP-1 RAs, can have a greater lowering effect on blood glucose and body weight in patients [1,19]. Clinical studies have confirmed their effectiveness in weight loss and some of them (LIR, SEM, and TIR) have been approved for chronic weight management [23,24].

LIR was the first GLP-1 RA approved for weight loss in patients without a history of T2DM. In 2014, it was approved by the FDA in adult patients with a body mass index (BMI) larger than 30 kg/m^2 on its own or with a BMI greater than 27 kg/m^2 associated with at least one comorbidity related to weight, such as hypertension, diabetes, or dyslipidaemia [25,34]. SEM only received approval from the FDA for weight control in 2021 [34]. In the clinical studies carried out in this respect, SEM was superior in comparison to other long-acting GLP-1 RAs from the same class, namely EXE [35] and DUL [36]. Moreover, in addition to its beneficial effects in T2DM and in controlling body weight, it also showed a significant decrease in the rates of deaths due to cardiovascular issues, non-fatal myocardial infarction and non-fatal stroke in T2DM patients at risk of cardiovascular diseases [34]. Thus, LIR could reduce body weight by up to 9.2% (56 weeks) [37,38], SEM up to 17.4% (68 weeks) [39,40], and TIR up to 20.9% (72 weeks) [39]. Compared to LIR (16%), SEM leads to a higher reduction in caloric intake vs placebo (35%) and reduces the food cravings, which suggests different mechanisms of energy intake regulation [41].

Real-world data are a valuable resource for healthcare research [42]. The information within is obtained from a heterogenous population [43,44] and is collected by various methods such as electronic health records, pharmacovigilance databases, and search engines, contributing to revealing the existing clinical aspects [45]. Appropriate analytical techniques are necessary to extract reliable results from the extensive raw data [46]. Both the research community [47] and several medicines regulatory authorities [48] have shown great interest in this domain and are preoccupied with setting quality standards in the field [49]. Real-world data complement the results of long-established research methods such as clinical trials, enhancing the accuracy of evidence-based clinical profile [50]. SEM is an adequate candidate for a real-world data assessment, due to the large interest of the population for this molecule. Although intended for diabetic patients, many non-diabetic ones have used it for aesthetic body adjustments [7,51]. The off-label use of SEM for weight loss was promoted by social media and heavily influenced by famous public figures [47]. This intense media coverage led to numerous shortages of this drug with major consequences for patients with T2DM. Beyond these shortages, the incorrect and inadequate use of GLP-1 RAs can have major consequences on the health status of the population. Until now, various studies have shown the negative impact of these drugs, mainly because of gastrointestinal disorders (pancreatitis, nausea, vomiting, etc.), renal failure, liver injury, allergic reactions etc. [52–55]. This study aimed to identify public interest in searching for information about SEM online and also to analyze the secondary real-world data regarding the use of inadequate doses (overdose, underdose or incorrect dose) or even the off-label use of SEM. In this respect, after the analysis of data presented on the Google Trends Tool, a detailed analysis of the Individual Case Safety Reports (ICSRs) uploaded in EudraVigilance (the European adverse reaction reporting database) was carried out. The evaluation of SEM popularity and the safety profile was performed through comparison with other GLP-1 RAs (including ALB, which was withdrawn from the market).

2. Materials and Methods

2.1. Study Design

In January 2021, Google had 91% of the market share of online searches worldwide, representing the main search engine [56]. Thus, the present study started with an analysis of the popularity of search queries that were entered into Google Search. A relative search volume (RSV) is generated from Google Trends. The RSV does not provide the actual number of searches but presents data on a relative scale. The numbers represent search interest relative to the highest point on the chart for the selected region and time. A value of 100 is the peak popularity for the term, while a value of 50 means that the term is half as popular [57–59]. In the present study, the data obtained from the Google Trends Tool were analyzed considering peoples' interest in searching for information about GLP-1 RAs. The terms used for comparison were the International Nonproprietary Names of each GLP-1 RA: "semaglutide", "liraglutide", "tirzepatide", "albiglutide", "dulaglutide", "lixisenatide", and "exenatide". The comparison was performed worldwide, between December 2005 and March 2024. The interest score is presented on a scale of 0 to 100, where 100 indicates the highest level of popularity and 0 represents the least amount of interest. Subsequently, the popularity by region of each GLP-1 RA was analyzed. For each molecule, 100 points were allocated to the country with the highest popularity, and, to the other countries, the number of points was allotted proportional to the number of searches. Furthermore, we identified the first 25 related queries which were searched for by the same consumers who performed the searches for GLP-1 Ras, and we analyzed the frequency of terms related to "side effects" and "weight loss".

The high popularity of SEM in the media could lead to self-medication and irrational or abusive consumption, potentially bringing on an increased number of ADRs, especially those which are severe or fatal. Thus, a retrospective pharmacovigilance analysis was performed based on the ICSRs uploaded in the EudraVigilance database until 31 March 2024 [60]. Firstly, a descriptive study of ICSRs reported for SEM was performed in comparison with other GLP-1 RAs (ALB, DUL, EXE, LIR, lixisenatide—LIX, TIR) or the entire group of all other GLP-1 RAs. ALB was withdrawn by the manufacturer because of commercial reasons, not for safety or efficiency reasons. In this context, we decided to use ALB for comparison, too. On the other hand, the ICSRs reported for the combination of LIR and degludec insulin were excluded from the present study. In the next step, a disproportionality analysis was performed to compare the reporting probability of ADRs for SEM with other GLP-1 RAs and with the entire group of all other GLP-1 RAs. No ethics approvals were required for the present study because no patients' personal information was included in the ICSRs [61]. Healthcare or non-healthcare professionals filled out the reports from the European Economic Area (EEA) or non-EEA [62].

2.2. Materials

The chronologic data from the Google Trends Tool reported for SEM were compared to the series of the other GLP-1 RAs. Regarding ALB and LIX, the search interest compared to SEM represents <1%. Thus, both molecules were excluded from this analysis.

According to the Medical Dictionary for Regulatory Activities (MedDRA) hierarchy, many preferred terms (PTs) were used for reported ADRs. Each PT can describe "a symptom, sign, disease diagnosis, therapeutic indication, investigation, surgical or medical procedure, and medical social or family history characteristic". In the next level, related PTs form the "High Level Terms" (HLTs) group, and related HLTs form "High Level Group Terms" (HLGTs). The final level for classification is represented by "System Organ Classes" (SOCs), with each SOC being formed from many related HLGTs [63]. At the moment, the total number of SOCs is 27.

In the present study, 4 HLTs were identified (modified dose, overdose, underdose, and off-label use) [62,64]. Thus, of a total of 35 Preferred terms (PTs), only 27 were identified in the ICSRs uploaded for the evaluated drugs (Table 1).

Table 1. The preferred terms used for analysis of ICSRs uploaded in EudraVigilance.

HLT	PT
modified dose	Dose calculation error Dose calculation error associated with device * Drug dose titration not performed Drug titration error Incorrect dosage administered Incorrect dose administered Incorrect dose administered by device Incorrect dose administered by product Incorrect product dosage form administered * Product dosage form confusion * Wrong dose
overdose	Accidental overdose Intentional overdose Extra dose administered Overdose Prescribed overdose
underdose	Accidental underdose Drug dose omission by device Incomplete dose administered * Intentional dose omission Intentional underdose Prescribed underdose Product dose omission * Product dose omission in error Product dose omission issue Underdose
Off-label use	Contraindicated product administered Contraindicated product prescribed Drug effective for unapproved indication * Off-label use Off-label use of device Product use in unapproved therapeutic environment * Product use in unapproved indication Product used for unknown indication * Unintentional use for unapproved indication

* PT with no reports.

2.3. Data Analysis

A descriptive analysis of cases reported in patients treated with SEM was performed. The data were compared to other GLP-1 RAs. The descriptive analysis was structured by taking into account the general characteristics such as age, sex, category of reporters, geographic origin, and seriousness. In the next step, the distribution of ADRs by SOC was compared for SEM with all other GLP-1 RAs.

To evaluate the risk of incorrect dosage or off-label use, many PTs were identified for each of the 4 HLTs (categories of ADRs): modified dose (11), overdose (5), underdose (10), and off-label use (9) (Table 1). The total number of ADRs for each HLT was determined and compared between SEM and all other GLP-1 RAs. Subsequently, the outcome of ADRs grouped in HLTs was also compared. According to the EMA rules, the outcomes of cases are classified into 6 categories: (i) fatal, (ii) not recovered/not resolved (NR/NRS), (iii) recovered/resolved with sequelae, (iv) recovering/resolving, (v) recovered/resolved, (vi) not specified, (vii) unknown [65].

A disproportionality analysis was performed to evaluate the probability of reporting adverse reactions included in the four categories. According to EMA recommendations, the reporting odds ratios (RORs) and 95% confidence intervals (95% CI) were calculated for each evaluated HLT [66], according to a previously published protocol [67,68]. The disproportionate signal was obtained when the number of ADRs was $\geq$5 for each HLT and the ROR was statistically >1 (lower limit of 95% CI > 1) [66]. The data calculated for SEM were compared with each other GLP-1 RA and with the entire group of all other GLP-1 RAs.

3. Results

3.1. Analysis of Searching Google Popularity

Based on the worldwide chronologic series obtained from Google Trends, starting with May 2019, the interest in SEM showed a constantly increasing tendency. Thus, for SEM, the highest level of interest was in March 2024. For other GLP-1 RAs the interest was lower than for SEM. For example, for LIR the highest number of searches was in June 2023 (~7% of total searches for SEM) and for DUL this was in February 2023 (~3% of the total searches for SEM). Since January 2022, the search interest has been increasing for TIR, the newest molecule approved on the market from the GLP-1 RA class. Thus, in March 2024, the inquiry proportion for TIR was about 29% of the total SEM searches (Figure 2). According to the same series, the search for ALB and LIX compared to SEM represents ~1%. Thus, both molecules were excluded from this analysis [46].

The searches for SEM were more frequent in Puerto Rico (100), the United States (71), Australia (32), United Kingdom (26), Ireland and Canada (22). The highest level of popularity for LIR was in Qatar, for DUL in New Zealand, for EXE in Qatar and Australia, and for TIR in the United States (Figure 3) [69].

Consumers who searched for GLP-1 RAs also searched for other related queries. The most frequent term used by consumers who also searched for "semaglutide", was "weight loss". Thus "weight loss semaglutide" was the most frequent related query for SEM. Also, another two terms that were identified as related queries for SEM were: "semaglutide for weight loss" and "ozempic weight loss". An interesting observation was in the TIR series, where "semaglutide weight loss" was one of the twenty-five most frequent terms associated with TIR queries. At the same time, people had a high interest in the side effects of SEM ("side effects semaglutide") (Table 2). The queries related to weight loss were more frequent than for the side effects for all other GLP-1 RAs, except EXE [69].

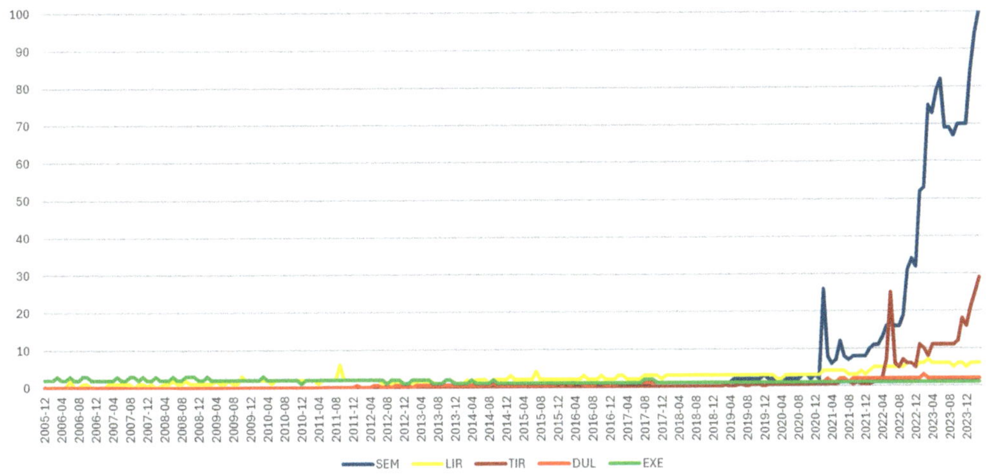

Figure 2. Comparison regarding the search interest related to GLP-1 RAs, according to Google Trends Tool (December 2005–March 2024) [69].

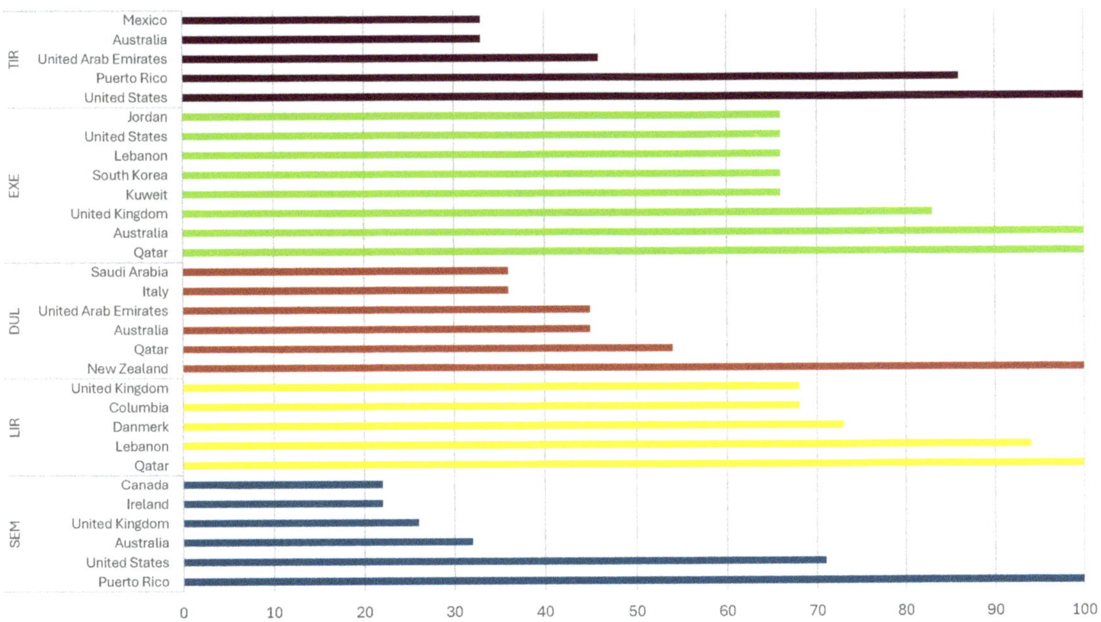

Figure 3. Comparison of interest in searching for information about GLP-1 RAs on Google by region [69].

Table 2. Comparison between the most frequent queries related to "side effects" and "weight loss" [69].

	Terms Associated with "Weight Loss"	Terms Associated with "Side Effects"
SEM	weight loss semaglutide semaglutide for weight loss ozempic weight loss	side effects semaglutide
LIR	liraglutide weight loss liraglutide for weight loss	liraglutide side effects
TIR	tirzepatide weight loss tirzepatide for weight loss semaglutide weight loss	tirzepatide side effects
DUL	dulaglutide weight loss	dulaglutide side effects
EXE	exenatide weight loss	exenatide side effects

3.2. Descriptive Analysis

3.2.1. Analysis of ICSRs

From a total number of 72,548 ICSRs uploaded in EV until 31 March 2024 for the GLP-1 RAs analyzed, 21,012 ICSRs have been reported for SEM. SEM had the largest share (29.0%) of the total, followed by LIR (25.0%) and DUL (23.9%) (Figure 4).

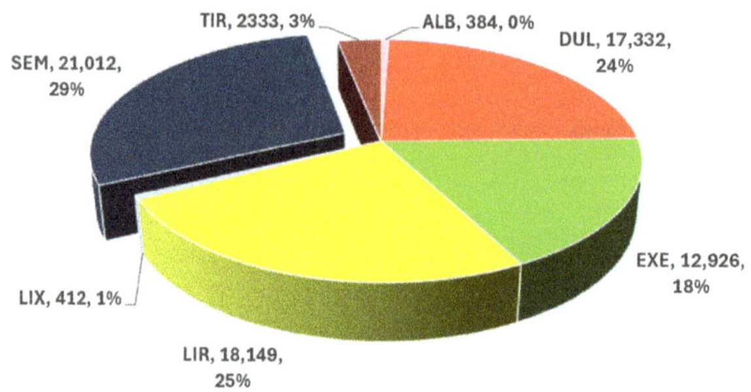

Figure 4. The shares of ICSRs that reported GLP-1 RAs. ALB—albiglutide; DUL—dulaglutide; EXE—exenatide; LIR—liraglutide; LIX—lixisenatide; SEM—semaglutide; TIR—tirzepatide.

The proportion of ADRs reported from total cases treated with SEM (1.99) is less than for the group of all other GLP-1 RAs (2.08). Also, higher proportions were observed for ALB (2.85), EXE (2.72), and LIX (2.08). Conversely, for LIR and DUL, other very prevalent GLP-1 RAs, the proportion of ADRs from the total ICSRs was lower (1.81, respectively 1.90). However, for TIR the proportion (1.98) was similar to SEM (Figure 5).

According to data published in EV, ADRs reported in the group of patients aged 18–64 years treated with SEM (39.7%) had a close frequency with all other GLP-1 RAs (41.8%), ALB (42.2%) and DUL (37.9%). Also, in the 65–85 years group, no great differences have been observed for SEM (21.6%) compared to the group of all other analogues (22.7%) and ALB (18.8%) (Table 3).

The most frequent cases have been reported in the female group that used SEM (57.7%) compared to the group of all other GLP-1 RAs (53.6%). Also, a similar frequency can be observed for LIR (59.8%). The most reported cases from EEA were for SEM (52.6%), similar to DUL (51.1%), but more frequent than the entire group of all other GLP-1 RAs. Healthcare professionals have been the ones to most often report ADRs related to SEM (61.3%). The same situation was noticed for all other GLP-1 RAs, except ALB (45.6%). Regarding the severity, the cases reported in EV as serious represented 74.2% (n = 38,215) of the total number related to all GLP-1 RAs. It can be noticed that serious cases reported for SEM (n = 12,029; 57.2%) had the lowest frequency compared to all other analogues (Table 3).

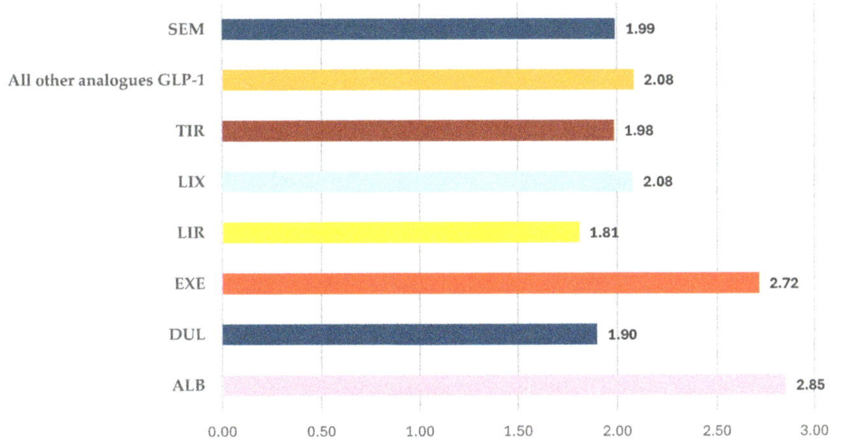

Figure 5. The proportion of ADRs reported from the total ICSRs. ALB—albiglutide; DUL—dulaglutide; EXE—exenatide; LIR—liraglutide; LIX—lixisenatide; SEM—semaglutide; TIR—tirzepatide.

Table 3. Characteristics of ICSRs reported for SEM. EEA—European Economic Area; HP—healthcare professional; NS—not specified; ALB—albiglutide; DUL—dulaglutide; EXE—exenatide; LIR—liraglutide; LIX—lixisenatide; SEM—semaglutide; TIR—tirzepatide.

	SEM	ALB	DUL	EXE	LIR	LIX	TIR	All Other GLP-1 RAs
	n (%)	n (%)	n (%)	n (%)	n (%)	n (%)	n (%)	n (%)
Total	21,012	384	17,332	12,926	18,149	412	2333	51,536
Age category								
NS	7942 (37.8)	148 (38.5)	5476 (31.6)	4160 (32.2)	6668 (36.7)	105 (25.5)	1138 (48.8)	17,695 (34.3)
0–1 Month	1 (0.0)	0 (0.0)	1 (0.0)	6 (0.0)	4 (0.0)	0 (0.0)	0 (0.0)	11 (0.0)
2 Months–2 Years	2 (0.0)	0 (0.0)	3 (0.0)	1 (0.0)	4 (0.0)	0 (0.0)	0 (0.0)	8 (0.0)
3–11 Years	9 (0.0)	0 (0.0)	2 (0.0)	1 (0.0)	9 (0.0)	0 (0.0)	0 (0.0)	12 (0.0)
12–17 Years	23 (0.1)	0 (0.0)	6 (0.0)	6 (0.0)	64 (0.4)	0 (0.0)	2 (0.0)	78 (0.2)
18–64 Years	8345 (39.7)	162 (42.2)	6576 (37.9)	5519 (42.7)	8236 (45.4)	186 (45.1)	863 (37.0)	21,542 (41.8)
65–85 Years	4546 (21.6)	72 (18.8)	4951 (28.6)	3153 (24.4)	3104 (17.1)	118 (28.6)	307 (13.2)	11,705 (22.7)
More than 85 Years	144 (0.7)	2 (0.5)	317 (1.8)	80 (0.6)	60 (0.3)	3 (0.7)	23 (1.0)	485 (0.9)
Sex								
Female	12,122 (57.7)	211 (54.9)	8443 (48.7)	6741 (52.2)	10,851 (59.8)	210 (51.0)	1180 (50.6)	27,636 (53.6)
Male	8206 (39.1)	158 (41.1)	7676 (44.3)	5825 (45.1)	6189 (34.1)	169 (41.0)	685 (29.4)	20,702 (40.2)

Table 3. *Cont.*

	SEM	ALB	DUL	EXE	LIR	LIX	TIR	All Other GLP-1 RAs
	n (%)	n (%)	n (%)	n (%)	n (%)	n (%)	n (%)	n (%)
NS	684 (3.3)	15 (3.9)	1213 (7.0)	360 (2.8)	1109 (6.1)	33 (8.0)	468 (20.1)	3198 (6.2)
Geographic origin								
EEA	11,060 (52.6)	12 (3.1)	8864 (51.1)	3226 (25.0)	7309 (40.3)	265 (64.3)	115 (4.9)	19,791 (38.4)
NON-EEA	9952 (47.4)	372 (96.9)	8468 (48.9)	9700 (75.0)	10,839 (59.7)	147 (35.7)	2218 (95.1)	31,744 (61.6)
NS	0 (0.0)	0 (0.0)	0 (0.0)	0 (0.0)	1 (0.0)	0 (0.0)	0 (0.0)	1 (0.0)
Reporter								
HP	12,877 (61.3)	175 (45.6)	11,001 (63.5)	8751 (67.7)	12,316 (67.9)	333 (80.8)	1470 (63.0)	34,046 (66.1)
NHP	8135 (38.7)	209 (54.4)	6331 (36.5)	4168 (32.2)	5832 (32.1)	79 (19.2)	863 (37.0)	17,482 (33.9)
NS	0 (0.0)	0 (0.0)	0 (0.0)	7 (0.1)	1 (0.0)	0 (0.0)	0 (0.0)	8 (0.0)
Seriousness								
Non serious	8983 (42.8)	5 (1.3)	7051 (40.7)	1383 (10.7)	4637 (25.5)	119 (28.9)	120 (5.1)	13,315 (25.8)
NS	0 (0.0)	0 (0.0)	0 (0.0)	3 (0.0)	3 (0.0)	0 (0.0)	0 (0.0)	6 (0.0)
Serious	12,029 (57.2)	379 (98.7)	10,281 (59.3)	11,540 (89.3)	13,509 (74.4)	293 (71.1)	2213 (94.9)	38,215 (74.2)

3.2.2. Comparative Evaluation of ADRs Grouped by SOC

Firstly, a comparison between the distribution of ADRs by SOC was conducted between SEM and all other GLP-1 RAs. Thus, it could be observed that the ADRs of SEM were most frequently reported in the following SOCs: "Gastrointestinal disorders" (25.0%; n = 10,468), "Injury, poisoning and procedural complications" (10.6%; n = 4414), "General disorders and administration site conditions" (10.2%; n = 4264). Similar situations were obtained for the ADRs reported in SOCs "Gastrointestinal disorders" and "General disorders and administration site conditions" for all comparators. Also, in the SOC "Injury, poisoning and procedural complications", similar situations were observed for ALB (11.8%) and TIR (10.0%). Among the SOCs with the lowest ADR reporting frequency were: "Congenital, familial and genetic disorders", "Pregnancy, puerperium and perinatal conditions", and "Social circumstances" (Figure 6).

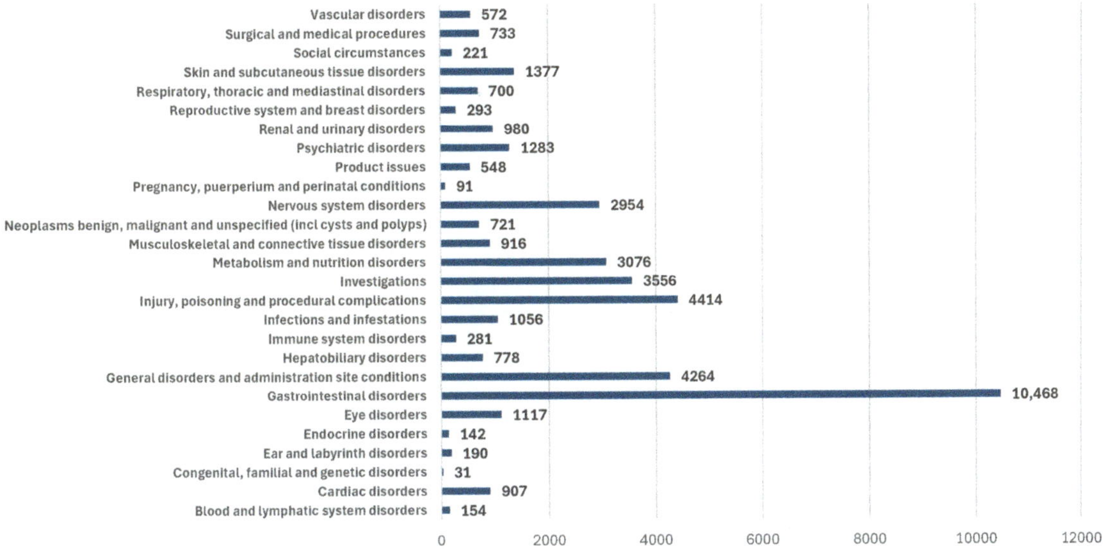

Figure 6. Distribution of ADRs reported for SEM by SOC.

3.2.3. ADRs Reported for Incorrect Dosage

Figure 7 presents the frequency of ADRs related to dosage in GLP-1 RAs class. Thus, for SEM, the most frequent are ADRs related to improper dose (0.79%), a percentage higher than that of DUL (0.68%), TIR (0.52%), and LIR (0.49%), but lower than that of EXE (1.90%), and the entire group of all other analogues (1.02%). Overdoses have been reported for SEM (0.59%) with a lower frequency than for DUL (0.66%), but higher than those reported for all other comparators. Underdoses have the lowest frequency (0.33%) in HLTs related to the dosage of SEM. This percentage is similar to LIR (0.32%) and inferior to all other comparators.

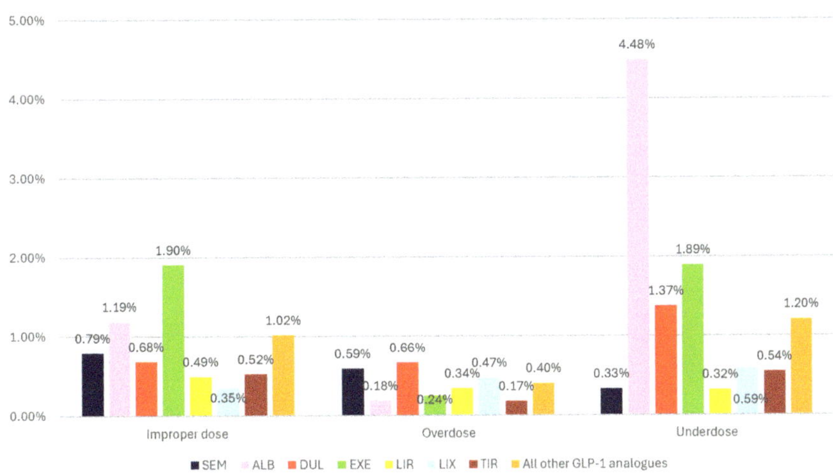

Figure 7. Frequency of ADRs related to dosage in GLP-1 RA series. ALB—albiglutide; DUL—dulaglutide; EXE—exenatide; LIR—liraglutide; LIX—lixisenatide; SEM—semaglutide; TIR—tirzepatide.

3.2.4. ADRs Reported as "Off-Label Use"

According to Figure 8, for the ADRs reported for off-label use, their frequency in the SEM series (6.16%) is similar to TIR (6.08%), but higher than other comparators, including the entire group of all other GLP-1 RAs.

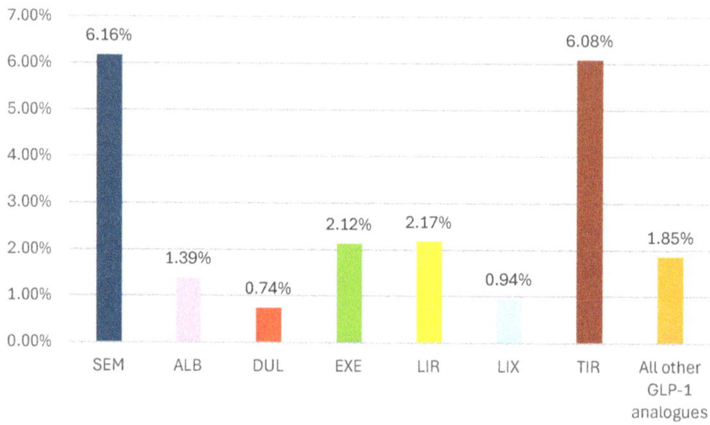

Figure 8. Frequency of ADRs related to off-label use in GLP-1 RA series. ALB—albiglutide; DUL—dulaglutide; EXE—exenatide; LIR—liraglutide; LIX—lixisenatide; SEM—semaglutide; TIR—tirzepatide.

3.2.5. Distribution of ADRs by Outcome

ADRs Reported for SEM

Regarding the outcomes, Figure 9 shows that unfavorable outcomes were reported as follows: (i) 4 cases related to overdoses were fatal; (ii) 41 cases related to incorrect dosage were not recovered or not resolved (23 for improper doses; 9 for overdosage, 9 for under dosage, respectively); (iii) 356 cases related to off-label use were not recovered or not resolved.

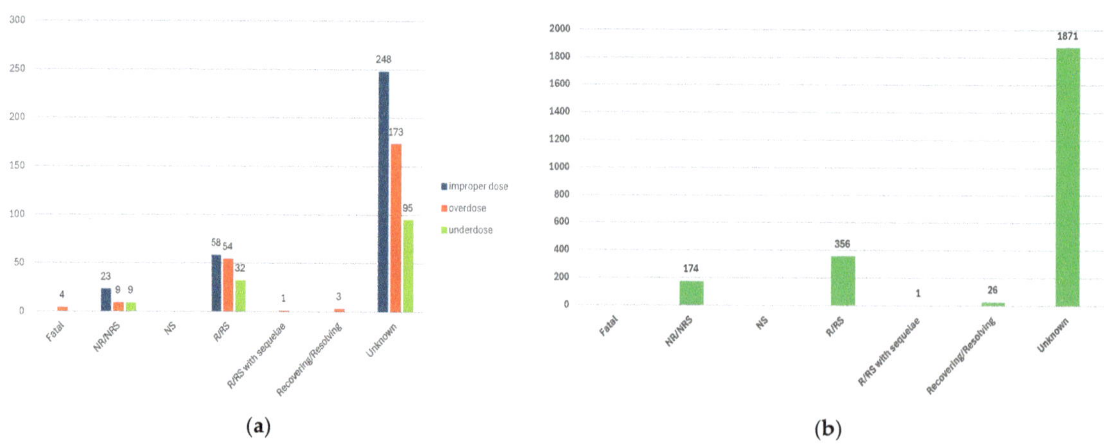

Figure 9. Distribution of ADRs of semaglutide by outcome: (**a**) related to dosage; (**b**) related to off-label use. NR/NRS—not recovered/not resolved; NS—not specified; R/RS—recovered/resolved; ALB—albiglutide; DUL—dulaglutide; EXE—exenatide; LIR—liraglutide; LIX—lixisenatide; SEM—semaglutide; TIR—tirzepatide.

The Frequency of ADRs with Unfavorable Outcomes Reported for SEM Compared to All Other GLP-1 RAs

The unfavorable outcomes of cases reported in EV (fatal or not recovered/not resolved) are represented below. Thus, Figure 10a presents the frequency of fatal ADRs reported for incorrect dosage. Fatal ADRs were reported only for overdosage, with a higher frequency in the LIR series (2.7%) than for SEM (1.6%). Also, for off-label use, no fatal ADRs were reported for any GLP-1 RAs.

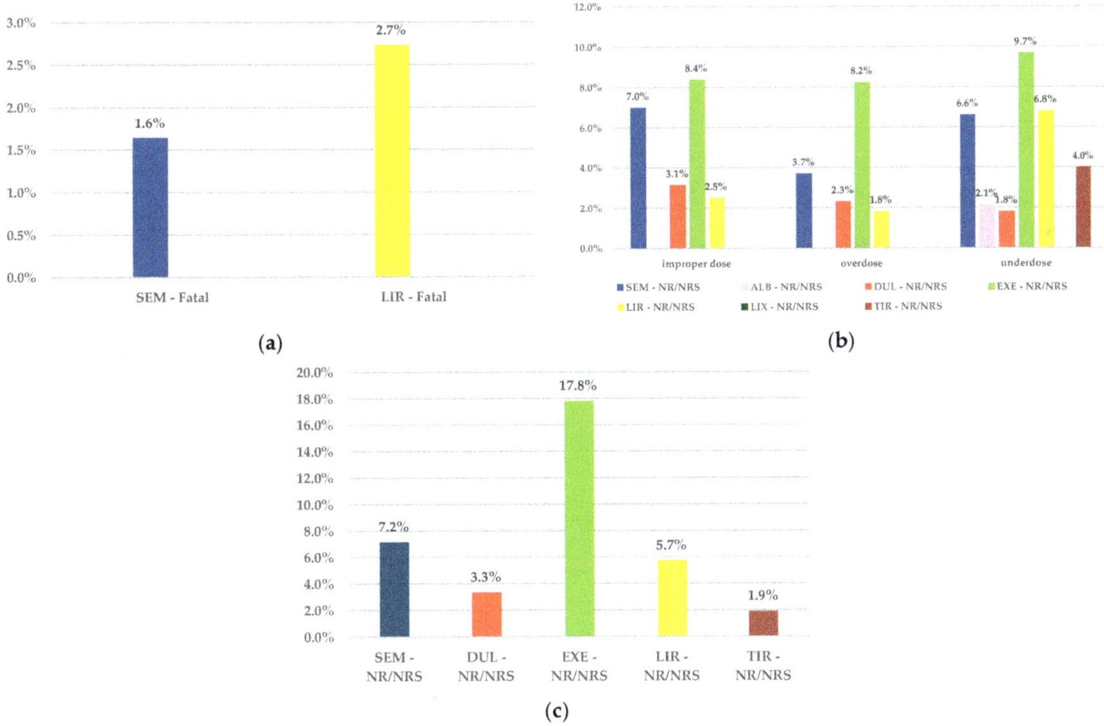

Figure 10. The frequency of ADRs with unfavorable outcomes. (**a**) Fatal outcomes of ADRs related to incorrect dosage; (**b**) not recovered/not resolved outcomes of ADRs related to incorrect dosage; (**c**) not recovered/not resolved outcomes of ADRs related to off-label use. NR/NRS—not recovered/not resolved; NS—not specified; R/RS—recovered/resolved; ALB—albiglutide; DUL—dulaglutide; EXE—exenatide; LIR—liraglutide; LIX—lixisenatide; SEM—semaglutide; TIR—tirzepatide.

The frequency of the not recovered/not resolved outcomes is presented in Figure 10b. According to this data, SEM presented a higher frequency in all three HLTs, compared with all other GLP-1 RAs, with the following exceptions (Figure 10b):

- improper doses: SEM—7.0% and EXE—8.4%
- overdose: SEM—3.7% and EXE—8.2%
- underdose: SEM—6.6%, EXE—9.7%, and LIR—6.8%

Regarding the frequency of the not recovered/not resolved ADRs related to off-label use, SEM (7.2%) also had a higher frequency of being reported compared to other GLP-1 RAs, except EXE (17.8%) (Figure 10c).

3.3. Disproportionality Analysis

3.3.1. Incorrect Doses

According to the data published in EV, the results of the disproportionality analysis show a higher probability of reporting ADRs related to improper doses for SEM compared to LIR (ROR: 1.6169, 95% CI: 1.3379–1.9542) and TIR (ROR: 1.5200, 95% CI: 1.0032–2.3031). Also, in Figure 11a, a lower probability of ADRs for SEM compared to EXE (ROR: 0.4087, 95% CI: 0.3579–0.4667) and the entire group of all other GLP-1 RAs (ROR: 0.7722, 95% CI: 0.6823–0.8740) could be observed. No difference could be observed for SEM compared to DUL and ALB.

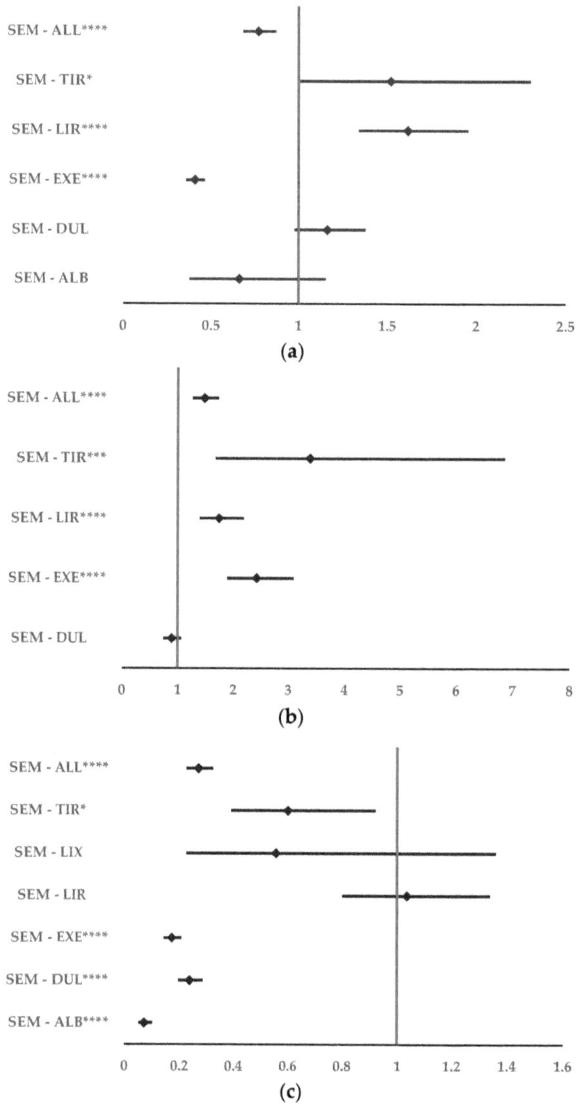

Figure 11. Disproportionality analysis for incorrect dosage of SEM: (**a**) improper dosage; (**b**) overdose; (**c**) underdose. ALB—albiglutide; DUL—dulaglutide; EXE—exenatide; LIR—liraglutide; LIX—lixisenatide; SEM—semaglutide; TIR—tirzepatide. * p <0.05; *** $p \leq 0.001$; **** $p \leq 0.0001$.

For ADRs related to overdose, SEM had a higher probability of being reported compared to EXE (ROR: 2.4174, 95% CI: 1.8878–3.0956), LIR (ROR: 1.7434, 95% CI: 1.3913–2.1845), and TIR (ROR: 3.3868, 95% CI: 1.6736–6.8535). The same results could be noticed through a comparison with the group of all other GLP-1 RAs (ROR: 1.4764, 95% CI: 1.2608–1.7288). Also, when compared to DUL, no difference could be noticed (Figure 11b).

For overdosage, SEM had a higher probability of being reported, but for underdosage the situation is reversed. Thus, no difference could be observed by comparison with LIR and LIX, but a lower probability of being reported could be observed by comparison with all other analogues and with the entire group of all other GLP-1 RAs (Figure 11c).

3.3.2. Off-Label Use

Figure 12 showed a higher probability of reporting off-label use for SEM compared to all other analogues, except TIR: ALB (ROR: 4.4375, 95% CI: 2.6615–7.3988), DUL (ROR: 8.3830, 95% CI: 7.3359–9.5796), EXE (ROR: 2.9018, 95% CI: 2.6680–3.1560), LIR (ROR: 2.8377, 95% CI: 2.6052–3.0910), and LIX (ROR: 6.5330, 95% CI: 3.2525–13.1221). Also, compared to the group of all other GLP-1 RAs the probability of being reported is higher (ROR: 3.3226; 95% CI: 3.1270–3.5304).

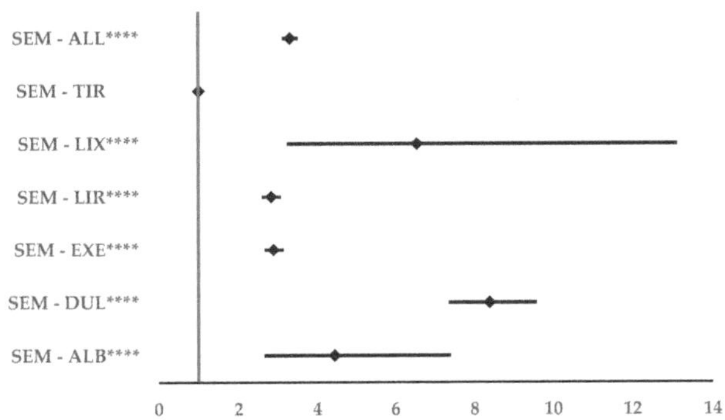

Figure 12. Disproportionality analysis for off-label use of SEM. ALB—albiglutide; DUL—dulaglutide; EXE—exenatide; LIR—liraglutide; LIX—lixisenatide; SEM—semaglutide; TIR—tirzepatide. **** $p \leq 0.0001$.

4. Discussion

A reduced appetite and food intake were observed after the administration of GLP-1 RAs. Thus, their benefits in weight loss are exploited by using them in obese patients with or without diabetes [70]. Improving the patients' adherence to GLP-1 RAs treatment through possible oral administration [71] was an important objective of the researchers following their approval on the market. Only a few years after the EXE approval in therapy, new molecules have been authorized. SEM presents some differences in pharmacokinetics due to the modifications in GLP-1 structure: (i) improved stability against dipeptide-peptidase-4 enzyme (DPP-4) through the substitution of alanine with aminoisobutyric acid; (ii) increased binding to albumin by the introduction of a linker and a C18 di-acid chain; (iii) preventing the binding of fatty acid at the wrong site through the substitution of Lys with Arg [72]. On the other hand, to improve the patients' adherence to SEM, its absorption across gastric mucosa was improved by obtaining a co-formulation with sodium N-(8-[2-hydroxybenzoyl]amino)caprylate. Based on this formulation, SEM was the first of the GLP-1 RAs suitable for oral administration [73]. Thus, SEM was expected to be very popular in the media and widely used in therapy, often as off-label or as auto medication. Because of this issue, the dosing errors were expected to be quite frequent.

The first item analyzed was the popularity of SEM in Google searches. The term "weight loss semaglutide" was the most frequently searched for by the people who also searched for the term "semaglutide". Also, the queries related to weight loss have a higher frequency than for the other GLP-1 RAs. Additionally, the search interest on Google for each molecule was related to a lower frequency with the side effects (Table 2). Based on this information, it could be considered that the people interested in these molecules had similar search behavior regarding the safety of the products. Our results are comparable to the ones in the study performed by Han et al., which showed that the greatest relative search was obtained for one of the SEM brand names [7]. Also, a study published in 2024 showed that SEM was one of the most popular pharmacological and surgical obesity methods searched on Google [74]. The popularity of SEM on TikTok (an online social media platform), is also very high. A total of 57 of the first 100 video searches under the hashtag "#Ozempic" were related to "weight loss" (44 million views), and 29 of 100 were related to "common side effects, toxicity" (24 million views). The "off-label" use was a search term only in 3 of 100 videos (2.8 million views) [75].

Although SEM was approved on the market more recently than LIR, DUL, EXE, and ALB, the descriptive analysis showed the highest number of ICSRs reported in EV (29% of the total) (Figure 4). Its popularity (Figure 2) and indication in obesity could contribute to an increase in the prescription numbers, as well as implicitly in its consumption. In 2022, the global market of SEM and LIR increased by 43% from 9.9 to 14.2 billion USD [76]. Moreover, according to a study published in 2023, prescriptions for SEM increased by 150%/year [77]. This increase could be justified by a higher efficiency of SEM in weight loss and by a lower cost of treatment [78,79]. Other studies showed the superior efficiency of SEM compared to LIX [80], EXE [80,81], DUL [81] and, LIR [82]. For example, SEM led to an average reduction in body weight of 12.4% in 68 weeks compared to LIR (−5.4% in 56 weeks) [82]. Therefore, SEM had an improved value for money in weight reduction compared with LIR (estimated cost of 1845 USD per 1% reduction in body weight for SEM, compared to 3256 USD for LIR) [82].

Regarding the demographic characteristics of patients, in the present study, most of the reports were in the 18–64 years group (Table 3). Also, the most frequent reports were for females (57.7%) (Table 3), similar to the results of another study performed on the data from the Food and Drug Administration Adverse Event Reporting System (FAERS) between 2018–2022 (54.4%) [9].

According to the present study, SEM had the lowest number of severe ADRs compared to the analyzed molecules (Table 3). These results are similar to other studies that reported a safety profile consistent with other GLP-1 RAs, with a low incidence of severe ADRs for SEM [81,83,84]. Generally, SEM is well tolerated, and most ADRs induced are mild-to-moderate and transient. The most frequent ADRs are related to the "Gastrointestinal disorders" SOC (nausea, vomiting, diarrhea, pancreatitis, etc.), or the "General disorders and administration site conditions" SOC (e.g., malaise). On the other hand, pathologies such as acute kidney injury from the "Renal and urinary disorders" SOC could have negative consequences on health status even if they are less frequent (Figure 6). Most probably, nausea and vomiting are caused by the inhibition of gastric emptying, and diarrhea could be induced by altering nutrient absorption or intestinal motility [83]. Additionally, malaise seems to be promoted by direct central GLP-1 R activation, primarily in the brainstem [85]. Regarding pancreatitis and pancreatic cancer, the FDA and EMA concluded that no causal association could be found between GLP-1 RAs and these pathologies. Only a few preclinical studies have shown a pancreatic inflammatory status after GLP-1 RA use [83,86]. Dehydration caused by nausea, vomiting or diarrhea, as well as increasing the sodium excretion after GLP-1 RA administration, could lead to renal failure [83,87]. To diminish gastrointestinal disturbances, different strategies could be applied: gradual dose titration, eating slowly, reducing the portion size per meal, avoiding high-fat food, and finishing eating before satiety. Also, it is recommended to avoid the risk factors for renal failure, such as dehydration or association with medication with a high renal risk [83].

Fatal outcomes were only reported for overdosing on SEM and LIR. Anyway, until now, no unexpected safety issues have been reported for SEM [83,84]. However, another interesting result of the present study suggests that SEM had a higher number of ADRs reported by each case than DUL and LIR, and was similar to those of TIR (Figure 5). Considering that TIR was recently authorized, it is expected that this situation will be different over time.

This study revealed a higher tendency to report ADRs related to overdosing of SEM (except DUL and EXE), and incorrect dosing compared to LIR and TIR (Figure 7). According to the American Association of Poison Control Centers, a total of 2941 cases related to SEM overdosing were reported between January–November 2023, more than double compared to 2022 [88]. The overdosing cases reported in the scientific literature were associated with notable gastrointestinal symptoms, and even with medical evaluation and treatment with antiemetics and intravenous fluids [89,90].

On the other hand, the off-label use of SEM was more frequently reported in EV than other GLP-1 RAs (except TIR) (Figure 8). Its advantages (high efficiency and safety, improved value for money in weight reduction, and increased benefits–risk ratio) probably represent factors for increasing the off-label use of SEM. According to the study performed by Chiappini et al., the off-label use of SEM was the fifth most frequent cause of reporting in FAERS (6%) [9].

Finally, media attention fuels the demand for this type of medication and, at the same time, generates an increase in illegal sales. Thus, the authorities in countries such as Austria, Denmark, United Kingdom, Ireland, Switzerland, etc., seek to repress illegal activity with these drugs, approaching different methods of social media monitoring, even reporting the confiscation of falsified pens with SEM in some EEA states [91]. Moreover, both manufacturers and regulatory agencies in the field of medicine issued warnings about the penetration of counterfeit products into the drug supply chain, finding them in retail pharmacies [92–94]. The warnings were issued by reglementary authorities such as the FDA, EMA, and the Medicines and Healthcare Products Regulatory Agency from the United Kingdom. These refer to using the unapproved salt forms of SEM or to online sales of fraudulent or unapproved products [95–97]. In this context, greater attention must be paid, both to the way of prescribing and also to the counselling of patients regarding the identification of fakes and the judicious use of medicines.

Limitations of the Study

Certain limitations should be considered for this study. Our searches in Google Trends only included active pharmaceutical ingredients. The online environment is extensive; besides Google, other search engines and social media platforms are widely used. We acknowledge that these results may not offer the full depiction of the off-label use for weight loss phenomenon. On the other hand, the use of the Internet, including the Google search engine, is reduced in different areas with limited access to internet or freedom of speech. Also, people with lower socioeconomic status or educational background, or old people, represent categories with low access to computers or internet [56,59]. Other limitations of this study are based on the analysis of ADRs from the EudraVigilance spontaneous reporting system, among which some are related to the phenomenon of underreporting, overreporting and reporting bias or to the inaccuracy of the information contained in the reports. The number of ADRs reported could be influenced by the extent of drug use, the awareness of the reporter, media coverage of the drug, the severity and outcome of the reaction, and the variability of reporting rates between different regions, etc. ADRs associated with newer drugs or severe cases might be reported more frequently compared with older drugs or minor adverse effects. Not least, off-label use could be a factor in the underreporting of adverse drug reactions. Moreover, information such as concomitant medication or other suspected drugs, comorbidities, medical status, etc., could be missing, thus affecting this analysis. Other limitations are the lack of a denominator or the lack of certainty of a causal relationship between the reported ADRs and the suspected drug. Furthermore, the ROR is a simple indicator that allows for the estimation of the relative risk of ADR reporting but could not be used to quantify the true risk. Further studies are needed for an extensive evaluation of the safety profile of SEM and other GLP-1 RAs.

5. Conclusions

Our study highlights the risk of the improper or off-label use of SEM based on an analysis of real-world data from Google Trends and the European spontaneous reporting system, EudraVigilance. To reduce these risks, especially of severe ADRs or unfavorable outcomes, stakeholders should promote the correct use and dispensing of drugs based on SEM. Also, an increased carefulness in patient counselling could improve healthcare outcomes. Likewise, new studies must be performed to obtain information regarding dosing errors or off-label use. Based on the results obtained following the analysis of ICSRs, useful information can be provided for a better monitoring and managing of adverse events related to abuse. Taking into consideration the limitations of spontaneous reporting of ADRs, a high level of standardization or more detailed reporting could improve the quality of data and strengthen the robustness of future analyses.

Author Contributions: Conceptualization A.B., C.M.D., A.M.A., C.M., A.F. and A.L.V.-T.; methodology, A.B., C.M.D., A.M.A., C.M., L.L.R., S.G., A.M.J., F.G.G. and A.L.V.-T.; software, A.B., C.M.D., A.M.A., A.C.M., A.E.L., C.M. and A.F. validation, A.B., C.M.D., A.M.A., S.G., C.M. and A.L.V.-T.; formal analysis, A.B., A.M.A., C.M.D., C.M., L.L.R., S.G., A.C.M., F.G.G. and A.L.V.-T.; investigation, A.B., A.C.M., A.A.C., A.M.J., A.E.L., C.M. and A.L.V.-T.; data curation, A.B., C.M.D., A.M.A., S.G., C.M., L.L.R. and A.L.V.-T.; resources, A.B., C.M.D., A.F. and A.L.V.-T.; writing—original draft preparation, A.B., C.M.D., A.M.A., A.F., A.A.C., C.M. and A.L.V.-T.; writing—review and editing, A.B., C.M.D., A.M.A., A.F., A.A.C., L.L.R., A.C.M., A.E.L., C.M. and A.L.V.-T.; visualization, A.B., C.M.D., A.M.A., A.F., A.A.C., L.L.R., A.M.J., A.C.M., S.G., A.E.L., F.G.G., C.M. and A.L.V.-T.; supervision, A.M.A., S.G., F.G.G., C.M. and A.L.V.-T. All authors have read and agreed to the published version of the manuscript.

Funding: Project financed by Lucian Blaga University of Sibiu through the research grant LBUS-IRG-2023/No. 3523, 24 July 2023.

Institutional Review Board Statement: Not applicable.

Informed Consent Statement: Not applicable.

Data Availability Statement: Data contained within the article.

Conflicts of Interest: The authors declare no conflicts of interest.

References

1. Prasad-Reddy, L.; Isaacs, D. A Clinical Review of GLP-1 Receptor Agonists: Efficacy and Safety in Diabetes and Beyond. *Drugs Context* **2015**, *4*, 212283. [CrossRef] [PubMed]
2. Wilding, J.P.H.; Batterham, R.L.; Calanna, S.; Davies, M.; Van Gaal, L.F.; Lingvay, I.; McGowan, B.M.; Rosenstock, J.; Tran, M.T.D.; Wadden, T.A.; et al. Once-Weekly Semaglutide in Adults with Overweight or Obesity. *N. Engl. J. Med.* **2021**, *384*, 989–1002. [CrossRef]
3. Stoicescu, L.; Crişan, D.; Morgovan, C.; Avram, L.; Ghibu, S. Heart Failure with Preserved Ejection Fraction: The Pathophysiological Mechanisms behind the Clinical Phenotypes and the Therapeutic Approach. *Int. J. Mol. Sci.* **2024**, *25*, 794. [CrossRef]
4. Pop, C.; Ștefan, M.G.; Muntean, D.M.; Stoicescu, L.; Gal, A.F.; Kiss, B.; Morgovan, C.; Loghin, F.; Rochette, L.; Lauzier, B.; et al. Protective Effects of a Discontinuous Treatment with Alpha-Lipoic Acid in Obesity-Related Heart Failure with Preserved Ejection Fraction, in Rats. *Antioxidants* **2020**, *9*, 1073. [CrossRef]
5. Qin, W.; Yang, J.; Deng, C.; Ruan, Q.; Duan, K. Efficacy and Safety of Semaglutide 2.4 Mg for Weight Loss in Overweight or Obese Adults without Diabetes: An Updated Systematic Review and Meta-Analysis Including the 2-Year STEP 5 Trial. *Diabetes. Obes. Metab.* **2024**, *26*, 911–923. [CrossRef]
6. Obesity and Overweight. Available online: https://www.who.int/news-room/fact-sheets/detail/obesity-and-overweight (accessed on 11 April 2024).
7. Han, S.H.; Safeek, R.; Ockerman, K.; Trieu, N.; Mars, P.; Klenke, A.; Furnas, H.; Sorice-Virk, S. Public Interest in the Off-Label Use of Glucagon-like Peptide 1 Agonists (Ozempic) for Cosmetic Weight Loss: A Google Trends Analysis. *Aesthetic Surg. J.* **2023**, *44*, 60–67. [CrossRef] [PubMed]
8. Morgovan, C.; Cosma, S.A.; Valeanu, M.; Juncan, A.M.; Rus, L.L.; Gligor, F.G.; Butuca, A.; Tit, D.M.; Bungau, S.; Ghibu, S. An Exploratory Research of 18 Years on the Economic Burden of Diabetes for the Romanian National Health Insurance System. *Int. J. Environ. Res. Public Health* **2020**, *17*, 4456. [CrossRef] [PubMed]

9. Chiappini, S.; Vickers-Smith, R.; Harris, D.; Papanti Pelletier, G.D.; Corkery, J.M.; Guirguis, A.; Martinotti, G.; Sensi, S.L.; Schifano, F. Is There a Risk for Semaglutide Misuse? Focus on the Food and Drug Administration's FDA Adverse Events Reporting System (FAERS) Pharmacovigilance Dataset. *Pharmaceuticals* **2023**, *16*, 994. [CrossRef] [PubMed]
10. Larsen, P.J. Mechanisms behind GLP-1 Induced Weight Loss. *Sage J.* **2008**, *8*, S34–S41. [CrossRef]
11. Onakpoya, I.J.; Heneghan, C.J.; Aronson, J.K. Post-Marketing Withdrawal of Anti-Obesity Medicinal Products Because of Adverse Drug Reactions: A Systematic Review. *BMC Med.* **2016**, *14*, 191. [CrossRef]
12. Czernichow, S.; Batty, D. Withdrawal of Sibutramine for Weight Loss: Where Does This Leave Clinicians? *Obes. Facts* **2010**, *3*, 155. [CrossRef]
13. EMA Confirms Recommendation to Withdraw Marketing Authorisations for Amfepramone Medicines | European Medicines Agency. Available online: https://www.ema.europa.eu/en/news/ema-confirms-recommendation-withdraw-marketing-authorisations-amfepramone-medicines-0 (accessed on 11 April 2024).
14. Waldrop, S.W.; Johnson, V.R.; Stanford, F.C. Inequalities in the Provision of GLP-1 Receptor Agonists for the Treatment of Obesity. *Nat. Med.* **2024**, *30*, 22–25. [CrossRef]
15. Rohani, P.; Malekpour Alamdari, N.; Bagheri, S.E.; Hekmatdoost, A.; Sohouli, M.H. The Effects of Subcutaneous Tirzepatide on Obesity and Overweight: A Systematic Review and Meta-regression Analysis of Randomized Controlled Trials. *Front. Endocrinol.* **2023**, *14*, 1230206. [CrossRef]
16. Sharma, D.; Verma, S.; Vaidya, S.; Kalia, K.; Tiwari, V. Recent Updates on GLP-1 Agonists: Current Advancements & Challenges. *Biomed. Pharmacother.* **2018**, *108*, 952–962. [CrossRef] [PubMed]
17. McLean, B.A.; Wong, C.K.; Campbell, J.E.; Hodson, D.J.; Trapp, S.; Drucker, D.J. Revisiting the Complexity of GLP-1 Action from Sites of Synthesis to Receptor Activation. *Endocr. Rev.* **2021**, *42*, 101–132. [CrossRef]
18. Vosoughi, K.; Salman Roghani, R.; Camilleri, M. Effects of GLP-1 Agonists on Proportion of Weight Loss in Obesity with or without Diabetes: Systematic Review and Meta-Analysis. *Obes. Med.* **2022**, *35*, 100456. [CrossRef]
19. Evolution of GLP-1 Receptor Agonists for Diabetes Treatment | Biopharma PEG. Available online: https://www.biochempeg.com/article/299.html (accessed on 11 April 2024).
20. Seufert, J.; Gallwitz, B. The Extra-Pancreatic Effects of GLP-1 Receptor Agonists: A Focus on the Cardiovascular, Gastrointestinal and Central Nervous Systems. *Diabetes, Obes. Metab.* **2014**, *16*, 673–688. [CrossRef]
21. Collins, L.; Costello, R.A. *Glucagon-Like Peptide-1 Receptor Agonists*; StatPearls: St. Petersburg, FL, USA, 2023.
22. Mishra, R.; Raj, R.; Elshimy, G.; Zapata, I.; Kannan, L.; Majety, P.; Edem, D.; Correa, R. Adverse Events Related to Tirzepatide. *J. Endocr. Soc.* **2023**, *7*, bvad016. [CrossRef] [PubMed]
23. Taylor, S.I. GLP-1 Receptor Agonists: Differentiation within the Class. *Lancet Diabetes Endocrinol.* **2018**, *6*, 83–85. [CrossRef]
24. Davies, M.J.; Aroda, V.R.; Collins, B.S.; Gabbay, R.A.; Green, J.; Maruthur, N.M.; Rosas, S.E.; Del Prato, S.; Mathieu, C.; Mingrone, G.; et al. Management of Hyperglycaemia in Type 2 Diabetes, 2022. A Consensus Report by the American Diabetes Association (ADA) and the European Association for the Study of Diabetes (EASD). *Diabetologia* **2022**, *65*, 1925–1966. [CrossRef]
25. Tilinca, M.C.; Tiuca, R.A.; Burlacu, A.; Varga, A. A 2021 Update on the Use of Liraglutide in the Modern Treatment of 'Diabesity': A Narrative Review. *Medicina* **2021**, *57*, 669. [CrossRef] [PubMed]
26. Blind, E.; Janssen, H.; Dunder, K.; de Graeff, P.A. The European Medicines Agency's Approval of New Medicines for Type 2 Diabetes. *Diabetes. Obes. Metab.* **2018**, *20*, 2059. [CrossRef] [PubMed]
27. Iepsen, E.W.; Torekov, S.S.; Holst, J.J. Liraglutide for Type 2 Diabetes and Obesity: A 2015 Update. *Expert Rev. Cardiovasc. Ther.* **2015**, *13*, 753–767. [CrossRef] [PubMed]
28. Acosta, A.; Camilleri, M.; Burton, D.; O'Neill, J.; Eckert, D.; Carlson, P.; Zinsmeister, A.R. Exenatide in Obesity with Accelerated Gastric Emptying: A Randomized, Pharmacodynamics Study. *Physiol. Rep.* **2015**, *3*, e12610. [CrossRef] [PubMed]
29. Chudleigh, R.A.; Platts, J.; Bain, S.C. Comparative Effectiveness of Long-Acting GLP-1 Receptor Agonists in Type 2 Diabetes: A Short Review on the Emerging Data. *Diabetes, Metab. Syndr. Obes. Targets Ther.* **2020**, *13*, 433. [CrossRef] [PubMed]
30. UK Government Letters Sent to Healthcare Professionals in September 2017—GOV.UK. Available online: https://www.gov.uk/drug-safety-update/letters-sent-to-healthcare-professionals-in-september-2017 (accessed on 11 April 2024).
31. Hughes, S.; Neumiller, J.J. Oral Semaglutide. *Clin. Diabetes* **2020**, *38*, 109. [CrossRef] [PubMed]
32. Blonde, L.; Umpierrez, G.E.; Reddy, S.S.; McGill, J.B.; Berga, S.L.; Bush, M.; Chandrasekaran, S.; DeFronzo, R.A.; Einhorn, D.; Galindo, R.J.; et al. American Association of Clinical Endocrinology Clinical Practice Guideline: Developing a Diabetes Mellitus Comprehensive Care Plan-2022 Update. *Endocr. Pract.* **2022**, *28*, 923–1049. [CrossRef] [PubMed]
33. Committee, A.D.A.P.P. Pharmacologic Approaches to Glycemic Treatment: Standards of Medical Care in Diabetes—2022. *Diabetes Care* **2022**, *45*, S125–S143. [CrossRef]
34. Singh, G.; Krauthamer, M.; Bjalme-Evans, M. Wegovy (Semaglutide): A New Weight Loss Drug for Chronic Weight Management. *J. Investig. Med.* **2022**, *70*, 5–13. [CrossRef]
35. Ahmann, A.J.; Capehorn, M.; Charpentier, G.; Dotta, F.; Henkel, E.; Lingvay, I.; Holst, A.G.; Annett, M.P.; Aroda, V.R. Efficacy and Safety of Once-Weekly Semaglutide Versus Exenatide ER in Subjects With Type 2 Diabetes (SUSTAIN 3): A 56-Week, Open-Label, Randomized Clinical Trial. *Diabetes Care* **2018**, *41*, 258–266. [CrossRef]
36. Pratley, R.E.; Aroda, V.R.; Lingvay, I.; Lüdemann, J.; Andreassen, C.; Navarria, A.; Viljoen, A. Semaglutide versus Dulaglutide Once Weekly in Patients with Type 2 Diabetes (SUSTAIN 7): A Randomised, Open-Label, Phase 3b Trial. *Lancet. Diabetes Endocrinol.* **2018**, *6*, 275–286. [CrossRef] [PubMed]

37. Pi-Sunyer, X.; Astrup, A.; Fujioka, K.; Greenway, F.; Halpern, A.; Krempf, M.; Lau, D.C.W.; le Roux, C.W.; Violante Ortiz, R.; Jensen, C.B.; et al. A Randomized, Controlled Trial of 3.0 Mg of Liraglutide in Weight Management. *N. Engl. J. Med.* **2015**, *373*, 11–22. [CrossRef]
38. Astrup, A.; Rössner, S.; Van Gaal, L.; Rissanen, A.; Niskanen, L.; Al Hakim, M.; Madsen, J.; Rasmussen, M.F.; Lean, M.E. Effects of Liraglutide in the Treatment of Obesity: A Randomised, Double-Blind, Placebo-Controlled Study. *Lancet* **2009**, *374*, 1606–1616. [CrossRef] [PubMed]
39. Rubino, D.; Abrahamsson, N.; Davies, M.; Hesse, D.; Greenway, F.L.; Jensen, C.; Lingvay, I.; Mosenzon, O.; Rosenstock, J.; Rubio, M.A.; et al. Effect of Continued Weekly Subcutaneous Semaglutide vs Placebo on Weight Loss Maintenance in Adults With Overweight or Obesity: The STEP 4 Randomized Clinical Trial. *JAMA* **2021**, *325*, 1414–1425. [CrossRef] [PubMed]
40. Wadden, T.A.; Bailey, T.S.; Billings, L.K.; Davies, M.; Frias, J.P.; Koroleva, A.; Lingvay, I.; O'Neil, P.M.; Rubino, D.M.; Skovgaard, D.; et al. Effect of Subcutaneous Semaglutide vs Placebo as an Adjunct to Intensive Behavioral Therapy on Body Weight in Adults With Overweight or Obesity: The STEP 3 Randomized Clinical Trial. *JAMA* **2021**, *325*, 1403–1413. [CrossRef] [PubMed]
41. Rubino, D.M.; Greenway, F.L.; Khalid, U.; O'Neil, P.M.; Rosenstock, J.; Sørrig, R.; Wadden, T.A.; Wizert, A.; Garvey, W.T. Effect of Weekly Subcutaneous Semaglutide vs Daily Liraglutide on Body Weight in Adults With Overweight or Obesity Without Diabetes: The STEP 8 Randomized Clinical Trial. *JAMA* **2022**, *327*, 138. [CrossRef] [PubMed]
42. Togo, K.; Yonemoto, N. Real World Data and Data Science in Medical Research: Present and Future. *Jpn. J. Stat. Data Sci.* **2022**, *5*, 769–781. [CrossRef] [PubMed]
43. Hsu, C.W.; Tseng, W.T.; Wang, L.J.; Yang, Y.H.; Kao, H.Y.; Lin, P.Y. Comparative Effectiveness of Antidepressants on Geriatric Depression: Real-World Evidence from a Population-Based Study. *J. Affect. Disord.* **2022**, *296*, 609–615. [CrossRef] [PubMed]
44. Lasky, T.; Chakravarty, A. Real World Data (RWD) in Pediatrics. *J. Biopharm. Stat.* **2023**, *33*, 875–880. [CrossRef]
45. Kim, H.S.; Lee, S.; Kim, J.H. Real-World Evidence versus Randomized Controlled Trial: Clinical Research Based on Electronic Medical Records. *J. Korean Med. Sci.* **2018**, *33*, e213. [CrossRef]
46. O'Leary, C.P.; Cavender, M.A. Emerging Opportunities to Harness Real World Data: An Introduction to Data Sources, Concepts, and Applications. *Diabetes Obes. Metab.* **2020**, *22*, 3–12. [CrossRef] [PubMed]
47. Gebrye, T.; Mbada, C.; Hakimi, Z.; Fatoye, F. Development of Quality Assessment Tool for Systematic Reviews and Meta-Analyses of Real-World Studies: A Delphi Consensus Survey. *Rheumatol. Int.* 2024; *Online ahead of print*. [CrossRef]
48. ICMRA Statement on International Collaboration to Enable Real-World Evidence (RWE) for Regulatory Decision-Making | International Coalition of Medicines Regulatory Authorities (ICMRA). Available online: https://www.icmra.info/drupal/sites/default/files/2022-07/icmra_statement_on_rwe.pdf (accessed on 11 April 2024).
49. ICH Reflection Paper: International Harmonisation of Real-World Evidence Terminology and Convergence of General Principles Regarding Planning and Reporting of Studies Using Real-World Data, with a Focus on Effectiveness of Medicines. 2023. Available online: https://admin.ich.org/sites/default/files/2023-06/ICH_ReflectionPaper_Harmonisation_RWE_Terminology_Endorsed-ForConsultation_2023_0613.pdf (accessed on 11 April 2024).
50. Blonde, L.; Khunti, K.; Harris, S.B.; Meizinger, C.; Skolnik, N.S. Interpretation and Impact of Real-World Clinical Data for the Practicing Clinician. *Adv. Ther.* **2018**, *35*, 1763–1774. [CrossRef] [PubMed]
51. Carboni, A.; Woessner, S.; Martini, O.; Marroquin, N.A.; Waller, J. Natural Weight Loss or "Ozempic Face": Demystifying A Social Media Phenomenon. *J. Drugs Dermatol.* **2024**, *23*, 1367–1368. [CrossRef] [PubMed]
52. Zhang, Z.; Zhang, Q.; Tan, Y.; Chen, Y.; Zhou, X.; Liu, S.; Yu, J. GLP-1RAs Caused Gastrointestinal Adverse Reactions of Drug Withdrawal: A System Review and Network Meta-Analysis. *Front. Endocrinol.* **2023**, *14*, 1149328. [CrossRef]
53. Sodhi, M.; Rezaeianzadeh, R.; Kezouh, A.; Etminan, M. Risk of Gastrointestinal Adverse Events Associated With Glucagon-Like Peptide-1 Receptor Agonists for Weight Loss. *JAMA* **2023**, *330*, 1795–1797. [CrossRef] [PubMed]
54. Shetty, R.; Basheer, F.T.; Poojari, P.G.; Thunga, G.; Chandran, V.P.; Acharya, L.D. Adverse Drug Reactions of GLP-1 Agonists: A Systematic Review of Case Reports. *Diabetes Metab. Syndr. Clin. Res. Rev.* **2022**, *16*, 102427. [CrossRef] [PubMed]
55. Filippatos, T.D.; Panagiotopoulou, T.V.; Elisaf, M.S. Adverse Effects of GLP-1 Receptor Agonists. *Rev. Diabet. Stud.* **2014**, *11*, 202. [CrossRef] [PubMed]
56. Sivesind, T.E.; Szeto, M.D.; Kim, W.; Dellavalle, R.P. Google Trends in Dermatology: Scoping Review of the Literature. *JMIR Dermatol.* **2021**, *4*, e27712. [CrossRef] [PubMed]
57. Mavragani, A.; Ochoa, G. Google Trends in Infodemiology and Infoveillance: Methodology Framework. *JMIR Public Health Surveill.* **2019**, *5*, e13439. [CrossRef]
58. Cohen, S.A.; Zhuang, T.; Xiao, M.; Michaud, J.B.; Amanatullah, D.F.; Kamal, R.N. Google Trend Analysis Shows Increasing Public Interest in Platelet-Rich Plasma Injections for Hip and Knee Osteoarthritis. *J. Arthroplast.* **2021**, *36*, 3616. [CrossRef]
59. Alibudbud, R. Google Trends for Health Research: Its Advantages, Application, Methodological Considerations, and Limitations in Psychiatric and Mental Health Infodemiology. *Front. Big Data* **2023**, *6*, 1132764. [CrossRef] [PubMed]
60. European Database of Suspected Adverse Drug Reaction Reports. Available online: https://www.adrreports.eu/ (accessed on 11 April 2024).
61. Postigo, R.; Brosch, S.; Slattery, J.; van Haren, A.; Dogné, J.M.; Kurz, X.; Candore, G.; Domergue, F.; Arlett, P. EudraVigilance Medicines Safety Database: Publicly Accessible Data for Research and Public Health Protection. *Drug Saf.* **2018**, *41*, 665–675. [CrossRef] [PubMed]

62. Medicines Agency, E. *Guideline on Good Pharmacovigilance Practices (GVP)—Product- or Population-Specific Considerations IV: Paediatric Population*; European Medicines Agency: London, UK, 2018.
63. Guo, Y.; Shen, Z.; Zhao, W.; Lu, J.; Song, Y.; Shen, L.; Lu, Y.; Wu, M.; Shi, Q.; Zhuang, W.; et al. Rational Identification of Novel Antibody-Drug Conjugate with High Bystander Killing Effect against Heterogeneous Tumors. *Adv. Sci.* **2024**, *11*, e2306309. [CrossRef] [PubMed]
64. Morgovan, C.; Dobrea, C.M.; Chis, A.A.; Juncan, A.M.; Arseniu, A.M.; Rus, L.L.; Gligor, F.G.; Ardelean, S.A.; Stoicescu, L.; Ghibu, S.; et al. A Descriptive Analysis of Direct Oral Anticoagulant Drugs Dosing Errors Based on Spontaneous Reports from the EudraVigilance Database. *Pharmaceuticals* **2023**, *16*, 455. [CrossRef] [PubMed]
65. European Medicines Agency. *Note for Guidance-EudraVigilance Human-Processing of Safety Messages and Individual Case Safety Reports (ICSRs)*; European Medicines Agency: Amsterdam, The Netherlands, 2010.
66. European Medicines Agency. *Guideline On The Use Of Statistical Signal Detection Methods In The Eudravigilance Data Analysis System*; European Medicines Agency: Amsterdam, The Netherlands, 2006.
67. Vintila, B.I.; Arseniu, A.M.; Butuca, A.; Sava, M.; Bîrluțiu, V.; Rus, L.L.; Axente, D.D.; Morgovan, C.; Gligor, F.G. Adverse Drug Reactions Relevant to Drug Resistance and Ineffectiveness Associated with Meropenem, Linezolid, and Colistin: An Analysis Based on Spontaneous Reports from the European Pharmacovigilance Database. *Antibiotics* **2023**, *12*, 918. [CrossRef] [PubMed]
68. Vintila, B.I.; Arseniu, A.M.; Morgovan, C.; Butuca, A.; Sava, M.; Bîrluțiu, V.; Rus, L.L.; Ghibu, S.; Bereanu, A.S.; Roxana Codru, I.; et al. A Pharmacovigilance Study Regarding the Risk of Antibiotic-Associated Clostridioides Difficile Infection Based on Reports from the EudraVigilance Database: Analysis of Some of the Most Used Antibiotics in Intensive Care Units. *Pharmaceuticals* **2023**, *16*, 1585. [CrossRef] [PubMed]
69. Google Trends: Semaglutide, Liraglutide, Tirzepatide, Dulaglutide, Exenatide. Available online: https://trends.google.com/trends/explore?date=2005-12-012024-03-31&q=semaglutide,liraglutide,tirzepatide,dulaglutide,exenatide&hl=ro (accessed on 20 April 2024).
70. Popoviciu, M.S.; Păduraru, L.; Yahya, G.; Metwally, K.; Cavalu, S. Emerging Role of GLP-1 Agonists in Obesity: A Comprehensive Review of Randomised Controlled Trials. *Int. J. Mol. Sci.* **2023**, *24*, 449. [CrossRef] [PubMed]
71. Isaacs, D.M.; Kruger, D.F.; Spollett, G.R. Optimizing Therapeutic Outcomes With Oral Semaglutide: A Patient-Centered Approach. *Diabetes Spectr.* **2021**, *34*, 7. [CrossRef] [PubMed]
72. Kalra, S.; Sahay, R. A Review on Semaglutide: An Oral Glucagon-Like Peptide 1 Receptor Agonist in Management of Type 2 Diabetes Mellitus. *Diabetes Ther.* **2020**, *11*, 1965–1982. [CrossRef]
73. Aroda, V.R.; Blonde, L.; Pratley, R.E. A New Era for Oral Peptides: SNAC and the Development of Oral Semaglutide for the Treatment of Type 2 Diabetes. *Rev. Endocr. Metab. Disord.* **2022**, *23*, 979–994. [CrossRef]
74. Kamiński, M.; Miętkiewska-Dolecka, M.; Kręgielska-Narożna, M.; Bogdański, P. Popularity of Surgical and Pharmacological Obesity Treatment Methods Searched by Google Users: The Retrospective Analysis of Google Trends Statistics in 2004–2022. *Obes. Surg.* **2024**, *34*, 882–891. [CrossRef] [PubMed]
75. Basch, C.H.; Narayanan, S.; Tang, H.; Fera, J.; Basch, C.E. Descriptive Analysis of TikTok Videos Posted under the Hashtag #Ozempic. *J. Med. Surg. Public Health* **2023**, *1*, 100013. [CrossRef]
76. Liraglutide and Semaglutide Market Share Report, 2023–2032. Available online: https://www.gminsights.com/industry-analysis/liraglutide-and-semaglutide-market (accessed on 14 April 2024).
77. Miriam, E. Tucker Semaglutide Prescribing Surged in the Past Year. Available online: https://www.medscape.com/viewarticle/997956?form=fpf (accessed on 14 April 2024).
78. Patoulias, D.; Popovic, D.S.; Stoian, A.P.; Janez, A.; Sahebkar, A.; Rizzo, M. Effect of Semaglutide versus Other Glucagon-like Peptide-1 Receptor Agonists on Cardio-Metabolic Risk Factors in Patients with Type 2 Diabetes: A Systematic Review and Meta-Analysis of Head-to-Head, Phase 3, Randomized Controlled Trials. *J. Diabetes Complicat.* **2023**, *37*, 108529. [CrossRef]
79. Ma, H.; Lin, Y.H.; Dai, L.Z.; Lin, C.S.; Huang, Y.; Liu, S.Y. Efficacy and Safety of GLP-1 Receptor Agonists versus SGLT-2 Inhibitors in Overweight/Obese Patients with or without Diabetes Mellitus: A Systematic Review and Network Meta-Analysis. *BMJ Open* **2023**, *13*, e061807. [CrossRef] [PubMed]
80. Chubb, B.; Gupta, P.; Gupta, J.; Nuhoho, S.; Kallenbach, K.; Orme, M. Once-Daily Oral Semaglutide Versus Injectable GLP-1 RAs in People with Type 2 Diabetes Inadequately Controlled on Basal Insulin: Systematic Review and Network Meta-Analysis. *Diabetes Ther.* **2021**, *12*, 1325. [CrossRef] [PubMed]
81. Chen, H.; Li, X.Z.; Chen, J.Q.; Ren, T.S.; Zhang, Y.S.; Wang, Y.N.; Zhao, Q.C. Comparative Efficacy and Safety of Glucagon-like Peptide 1 Receptor Agonists for the Treatment of Type 2 Diabetes: A Network Meta-Analysis. *Medicine* **2023**, *102*, E34122. [CrossRef] [PubMed]
82. Azuri, J.; Hammerman, A.; Aboalhasan, E.; Sluckis, B.; Arbel, R. Liraglutide versus Semaglutide for Weight Reduction—A Cost Needed to Treat Analysis. *Obesity* **2023**, *31*, 1510–1513. [CrossRef]
83. Smits, M.M.; Van Raalte, D.H. Safety of Semaglutide. *Front. Endocrinol.* **2021**, *12*, 645563. [CrossRef] [PubMed]
84. Amaro, A.; Sugimoto, D.; Wharton, S. Efficacy and Safety of Semaglutide for Weight Management: Evidence from the STEP Program. *Postgrad. Med.* **2022**, *134*, 5–17. [CrossRef]
85. Borner, T.; Workinger, J.L.; Tinsley, I.C.; Fortin, S.M.; Stein, L.M.; Chepurny, O.G.; Holz, G.G.; Wierzba, A.J.; Gryko, D.; Nexø, E.; et al. Corrination of a GLP-1 Receptor Agonist for Glycemic Control without Emesis. *Cell Rep.* **2020**, *31*, 107768. [CrossRef]

86. Gier, B.; Matveyenko, A.V.; Kirakossian, D.; Dawson, D.; Dry, S.M.; Butler, P.C. Chronic GLP-1 Receptor Activation by Exendin-4 Induces Expansion of Pancreatic Duct Glands in Rats and Accelerates Formation of Dysplastic Lesions and Chronic Pancreatitis in the Kras G12D Mouse Model. *Diabetes* **2012**, *61*, 1250–1262. [CrossRef] [PubMed]
87. Winzeler, B.; da Conceição, I.; Refardt, J.; Sailer, C.O.; Dutilh, G.; Christ-Crain, M. Effects of Glucagon-like Peptide-1 Receptor Agonists on Fluid Intake in Healthy Volunteers. *Endocrine* **2020**, *70*, 292–298. [CrossRef] [PubMed]
88. Poison Centers See Nearly 1500% Increase in Calls Related to Injected Weight-Loss Drugs as People Accidentally Overdose | CNN. Available online: https://edition.cnn.com/2023/12/13/health/semaglutide-overdoses-wellness/index.html (accessed on 14 April 2024).
89. Lambson, J.E.; Flegal, S.C.; Johnson, A.R. Administration Errors of Compounded Semaglutide Reported to a Poison Control Center—Case Series. *J. Am. Pharm. Assoc.* **2023**, *63*, 1643–1645. [CrossRef]
90. Wiener, B.G.; Gnirke, M.; Vassallo, S.; Smith, S.W.; Su, M.K. Challenges with Glucagon-like Peptide-1 (GLP-1) Agonist Initiation: A Case Series of Semaglutide Overdose Administration Errors. *Clin. Toxicol.* **2024**, *62*, 131–133. [CrossRef] [PubMed]
91. Surge in Fake Ozempic Reveals Dark Side of Weight-Loss Frenzy. Available online: https://medwatch.com/News/other/article16935969.ece (accessed on 16 April 2024).
92. News Details. Available online: https://www.novonordisk-us.com/media/news-archive/news-details.html?id=166119 (accessed on 16 April 2024).
93. Counterfeit Ozempic Found in US Retail Pharmacy—National Association of Boards of Pharmacy. Available online: https://nabp.pharmacy/news/blog/regulatory_news/counterfeit-ozempic-found-in-us-retail-pharmacy/ (accessed on 16 April 2024).
94. EMA Alerts EU Patients and Healthcare Professionals to Reports of Falsified Ozempic Pens | European Medicines Agency. Available online: https://www.ema.europa.eu/en/news/ema-alerts-eu-patients-healthcare-professionals-reports-falsified-ozempic-pens (accessed on 16 April 2024).
95. Medications Containing Semaglutide Marketed for Type 2 Diabetes or Weight Loss | FDA. Available online: https://www.fda.gov/drugs/postmarket-drug-safety-information-patients-and-providers/medications-containing-semaglutide-marketed-type-2-diabetes-or-weight-loss (accessed on 11 May 2024).
96. FDA Warns Consumers Not to Use Counterfeit Ozempic (Semaglutide) Found in U.S. Drug Supply Chain | FDA. Available online: https://www.fda.gov/drugs/drug-safety-and-availability/fda-warns-consumers-not-use-counterfeit-ozempic-semaglutide-found-us-drug-supply-chain (accessed on 11 May 2024).
97. Ozempic▼(Semaglutide) and Saxenda (Liraglutide): Vigilance Required Due to Potentially Harmful Falsified Products—GOV.UK. Available online: https://www.gov.uk/drug-safety-update/ozempicv-semaglutide-and-saxenda-liraglutide-vigilance-required-due-to-potentially-harmful-falsified-products (accessed on 11 May 2024).

biomedicines

MDPI

Article

Depressive Symptoms Associated with Peripheral Artery Disease and Predicting Mortality in Type 2 Diabetes

Yu-Hsuan Li [1,2,3], Yu-Cheng Cheng [1,2,4], Hsiu-Chen Liu [5], Junyi Wu [1] and I-Te Lee [1,2,6,*]

1 Division of Endocrinology and Metabolism, Department of Internal Medicine, Taichung Veterans General Hospital, Taichung 40705, Taiwan; brightlight720720@gmail.com (Y.-H.L.); fererro1552@hotmail.com (Y.-C.C.); meganjunyiwu@gmail.com (J.W.)

2 School of Medicine, National Yang Ming Chiao Tung University, Taipei 11221, Taiwan

3 Department of Computer Science & Information Engineering, National Taiwan University, Taipei 10617, Taiwan

4 Institute of Biomedical Sciences, National Chung Hsing University, Taichung 40227, Taiwan

5 Department of Nursing, Taichung Veterans General Hospital, Taichung 40705, Taiwan; jane@vghtc.gov.tw

6 School of Medicine, Chung Shan Medical University, Taichung 40201, Taiwan

* Correspondence: itlee@vghtc.gov.tw

Abstract: This retrospective cohort study aimed to assess the mortality risk in patients with type 2 diabetes mellitus (DM) by screening for depressive symptoms and peripheral artery disease (PAD). We enrolled patients aged ≥60 years who had undergone assessments of both the ankle–brachial index (ABI) and the five-item Geriatric Depression Scale (GDS-5). PAD and depression were defined as ABI ≤ 0.90 and GDS-5 ≥ 1, respectively. The primary endpoint was total mortality. In 1673 enrolled patients, the prevalence of PAD was higher in those with depression than in those without depression (8.9% vs. 5.7%, p = 0.021). After a median follow-up of 56.6 months (interquartile range: 47.0–62.3 months), a total of 168 (10.0%) deaths occurred. The patients in the depression and PAD subgroup had the highest hazard ratio of mortality, followed by the PAD without depression subgroup and the depression without PAD subgroup (2.209, 95%CI: 1.158–4.217; 1.958, 95%CI: 1.060–3.618; and 1.576, 95%CI: 1.131–2.196; respectively) in comparison to the patients without depression and PAD after adjustment for associated factors. In conclusion, a combination of depression and PAD predicted the highest mortality risk. Screening for depression and PAD is recommended in patients aged ≥60 years with type 2 DM.

Keywords: ankle–brachial index; geriatric depression scale; depression; mortality; peripheral artery disease; type 2 diabetes

1. Introduction

Depression has become an important health burden worldwide [1]. According to data from the Global Burden of Disease study between 1990 and 2017, the prevalence of depression has been increasing in the Chinese population aged over 55 years [2]. According to population-based data by questionnaire screening in the Healthy Aging Longitudinal Study, the prevalence of minor depression was 3.7%, and the prevalence of major depression was 1.5% in people aged over 55 years in Taiwan [3]. There is strong evidence that depression increases the risk of cardiovascular disease, disability, and mortality [2,4,5].

In particular, the presence of depressive symptoms is associated with an increased prevalence of diabetes mellitus (DM) [6]. Based on data from the UK Biobank, 5.5% of patients with type 2 DM developed major depression, and the risk, with a hazard ratio (HR) of 1.6, was significantly increased compared to patients without type 2 DM during a longitudinal follow-up for a median of 12.7 years; patients with type 2 DM also had a significantly higher risk of developing depressive symptoms than people without DM during a follow-up for a median of 7.5 years [7]. According to the National Health Insurance

(NHI) research database regarding people in Taiwan between 2000 and 2007, the incidence of depression was 7.03 per 1000 person-years in patients with type 2 DM, and the HR of 1.43 was significantly higher than that in people without DM [8].

In addition to the association between the presence of DM and depression, there is a synergistic effect of depression and DM on mortality risk. Compared with people with neither DM nor depression, patients with a combination of DM and depression had an increased risk of mortality, and the corresponding HR of 2.16 was higher than that of patients with DM alone or depression alone according to the UK Biobank dataset for a median 6.8 years of follow-up [9]. Similarly, having a combination of DM and depressive symptoms is associated with a higher risk of mortality than DM alone or depression alone according to Taiwan population-based data for a longitudinal follow-up of 10 years [10]. The increased mortality risk might be contributed to the link between depression and cardiovascular risk in patients with type 2 DM [7].

Peripheral artery disease (PAD) is a well-known risk factor for cardiovascular events and mortality [11]. PAD is also a prevalent macrovascular complication in patients with DM [12], and DM was reported to confer a 1.4-fold increased risk of mortality in patients with PAD in a mean follow-up of 5.9 years [13]. However, the prevalence of PAD might be underestimated. Hong et al. [14] reported that only 34.7% of patients with an ankle–brachial index (ABI) $\leq$ 0.9 had been previously diagnosed with PAD based on administrative data. Measurement of the ABI can detect PAD early and is recommended by guidelines for clinical practice [15,16].

Depression is also an important risk factor for PAD. A meta-analysis study suggested that depression increases the mortality risk by 24% in patients with PAD [17]. However, depression might be underdiagnosed in patients with PAD. Welch et al. [18] reported that 28.4% of 148 patients undergoing interventions for PAD were diagnosed with depression based on screening with the 15-item Geriatric Depression Scale (GDS), but only 3.3% had a documented history of depression. Therefore, a simple questionnaire with high sensitivity is warranted to screen depression in patients at high risk. The five-item GDS (GDS-5), extracted from the 15-item GDS, has been developed and validated for screening depressive symptoms [19,20], but data on long-term mortality are scarce. We hypothesized that depressive symptoms are not only associated with PAD but are also predictive of long-term mortality in patients with type 2 DM. Therefore, we conducted a retrospective cohort study to assess the mortality risk categorized by GDS-5 and ABI in patients with type 2 DM.

2. Materials and Methods

2.1. Study Design and Population

This retrospective cohort study was conducted at Taichung Veterans General Hospital. The diabetic pay-for-performance (P4P) program has been an important policy launched by the NHI administration in Taiwan [21], and an annual comprehensive assessment including screening for PAD and mental health is recommended in this program [22]. In addition to ABI, the screening of GDS-5 has been included in the annual comprehensive assessment of diabetic P4P program in patients aged $\geq$60 years at Taichung Veterans General Hospital since 1 August 2016.

We screened candidates from outpatients of the Division of Endocrinology and Metabolism. The inclusion criteria were (1) individuals aged $\geq$60 years, (2) patients with DM, and (3) patients who had received assessments of both ABI and GDS-5 in the same annual comprehensive assessment between August 2016 and July 2020. The exclusion criteria were (1) current use of antidepressant or dementia drugs at the time of interview for answering the questionnaire, (2) DM other than type 2, (3) estimated glomerular filtration rate (eGFR) < 15 mL/min/1.73 m^2, (4) unreliable ABI data, including ABI value $\geq$ 1.4, history of lower-limb surgery, or systolic blood pressure not detected in any of the four limbs, and (5) death within 30 days after enrollment.

2.2. Assessment of Risk Factors

The clinical data in the same annual comprehensive assessment were extracted from the electronic medical records. For patients who had undergone repeated comprehensive assessments during this study period, only the data from the first completed assessment were recorded. The characteristics of patients were age, sex, body height, body weight, blood pressure, smoking status, history of cardiovascular disease and hypertension, and current use of medication. The laboratory data comprised hemoglobin A1c (HbA1c), plasma glucose, serum levels of total cholesterol, high-density lipoprotein (HDL) cholesterol, triglycerides and creatinine, and urinary albumin and creatinine. HbA1c was measured using cation-exchange high-performance liquid chromatography (NGSP certified; G8, TOSOH, Tokyo, Japan). Serum lipid profiles and creatinine levels were measured by commercial kits (Beckman Coulter, Fullerton, CA, USA).

Overweight in Taiwan was defined as a body mass index (BMI) $\geq$ 24 kg/m^2 [23]. Hypertension was defined as a systolic blood pressure $\geq$ 130 mmHg, a diastolic blood pressure $\geq$ 80 mmHg, or the current use of an antihypertensive drug. Low HDL cholesterol was defined as an HDL cholesterol level < 50 mg/dL (1.29 mmol/L) in women or <40 mg/dL (1.03 mmol/L) in men. The eGFR was calculated using the Chronic Kidney Disease Epidemiology Collaboration (CKD-EPI) equation for Chinese individuals with type 2 DM [24]. CKD was defined as an index eGFR < 60 mL/min/1.73 m^2. The urinary albumin-to-creatinine ratio (UACR) was calculated using the ratio of urine albumin (mg/dL) to urine creatinine (g/dL), and increased albuminuria was defined as a UACR $\geq$ 30 mg/g. Diabetic kidney disease (DKD) was defined as CKD and/or increased albuminuria.

2.3. Assessments of GDS-5 and ABI

GDS-5 comprises 5 items reported by patients themselves. Item 1 received a score of 1 when a participant answered "No", and Items 2 to 5 received a score of 1 when a participant answered "Yes". The total score for GDS-5 ranges from 0 to 5, and a score $\geq$ 1 has a high sensitivity for the diagnosis of depression [19,20]. Therefore, depression is defined as a reported GDS-5 core $\geq$ 1 in the present study. The Mandarin Chinese version of GDS-5 has been reported in previous studies [25,26].

To measure ABI, blood pressure was detected at the bilateral brachial arteries and at the bilateral ankles using a validated automatic device (VP-1000 Plus; Omron healthcare Co. Ltd., Kyoto, Japan) after patients had rested in the supine position for at least 5 min. The ABI value was calculated as the ratio of the systolic blood pressure at each ankle to the higher systolic blood pressure of the bilateral brachial pressures [27]. The lower value of bilateral ABI in the same patient was recorded for the analyses. The reproducibility of ABI was reported in our previous study. Briefly, based on the Bland–Altman plots, the 95% confidence interval (CI) for the bias of ABI was 0.02 $\pm$ 0.01 between the repeated measurements in a group of 20 subjects [28]. PAD is defined as a recorded ABI value $\leq$ 0.90 [15,27].

2.4. Statistical Analysis

The total mortality served as the primary outcome. After collection of all the clinical data, the occurrence of mortality was recorded through 31 March 2022. Information on registered deaths was obtained from the Ministry of Health and Welfare, Executive Yuan, Taiwan. This research protocol was approved by the Institutional Review Board of Taichung Veterans General Hospital, and the need for informed consent was waived due to the retrospective cohort study design.

Continuous data are presented as the mean $\pm$ standard deviation, and categorical data are summarized as numbers with percentages (%). The statistical significance of differences in continuous data was examined using Student's t tests between patients with and without any depressive symptom and by using one-way analysis of variance tests among the four study subgroups. The statistical significance of differences in categorized data was examined using chi-square tests.

The cumulative risk of total mortality was assessed using the Kaplan–Meier analysis; the log-rank test was used to examine the statistical significance of differences in survival rates among groups. Cox proportional hazards regression analysis was conducted to examine the independent predictors of mortality, and HR values with a 95% CI are presented. Because age and sex were important confounding factors, we included age, sex, and other assessed variables that were significantly associated with a GDS-5 score or PAD in the multivariable models. A two-sided p value < 0.05 indicated statistical significance. Statistical analysis was performed using SPSS v22.0 (IBM Corp., Armonk, NY, USA).

3. Results

In total, 1673 patients who met the study criteria were enrolled in this study (Figure 1). According to the self-reported GDS-5 questionnaire, 539 (32.2%) patients had at least one depressive symptom (GDS-5 $\geq$ 1), and 1134 patients had none of the five depressive symptoms (GDS-5 = 0). The baseline characteristics of patients with or without depressive symptoms are shown in Table 1. The patients with GDS-5 $\geq$ 1 had a significantly older age (73 $\pm$ 8 vs. 71 $\pm$ 7 years, $p < 0.001$) and significantly higher proportions of current smoking (8.3% vs. 4.9%, $p = 0.009$) and cardiovascular disease (27.8% vs. 20.7%, $p = 0.002$) than those with GDS-5 = 0. However, there was no significant difference in proportions of sex ($p = 0.832$), DKD ($p = 0.999$), hypertension ($p = 0.181$), and use of antihypertensive drugs ($p = 0.167$), antiplatelet drugs ($p = 0.138$), antidiabetic drugs ($p > 0.05$), and statins ($p = 0.051$) between patients with GDS-5 $\geq$ 1 and those with GDS-5 = 0. There was no significant difference in BMI ($p = 0.664$), systolic blood pressure ($p = 0.152$), diastolic blood pressure ($p = 0.343$), fasting plasma glucose ($p = 0.653$), HbA1c ($p = 0.382$), eGFR ($p = 0.246$), UACR ($p = 0.062$), and serum levels of total cholesterol ($p = 0.618$), HDL cholesterol ($p = 0.426$), triglycerides ($p = 0.154$), and ALT ($p = 0.129$) between patients with a GDS-5 $\geq$ 1 and those with GDS-5 = 0.

Based on the definition of PAD as ABI $\leq$ 0.90, there were 113 (6.8%) patients with PAD in all enrolled patients. Notably, the ABI value was significantly lower in the patients with GDS-5 $\geq$ 1 than in those with GDS-5 = 0 (1.07 $\pm$ 0.13 vs. 1.09 $\pm$ 0.12, $p = 0.007$). The prevalence of PAD was also significantly higher in the patients with GDS-5 $\geq$ 1 than in those with GDS-5 = 0 (8.9% vs. 5.7%, $p = 0.021$, Figure 2).

During a median follow-up period of 56.6 months (interquartile range: 47.0–62.3 months), a total of 168 (10.0%) deaths occurred among all 1673 enrolled patients, including 72 in 539 patients (13.4%) with GDS-5 $\geq$ 1 and 96 in 1134 patients (8.5%) with GDS-5 = 0 ($p = 0.002$). The incidence of mortality was significantly higher in patients with GDS-5 $\geq$ 1 than in those with GDS-5 = 0 (3.1 vs. 1.9 per 100 person-years, log-rank test $p = 0.002$).

To assess the synergistic effect between GDS-5 and PAD on long-term mortality, we further divided all patients into four subgroups based on a cutoff value of 1 for GDS-5 and 0.90 for ABI. There were 1069 patients in the ABI > 0.90 and GDS-5 = 0 group, 491 patients in the ABI > 0.90 and GDS-5 $\geq$ 1 group, 65 patients in the ABI $\leq$ 0.90 and GDS-5 = 0 group, and 48 patients in the ABI $\leq$ 0.90 and GDS-5 $\geq$ 1 group. The baseline characteristics among these four groups are presented in Table 2. Patients with PAD and depression had a trend toward a higher proportion of age $\geq$ 70 years ($p = 0.012$), current smokers ($p < 0.001$), cardiovascular disease ($p < 0.001$), hypertension ($p = 0.012$), DKD ($p < 0.001$), CKD ($p < 0.001$), increased UACR ($p < 0.001$), and use of antiplatelet drugs ($p < 0.001$).

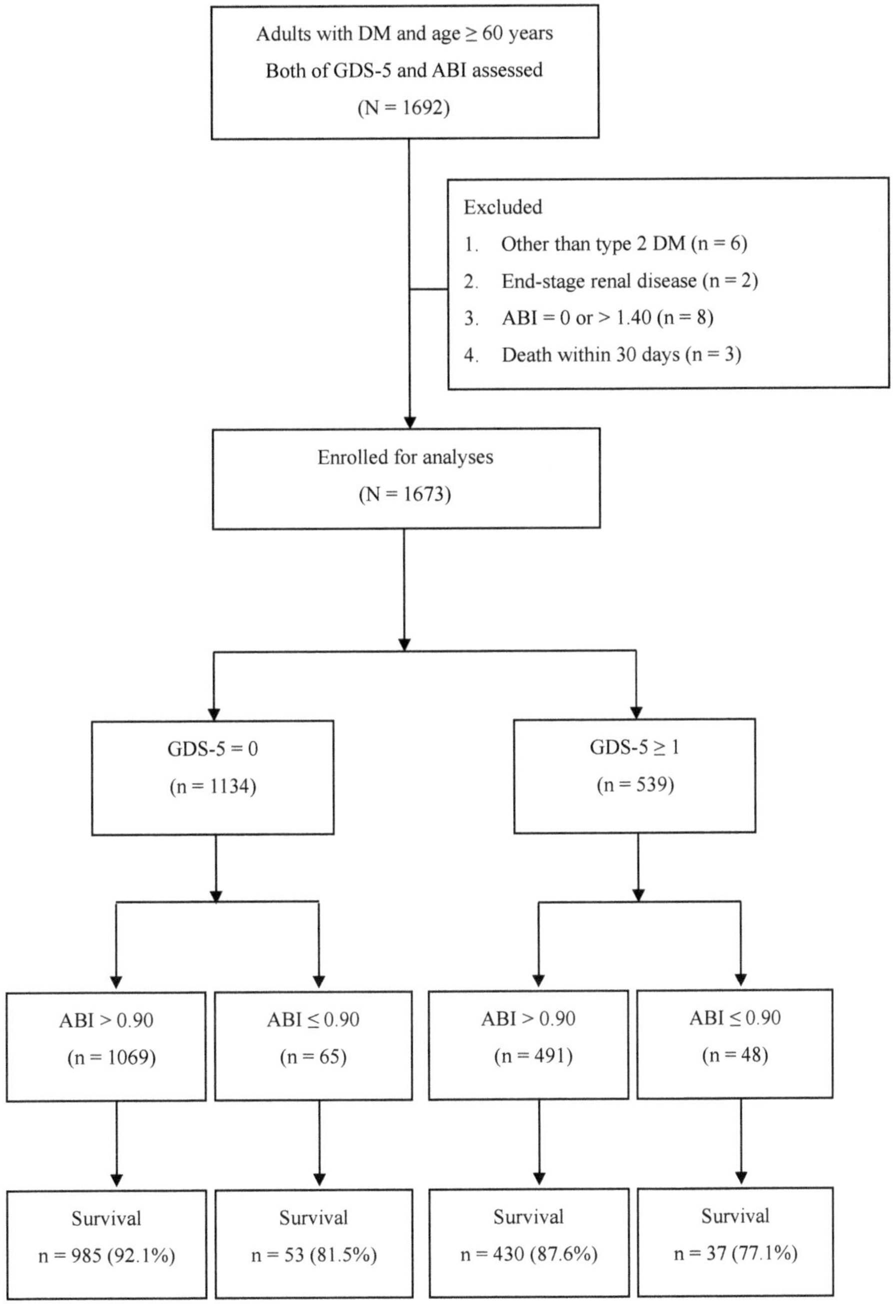

Figure 1. Flow diagram of the enrollment of study subjects (abbreviations: GDS-5, five-item Geriatric Depression Scale; ABI, ankle–brachial index; DM, diabetes mellitus).

Table 1. Baseline characteristics and mortality rate of enrolled patients categorized by GDS-5 score.

	GDS-5 = 0 (*n* = 1134)		GDS-5 ≥ 1 (*n* = 539)		*p*
Age (years)	71	± 7	73	± 8	<0.001
Male, *n* (%)	556	(49.0%)	268	(49.7%)	0.832
Current smoker, *n* (%)	56	(4.9%)	45	(8.3%)	0.009
CVD, *n* (%)	235	(20.7%)	150	(27.8%)	0.002
BMI (kg/m^2)	25.4	± 3.8	25.3	± 4.0	0.664
Hypertension, *n* (%)	948	(83.6%)	465	(86.3%)	0.181
Systolic BP (mmHg)	138	± 20	139	± 20	0.152
Diastolic BP (mmHg)	75	± 10	76	± 11	0.343
Use of antihypertensive agents, *n* (%)	678	(59.8%)	342	(63.5%)	0.167
Fasting glucose (mmol/L)	7.7	± 2.5	7.8	± 2.6	0.635
HbA1c (%)	7.3	± 1.2	7.4	± 1.4	0.382
HbA1c (mmol/mol)	56.6	± 13.5	57.3	± 15.5	
Total cholesterol (mmol/L)	4.0	± 0.8	4.0	± 0.8	0.618
HDL cholesterol (mmol/L)	1.3	± 0.4	1.3	± 0.4	0.426
Triglycerides (mmol/L)	1.4	± 1.0	1.5	± 1.0	0.154
ALT (U/L)	24	± 17	25	± 19	0.129
Diabetic kidney disease, *n* (%)	604	(53.3%)	287	(53.2%)	0.999
eGFR (mL/min/1.73 m^2)	67	± 15	66	± 15	0.246
UACR (mg/g)	184	± 554	247	± 795	0.062
ABI	1.09	± 0.12	1.07	± 0.13	0.007
Use of antiplatelet drugs, *n* (%)	363	(32.0%)	193	(35.8%)	0.138
Use of statins, *n* (%)	856	(75.5%)	382	(70.9%)	0.051
Use of antidiabetic drugs					
Insulin or insulin secretagogues, *n* (%)	656	(57.8%)	328	(60.9%)	0.265
Metformin, *n* (%)	400	(35.3%)	191	(35.4%)	0.992
Thiazolidinediones, *n* (%)	292	(25.7%)	120	(22.3%)	0.137
α-Glucosidase inhibitors, *n* (%)	131	(11.6%)	64	(11.9%)	0.912
DPP4 inhibitors, *n* (%)	733	(64.6%)	324	(60.1%)	0.082
SGLT2 inhibitors, *n* (%)	90	(7.9%)	49	(9.1%)	0.481
Mortality, *n* (%)	96	(8.5%)	72	(13.4%)	0.002

Continuous data are presented as the mean ± standard deviation, and categorical data are presented as numbers (percentages). Abbreviations: ABI = ankle–brachial index, ALT = alanine aminotransferase, BMI = body mass index, BP = blood pressure, CVD = cardiovascular disease, DPP4 = dipeptidyl peptidase-4, eGFR = estimated glomerular filtration rate, GDS-5 = five-item Geriatric Depression Scale, HbA1c = hemoglobin A1c, HDL = high-density lipo-protein, SGLT2 = sodium glucose cotransporter 2, UACR = urine albumin-to-creatinine ratio.

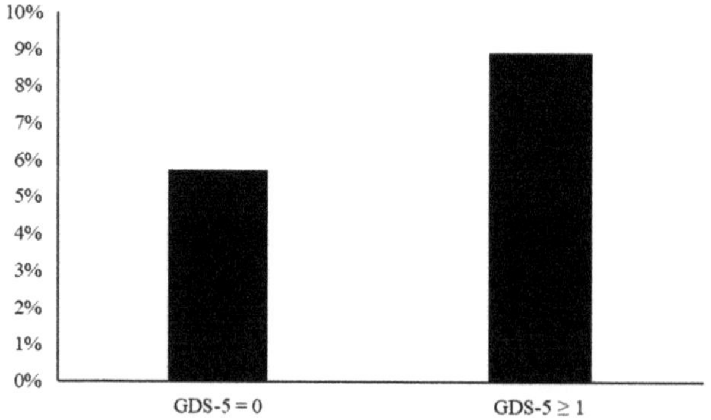

Figure 2. Prevalence of peripheral artery disease defined by ankle–brachial index ≤ 0.90 in the GDS-5 = 0 and GDS-5 ≥ 1 groups (8.9% vs. 5.7%, $p = 0.021$). (Abbreviation: GDS-5, five-item Geriatric Depression Scale).

Table 2. Characteristics of enrolled patients categorized based on GDS and ABI.

	Group	*N*	ABI > 0.90 GDS-5 = 0 (*n* = 1069)		ABI > 0.90 GDS-5 ≥ 1 (*n* = 491)		ABI ≤ 0.90 GDS-5 = 0 (*n* = 65)		ABI ≤ 0.90 GDS-5 ≥ 1 (*n* = 48)		*p*
Age (years)	<70	797	534	(50.0%)	224	(45.6%)	22	(33.8%)	17	(35.4%)	0.012
	≥70	876	535	(50.0%)	267	(54.4%)	43	(66.2%)	31	(64.6%)	
Sex	Female	849	540	(50.5%)	251	(51.1%)	38	(58.5%)	20	(41.7%)	0.364
	Male	824	529	(49.5%)	240	(48.9%)	27	(41.5%)	28	(58.3%)	
Current smoker	No	1572	1020	(95.4%)	454	(92.5%)	58	(89.2%)	40	(83.3%)	<0.001
	Yes	101	49	(4.6%)	37	(7.5%)	7	(10.8%)	8	(16.7%)	
CVD	No	1288	853	(79.8%)	368	(74.9%)	46	(70.8%)	21	(43.8%)	<0.001
	Yes	385	216	(20.2%)	123	(25.1%)	19	(29.2%)	27	(56.3%)	
BMI (kg/m^2)	<24	662	417	(39.0%)	201	(40.9%)	26	(40.0%)	18	(37.5%)	0.893
	≥24	1011	652	(61.0%)	290	(59.1%)	39	(60.0%)	30	(62.5%)	
Hypertension	No	243	170	(15.9%)	67	(13.6%)	2	(3.1%)	4	(8.3%)	0.016
	Yes	1430	899	(84.1%)	424	(86.4%)	63	(96.9%)	44	(91.7%)	
Systolic BP (mmHg)	<130	596	387	(36.2%)	181	(36.9%)	17	(26.2%)	11	(22.9%)	0.093
	≥130	1077	682	(63.8%)	310	(63.1%)	48	(73.8%)	37	(77.1%)	
Diastolic BP (mmHg)	<80	1167	747	(69.9%)	347	(70.7%)	44	(67.7%)	29	(60.4%)	0.509
	≥80	506	322	(30.1%)	144	(29.3%)	21	(32.3%)	19	(39.6%)	
Fasting glucose (mmol/L)	<7.2	802	506	(47.3%)	240	(48.9%)	36	(55.4%)	20	(41.7%)	0.470
	≥7.2	871	563	(52.7%)	251	(51.1%)	29	(44.6%)	28	(58.3%)	
HbA1c	<7%	739	476	(44.5%)	218	(44.4%)	24	(36.9%)	21	(43.8%)	0.693
	>7%	934	593	(55.5%)	273	(55.6%)	41	(63.1%)	27	(56.3%)	
Total cholesterol (mmol/L)	<4.1	1029	661	(61.8%)	297	(60.5%)	37	(56.9%)	34	(70.8%)	0.457
	≥4.1	644	408	(38.2%)	194	(39.5%)	28	(43.1%)	14	(29.2%)	
Low HDL cholesterol	No	1086	696	(65.1%)	327	(66.6%)	35	(53.8%)	28	(58.3%)	0.169
	Yes	587	373	(34.9%)	164	(33.4%)	30	(46.2%)	20	(41.7%)	
Triglycerides (mmol/L)	<1.7	1231	807	(75.5%)	349	(71.1%)	41	(63.1%)	34	(70.8%)	0.059
	≥1.7	442	262	(24.5%)	142	(28.9%)	24	(36.9%)	14	(29.2%)	
Diabetic kidney disease	No	782	514	(48.1%)	239	(48.7%)	16	(24.6%)	13	(27.1%)	<0.001
	Yes	891	555	(51.9%)	252	(51.3%)	49	(75.4%)	35	(72.9%)	
eGFR (mL/min/1.73 m^2)	≥60	1130	739	(69.1%)	336	(68.4%)	32	(49.2%)	23	(47.9%)	<0.001
	<60	543	330	(30.9%)	155	(31.6%)	33	(50.8%)	25	(52.1%)	
UACR (mg/g)	<30	980	648	(60.6%)	292	(59.5%)	24	(36.9%)	16	(33.3%)	<0.001
	≥30	693	421	(39.4%)	199	(40.5%)	41	(63.1%)	32	(66.7%)	
ALT (U/L)	<20	806	520	(48.6%)	222	(45.2%)	33	(50.8%)	31	(64.6%)	0.067
	≥20	867	549	(51.4%)	269	(54.8%)	32	(49.2%)	17	(35.4%)	
Use of antiplatelet	No	1117	744	(69.6%)	328	(66.8%)	27	(41.5%)	18	(37.5%)	<0.001
	Yes	556	325	(30.4%)	163	(33.2%)	38	(58.5%)	30	(62.5%)	
Use of statins	No	435	267	(25.0%)	146	(29.7%)	11	(16.9%)	11	(22.9%)	0.067
	Yes	1238	802	(75.0%)	345	(70.3%)	54	(83.1%)	37	(77.1%)	
Use of antidiabetic drugs											
Insulin or insulin secretagogues	No	689	454	(42.5%)	196	(39.9%)	24	(36.9%)	15	(31.3%)	0.321
	Yes	984	615	(57.5%)	295	(60.1%)	41	(63.1%)	33	(68.8%)	
Metformin	No	1082	691	(64.6%)	312	(63.5%)	43	(66.2%)	36	(75.0%)	0.461
	Yes	591	378	(35.4%)	179	(36.5%)	22	(33.8%)	12	(25.0%)	
Thiazolidinediones	No	1261	794	(74.3%)	380	(77.4%)	48	(73.8%)	39	(81.3%)	0.432
	Yes	412	275	(25.7%)	111	(22.6%)	17	(26.2%)	9	(18.8%)	
α-Glucosidase inhibitors	No	1478	944	(88.3%)	434	(88.4%)	59	(90.8%)	41	(85.4%)	0.856
	Yes	195	125	(11.7%)	57	(11.6%)	6	(9.2%)	7	(14.6%)	
DPP4 inhibitors	No	616	380	(35.5%)	199	(40.5%)	21	(32.3%)	16	(33.3%)	0.215
	Yes	1057	689	(64.5%)	292	(59.5%)	44	(67.7%)	32	(66.7%)	
SGLT2 inhibitors	No	1534	981	(91.8%)	446	(90.8%)	63	(96.9%)	44	(91.7%)	0.421
	Yes	139	88	(8.2%)	45	(9.2%)	2	(3.1%)	4	(8.3%)	

ABI = ankle–brachial index, ALT = alanine aminotransferase, BMI = body mass index, CVD = cardiovascular disease, DPP4 = dipeptidyl peptidase-4, eGFR = estimated glomerular filtration rate, GDS-5 = five-item Geriatric Depression Scale, HbA1c = hemoglobin A1c, HDL = high-density lipoprotein, SGLT2 = sodium glucose cotransporter 2, UACR = urine albumin-to-creatinine ratio.

During the follow-up period, 84 (7.9%) deaths occurred in the ABI > 0.90 and GDS-5 = 0 group, 61 (12.4%) deaths occurred in the ABI > 0.90 and GDS-5 ≥ 1 group, 12 (18.5%) deaths occurred in the ABI ≤ 0.90 and GDS-5 = 0 group, and 11 (22.9%) deaths occurred in the ABI ≤ 0.90 and GDS-5 ≥ 1 group. The incidences of mortality were 1.8 per 100 person-years in the ABI > 0.90 and GDS-5 = 0 group, 2.8 per 100 person-years in the ABI > 0.90 and GDS-5 ≥ 1 group, 4.5 per 100 person-years in the ABI ≤ 0.90 and GDS-5 = 0 group, and 5.7 per 100 person-years in the ABI ≤ 0.90 and GDS-5 ≥ 1 group. The survival rates were significantly different among these four groups (log-rank test $p < 0.001$, Figure 3). In addition to age and sex, we selected the factors associated with GDS-5 and PAD, including smoking status, cardiovascular disease, hypertension, DKD, and use of antiplatelet drugs, which showed significant between-group differences (in Tables 1 and 2) for the multivariable model. The mortality risks were still significantly different among these four groups after adjusting for the selected factors using multivariable Cox regression analysis. Compared to the mortality risk of the ABI > 0.90 and GDS-5 = 0 group, a significantly higher HR of 1.576 (95% CI: 1.131–2.196, $p = 0.007$) was observed in the ABI > 0.90 and GDS-5 ≥ 1 group, a significantly higher HR of 1.958 (95% CI: 1.060–3.618, $p = 0.032$) was observed in the ABI ≤ 0.90 and GDS-5 = 0 group, and the highest HR of 2.209 (95% CI: 1.158–4.217, $p = 0.016$) was observed in the ABI ≤ 0.90 and GDS-5 ≥ 1 group (Table 3). In the post hoc analyses between subgroups, patients in the ABI ≤ 0.90 and GDS-5 ≥ 1 group had a significantly higher mortality risk than those in the ABI > 0.90 and GDS-5 ≥ 1 group (HR = 1.924, 95% CI: 1.034–3.578; $p = 0.039$), but it was not significantly different from those in the ABI ≤ 0.90 and GDS-5 = 0 group (HR = 1.291, 95% CI: 0.577–2.892; $p = 0.534$) after adjusting for age and sex. Furthermore, there was no significant difference in the mortality risk between patients in the ABI > 0.90 and GDS-5 ≥ 1 group and those in the ABI ≤ 0.90 and GDS-5 = 0 group ($p = 0.241$).

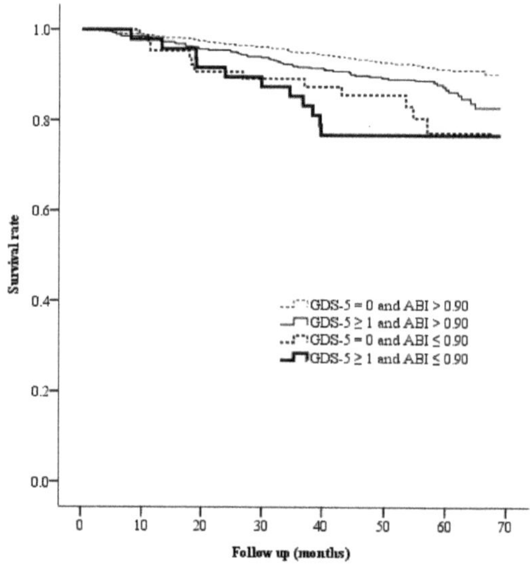

Figure 3. Kaplan–Meier curves presenting the survival rates across the four groups categorized based on GDS-5 and ABI. The median follow-up period was 56.6 months (interquartile range: 47.0–62.3 months). Abbreviations: GDS-5, five-item Geriatric Depression Scale; ABI, ankle–brachial index.

Table 3. Cox regression analysis for the risk of mortality.

	Crude				Model 1				Model 2			
	HR	95%	CI	p	HR	95%	CI	p	HR	95%	CI	p
GDS-5 = 0 and ABI > 0.90	1.000				1.000				1.000			
GDS-5 ≥ 1 and ABI > 0.90	1.628	(1.171,	2.264)	0.004	1.558	(1.120,	2.167)	0.008	1.576	(1.131,	2.196)	0.007
GDS-5 = 0 and ABI ≤ 0.90	2.604	(1.422,	4.770)	0.002	2.238	(1.220,	4.105)	0.009	1.958	(1.060,	3.618)	0.032
GDS-5 ≥ 1 and ABI ≤ 0.90	3.294	(1.756,	6.177)	<0.001	2.758	(1.469,	5.178)	0.002	2.209	(1.158,	4.217)	0.016
Age ≥ 70 years					3.245	(2.257,	4.666)	<0.001	2.519	(1.733,	3.662)	<0.001

Table 3. *Cont.*

	Crude				Model 1				Model 2			
	HR	95%	CI	*p*	HR	95%	CI	*p*	HR	95%	CI	*p*
Male					1.776	(1.302,	2.424)	<0.001	1.488	(1.074,	2.062)	0.017
Current smoker									0.942	(0.502,	1.768)	0.853
Cardiovascular disease									1.442	(0.991,	2.096)	0.056
Hypertension									1.501	(0.840,	2.680)	0.170
Diabetic kidney disease									2.469	(1.656,	3.680)	<0.001
Use of antiplatelet drugs									0.826	(0.575,	1.185)	0.299

Abbreviations: ABI = ankle–brachial index, CI = confidence interval, GDS = five-item Geriatric Depression Scale.

4. Discussion

Our main finding in this study is that when depression was screened using GDS-5, it was significantly associated with PAD, which was screened using the ABI in patients with type 2 DM and aged ≥60 years. Patients with depression and PAD had the highest mortality risk, followed by those with PAD alone and those with depression alone, compared to those without depression or PAD during a median follow-up of 56.6 months. It is well known that depression is associated with mortality in patients with DM [9,10,29]. Depression has also been reported to be associated with mortality in patients with PAD [17]. The strength of the present study is that an increased risk of mortality could be predicted using both GDS-5 and ABI in patients aged ≥60 years with type 2 DM.

Only 2.7% of patients with DM had a diagnosis of depression in 2005 according to the international classification of diseases code based on the NHI research database [30], but the prevalence of depression might be 25.9% when screened by questionnaires in patients with type 2 DM and 29.5% in those aged ≥60 years based on meta-analyses of population-based studies, although the results were various and dependent on the questionnaire [31]. Based on the hospital-based population of the Indian Depression in Diabetes Study, the prevalence of depression was 35% in outpatients aged >60 years with type 2 DM according to questionnaire screenings [32]. In the present study, the prevalence of depression based on GDS-5 ≥ 1 was 32.2% in outpatients with type 2 DM and age ≥ 60 years. Compared to the 491 (31.5%) patients with depression in the 1560 patients without PAD, the prevalence of depression was significantly increased to 42.5% in the 113 patients with PAD.

PAD is prevalent in patients with depression [33]. Seldenrijk et al. [34] reported a higher prevalence of ABI < 0.9 in patients with an established diagnosis of depression than in those without depression; however, the prevalence of an ABI > 1.4 was not significantly associated with depression. Interestingly, Grenon et al. [33] reported that depressive symptoms were predictive of PAD development during a mean 7.2 years of follow-up, but the increased PAD incidence might be contributed to by comorbid cardiovascular risks in patients with depressive symptoms. However, in the prospective study of Atherosclerosis Risk in Communities (ARIC) with a mean 9.7 years of follow-up, a high depressive score was an independent predictor for PAD development after adjusting for cardiovascular risks [35]. McDermott et al. [36] also reported that patients with PAD developed more depressive symptoms assessed by GDS-15 than those without PAD during 2.7 years of follow-up. Therefore, the screening of ABI is suggested for patients with depressive symptoms, and vice versa.

It has been reported that the GDS-15 score is associated with mortality in older people [37]. In the present study, we detected depressive symptoms using GDS-5. Although a GDS-5 score cutoff value of 2 was suggested for depression diagnosis, a cutoff value of 1 can provide better sensitivity than other cutoff values [20], and we can further categorize the mortality risk by using ABI. There are several potential mechanisms involved in depression, PAD, and mortality in patients with type 2 DM. Depressive symptoms have been reported to be associated with chronic systemic inflammation reflected by an increase in inflammatory biomarkers in patients with PAD [38]. Depressive symptoms are also associated with the dysregulation of cortisol rhythm controlled by the hypothalamic–pituitary–adrenal axis [39]. The unsuppressed cortisol and autonomic dysfunction might induce insulin resistance and advanced atherosclerosis [40,41]. Moreover, ischemic heart disease and endothelial dysfunction are associated with a reduction in brain-derived neurotrophic factor (BDNF), which supports the functions and survival of neurons [42]. A reduction in BDNF, a bridge between atherosclerotic cardiovascular disease and depression [43], is predictive of long-term mortality [44]. Recently, a decrease in circulating BDNF was reported to be associated with CKD [45]. At present, DKD is not only a risk factor for dementia but also a predictor for mortality. BDNF, as a protective biomarker for depression, was shown to be a significant predictor for survival in patients with CAD and CKD [46]. Novak et al. [47] also reported that depression increased the risk of CKD and mortality.

In addition to CKD, age is a well-known factor for depression in community studies. In line with our study, Liu et al. [31] reported that a higher prevalence of depression was associated with older age in a population with type 2 DM. However, older age is also associated with more comorbidities. In the present study, the prevalence of depression was not significantly different between patients aged ≥70 years and <70 years (41.9% vs. 43.6%, $p > 0.05$) in the subgroup of patients with PAD. In contrast, in a hospital-based investigation, Majumdar et al. [32] reported that a higher prevalence of depression was associated with a younger age in outpatients with type 2 DM. Generally, female sex is a risk factor for depression [30–32]; however, there was no significant difference in depression prevalence between sexes in the present study. In line with our study, a hospital-based study reported that no significant difference in depression prevalence was observed between sexes in inpatients with type 2 DM [48]. According to the NHI research database, Chen et al. [22] reported that the proportion of female patients (52.3%) was higher than that of male patients with type 2 DM who were newly enrolled into the P4P program in 2004, but the trend of the female proportion in the P4P program decreased from 51.8% in 2005 to 50.0% in 2014 [21]. According to the NHI research database between 2005 and 2014, the mortality risk in male patients was higher than that in female patients with DM [49]. Similarly, male sex was still a significant predictor of mortality in the present study.

The categories of antidiabetic drugs were not significantly associated with depressive symptoms or PAD at baseline in the present study. Impaired insulin signaling in the brain plays a role in mood disorders in patients with type 2 DM [50]. As a technological improvement, intranasal delivery is a convenient method for providing insulin to the brain [51]. Despite an anxiolytic-like effect in mice [50], intranasal insulin delivery might not have a significant effect on depressive symptoms in the clinical study [52].

The present study has several limitations. First, all of the study data were collected from a single medical center. Second, we did not investigate the causal effects between PAD and depression. Third, we did not investigate the mechanisms of increased mortality risk caused by PAD and depression. Fourth, we only enrolled patients with type 2 DM in the P4P program, and the results could not be applied to other populations because it has been reported that the P4P program might reduce depression risk [53]. Fifth, we did not collect other demographic characteristics such as religion, education, occupation, and socio-economic level or personal habits such as alcohol intake and exercise. A lower socioeconomic status might be associated with not only depression but also PAD [54]. Finally, we only enrolled patients aged ≥60 years because the GDS-5 was clinically applied for screening in this population. The results of our study could not be applied to other age populations because the depressive risk might depend on age in patients with type 2 DM [31].

5. Conclusions

The use of GDS-5 and ABI is helpful for predicting long-term mortality in patients with type 2 DM aged ≥60 years in a regular diabetes management program. The prevalence of PAD was increased in patients with depressive symptoms, and vice versa. Screening of the self-report GDS-5 questionnaire and ABI is recommended in patients aged ≥60 years with type 2 DM. Further studies of early interventions in depression and PAD are warranted for patients with type 2 DM.

Author Contributions: Conceptualization, Y.-H.L., Y.-C.C., H.-C.L., J.W. and I.-T.L.; data curation, I.-T.L.; formal analysis, I.-T.L.; funding acquisition, I.-T.L.; investigation, Y.-H.L., Y.-C.C., H.-C.L., J.W. and I.-T.L.; methodology, Y.-H.L., Y.-C.C., H.-C.L. and I.-T.L.; project administration, Y.-C.C. and I.-T.L.; resources, H.-C.L. and I.-T.L.; software, I.-T.L.; supervision, I.-T.L.; validation, I.-T.L.; visualization, I.-T.L.; writing—original draft, Y.-H.L.; writing—review and editing, I.-T.L. All authors have read and agreed to the published version of the manuscript.

Funding: This research was funded by Taichung Veterans General Hospital, Taichung, Taiwan, grant number TCVGH-1123501C and the Ministry of Science and Technology, Taiwan, grant number MOST 110-2314-B-075A-004-MY3. The APC was funded by the Ministry of Science and Technology, Taiwan, grant number MOST 110-2314-B-075A-004-MY3.

Institutional Review Board Statement: This study was reviewed and approved by the Institutional Review Board of Taichung Veterans General Hospital (TCVGH-IRB No. CE21376A-1, date of approval: 22 September 2022).

Informed Consent Statement: Patient consent was waived due to a retrospective cohort study design with the endpoint of death.

Data Availability Statement: The data presented in this study are available on request from the corresponding author.

Acknowledgments: We thank the Clinical Informatics Research and Development Center of Taichung Veterans General Hospital for their support. Statistical analysis was performed by the Biostatistics Task Force of Taichung Veterans General Hospital.

Conflicts of Interest: The authors declare no conflict of interest. The funders had no role in the design of the study; in the collection, analyses, or interpretation of data; in the writing of the manuscript; or in the decision to publish the results.

References

1. Liu, Q.; He, H.; Yang, J.; Feng, X.; Zhao, F.; Lyu, J. Changes in the global burden of depression from 1990 to 2017: Findings from the Global Burden of Disease study. *J. Psychiatr. Res.* **2019**, *126*, 134–140. [CrossRef]
2. Ren, X.; Yu, S.; Dong, W.; Yin, P.; Xu, X.; Zhou, M. Burden of depression in China, 1990–2017: Findings from the global burden of disease study 2017. *J. Affect. Disord.* **2020**, *268*, 95–101. [CrossRef]
3. Wu, C.-S.; Yu, S.-H.; Lee, C.-Y.; Tseng, H.-Y.; Chiu, Y.-F.; Hsiung, C.A. Prevalence of and risk factors for minor and major depression among community-dwelling older adults in Taiwan. *Int. Psychogeriatr.* **2017**, *29*, 1113–1121. [CrossRef]
4. Yang, H.; Sun, D.; Yang, Y.; Lin, R.; Xu, J.; Wu, J.; Cui, X.; Li, J.; Qin, G.; Han, X.; et al. Association of depression with all-cause and cardiovascular mortality among US adults with high and low baseline risk of cardiovascular disease. *Psychiatry Res.* **2023**, *320*, 115051. [CrossRef]
5. Charlson, F.J.; Moran, A.; Freedman, G.; Norman, R.; Stapelberg, N.J.; Baxter, A.J.; Vos, T.; A Whiteford, H. The contribution of major depression to the global burden of ischemic heart disease: A comparative risk assessment. *BMC Med.* **2013**, *11*, 250. [CrossRef]
6. Lee, J.; Kim, K.H.; Ahn, J.C.; Kim, J.A.; Lee, G.; Son, J.S.; Park, S.M. Prevalence, awareness, treatment, and control of diabetes mellitus by depressive symptom severity: A cross-sectional analysis of NHANES 2011–2016. *BMJ Open Diabetes Res. Care* **2021**, *9*, e002268. [CrossRef]
7. van Gennip, A.C.; Schram, M.T.; Köhler, S.; Kroon, A.A.; Koster, A.; Eussen, S.J.; de Galan, B.; van Sloten, T.T.; Stehouwer, C.D. Association of type 2 diabetes according to the number of risk factors within the recommended range with incidence of major depression and clinically relevant depressive symptoms: A prospective analysis. *Lancet Healthy Longev.* **2023**, *4*, e63–e71. [CrossRef]
8. Chen, P.-C.; Chan, Y.-T.; Chen, H.-F.; Ko, M.-C.; Li, C.-Y. Population-Based Cohort Analyses of the Bidirectional Relationship Between Type 2 Diabetes and Depression. *Diabetes Care* **2013**, *36*, 376–382. [CrossRef]
9. Prigge, R.; Wild, S.H.; Jackson, C.A. Depression, diabetes, comorbid depression and diabetes and risk of all-cause and cause-specific mortality: A prospective cohort study. *Diabetologia* **2022**, *65*, 1450–1460. [CrossRef]
10. Chen, V.C.-H.; Wang, T.-N.; Hsieh, M.-C.; Chou, S.-Y.; Lee, M.-C.; McIntyre, R.S.; Lu, M.-L.; Liao, Y.-T.; Yeh, C.-J. Depression, Diabetes Mellitus and Mortality in Older Adults: A National Cohort Study in Taiwan. *Neuropsychiatr. Dis. Treat.* **2022**, *18*, 2639–2648. [CrossRef]

11. Agnelli, G.; Belch, J.J.F.; Baumgartner, I.; Giovas, P.; Hoffmann, U. Morbidity and mortality associated with atherosclerotic peripher-al artery disease: A systematic review. *Atherosclerosis* **2020**, *293*, 94–100. [CrossRef] [PubMed]
12. Tavintharan, S.; Cheung, N.; Lim, S.C.; Tay, W.; Shankar, A.; Shyong Tai, E.; Wong, T.Y. Prevalence and risk factors for peripheral artery dis-ease in an Asian population with diabetes mellitus. *Diabetes Vasc. Dis. Res.* **2009**, *6*, 80–86. [CrossRef] [PubMed]
13. Caro, J.; Migliaccio-Walle, K.; Ishak, K.J.; Proskorovsky, I. The morbidity and mortality following a diagnosis of peripheral arterial disease: Long-term follow-up of a large database. *BMC Cardiovasc. Disord.* **2005**, *5*, 14. [CrossRef] [PubMed]
14. Hong, Y.; Sebastianski, M.; Makowsky, M.; Tsuyuki, R.; McMurtry, M.S. Administrative data are not sensitive for the detection of peripheral artery disease in the community. *Vasc. Med.* **2016**, *21*, 331–336. [CrossRef] [PubMed]
15. Aboyans, V.; Ricco, J.B.; Bartelink, M.E.L.; Bjorck, M.; Brodmann, M.; Cohnert, T.; Collet, J.P.; Czerny, M.; De Carlo, M.; Debus, S.; et al. 2017 ESC Guidelines on the Diagnosis and Treatment of Peripheral Arterial Diseases, in collaboration with the European Society for Vascular Surgery (ESVS): Document covering atherosclerotic disease of extracranial carotid and vertebral, mesenteric, renal, upper and lower extremity arter-iesEndorsed by: The European Stroke Organization (ESO)The Task Force for the Diagnosis and Treatment of Peripheral Arte-rial Diseases of the European Society of Cardiology (ESC) and of the European Society for Vascular Surgery (ESVS). *Eur. Heart J.* **2018**, *39*, 763–816. [PubMed]
16. Gerhard-Herman, M.D.; Gornik, H.L.; Barrett, C.; Barshes, N.R.; Corriere, M.A.; Drachman, D.E.; Walsh, M.E. 2016 AHA/ACC Guideline on the Management of Patients With Lower Extremity Peripheral Artery Disease: A Report of the American College of Cardiolo-gy/American Heart Association Task Force on Clinical Practice Guidelines. *Circulation* **2017**, *135*, e686–e725. [PubMed]
17. Scierka, L.E.; Mena-Hurtado, C.; Ahmed, Z.V.; Yousef, S.; Arham, A.; Grimshaw, A.A.; Smolderen, K.G. The association of depression with mortal-ity and major adverse limb event outcomes in patients with peripheral artery disease: A systematic review and meta-analysis. *J. Affect. Disord.* **2023**, *320*, 169–177. [CrossRef] [PubMed]
18. Welch, K.G.; Faria, I.; Browder, S.E.; Drudi, L.M.; McGinigle, K.L. Depression in Patients with Peripheral Artery Disease: An Underdi-agnosis with Increased Mortality. *Ann. Vasc. Surg.* **2023**, *95*, 80–86. [CrossRef]
19. Weeks, S.K.; McGann, P.E.; Michaels, T.K.; Penninx, B.W. Comparing various short-form Geriatric Depression Scales leads to the GDS-5/15. *J. Nurs. Scholarsh.* **2003**, *35*, 133–137. [CrossRef]
20. Brañez-Condorena, A.; Soriano-Moreno, D.R.; Navarro-Flores, A.; Solis-Chimoy, B.; Diaz-Barrera, M.E.; Taype-Rondan, A. Accuracy of the Geriatric Depression Scale (GDS)-4 and GDS-5 for the screening of depression among older adults: A systematic review and meta-analysis. *PLoS ONE* **2021**, *16*, e0253899. [CrossRef]
21. Lee, I.-T.; Hsu, C.-C.; Sheu, W.H.-H.; Su, S.-L.; Wu, Y.-L.; Lin, S.-Y. Pay-for-performance for shared care of diabetes in Taiwan. *J. Formos. Med. Assoc.* **2019**, *118*, S122–S129. [CrossRef] [PubMed]
22. Chen, Y.C.; Lee, C.T.; Lin, B.J.; Chang, Y.Y.; Shi, H.Y. Impact of pay-for-performance on mortality in diabetes patients in Taiwan: A population-based study. *Medicine* **2016**, *95*, e4197. [CrossRef]
23. Pan, W.H.; Flegal, K.M.; Chang, H.Y.; Yeh, W.T.; Yeh, C.J.; Lee, W.C. Body mass index and obesity-related metabolic disorders in Tai-wanese and US whites and blacks: Implications for definitions of overweight and obesity for Asians. *Am. J. Clin. Nutr.* **2004**, *79*, 31–99. [CrossRef] [PubMed]
24. Lee, C.H.; Shih, A.Z.L.; Woo, Y.C.; Fong, C.H.Y.; Yuen, M.M.A.; Chow, W.S.; Lam, K.S.L. Which creatinine-based estimated glomerular filtration rate equation best predicts all-cause mortality in Chinese subjects with type 2 diabetes? *Diabetes Res. Clin. Pract.* **2017**, *126*, 25–29. [CrossRef] [PubMed]
25. Wu, L.F.; Yang, S.H.; Koo, M. Psychometric properties of the Chinese version of Spiritual Index of Well-Being in elderly Taiwan-ese. *BMC Geriatr.* **2017**, *17*, 3. [CrossRef] [PubMed]
26. Huang, C.H.; Hsu, C.C.; Yu, P.C.; Peng, L.N.; Lin, M.H.; Chen, L.K. Hospitalization-associated muscle weakness and functional out-comes among oldest old patients: A hospital-based cohort study. *Exp. Gerontol.* **2021**, *150*, 111353. [CrossRef]
27. Hiatt, W.R. Medical Treatment of Peripheral Arterial Disease and Claudication. *N. Engl. J. Med.* **2001**, *344*, 1608–1621. [CrossRef]
28. Lee, I.-T. Mean and variability of annual haemoglobin A1c are associated with high-risk peripheral artery disease. *Diabetes Vasc. Dis. Res.* **2020**, *17*, 1479164120909030. [CrossRef]
29. Salinero-Fort, M.; Gómez-Campelo, P.; Cárdenas-Valladolid, J.; Andrés-Rebollo, F.S.; de Miguel-Yanes, J.; de Burgos-Lunar, C. Effect of depression on mortality in type 2 diabetes mellitus after 8 years of follow-up. The DIADEMA study. *Diabetes Res. Clin. Pract.* **2021**, *176*, 108863. [CrossRef]
30. Lin, C.; Lee, Y.; Liu, C.; Chen, H.; Ko, M.; Li, C. Urbanization and prevalence of depression in diabetes. *Public Health* **2012**, *126*, 104–111. [CrossRef]
31. Liu, X.; Li, Y.; Guan, L.; He, X.; Zhang, H.; Zhang, J.; Li, J.; Zhong, D.; Jin, R. A Systematic Review and Meta-Analysis of the Prevalence and Risk Factors of Depression in Type 2 Diabetes Patients in China. *Front. Med.* **2022**, *9*, 759499. [CrossRef] [PubMed]
32. Majumdar, S.; Sinha, B.; Dastidar, B.G.; Gangopadhyay, K.K.; Ghoshal, S.; Mukherjee, J.J.; Mazumdar, A.; Ray, S.; Dasgupta, S.; Bhattacharjee, K. Assessing prevalence and predictors of depression in Type 2 Diabetes Mellitus (DM) patients—The DEPDIAB study. *Diabetes Res. Clin. Pract.* **2021**, *178*, 108980. [CrossRef] [PubMed]
33. Grenon, S.M.; Hiramoto, J.; Smolderen, K.G.; Vittinghoff, E.; Whooley, M.A.; Cohen, B.E. Association between depression and periph-eral artery disease: Insights from the heart and soul study. *J. Am. Heart Assoc.* **2012**, *1*, e002667. [CrossRef] [PubMed]
34. Seldenrijk, A.; Vogelzangs, N.; van Hout, H.P.; van Marwijk, H.W.; Diamant, M.; Penninx, B.W. Depressive and anxiety disorders and risk of subclinical atherosclerosis Findings from the Netherlands Study of Depression and Anxiety (NESDA). *J. Psychosom. Res.* **2010**, *69*, 203–210. [CrossRef]

35. Wattanakit, K.; E Williams, J.; Schreiner, P.J.; Hirsch, A.T.; Folsom, A.R. Association of anger proneness, depression and low social support with peripheral arterial disease: The Atherosclerosis Risk in Communities Study. *Vasc. Med.* **2005**, *10*, 199–206. [CrossRef]
36. McDermott, M.M.; Guralnik, J.M.; Tian, L.; Kibbe, M.R.; Ferrucci, L.; Zhao, L.; Liu, K.; Liao, Y.; Gao, Y.; Criqui, M.H. Incidence and Prognostic Significance of Depressive Symptoms in Peripheral Artery Disease. *J. Am. Heart Assoc.* **2016**, *5*, e002959. [CrossRef]
37. Wada, T.; Kasahara, Y.; Ishimoto, Y.; Fukutomi, E.; Kimura, Y.; Imai, H.; Chen, W.-L.; Sakamoto, R.; Ishine, M.; Fujisawa, M.; et al. Fifteen-Item Geriatric Depression Scale Predicts 8-Year Mortality in Older Japanese. *J. Am. Geriatr. Soc.* **2011**, *59*, 2159–2160. [CrossRef]
38. Miller, A.H.; Raison, C.L. The role of inflammation in depression: From evolutionary imperative to modern treatment target. *Nat. Rev. Immunol.* **2015**, *16*, 22–34. [CrossRef]
39. Bhattacharyya, M.R.; Molloy, G.J.; Steptoe, A. Depression is associated with flatter cortisol rhythms in patients with coronary ar-tery disease. *J. Psychosom. Res.* **2008**, *65*, 107–113. [CrossRef]
40. Otte, C.; Neylan, T.C.; Pipkin, S.S.; Browner, W.S.; Whooley, M.A. Depressive symptoms and 24-hour urinary norepinephrine excre-tion levels in patients with coronary disease: Findings from the Heart and Soul Study. *Am. J. Psychiatry* **2005**, *162*, 2139–2145. [CrossRef]
41. Ramirez, J.L.; Drudi, L.M.; Grenon, S.M. Review of biologic and behavioral risk factors linking depression and peripheral artery disease. *Vasc. Med.* **2018**, *23*, 478–488. [CrossRef]
42. Lee, I.T.; Wang, J.S.; Lee, W.J.; Lin, S.Y.; Fu, C.P.; Liang, K.W.; Sheu, W.H.H. The synergistic effect of vascular cell adhesion molecule-1 and coro-nary artery disease on brain-derived neurotrophic factor. *Clin. Chim. Acta.* **2017**, *466*, 194–200. [CrossRef]
43. Cavaleri, D.; Moretti, F.; Bartoccetti, A.; Mauro, S.; Crocamo, C.; Carrà, G.; Bartoli, F. The role of BDNF in major depressive disorder, related clinical features, and antidepressant treatment: Insight from meta-analyses. *Neurosci. Biobehav. Rev.* **2023**, *149*, 105159. [CrossRef]
44. Lee, I.-T.; Li, Y.-H.; Sheu, W.H.-H. Brain-Derived Neurotrophic Factor during Oral Glucose Tolerance Test Predicts Cardiovascular Outcomes. *Int. J. Mol. Sci.* **2020**, *21*, 5008. [CrossRef]
45. Hsu, C.-Y.; Sheu, W.H.-H.; Lee, I.-T. Brain-derived neurotrophic factor associated with kidney function. *Diabetol. Metab. Syndr.* **2023**, *15*, 1–10. [CrossRef]
46. Hsu, C.Y.; Sheu, W.H.; Lee, I.T. Brain-Derived Neurotrophic Factor Reduces Long-Term Mortality in Patients with Coronary Ar-tery Disease and Chronic Kidney Disease. *Front Cardiovasc. Med.* **2022**, *9*, 881441. [CrossRef]
47. Novak, M.; Mucsi, I.; Rhee, C.M.; Streja, E.; Lu, J.L.; Kalantar-Zadeh, K.; Molnar, M.Z.; Kovesdy, C.P. Increased Risk of Incident Chronic Kidney Disease, Cardiovascular Disease, and Mortality in Patients with Diabetes with Comorbid Depression. *Diabetes Care* **2016**, *39*, 1940–1947. [CrossRef]
48. Maimaitituerxun, R.; Chen, W.; Xiang, J.; Kaminga, A.C.; Wu, X.Y.; Chen, L.; Yang, J.; Liu, A.; Dai, W. Prevalence of comorbid depression and associated factors among hospitalized patients with type 2 diabetes mellitus in Hunan, China. *BMC Psychiatry* **2023**, *23*, 1–11. [CrossRef]
49. Li, H.-Y.; Wu, Y.-L.; Tu, S.T.; Hwu, C.-M.; Liu, J.-S.; Chuang, L.-M. Trends of mortality in diabetic patients in Taiwan: A nationwide survey in 2005–2014. *J. Formos. Med. Assoc.* **2019**, *118* (Suppl. S2), S83–S89. [CrossRef]
50. Martin, H.; Bullich, S.; Martinat, M.; Chataigner, M.; Di Miceli, M.; Simon, V.; Clark, S.; Butler, J.; Schell, M.; Chopra, S.; et al. Insulin modulates emotional behavior through a serotonin-dependent mechanism. *Mol. Psychiatry*, 2022. (in press) [CrossRef]
51. Sabbagh, F.; Muhamad, I.I.; Niazmand, R.; Dikshit, P.K.; Kim, B.S. Recent progress in polymeric non-invasive insulin delivery. *Int. J. Biol. Macromol.* **2022**, *203*, 222–243. [CrossRef]
52. Cha, D.S.; Best, M.W.; Bowie, C.R.; Gallaugher, L.A.; Woldeyohannes, H.O.; Soczynska, J.K.; McIntyre, R.S. A randomized, double-blind, place-bo-controlled, crossover trial evaluating the effect of intranasal insulin on cognition and mood in individuals with treat-ment-resistant major depressive disorder. *J. Affect Disord.* **2017**, *210*, 57–65. [CrossRef] [PubMed]
53. Lian, W.-C.; Livneh, H.; Huang, H.-J.; Lu, M.-C.; Guo, H.-R.; Tsai, T.-Y. Adding Pay-for-Performance Program to Routine Care Was Related to a Lower Risk of Depression Among Type 2 Diabetes Patients in Taiwan. *Front. Public Health* **2021**, *9*, 650452. [CrossRef] [PubMed]
54. Chang, P.; Nead, K.T.; Olin, J.W.; Cooke, J.P.; Leeper, N.J. Clinical and socioeconomic factors associated with unrecognized peripheral artery disease. *Vasc. Med.* **2014**, *19*, 289–296. [CrossRef] [PubMed]

biomedicines

MDPI

Article

Serum Cytokines and Growth Factors in Subjects with Type 1 Diabetes: Associations with Time in Ranges and Glucose Variability

Vadim V. Klimontov [1,*], Kamilla R. Mavlianova [1], Nikolai B. Orlov [2], Julia F. Semenova [1] and Anton I. Korbut [1]

[1] Laboratory of Endocrinology, Research Institute of Clinical and Experimental Lymphology—Branch of the Institute of Cytology and Genetics, Siberian Branch of Russian Academy of Sciences (RICEL—Branch of IC&G SB RAS), 630060 Novosibirsk, Russia

[2] Laboratory of Clinical Immunogenetics, Research Institute of Clinical and Experimental Lymphology—Branch of the Institute of Cytology and Genetics, Siberian Branch of Russian Academy of Sciences (RICEL—Branch of IC&G SB RAS), 630060 Novosibirsk, Russia

* Correspondence: klimontov@mail.ru

Abstract: The detrimental effect of hyperglycemia and glucose variability (GV) on target organs in diabetes can be implemented through a wide network of regulatory peptides. In this study, we assessed a broad panel of serum cytokines and growth factors in subjects with type 1 diabetes (T1D) and estimated associations between concentrations of these molecules with time in ranges (TIRs) and GV. One hundred and thirty subjects with T1D and twenty-seven individuals with normal glucose tolerance (control) were included. Serum levels of 44 cytokines and growth factors were measured using a multiplex bead array assay. TIRs and GV parameters were derived from continuous glucose monitoring. Subjects with T1D compared to control demonstrated an increase in concentrations of IL-1β, IL-1Ra, IL-2Rα, IL-3, IL-6, IL-7, IL-12 p40, IL-16, IL-17A, LIF, M-CSF, IFN-α2, IFN-γ, MCP-1, MCP-3, and TNF-α. Patients with TIR $\leq$ 70% had higher levels of IL-1α, IL-1β, IL-6, IL-12 p70, IL-16, LIF, M-CSF, MCP-1, MCP-3, RANTES, TNF-α, TNF-β, and b-NGF, and lower levels of IL-1α, IL-4, IL-10, GM-CSF, and MIF than those with TIR > 70%. Serum IL-1β, IL-10, IL-12 p70, MCP-1, MCP-3, RANTES, SCF, and TNF-α correlated with TIR and time above range. IL-1β, IL-8, IL-10, IL-12 p70, MCP-1, RANTES, MIF, and SDF-1α were related to at least one amplitude-dependent GV metric. In logistic regression models, IL-1β, IL-4, IL-10, IL-12 p70, GM-CSF, HGF, MCP-3, and TNF-α were associated with TIR $\leq$ 70%, and MIF and PDGF-BB demonstrated associations with coefficient of variation values $\geq$ 36%. These results provide further insight into the pathophysiological effects of hyperglycemia and GV in people with diabetes.

Keywords: type 1 diabetes; inflammation; cytokines; growth factors; hyperglycemia; time in range; glucose variability; continuous glucose monitoring

1. Introduction

The burden of type 1 diabetes (T1D) is enormous and is expected to increase. In 2021, there were about 8.4 million individuals worldwide living with T1D. The remaining life expectancy of a 10-year-old diagnosed with T1D ranges from a mean of 13 years in low-income countries to 65 years in high-income ones [1]. Vascular diabetes complications remain an important determinant of mortality in subjects with T1D [2–4]. The Diabetes Control and Complications Trial (DCCT) and its longitudinal observational follow-up study, the Epidemiology of Diabetes Interventions and Complications (EDIC) study, clearly showed a reduction in the incidence of diabetic retinopathy, diabetic nephropathy, diabetic neuropathy, and cardiovascular disease (CVD) outcomes, following the optimization of glycemic control in people with T1D [5,6]. However, the benefits of intensive insulin treatment in terms of the risk of major adverse cardiovascular events vary substantially between individuals with T1D [7]. Age, diabetes duration, and glucose level do not completely explain the associations between complications and mortality [4]. This underlines the necessity for a better understanding of the drivers of diabetic complications.

Clinicians noticed a long time ago that many patients with excessive glucose fluctuations and unstable glycemic control rapidly develop complications. One of the first experimental studies testing the deteriorating effect of glucose fluctuations on the kidneys was published in 1957: it showed the rapid development of glomerulosclerosis in rats when excessive blood glucose fluctuations were induced by the intermittent administration of glucose and insulin [8]. In recent years, the role of glucose variability (GV) as a trigger of diabetic vascular complications has attracted increasing attention [9,10]. In the observational Finnish Diabetic Nephropathy (FinnDiane) study, glycated hemoglobin A1c (HbA1c) variability predicts incident cardiovascular events, microalbuminuria, and overt diabetic nephropathy in subjects with T1D [11]. A recent analysis of 14 studies with 254,017 patients with diabetes revealed that the highest HbA1c variability is associated with increased risks of CVD. The CVD risk associated with HbA1c variability might be even higher among patients with T1D [12]. However, the role of short-term GV as a trigger of diabetic complications remains to be clarified.

Continuous glucose monitoring (CGM) opened the way for the comprehensive assessment of short-term GV in patients with diabetes. Two principal dimensions of GV, amplitude and time, can be assessed and visualized from CGM data [9]. Time in range (TIR), time above range (TAR), and time below range (TBR) became standardized CGM metrics for clinical care [13]. Accumulating evidence suggests a negative association between time in range (TIR) and microvascular complications in subjects with T1D [14,15]. In addition, associations of coefficient of variation (CV) and the mean amplitude of glycemic excursions (MAGE) with diabetic microvascular complications [16] and cardiovascular autonomic neuropathy [17] were reported.

The mechanisms of the harmful effects of excessive GV on target organs in diabetes have been intensively studied in recent years. The cardiovascular system, pancreas, adipose and muscle tissues, gastrointestinal tract, and kidney have been recognized as the loci with the highest expression of GV-related genes [18]. Current data indicate that GV effects can be realized through oxidative stress, non-enzymatic glycation, chronic low-grade inflammation, endothelial dysfunction, platelet activation, impaired angiogenesis, and renal fibrosis. At the molecular level, these pathophysiological processes may be mediated through shifts in the production of cytokines and growth factors playing an important role in intercellular interactions [19]. At present, the relationships between GV and changes in the production of these regulators are not well understood.

The large number of secreted cytokines and their interactions make it difficult to assess changes in the cytokine response during stress and disease. Moreover, measuring individual regulators can lead to a one-sided or even incorrect interpretation of the response. In such situations, multiplex platforms, widely used to measure multiple biomarkers from a single assay, may have advantages over single assay-based detection methods [20,21]. In recent years, a multiplex bead assay has become increasingly popular in studies of cytokine panels in various diseases, including diabetes [22–24].

Therefore, we aimed to assess a broad panel of circulating cytokines and growth factors in subjects with T1D via a multiplex bead array assay and to determine the associations of these regulators with CGM-derived TIR and GV parameters.

2. Materials and Methods

2.1. Design

We performed a cross-sectional observational single-center comparative study.

Caucasian male and female patients with T1D aged 18 to 70 years were included. Acute infections within three months prior to the study, pregnancy, malignant neoplasm, chronic inflammatory or autoimmune diseases, current diabetic ketoacidosis or hyperglycemic hyperosmolar state, end-stage renal disease, and diabetic foot syndrome were established as the principal exclusion criteria. Subjects without the above-mentioned diseases and conditions who had normal glucose tolerance (NGT) verified by the results of the oral glucose tolerance test and HbA1c measurement were included in the control group.

All study participants underwent a detailed clinical examination with real-time CGM. Digital CGM data were used for the calculation of TIRs and GV parameters. The panel of serum cytokines and growth factors was assessed with a multiplex bead array assay.

The study design is shown in Figure 1.

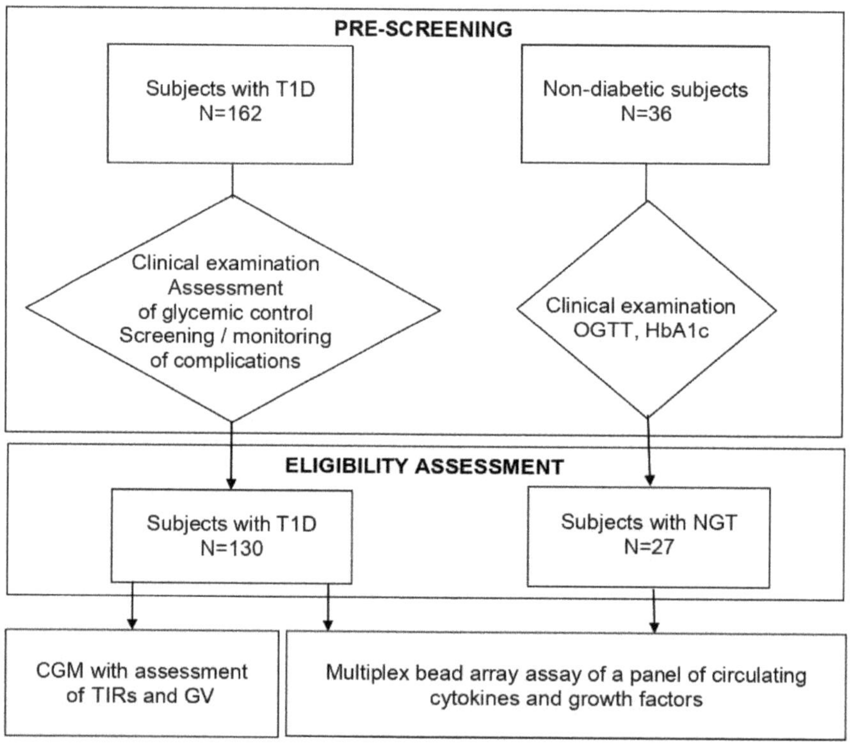

Figure 1. Study design. CGM, continuous glucose monitoring; GV, glucose variability; HbA1c, glycated hemoglobin A1c; NGT, normal glucose tolerance; OGTT, oral glucose tolerance test; T1D, type 1 diabetes; TIRs, time in ranges.

2.2. Methods

General clinical tests. The levels of HbA1c, serum biochemical parameters, and urinary albumin were assessed in patients with T1D with the use of a AU480 Chemical Analyzer (Beckman Coulter, Brea, CA, USA) and commercially available cartridges. A complete blood count was performed on a hematology analyzer (Analyticon Biotechnologies AG, Lichtenfels, Germany). The fasting C-peptide was determined using chemiluminescent immunoassay with an Immulite 2000 XPi immunological analyzer (Siemens Healthineers, Erlangen, Germany).

A standard oral glucose tolerance test with 75 g of glucose was performed in non-diabetic subjects. Blood samples for the measurement of glucose were taken from the cubital vein at 0 and 120 min of the test.

CGM parameters. Patients with T1D underwent real-time CGM within 3–13 days (median 5.4 days) with MMT-722 or MMT-754 monitoring systems and CareLink® Pro software 2.5.524.0 (version 2.5A, Medtronic, Minneapolis, MN, USA). Study participants were instructed to calibrate the system at least three times a day. The results of the CGM of each subject were reviewed individually and recording defects were eliminated.

TIRs were defined according to the International Consensus on Use of Continuous Glucose Monitoring [25] and the International Consensus on Time in Range [13]. Specifically, we assessed TIR: 70–180 mg/dL (3.9–10.0 mmol/L), time above range, level 1 (TAR L-1: 181–250 mg/dL [10.1–13.9 mmol/L]), time above range, level 2 (TAR L-2: >250 mg/dL [>13.9 mmol/L]), time below range, level 1 (TBR L-1: 54–69 mg/dL [3.0–3.8 mmol/L]), and time below range, level 2 (TBR L-2: <54 mg/dL [<3.0 mmol/L]). In addition, the following GV parameters were calculated: CV, MAGE, and mean absolute glucose (MAG) changes. Among these parameters, CV is an indicator of variations around the mean glucose, MAGE is the mean differences from peaks to nadirs, and MAG is the absolute differences between sequential readings divided by the time [9,10]. The GV parameters were estimated with the use of EasyGV v. 9.0.R2 software [26]. The values of TIR > 70% were considered as targets [13] and values of CV < 36% as indicators of stable glucose level [25].

Serum cytokines and growth factors. Serum samples for the assay of cytokines and growth factors were obtained from the fasting blood and stored at −80 °C until the analysis. Repeated freeze–thaw cycles were avoided.

The concentrations of interleukin 1 alpha (IL-1α), interleukin 1 beta (IL-1β), interleukin-1 receptor antagonist (IL-1Ra), interleukin 2 (IL-2), interleukin-2 receptor alpha chain (IL-2Rα), interleukin 3 (IL-3), interleukin 4 (IL-4), interleukin 5 (IL-5), interleukin 6 (IL-6), interleukin 7 (IL-7), interleukin 8 (IL-8), interleukin 9 (IL-9), interleukin 10 (IL-10), interleukin-12 subunit beta (IL-12 p40), interleukin 12 active heterodimer (IL-12 p70), interleukin 16 (IL-16), interleukin 17A (IL-17A), interleukin 18 (IL-18), leukemia inhibitory factor (LIF), granulocyte colony-stimulating factor (G-CSF), granulocyte-macrophage colony-stimulating factor (GM-CSF), macrophage colony-stimulating factor (M-CSF), chemokine growth-regulated protein alpha (GRO-α), interferon alpha 2 (IFN-α2), interferon gamma (IFN-γ), interferon gamma-induced protein 10 (IP-10), monocyte chemoattractant protein 1 (MCP-1), monocyte chemoattractant protein 3 (MCP-3), macrophage migration inhibitory factor (MIF), monokine induced by interferon-γ (MIG), macrophage inflammatory protein 1 alpha (MIP-1α), macrophage inflammatory protein 1 beta (MIP-1β), regulated on activation, normal T cell expressed and secreted (RANTES), tumor necrosis factor alpha (TNF-α), tumor necrosis factor-beta (TNF-β), TNF-related apoptosis-inducing ligand (TRAIL), soluble cytotoxic factor (SCF), stem cell growth factor beta (SCGF beta), stromal cell-derived factor-1 alpha (SDF-1α), basic fibroblast growth factor (bFGF), platelet-derived growth factor subunit B (PDGF-BB), hepatocyte growth factor (HGF), beta subunit of nerve growth factor (β-NGF), and vascular endothelial growth factor (VEGF) were assessed with the use of Bio-Plex Pro™ Human Cytokine Screening Panel Assay (Bio-Rad Laboratories, Hercules, CA, USA).

A multiplex bead array assay was performed according to the manufacturer's instructions. Serum samples were centrifuged at 10,000× *g* for 10 min at 4 °C, diluted 1:4 with Bio-Plex Sample Diluent, and incubated with antibody-coupled beads, detection antibody, and streptavidin for 30 min, 30 min, and 10 min, respectively. After each coating with antigen, the plate was washed with a Bio-Plex Handheld Magnetic Washer, resuspended, and vortexed. Fluorescence was measured on a two-beam laser automated analyzer Bio-Plex® 200 system. Data were acquired with Bio-Plex Manager Software 4.0. The values below the detection limit were set to zero.

2.3. Statistical Analysis

Statistics 12.0 software package (Dell, Round Rock, TX, USA) was used for analysis. The outliers were excluded with Dixon's Q test. Quantitative data are presented as medians (lower quartiles; upper quartiles); frequencies are presented as percentages (%). The Kolmogorov–Smirnov (KS) test was applied to test the normality of data distribution. As most of the studied parameters were not distributed normally, a non-parametric Mann–Whitney U-test was used for group comparisons. Spearman's rank correlation analysis and logistic regression analysis were applied to test the associations between studied parameters. *p*-values less than 0.05 were considered significant.

3. Results

3.1. Clinical Characteristics of the Study Participants

One hundred and thirty subjects with T1D, fifty-five men and seventy-five women, aged from 18 to 70 years (median 33 years), with diabetes duration from 0.5 to 55 years (median 15 years), were included in the study. Eighty eight patients had normal body mass index (BMI), twenty-four were overweight, and eighteen individuals had obesity. The level of fasting C-peptide in most patients was below the sensitivity limit (<0.1 ng/mL); however, 19 subjects had detectable C-peptide (range: 0.102–1.3 ng/mL). Eighty-two individuals received multiple daily injections of insulin and forty-eight were on continuous subcutaneous insulin infusion. Clinical characteristics are presented in Table 1.

Table 1. Clinical characteristics of the study participants with T1D.

Parameter	Median (25; 75 Percentile)
Demographic and general clinical parameters	
Age, years	33 (24; 43)
Smokers, *n* (%)	23 (18%)
BMI, kg/m^2	23 (20; 26)
Waist-to-hip ratio	0.81 (0.76; 0.91)
Diabetes-related parameters and associated diseases	
Diabetes duration, years	15 (10; 23)
Daily insulin dose, IU/kg	0.7 (0.5; 0.9)
Diabetic retinopathy, *n* (%)	79 (61%)
Chronic kidney disease, *n* (%)	75 (58%)
Diabetic neuropathy, *n* (%)	96 (74%)
Arterial hypertension, *n* (%)	39 (30%)
Coronary artery disease, *n* (%)	7 (5.3%)
Peripheral artery disease, *n* (%)	18 (14%)
Laboratory parameters	
HbA1c, %	7.9 (6.8; 9.6)
HbA1c, mmol/L	67 (51; 81)
Total cholesterol, mmol/L	5.1 (4.2; 6.3)
LDL-cholesterol, mmol/L	3.0 (2.4; 3.7)
HDL-cholesterol, mmol/L	1.5 (1.3; 1.8)
Triglycerides, mmol/L	1.0 (0.7; 1.3)
hsCRP, mmol/L	1.3 (0.7; 2.8)
eGFR (CKD-EPI formula, 2009), mL/min/1.73 m^2	94 (82; 105)
UACR, mg/mmol	0.5 (0.3; 1.1)
Hemoglobin, g/L	139 (125; 150)
RBC, $\times 10^{12}$	4.7 (4.4; 5.0)
WBC, $\times 10^{9}$	5.4 (4.8; 6.9)

Continuous data are presented as medians (lower quartile; upper quartile), and frequencies are presented as number of patients (percentage). BMI, body mass index; eGFR, estimated glomerular filtration rate; HbA1c, glycated hemoglobin A1c; HDL, high density lipoprotein; hsCRP, high sensitivity C-reactive protein; LDL, low-density lipoprotein; RBC, red blood cells; UACR, urinary albumin-to-creatinine ratio; WBC, white blood cells.

Twenty-seven non-obese individuals with NGT, twelve men and fifteen women, from 19 to 62 years of age (median 32 years), were included in the control group.

Mean monitoring glucose, CGM-derived TIRs, and GV parameters in subjects with T1D are presented in Table 2.

Table 2. CGM-derived TIRs and GV parameters in subjects with T1D.

Parameter	Median (25; 75 Percentile)
Mean glucose, mmol/L	7.7 (6.6; 9.3)
TIR, %	72 (57; 88)
TAR L-1, %	17 (7.4; 25)
TAR L-2, %	3.5 (0.3; 11)
TBR L-1, %	1.5 (0; 2.1)
TBR L-2, %	0.2 (0; 1.2)
CV, %	33 (27; 38)
MAGE, mmol/L	4.3 (3.1; 5.2)
MAG, mmol $\times$ h^{-1} $\times$ L^{-1}	1.7 (2.1; 2.4)

Data are presented as median (lower quartile; upper quartile). TIR, time in range; TAR L-1, time above range, level 1; TAR L-2, time above range, level 2; TBR L-1, time below range, level 1; TBR L-2, time below range, level 2; CV, coefficient of variation; MAGE, mean amplitude of glycemic excursions; MAG, mean absolute glucose change.

3.2. Serum Cytokines and Growth Factors in Subjects with NGT and T1D

Patients with T1D as compared to subjects with NGT demonstrated significant increases in serum levels of IL-1β, IL-1Ra, IL-2Rα, IL-3, IL-6, IL-7, IL-12 p70, IL-16, IL-17A, LIF, M-CSF, IFN-α2, IFN-γ, MCP-1, MCP-3, and TNF-α (Figure 2).

In addition, there were trends towards an increase in the levels of G-CSF, SCF, TRAIL, and HGF. On the other hand, concentrations of IL-1α, IL-4, and GM-CSF were decreased and MIF demonstrated a tendency to decrease. Other molecules showed no significant changes (Figure 2).

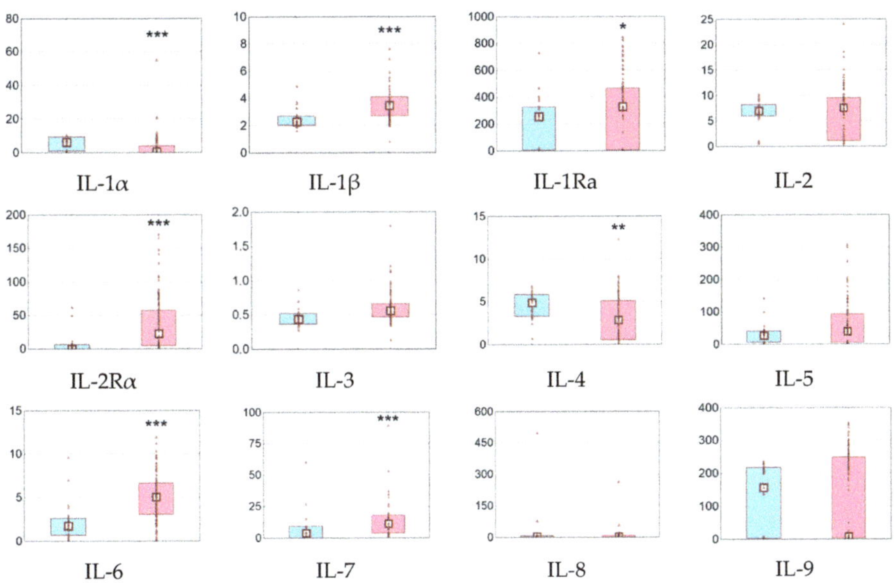

Figure 2. *Cont.*

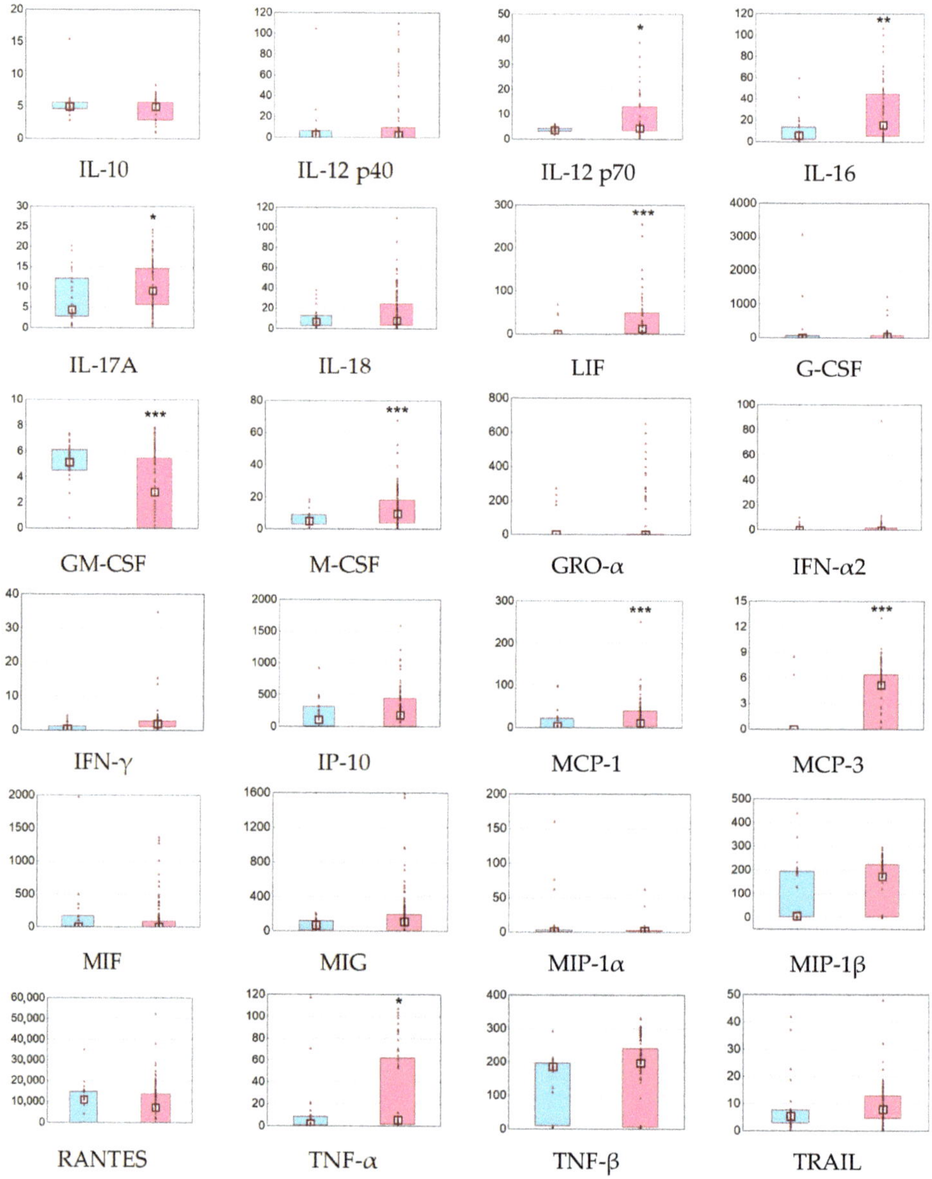

Figure 2. *Cont.*

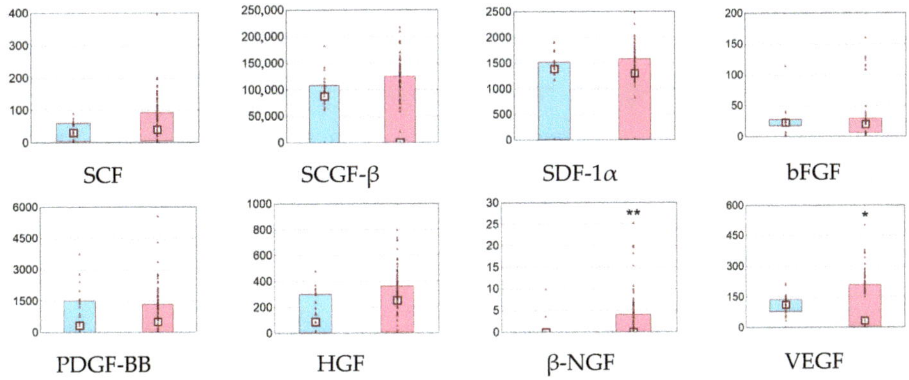

Figure 2. Serum concentrations of cytokines and growth factors in subjects with NGT and T1D. Data are presented as raw data (dots), medians (squares), and interquartile ranges (boxes). NGT subjects are marked in blue and patients with T1D are marked in pink. The concentrations are expressed in pg/mL. * $p < 0.05$, ** $p < 0.01$, *** $p < 0.001$ vs. subjects with NGT. NGT, normal glucose tolerance; T1D, type 1 diabetes.

3.3. Serum Cytokines and Growth Factors in Subjects with T1D: Relationships with TIRs

The changes in the levels of the most studied molecules were more pronounced in subjects with TIR < 70%; in this group we found significant increases in the levels of IL-1β, IL-1Ra, IL-2Rα, IL-3, IL-6, IL-7, IL-12 p40, IL-16, IL-17A, G-CSF, M-CSF, IFN-γ, MCP-1, MCP-3, TNF-α, TNF-β, SCF, and HGF, and decreases in the levels of IL-1α, IL-4, IL-8, IL-10, GM-CSF, and MIF when compared to control (Table 3). In patients with TIR > 70%, concentrations of IL-1α, IL-1β, IL-2Rα, IL-3, IL-4, IL-7, IL-16, IL-17A, LIF, G-CSF, IFN-α2, IFN-γ, MCP-1, MCP-3, and β-NGF were significantly different from control.

Table 3. Serum concentrations (pg/mL) of cytokines and growth factors in T1D subjects depending on TIR.

Molecule	Group		p
	TIR > 70% (n = 69)	**TIR ≤ 70% (n = 61)**	
IL-1α	0.93 (0; 6.42) **	0 (0; 3.82) ***	**0.01**
IL-1β	3.07 (2.53; 3.90) ***	3.79 (3.06; 4.31) ***	**0.0004**
IL-1Ra	296 (4.46; 461)	405 (7.25; 478) **	0.08
IL-2	7.94 (3.42; 9.55)	6.12 (1.07; 9.56)	0.09
IL-2Rα	18 (3.24; 63) ***	30 (4.96; 54) ***	0.68
IL-3	0.53 (0.45; 0.65) ***	0.56 (0.49; 0.70)***	0.07
IL-4	3.82 (1.10; 5.88) ***	1.53 (0.42; 3.95) ***	**0.01**
IL-5	42 (5.14; 77)	9.89 (4.14; 117)	0.96
IL-6	4.32 (2.40; 5.86)	5.54 (3.84; 7.03) ***	**0.007**
IL-7	10 (3.91; 18) **	11 (3.78; 18) ***	0.78
IL-8	6.53 (2.28; 9.38)	3.83 (1.52; 6.90) *	0.07
IL-9	182 (5.22; 251)	6.64 (2.92; 235)	0.07
IL-10	5.29 (3.83; 6.05)	4.75 (2.90; 5.29) *	**0.001**
IL-12 p40	3.62 (0; 9.66)	0.28 (0; 9.42)	0.25
IL-12 p70	4.10 (3.41; 5.41)	6.56 (3.41; 14) **	**0.02**
IL-16	9.12 (3.74; 36) *	34 (6.08; 490) ***	**0.02**
IL-17A	10 (4.46; 15) *	8.95 (6.09; 13) **	0.94
IL-18	8.34 (3.29; 23)	8.01 (4.02; 32)	0.35
LIF	8.58 (0; 49) ***	26 (8.58; 59)	**0.02**
G-CSF	14 (2.46; 72) **	38 (5.48; 74) *	0.16
GM-CSF	4.66 (0.83; 6.04)	1.08 (0; 5.08) ***	**0.002**
M-CSF	9.29 (3.67; 18)	12 (4.4; 21) ***	0.25

Table 3. *Cont.*

Molecule	Group		p
	TIR > 70% (n = 69)	**TIR ≤ 70% (n = 61)**	
GRO-α	0 (0; 5.46)	0 (0; 0.75)	0.2
IFN-α2	0 (0; 1.62) *	0 (0; 1.62)	0.71
IFN-γ	1.79 (1.09; 3.06) ***	1.94 (1.07; 2.53) ***	0.87
IP-10	145 (4.57; 333)	235 (6.09; 471)	0.13
MCP-1	6.83 (3.11; 30) *	24.39 (6.48; 41) ***	**0.01**
MCP-3	0 (0; 5.70) **	6.05 (0.91; 6.74) ***	**0.0006**
MIF	8.44 (0; 149)	0.44 (0; 28) **	**0.005**
MIG	110 (6.23; 177)	117 (5.95; 200)	0.84
MIP-1α	1.54 (1.18; 2.22)	1.81 (1.50; 2.58)	0.07
MIP-1β	193 (4.51; 224)	7.98 (4.07; 232)	0.61
RANTES	2437 (3.14; 11,840)	9590 (6.99; 14,106)	**0.02**
TNF-α	4.25 (0; 12)	6.77 (3.29; 79) ***	**0.002**
TNF-β	176 (4.30; 226)	208 (6.72; 289) *	**0.04**
TRAIL	7.47 (5.35; 13)	8.49 (3.79; 13)	0.95
SCF	19 (3.10; 78)	69 (6.48; 99) *	0.06
SCGF-β	9.01 (4.57; 117,138)	9.85 (3.87; 126,518)	0.92
SDF-1α	1276 (4.63; 1611)	1339 (1132; 1543)	0.26
bFGF	20 (3.82; 28)	8.33 (7.06; 108)	0.75
PDGF-BB	385 (5.66; 1307)	730 (4.78; 1402)	0.58
HGF	159 (5.42; 326)	291 (6.28; 407) *	0.06
β-NGF	0 (0; 1.24) *	1.24 (0; 4.69)	**0.02**
VEGF	152 (6.11; 208)	6.11 (2.87; 214)	0.22

Data are presented as medians (lower quartile; upper quartile). * $p < 0.05$, ** $p < 0.01$, *** $p < 0.001$ vs. subjects with NGT. Significant differences between diabetic groups are highlighted in bold. NGT, normal glucose tolerance; T1D, type 1 diabetes; TIR, time in range.

Among subjects with diabetes, those with TIR ≤ 70% had higher levels of IL-1α, IL-1β, IL-6, IL-12 p70, IL-16, LIF, M-CSF, MCP-1, MCP-3, RANTES, TNF-α, TNF-β, and b-NGF, and lower levels of IL-1α, IL-4, IL-10, GM-CSF, and MIF than individuals with TIR > 70% (Table 3).

We found weak correlations between TIR and concentrations of IL-1β (r = −0.21, p = 0.02), IL-10 (r = 0.23, p = 0.008), IL-12 p70 (r = −0.26, p = 0.004), MCP-1 (r = −0.32, p = 0.0002), MCP-3 (r = −0.19, p = 0.03), RANTES (r = −0.24, p = 0.006), SCF (r = −0.18, p = 0.04), and TNF-α (r = −0.23, p = 0.008). Most of these cytokines demonstrated correlations with TAR L1: IL-1β (r = 0.23, p = 0.008), IL-10 (r = −0.21, p = 0.02), IL-12 p70 (r = 0.28, p = 0.001), MCP-1 (r = 0.32, p = 0.0002), MCP-3 (r = 0.21, p = 0.02), RANTES (r = 0.30, p = 0.0005), TNF-α (r = 0.29, p = 0.0008), and TAR L2: IL-1β (r = 0.24, p = 0.006), IL-10 (r = −0.24, p = 0.006), IL-12 p70 (r = 0.24, p = 0.006), IL-16 (r = 0.20, p = 0.02), MCP-1 (r = 0.28, p = 0.001), MCP-3 (r = 0.19, p = 0.03), MIF (r = −0.20, p = 0.02), RANTES (r = 0.21, p = 0.02), SCF (r = 0.22, p = 0.01), and TNF-α (r = 0.22, p = 0.01).

There were negative correlations between TBR L1 and IL-1β (r = −0.29, p = 0.0008), IL-3 (r = −0.23, p = 0.008), IL-4 (r = −0.24, p = 0.006), IL-16 (r = −0.23, p = 0.008), IL-18 (r = −0.20, p = 0.02), LIF (r = −0.21, p = 0.02), MCP-3 (r = −0.34, p < 0.0001), MIP-1α (r = −0.23, p = 0.008), β-NGF (r = −0.26, p = 0.004), and TNF-α (r = −0.23, p = 0.008). Additionally, we found negative correlations between TBR L2 and IL-1Ra (r = −0.21, p = 0.02), IL-3 (r = −0.22, p = 0.01), IL-16 (r = −0.20, p = 0.02), MCP-3 (r = −0.22, p = 0.01), and G-CSF (r = −0.23, p = 0.008), and a positive correlation between TBR L2 and PDGF-BB (r = 0.23, p = 0.008).

3.4. Serum Concentrations of Cytokines and Growth Factors in Subjects with T1D: Relationships with GV

We compared the concentrations of the studied cytokines and growth factors in patients with CV values < 36% and in those with CV ≥ 36%. Most of the molecules demonstrated no significant differences between the groups (Table 4). However, MCP-1 and RANTES were markedly higher and the MIF level was decreased in patients with unstable glucose levels. Both diabetic groups showed significant differences with the control group in concentrations of IL-1α, IL-1β, IL-2Rα, IL-3, IL-4, IL-6, IL-7, IL-16, IL-17A, LIF, GM-CSF, M-CSF, IFN-γ, MCP-1, MCP-3, and β-NGF.

Table 4. Serum concentrations (pg/mL) of cytokines and growth factors in T1D subjects depending on CV.

Molecule	Group		p
	CV < 36% (n = 72)	**CV ≥ 36% (n = 58)**	
IL-1α	0.46 (0; 4.85) ***	0.51 (0; 4.05) ***	0.74
IL-1β	3.60 (2.62; 4.10) ***	3.48 (2.71; 4.10) ***	0.94
IL-1Ra	324 (5.81; 464)	376 (5.81; 478) *	0.69
IL-2	7.78 (2.35; 9.93)	7.20 (1.07; 9.24)	0.16
IL-2Rα	21 (4.96; 59) ***	25 (4.96; 54) ***	0.99
IL-3	0.57 (0.46; 0.69) ***	0.53 (0.49; 0.63) ***	0.23
IL-4	4.89 (2.40; 6.26) ***	5.17 (3.33; 6.69) ***	0.33
IL-5	39 (5.03; 98)	38 (4.63; 90)	0.40
IL-6	3.08 (0.90; 4.86) **	2.73 (0.17; 5.29) **	0.76
IL-7	11 (4.03; 18) ***	10 (3.78; 18) **	0.63
IL-8	5.69 (2.43; 9.26)	4.41 (1.52; 8.10)	0.15
IL-9	7.85 (3.71; 244)	11 (4.35; 258)	0.55
IL-10	4.96 (3.83; 5.66)	4.75 (2.90; 5.66)	0.45
IL-12 p40	2.92 (0; 14)	0.38 (0; 6.09) *	0.33
IL-12 p70	4.33 (3.41; 13)	4.45 (3.41; 13)	0.73
IL-16	31 (5.74; 45) **	9.12 (4.87; 38) *	0.26
IL-17A	9.15 (4.85; 15) *	9.36 (5.77; 15) **	0.57
IL-18	8.85 (3.86; 24)	7.37 (3.89; 25)	0.98
LIF	8.58 (0.43; 49) ***	22 (4.92; 54) ***	0.29
G-CSF	38 (3.30; 87)	22 (3.37; 60)	0.53
GM-CSF	2.85 (0.24; 5.40) ***	2.94 (0; 6.28) *	0.96
M-CSF	9.78 (3.89; 18) **	9.66 (3.89; 20) **	0.77
GRO-α	0 (0; 4.34)	0 (0; 0.75)	0.45
IFN-α2	0 (0; 1.62)	0 (0; 3.35) *	0.27
IFN-γ	1.87 (1.08; 2.98) ***	1.94 (1.07; 2.48) ***	0.67
IP-10	180 (5.62; 442)	193 (6.09; 448)	0.87
MCP-1	6.91 (3.18; 30) *	24 (6.75; 43) ***	**0.007**
MCP-3	5.34 (0; 6.63) ***	4.74 (0; 6.28) ***	0.72
MIF	14 (0; 144)	1.59 (0; 20) **	**0.04**
MIG	115 (6.23; 217)	112 (6.11; 193)	0.79
MIP-1α	1.63 (1.35; 3.06)	1.74 (1.41; 2.24)	0.65
MIP-1β	173 (3.95; 224)	96 (4.99; 230)	0.58
RANTES	9.85 (4.07; 12,458)	9868 (7.22; 13,970)	**0.03**
TNF-α	5.21 (0.67; 62)	6.53 (2.77; 60) *	0.61
TNF-β	170 (4.77; 236)	208 (6.96; 266) *	0.18
TRAIL	7.78 (5.12; 12)	7.98 (3.79; 13)	0.93
SCF	14 (3.65; 88)	69 (6.68; 99) *	0.18
SCGF-β	10,314 (4.04; 115,521)	8.39 (4.65; 130,694)	0.64
SDF-1α	1298 (6.48; 1580)	1314 (8.44; 1569)	0.55
bFGF	20 (5.26; 34)	8.33 (5.64; 28)	0.36
PDGF-BB	190 (3.80; 1212)	794 (5.38; 1544)	0.11
HGF	219 (5.33; 328)	288 (6.72; 403) *	0.19
β-NGF	0.00 (0; 4.07) **	0 (0; 3.18) **	0.53
VEGF	167 (3.39; 226)	6.18 (3.31; 198)	0.21

Data are presented as medians (lower quartile; upper quartile). * $p < 0.05$, ** $p < 0.01$, *** $p < 0.001$ vs. subjects with NGT. Significant differences between diabetic groups are highlighted in bold. CV, coefficient of variation; NGT, normal glucose tolerance; T1D, type 1 diabetes.

In subjects with T1D, CV correlated positively with concentrations of MCP-1 (r = 0.18, $p = 0.04$) and RANTES (r = 0.27, $p = 0.002$). There were negative correlations between CV and IL-10 (r = −0.23, $p = 0.008$) and MIF (r = −0.26, $p = 0.003$). MAGE demonstrated positive correlations with IL-1β (r = 0.19, $p = 0.03$), IL-12 p70 (r = 0.29, $p = 0.0008$), MCP-1 (r = 0.21, $p = 0.02$), RANTES (r = 0.27, $p = 0.02$), and SDF-1α (r = 0.21, $p = 0.02$). There were negative correlations between MAGE and IL-8 (r = −0.19, $p = 0.03$), IL-10 (r = −0.22, $p = 0.01$), and MIF (r = −0.25, $p = 0.004$). MAG showed positive correlations with IL-12 p70 (r = 0.39, $p < 0.0001$), MCP-1 (r = 0.31, $p = 0.0003$), and SDF-1α (r = 0.26, $p = 0.003$).

3.5. Serum Concentrations of Cytokines and Growth Factors in Subjects with T1D: Other Relationships

In the panel of studied molecules, IL-1β, MCP-3, and TNF-α only showed weak positive correlations with HbA1c (r = 0.23, $p = 0.008$; r = 0.19, $p = 0.03$; r = 0.21, $p = 0.02$, respectively). Additionally, IL-1β, IL-2Rα, and IL-16 demonstrated negative correlations with C-peptide (r = −0.25, $p = 0.004$; r = −0.19, $p = 0.03$; r = −0.26, $p = 0.003$, respectively). None of the cytokines were associated with age.

Patients with BMI ≥ 25 kg/m^2 when compared to those with BMI < 25 kg/m^2 demonstrated higher levels of IL-1β (3.9, 3.0–4.4 vs. 3.3, 2.5–3.9 pg/mL, $p = 0.003$), IL-12 p70 (7.0, 3.9–13.7 vs. 4.1, 2.7–5.7 pg/mL, $p = 0.005$), IP-10 (257, 7.5–490 vs. 88, 4.5–372 pg/mL, $p = 0.03$), LIF (26.5, 8.6–59.3 vs. 8.6, 0–49.4 pg/mL, $p = 0.006$), MCP-3 (6.0, 0–6.8 vs. 1.0, 0–6.2 pg/mL, $p = 0.02$), β-NGF (0, 0–1.9 vs. 1.4, 0–4.7 pg/mL, $p = 0.002$), and TNF-α (7.4, 3.0–75 vs. 4.8, 0.56–54 pg/mL, $p = 0.02$) and lower levels of IL-10 (4.3, 2.9–5.3 vs. 5.2, 3.8–6.0 pg/mL, $p = 0.049$). Other cytokines did not demonstrate statistically significant differences (data are not shown). BMI correlated positively with IL-1β (r = 0.20, $p = 0.02$), IL-16 (r = 0.23, $p = 0.008$), IP-10 (r = 0.20, $p = 0.02$), LIF (r = 0.19, $p = 0.03$), MCP-3 (r = 0.20, $p = 0.02$), and β-NGF (r = 0.21, $p = 0.02$). There was a negative correlation between BMI and IL-10 (r = −0.20, $p = 0.02$).

3.6. Multiple Regression Models

In logistic regression models, the levels of IL-1β, IL-4, IL-10, IL-12 (p70), GM-CSF, HGF, MCP-3, MIF, and TNF-α were associated with TIR ≤ 70% (Table 5). All these molecules, excluding MIF, demonstrated significant associations with TIR ≤ 70% after adjustments for age, sex, BMI, diabetes duration, and eGFR. The concentrations of MIF and PDGF-BB were associated with CV ≥ 36%.

Table 5. Serum cytokines and growth factors associated with TIR ≤ 70% and CV ≥ 36% in subjects with T1D.

Molecule	Crude OR (95% CI), *p*-Value	Adjusted OR (95% CI), *p*-Value
	TIR ≤ 70%	
IL-1β, 1 pg/mL	1.78 (1.18–2.67), $p = 0.006$	1.69 (1.12–2.55), $p = 0.01$
IL-4, 1 pg/mL	0.82 (0.71–0.95), $p = 0.007$	0.82 (0.7–0.96), $p = 0.01$
IL-10, 1 pg/mL	0.7 (0.56–0.89), $p = 0.003$	0.73 (0.56–0.94), $p = 0.01$
IL-12 (p70), 1 pg/mL	1.08 (1.02–1.15), $p = 0.006$	1.08 (1.01–1.15), $p = 0.02$
MCP-3, 1 pg/mL	1.16 (1.04–1.29), $p = 0.006$	1.14 (1.02–1.28), $p = 0.03$
MIF, 100 pg/mL	0.76 (0.6–0.97), $p = 0.03$	0.79 (0.62–1.01), $p = 0.06$
TNF-α, 10 pg/mL	1.14 (1.03–1.27), $p = 0.01$	1.12 (1–1.25), $p = 0.04$
GM-CSF, 1 pg/mL	0.82 (0.72–0.94), $p = 0.005$	0.84 (0.73–0.97), $p = 0.02$
HGF, 100 pg/mL	1.21 (1.02–1.44), $p = 0.03$	1.23 (1.02–1.47), $p = 0.03$
	CV ≥ 36%	
MIF, 100 pg/mL	0.78 (0.62–0.99), $p = 0.04$	0.78 (0.61–0.99), $p = 0.04$
PDGF-BB, 1000 pg/mL	1.56 (1.05–2.32), $p = 0.03$	1.58 (1.05–2.37), $p = 0.03$

Logistic regression models. Adjustment to age, sex, BMI, diabetes duration, and eGFR. CV, coefficient of variation; T1D, type 1 diabetes; TIR, time in range.

4. Discussion

In this study, we assessed serum levels of 44 cytokines and growth factors that are discussed as mediators of diabetic complications in subjects with T1D depending on CGM-derived TIRs and GV metrics. To determine the circulating regulators, we used multiplex analysis, or multiplex bead array assay. This method makes it possible to simultaneously determine a large number of biomarkers in one biological sample [20,21]. Moreover, we performed a comprehensive analysis of the GV [10,27] that included an assessment of time-dependent parameters (TIR, TAR L1, TAR L2, TBR L1, TBR L2), the dispersion of glucose values (CV), the amplitude of glucose fluctuations (MAGE), and the rate of glucose changes (MAG).

The results demonstrate significant changes in the levels of the studied regulators in subjects with T1D as compared with normoglycemic individuals. In particular, we recorded an increase in the levels of pro-inflammatory cytokines (IL-1β, IL-6, IL-12 p70, IL-16, IL-17A, IFN-γ, TNF-α), monocyte chemoattractant proteins (MCP-1, MCP-3), a depletion of an anti-inflammatory cytokine (IL-4), an imbalance among hematopoietic growth factors (IL-3, IL-7, M-CSF, GM-CSF), and changes in the concentrations of other regulators of the immune system and cell differentiation (IL-1α, IL-1Ra, IL-2Rα, IFN-α2, LIF). In general, these findings are consistent with the literature data on an increase in the levels of circulating IL-1β [28–30], IL-6 [29,31,32], IL-12 [29], IL-17A [30,33], IFN-γ [32,34], MCP-1 [29,35], TNF-α [28,29,32,36], and a decrease in IL-4 concentrations [37] in patients with T1D. However, decreased concentrations of IL-6 [28] and MCP-1 [38,39] in T1D patients were also reported. Other authors demonstrated no differences between healthy individuals and people with diabetes in serum IL-4 [40] and MCP-1 [41]. The discrepancies in the data can be explained by the heterogeneity of the included patients in terms of age, diabetes duration, the presence of complications, and the quality of glycemic control.

When interpreting the levels of cytokines in subjects with T1D, the autoimmune nature of the disease should be taken into account. Some studies have matched the levels of circulating cytokines with markers of the autoimmune process in patients with T1D. It was reported that children with one or two diabetes-related antibodies (IA-2 and/or GAD65) have significantly higher levels of IL-1β and IL-2 and lower levels of IL-4 than children with diabetes who were negative for these markers [40]. In patients with recent-onset T1D, an increase in IL-18 and decrease in MIF and MCP-1 levels were associated with IA-2 and GAD65 antibody positivity [42]. Another study showed a dependency of accelerated autoimmunity and beta cell destruction on increased IFN-γ, IL-12, and IL-17 and decreased IL-4, IL-6, and IL-13 in pediatric patients with T1D [37]. The onset of T1D in children was characterized by the upregulation of GM-CSF, IL-1β, IL-7, IL-8, IL-10, IL-17F, IL-21, IL-23, and IL-27, but not IL-6 or TNF-α; the presence of autoantibodies (anti-IA-2 and -ZnT8) influenced the blood cytokine levels [43]. In this study, we did not test patients for autoimmune markers of diabetes but assessed fasting C-peptide levels. Though we found negative correlations between fasting C-peptide and IL-1β, IL-2Rα, and IL-16 concentrations, it should be emphasized that the majority of patients in our study had long-term diabetes with undetectable beta-cell function. Therefore, the autoimmune process hardly played a significant role in changing the cytokine profile in our cohort.

The greatest changes in the levels of the studied molecules were revealed in patients with TIR values < 70%. Compared to individuals with target TIR, these patients showed higher concentrations of IL-1β, IL-1Ra, IL-2Rα, IL-3, IL-6, IL-7, IL-12 p70, IL-16, IL-17A, G-CSF, M-CSF, IFN-γ, MCP-1, MCP-3, TNF-α, TNF-β, SCF, and HGF, and lower levels of IL-1α, IL-4, IL-8, IL-10, GM-CSF, and MIF. Associations of IL-1β, IL-4, IL-10, IL-12 (p70), GM-CSF, HGF, MCP-3, and TNF-α with target TIR were confirmed in a multivariate logistic analysis. It is interesting to note that many of the studied molecules showed associations with TIR, but not with HbA1c. Naturally, TIR reflects glucose levels over a much shorter period than HbA1c. Therefore, it can be hypothesized that recent glucose fluctuations may have a greater impact on cytokine production than long-term glycemic control. Our data on the associations of TIR with the levels of important biological regulators represent another argument for the widespread use of TIR in assessing glycemic control in people with diabetes.

Most of the TIR-associated molecules also showed correlations with TAR L1 and TAR L2. This is consistent with the literature data on the pro-inflammatory effect of hyperglycemia in diabetes. In vitro experiments showed a stimulating effect of high glucose on the production of principal proinflammatory cytokines in cultured human mononuclear cells [44–46], B cells [47], human umbilical vein endothelial cells [48], aortic endothelial cells [49], glomerular endothelial cells [50], cardiomyocytes [51], and beta cells [52]. According to these data, a high glucose level increases the secretion of IL-1β [46,50,52], IL-6 [46,51], IL-12 [44], IFN-γ [46], TNF-α [45,46,49,51], MCP-1 [48,49], and other proinflammatory cytokines. These findings are consistent with our results. Moreover, we found a depletion in the levels of anti-inflammatory cytokines (IL-4, IL-10) in patients with non-target TIR, which confirmed the imbalance between inflammatory and anti-inflammatory cytokines under hyperglycemic conditions.

In our study, many molecules were associated with time-dependent parameters reflecting hyperglycemic fluctuations (TAR L1 and TAR L2), and some molecules (IL-1β, IL-8, IL-12 p70, MCP-1, RANTES, MIF, SDF-1α) demonstrated correlation(s) with at least one amplitude-dependent GV metric (CV, MAGE, and/or MAG indices). It has previously been shown that intermittently high glucose enhances the secretion of IL-6 and TNF-α by activated monocytes [53]. Moreover, it has been demonstrated that glucose oscillations stimulate IL-6 production in endothelial cells to a greater extent than persistently high glucose [54,55]. Similarly, acute glucose fluctuations were a more potent inducer of IL-1β and TNF-α in rat podocytes than constantly high glucose [56]. In adipocytes, oscillating glucose induced a greater increase in MCP-1 secretion than constantly high glucose [57]. In rats, blood glucose fluctuations induced by intermittent glucose infusions increased the expression of IL-6 and TNF-α in vascular endothelial cells [58]. Therefore, the effect of hyperglycemia on cytokine synthesis may be exacerbated by that of GV.

Hypoglycemia may act as an additional trigger of inflammation in individuals with high GV. In cultured macrophages, intermittent episodes of hypoglycemia and hyperglycemia promote M1 polarization and enhance IL-1β, TNF-α, IL-6, and MCP-1 secretion [59]. In healthy individuals and those with T1D, hypoglycemia promotes leukocyte mobilization into the bloodstream and induces proinflammatory changes in these cells [60]. In individuals with T1D, an episode of two-hour hypoglycemia was followed by an increase in the levels of IL-6 [61]. High blood glucose, replacing hypoglycemia, caused a further increase in the concentrations of IL-6 [62]. Contrary to these data, we found weak negative correlations between TBR and some studied cytokines. This can be explained by associations of these molecules with TIR and TAR, which are in reciprocal relationships in TBR. It should also be noted that all hypoglycemic episodes in our study were non-severe and may not have affected cytokine levels.

When discussing possible confounders affecting cytokine levels in patients with T1D, BMI should be taken into account [63]. The prevalence of obesity among people with T1D is increasing [64] and nearly a quarter of T1D patients are affected by metabolic syndrome [65]. In our study, patients with excessive BMI had higher levels of IL-1β, IL-12 p70, IP-10, LIF, MCP-3, β-NGF, and TNF-α, and lower levels of IL-10. However, associations of IL-1β, IL-10, IL-12 p70, MCP-3, and TNF-α with TIR remained significant after adjustment to BMI, as well as other possible confounders (age, sex, diabetes duration, and eGFR). This demonstrates an independent association of excessive glucose oscillations with the changes in cytokine levels.

Our study is not without limitations. The recruitment of patients in one center could lead to some bias in the sample selection. A cross-sectional design does not prove the causality. The CGM duration was rather short. However, to the best of our knowledge, this is the first study that examined a panel of circulating cytokines and growth factors depending on GV parameters in T1D patients. The strengths of the study are a comprehensive analysis of GV with time-dependent and amplitude-dependent metrics and a determination of the relationship of these parameters with the levels of a large number of cytokines and growth factors. As a result, we have identified the regulators most associated with off-target glucose values and GV. Further studies are needed to explore the effect of glucose fluctuations on their production and signaling. At the same time, identified molecules can be considered to be perspective biomarkers of GV-related immune dysfunction in T1D.

5. Conclusions

Subjects with T1D demonstrated an increase in serum concentrations of IL-1β, IL-1Ra, IL-2Rα, IL-3, IL-6, IL-7, IL-12 p40, IL-16, IL-17A, LIF, M-CSF, IFN-α2, IFN-γ, MCP-1, MCP-3, and TNF-α compared to normoglycemic individuals. The changes in the levels of these cytokines and growth factors are related to the time-dependent and amplitude-dependent GV characteristics. Specifically, the levels of IL-1β, IL-10, IL-12 p70, IL-16, MCP-1, MCP-3, RANTES, TNF-α, SCF, and MIF are associated with TAR, while IL-1β, IL-8, IL-12 p70, MCP-1, RANTES, MIF, and SDF-1α show association with at least one amplitude-dependent GV parameter (CV, MAGE, and MAG). Therefore, the pro-inflammatory effect of hyperglycemia and GV in diabetes may be realized through the shifts in cytokine and chemokine production. The study results provide further support for the notion that GV may be a therapeutic target in the management of diabetes.

Author Contributions: Conceptualization, V.V.K.; methodology, V.V.K.; software, J.F.S.; formal analysis, V.V.K., K.R.M. and A.I.K.; investigation, K.R.M., N.B.O. and J.F.S.; visualization—A.I.K.; resources, V.V.K.; data curation, J.F.S. and A.I.K.; writing—original draft preparation, V.V.K. and K.R.M.; writing—review and editing, V.V.K.; supervision, V.V.K.; project administration, V.V.K.; funding acquisition, V.V.K. All authors have read and agreed to the published version of the manuscript.

Funding: This study was funded by the Russian Science Foundation (grant 20-15-00057-П).

Institutional Review Board Statement: The study protocol was approved by the Ethical Committee of RICEL—Branch of IC&G SB RAS (Approval: 158, 1 June 2020).

Informed Consent Statement: Informed consent was obtained from all subjects involved in the study.

Data Availability Statement: The data that support the findings of this study are available from the corresponding author [V.V.K.] upon reasonable request.

Conflicts of Interest: The authors declare no conflict of interest.

References

1. Gregory, G.A.; Robinson, T.I.G.; Linklater, S.E.; Wang, F.; Colagiuri, S.; De Beaufort, C.; Donaghue, K.C.; Magliano, D.J.; Maniam, J.; Orchard, T.J.; et al. Global Incidence, Prevalence, and Mortality of Type 1 Diabetes in 2021 with Projection to 2040: A Modelling Study. *Lancet Diabetes Endocrinol.* **2022**, *10*, 741–760. [CrossRef] [PubMed]
2. Garofolo, M.; Gualdani, E.; Giannarelli, R.; Aragona, M.; Campi, F.; Lucchesi, D.; Daniele, G.; Miccoli, R.; Francesconi, P.; Del Prato, S.; et al. Microvascular Complications Burden (Nephropathy, Retinopathy and Peripheral Polyneuropathy) Affects Risk of Major Vascular Events and All-Cause Mortality in Type 1 Diabetes: A 10-Year Follow-up Study. *Cardiovasc. Diabetol.* **2019**, *18*, 159. [CrossRef] [PubMed]
3. Bjerg, L.; Gudbjörnsdottir, S.; Franzén, S.; Carstensen, B.; Witte, D.R.; Jørgensen, M.E.; Svensson, A.-M. Duration of Diabetes-Related Complications and Mortality in Type 1 Diabetes: A National Cohort Study. *Int. J. Epidemiol.* **2021**, *50*, 1250–1259. [CrossRef]
4. Bebu, I.; Braffett, B.H.; De Boer, I.H.; Aiello, L.P.; Bantle, J.P.; Lorenzi, G.M.; Herman, W.H.; Gubitosi-Klug, R.A.; Perkins, B.A.; Lachin, J.M.; et al. Relationships Between the Cumulative Incidences of Long-Term Complications in Type 1 Diabetes: The DCCT/EDIC Study. *Diabetes Care* **2023**, *46*, 361–368. [CrossRef]
5. Diabetes Control and Complications Trial Research Group; Nathan, D.M.; Genuth, S.; Lachin, J.; Cleary, P.; Crofford, O.; Davis, M.; Rand, L.; Siebert, C. The Effect of Intensive Treatment of Diabetes on the Development and Progression of Long-Term Complications in Insulin-Dependent Diabetes Mellitus. *N. Engl. J. Med.* **1993**, *329*, 977–986. [CrossRef]
6. The Diabetes Control and Complications Trial (DCCT)/Epidemiology of Diabetes Interventions and Complications (EDIC) Study Research Group. Intensive Diabetes Treatment and Cardiovascular Outcomes in Type 1 Diabetes: The DCCT/EDIC Study 30-Year Follow-Up. *Diabetes Care* **2016**, *39*, 686–693. [CrossRef]
7. Helmink, M.A.G.; Hageman, S.H.J.; Visseren, F.L.J.; De Ranitz-Greven, W.L.; De Valk, H.W.; Van Sloten, T.T.; Westerink, J. Variability in Benefit from Intensive Insulin Therapy on Cardiovascular Events in Individuals with Type 1 Diabetes: A Post Hoc Analysis of the DCCT/EDIC Study. *Diabet. Med.* **2023**, *40*, e15183. [CrossRef]

8. Goth, A.; Lengyel, L.; Nadasdi, N.; Savely, C. Renal Lesions Due to Fluctuations in Blood Sugar Levels. *Acta Med. Scand.* **1957**, *158*, 475–480. [CrossRef] [PubMed]
9. Kovatchev, B. Glycemic Variability: Risk Factors, Assessment, and Control. *J. Diabetes Sci. Technol.* **2019**, *13*, 627–635. [CrossRef]
10. Sun, B.; Luo, Z.; Zhou, J. Comprehensive Elaboration of Glycemic Variability in Diabetic Macrovascular and Microvascular Complications. *Cardiovasc. Diabetol.* **2021**, *20*, 9. [CrossRef]
11. Wadén, J.; Forsblom, C.; Thorn, L.M.; Gordin, D.; Saraheimo, M.; Groop, P.-H.; Finnish Diabetic Nephropathy Study Group A1C. Variability Predicts Incident Cardiovascular Events, Microalbuminuria, and Overt Diabetic Nephropathy in Patients with Type 1 Diabetes. *Diabetes* **2009**, *58*, 2649–2655. [CrossRef]
12. Li, F.; Zhang, L.; Shen, Y.; Liu, H.-H.; Zhang, Z.-Y.; Hu, G.; Wang, R.-X. Higher Glucose Fluctuation Is Associated with a Higher Risk of Cardiovascular Disease: Insights from Pooled Results among Patients with Diabetes. *J. Diabetes* **2023**, *15*, 368–381. [CrossRef]
13. Battelino, T.; Danne, T.; Bergenstal, R.M.; Amiel, S.A.; Beck, R.; Biester, T.; Bosi, E.; Buckingham, B.A.; Cefalu, W.T.; Close, K.L.; et al. Clinical Targets for Continuous Glucose Monitoring Data Interpretation: Recommendations From the International Consensus on Time in Range. *Diabetes Care* **2019**, *42*, 1593–1603. [CrossRef]
14. El Malahi, A.; Van Elsen, M.; Charleer, S.; Dirinck, E.; Ledeganck, K.; Keymeulen, B.; Crenier, L.; Radermecker, R.; Taes, Y.; Vercammen, C.; et al. Relationship Between Time in Range, Glycemic Variability, HbA1c, and Complications in Adults with Type 1 Diabetes Mellitus. *J. Clin. Endocrinol. Metab.* **2022**, *107*, e570–e581. [CrossRef]
15. Ranjan, A.G.; Rosenlund, S.V.; Hansen, T.W.; Rossing, P.; Andersen, S.; Nørgaard, K. Improved Time in Range Over 1 Year Is Associated With Reduced Albuminuria in Individuals With Sensor-Augmented Insulin Pump-Treated Type 1 Diabetes. *Diabetes Care* **2020**, *43*, 2882–2885. [CrossRef]
16. Šoupal, J.; Škrha, J., Jr.; Fajmon, M.; Horová, E.; Mráz, M.; Škrha, J.; Prázný, M. Glycemic variability is higher in type 1 diabetes patients with microvascular complications irrespective of glycemic control. *Diabetes Technol. Ther.* **2014**, *16*, 198–203. [CrossRef]
17. Naaman, S.H.; Mizrak, H.I.; Lind, N.; Laursen, J.C.; Kufaishi, H.; Christensen, M.M.B.; Ranjan, A.G.; Nørgaard, K.; Hansen, C.S. Cardiovascular Autonomic Neuropathy Is Associated With Increased Glucose Variability in People With Type 1 Diabetes. *Diabetes Care* **2022**, *45*, 2461–2465. [CrossRef]
18. Saik, O.V.; Klimontov, V.V. Bioinformatic Reconstruction and Analysis of Gene Networks Related to Glucose Variability in Diabetes and Its Complications. *Int. J. Mol. Sci.* **2020**, *21*, 8691. [CrossRef]
19. Klimontov, V.V.; Saik, O.V.; Korbut, A.I. Glucose Variability: How Does It Work? *Int. J. Mol. Sci.* **2021**, *22*, 7783. [CrossRef]
20. Capone, F.; Guerriero, E.; Sorice, A.; Colonna, G.; Ciliberto, G.; Costantini, S. Serum Cytokinome Profile Evaluation: A Tool to Define New Diagnostic and Prognostic Markers of Cancer Using Multiplexed Bead-Based Immunoassays. *Mediat. Inflamm.* **2016**, *2016*, 3064643. [CrossRef]
21. Zhang, Y.; Li, X.; Di, Y.P. Fast and efficient measurement of clinical and biological samples using immunoassay-based multiplexing systems. *Methods Mol. Biol.* **2020**, *2102*, 129–147. [CrossRef]
22. Chen, H.; Zhang, X.; Liao, N.; Wen, F. Assessment of biomarkers using multiplex assays in aqueous humor of patients with diabetic retinopathy. *BMC Ophthalmol.* **2017**, *17*, 176. [CrossRef]
23. Klimontov, V.V.; Korbut, A.I.; Orlov, N.B.; Dashkin, M.V.; Konenkov, V.I. Multiplex Bead Array Assay of a Panel of Circulating Cytokines and Growth Factors in Patients with Albuminuric and Non-AlbuminuricDiabetic Kidney Disease. *J. Clin. Med.* **2020**, *9*, 3006. [CrossRef]
24. Lee, M.Y.; Park, S.; Song, J.Y.; Ra, H.; Baek, J.U.; Baek, J. Inflammatory cytokines and retinal nonperfusion area in quiescent proliferative diabetic retinopathy. *Cytokine* **2022**, *154*, 155774. [CrossRef]
25. Danne, T.; Nimri, R.; Battelino, T.; Bergenstal, R.M.; Close, K.L.; DeVries, J.H.; Garg, S.; Heinemann, L.; Hirsch, I.; Amiel, S.A.; et al. International Consensus on Use of Continuous Glucose Monitoring. *Diabetes Care* **2017**, *40*, 1631–1640. [CrossRef]
26. Hill, N.R.; Oliver, N.S.; Choudhary, P.; Levy, J.C.; Hindmarsh, P.; Matthews, D.R. Normal Reference Range for Mean Tissue Glucose and Glycemic Variability Derived from Continuous Glucose Monitoring for Subjects without Diabetes in Different Ethnic Groups. *Diabetes Technol. Ther.* **2011**, *13*, 921–928. [CrossRef]
27. Kovatchev, B.; Cobelli, C. Glucose Variability: Timing, Risk Analysis, and Relationship to Hypoglycemia in Diabetes. *Diabetes Care* **2016**, *39*, 502–510. [CrossRef]
28. Dogan, Y.; Akarsu, S.; Ustundag, B.; Yilmaz, E.; Gurgoze, M.K. Serum IL-1beta, IL-2, and IL-6 in Insulin-Dependent Diabetic Children. *Mediat. Inflamm.* **2006**, *2006*, 59206. [CrossRef]
29. Gabbay, M.A.L.; Sato, M.N.; Duarte, A.J.S.; Dib, S.A. Serum Titres of Anti-Glutamic Acid Decarboxylase-65 and Anti-IA-2 Autoantibodies Are Associated with Different Immunoregulatory Milieu in Newly Diagnosed Type 1 Diabetes Patients. *Clin. Exp. Immunol.* **2012**, *168*, 60–67. [CrossRef]
30. Fatima, N.; Faisal, S.M.; Zubair, S.; Ajmal, M.; Siddiqui, S.S.; Moin, S.; Owais, M. Role of Pro-Inflammatory Cytokines and Biochemical Markers in the Pathogenesis of Type 1 Diabetes: Correlation with Age and Glycemic Condition in Diabetic Human Subjects. *PLoS ONE* **2016**, *11*, e0161548. [CrossRef]
31. Chen, Y.-L.; Qiao, Y.-C.; Pan, Y.-H.; Xu, Y.; Huang, Y.-C.; Wang, Y.-H.; Geng, L.-J.; Zhao, H.-L.; Zhang, X.-X. Correlation between Serum Interleukin-6 Level and Type 1 Diabetes Mellitus: A Systematic Review and Meta-Analysis. *Cytokine* **2017**, *94*, 14–20. [CrossRef]

32. Tangjittipokin, W.; Umjai, P.; Khemaprasit, K.; Charoentawornpanich, P.; Chanprasert, C.; Teerawattanapong, N.; Narkdontri, T.; Santiprabhob, J. Vitamin D Pathway Gene Polymorphisms, Vitamin D Level, and Cytokines in Children with Type 1 Diabetes. *Gene* **2021**, *791*, 145691. [CrossRef] [PubMed]
33. Li, J.; Xu, L.; Zhao, W.; Pan, J.; Lu, J.; Lu, H.; Yan, J.; Weng, J.; Liu, F. Serum IL-17A Concentration and a IL17RA Single Nucleotide Polymorphism Contribute to the Risk of Autoimmune Type 1 Diabetes. *Diabetes Metab. Res. Rev.* **2022**, *38*, e3547. [CrossRef] [PubMed]
34. Alizadeh, B.Z.; Hanifi-Moghaddam, P.; Eerligh, P.; van der Slik, A.R.; Kolb, H.; Kharagjitsingh, A.V.; Pereira Arias, A.M.; Ronkainen, M.; Knip, M.; Bonfanti, R.; et al. Association of Interferon-Gamma and Interleukin 10 Genotypes and Serum Levels with Partial Clinical Remission in Type 1 Diabetes. *Clin. Exp. Immunol.* **2006**, *145*, 480–484. [CrossRef]
35. Ismail, N.A.; Abd El Baky, A.N.; Ragab, S.; Hamed, M.; Hashish, M.A.; Shehata, A. Monocyte Chemoattractant Protein 1 and Macrophage Migration Inhibitory Factor in Children with Type 1 Diabetes. *J. Pediatr. Endocrinol. Metab.* **2016**, *29*, 641–645. [CrossRef]
36. Qiao, Y.-C.; Chen, Y.-L.; Pan, Y.-H.; Tian, F.; Xu, Y.; Zhang, X.-X.; Zhao, H.-L. The Change of Serum Tumor Necrosis Factor Alpha in Patients with Type 1 Diabetes Mellitus: A Systematic Review and Meta-Analysis. *PLoS ONE* **2017**, *12*, e0176157. [CrossRef] [PubMed]
37. Abdel-Latif, M.; Abdel-Moneim, A.A.; El-Hefnawy, M.H.; Khalil, R.G. Comparative and Correlative Assessments of Cytokine, Complement and Antibody Patterns in Paediatric Type 1 Diabetes. *Clin. Exp. Immunol.* **2017**, *190*, 110–121. [CrossRef]
38. Jamali, Z.; Nazari, M.; Khoramdelazad, H.; Hakimizadeh, E.; Mahmoodi, M.; Karimabad, M.N.; Hassanshahi, G.; Rezaeian, M.; Balaei, P.; Darakhshan, S.; et al. Expression of CC Chemokines CCL2, CCL5, and CCL11 Is Associated with Duration of Disease and Complications in Type-1 Diabetes: A Study on Iranian Diabetic Patients. *Clin. Lab.* **2013**, *59*, 993–1001. [CrossRef]
39. Purohit, S.; Sharma, A.; Hopkins, D.; Steed, L.; Bode, B.; Anderson, S.W.; Reed, J.C.; Steed, R.D.; Yang, T.; She, J.-X. Large-Scale Discovery and Validation Studies Demonstrate Significant Reductions in Circulating Levels of IL8, IL-1Ra, MCP-1, and MIP-1β in Patients With Type 1 Diabetes. *J. Clin. Endocrinol. Metab.* **2015**, *100*, E1179–E1187. [CrossRef]
40. Pérez, F.; Oyarzún, A.; Carrasco, E.; Angel, B.; Albala, C.; Santos, J.L. Plasma levels of interleukin-1beta, interleukin-2 and interleukin-4 in recently diagnosed type 1 diabetic children and their association with beta-pancreatic autoantibodies. *Rev. Med. Chil.* **2004**, *132*, 413–420. [CrossRef]
41. Antonelli, A.; Fallahi, P.; Ferrari, S.M.; Pupilli, C.; d'Annunzio, G.; Lorini, R.; Vanelli, M.; Ferrannini, E. Serum Th1 (CXCL10) and Th2 (CCL2) Chemokine Levels in Children with Newly Diagnosed Type 1 Diabetes: A Longitudinal Study. *Diabet Med.* **2008**, *25*, 1349–1353. [CrossRef] [PubMed]
42. Hanifi-Moghaddam, P.; Schloot, N.C.; Kappler, S.; Seissler, J.; Kolb, H. An Association of Autoantibody Status and Serum Cytokine Levels in Type 1 Diabetes. *Diabetes* **2003**, *52*, 1137–1142. [CrossRef] [PubMed]
43. Alnek, K.; Kisand, K.; Heilman, K.; Peet, A.; Varik, K.; Uibo, R. Increased Blood Levels of Growth Factors, Proinflammatory Cytokines, and Th17 Cytokines in Patients with Newly Diagnosed Type 1 Diabetes. *PLoS ONE* **2015**, *10*, e0142976. [CrossRef]
44. Wu, H.-P.; Kuo, S.-F.; Wu, S.-Y.; Chuang, D.-Y. High Interleukin-12 Production from Stimulated Peripheral Blood Mononuclear Cells of Type 2 Diabetes Patients. *Cytokine* **2010**, *51*, 298–304. [CrossRef]
45. Gonzalez, Y.; Herrera, M.T.; Soldevila, G.; Garcia-Garcia, L.; Fabián, G.; Pérez-Armendariz, E.M.; Bobadilla, K.; Guzmán-Beltrán, S.; Sada, E.; Torres, M. High Glucose Concentrations Induce TNF-α Production through the down-Regulation of CD33 in Primary Human Monocytes. *BMC Immunol.* **2012**, *13*, 19. [CrossRef] [PubMed]
46. Hu, R.; Xia, C.-Q.; Butfiloski, E.; Clare-Salzler, M. Effect of High Glucose on Cytokine Production by Human Peripheral Blood Immune Cells and Type I Interferon Signaling in Monocytes: Implications for the Role of Hyperglycemia in the Diabetes Inflammatory Process and Host Defense against Infection. *Clin. Immunol.* **2018**, *195*, 139–148. [CrossRef] [PubMed]
47. Li, Z.; Zhao, M.; Li, J.; Luo, W.; Huang, J.; Huang, G.; Xie, Z.; Xiao, Y.; Huang, J.; Li, X.; et al. Elevated Glucose Metabolism Driving Pro-Inflammatory Response in B Cells Contributes to the Progression of Type 1 Diabetes. *Clin. Immunol.* **2023**, *255*, 109729. [CrossRef]
48. Wu, M.; Wu, Y.; Xu, K.; Lin, L. Protective Effects of 1,25 Dihydroxyvitamin D3 against High-Glucose-Induced Damage in Human Umbilical Vein Endothelial Cells Involve Activation of Nrf2 Antioxidant Signaling. *J. Vasc. Res.* **2021**, *58*, 267–276. [CrossRef]
49. Zhang, M.; Jin, X.; Zhang, Z.; Li, B.; Yang, G. Vildagliptin Protects Endothelial Cells against High Glucose-Induced Damage. *Biomed. Pharmacother.* **2018**, *108*, 1790–1796. [CrossRef]
50. Xu, L.; Shao, F. Sitagliptin Protects Renal Glomerular Endothelial Cells against High Glucose-Induced Dysfunction and Injury. *Bioengineered* **2022**, *13*, 655–666. [CrossRef]
51. Cheng, G.; Li, L. High-Glucose-Induced Apoptosis, ROS Production and pro-Inflammatory Response in Cardiomyocytes Is Attenuated by Metformin Treatment via PP2A Activation. *J. Biosci.* **2020**, *45*, 126. [CrossRef]
52. Maedler, K.; Sergeev, P.; Ris, F.; Oberholzer, J.; Joller-Jemelka, H.I.; Spinas, G.A.; Kaiser, N.; Halban, P.A.; Donath, M.Y. Glucose-Induced Beta Cell Production of IL-1beta Contributes to Glucotoxicity in Human Pancreatic Islets. *J. Clin. Investig.* **2002**, *110*, 851–860. [CrossRef] [PubMed]
53. Li-Bo, Y.; Wen-Bo, Q.; Xiao-Hong, L.; You-Lun, F.; Tie, Z. Intermittent High Glucose Promotes Expression of Proinflammatory Cytokines in Monocytes. *Inflamm. Res.* **2011**, *60*, 367–370. [CrossRef] [PubMed]

54. Piconi, L.; Quagliaro, L.; Assaloni, R.; Da Ros, R.; Maier, A.; Zuodar, G.; Ceriello, A. Constant and Intermittent High Glucose Enhances Endothelial Cell Apoptosis through Mitochondrial Superoxide Overproduction. *Diabetes Metab. Res. Rev.* **2006**, *22*, 198–203. [CrossRef] [PubMed]
55. Quagliaro, L.; Piconi, L.; Assaloni, R.; Da Ros, R.; Maier, A.; Zuodar, G.; Ceriello, A. Intermittent High Glucose Enhances ICAM-1, VCAM-1 and E-Selectin Expression in Human Umbilical Vein Endothelial Cells in Culture: The Distinct Role of Protein Kinase C and Mitochondrial Superoxide Production. *Atherosclerosis* **2005**, *183*, 259–267. [CrossRef]
56. Hu, Z.; Fang, W.; Liu, Y.; Liang, H.; Chen, W.; Wang, H. Acute Glucose Fluctuation Promotes RAGE Expression via Reactive Oxygen Species-mediated NF-κB Activation in Rat Podocytes. *Mol. Med. Rep.* **2021**, *23*, 330. [CrossRef] [PubMed]
57. Sun, J.; Xu, Y.; Dai, Z.; Sun, Y. Intermittent High Glucose Stimulate MCP-l, IL-18, and PAI-1, but Inhibit Adiponectin Expression and Secretion in Adipocytes Dependent of ROS. *Cell Biochem. Biophys.* **2009**, *55*, 173–180. [CrossRef]
58. Wu, N.; Shen, H.; Liu, H.; Wang, Y.; Bai, Y.; Han, P. Acute Blood Glucose Fluctuation Enhances Rat Aorta Endothelial Cell Apoptosis, Oxidative Stress and pro-Inflammatory Cytokine Expression in Vivo. *Cardiovasc. Diabetol.* **2016**, *15*, 109. [CrossRef]
59. Al-Rashed, F.; Sindhu, S.; Arefanian, H.; Al Madhoun, A.; Kochumon, S.; Thomas, R.; Al-Kandari, S.; Alghaith, A.; Jacob, T.; Al-Mulla, F.; et al. Repetitive Intermittent Hyperglycemia Drives the M1 Polarization and Inflammatory Responses in THP-1 Macrophages Through the Mechanism Involving the TLR4-IRF5 Pathway. *Cells* **2020**, *9*, 1892. [CrossRef]
60. Ratter, J.M.; Rooijackers, H.M.M.; Tack, C.J.; Hijmans, A.G.M.; Netea, M.G.; de Galan, B.E.; Stienstra, R. Proinflammatory Effects of Hypoglycemia in Humans With or Without Diabetes. *Diabetes* **2017**, *66*, 1052–1061. [CrossRef] [PubMed]
61. Ceriello, A.; Novials, A.; Ortega, E.; Canivell, S.; La Sala, L.; Pujadas, G.; Esposito, K.; Giugliano, D.; Genovese, S. Glucagon-like Peptide 1 Reduces Endothelial Dysfunction, Inflammation, and Oxidative Stress Induced by Both Hyperglycemia and Hypoglycemia in Type 1 Diabetes. *Diabetes Care* **2013**, *36*, 2346–2350. [CrossRef] [PubMed]
62. Ceriello, A.; Novials, A.; Ortega, E.; Canivell, S.; Pujadas, G.; La Sala, L.; Bucciarelli, L.; Rondinelli, M.; Genovese, S. Vitamin C Further Improves the Protective Effect of GLP-1 on the Ischemia-Reperfusion-like Effect Induced by Hyperglycemia Post-Hypoglycemia in Type 1 Diabetes. *Cardiovasc. Diabetol.* **2013**, *12*, 97. [CrossRef] [PubMed]
63. Fleiner, H.F.; Radtke, M.; Ryan, L.; Moen, T.; Grill, V. Circulating Immune Mediators Are Closely Linked in Adult-Onset Type 1 Diabetes as Well as in Non-Diabetic Subjects. *Autoimmunity* **2014**, *47*, 530–537. [CrossRef] [PubMed]
64. Wallace, A.S.; Chang, A.R.; Shin, J.-I.; Reider, J.; Echouffo-Tcheugui, J.B.; Grams, M.E.; Selvin, E. Obesity and Chronic Kidney Disease in US Adults With Type 1 and Type 2 Diabetes Mellitus. *J. Clin. Endocrinol. Metab.* **2022**, *107*, 1247–1256. [CrossRef] [PubMed]
65. Belete, R.; Ataro, Z.; Abdu, A.; Sheleme, M. Global Prevalence of Metabolic Syndrome among Patients with Type I Diabetes Mellitus: A Systematic Review and Meta-Analysis. *Diabetol. Metab. Syndr.* **2021**, *13*, 25. [CrossRef]

biomedicines

MDPI

Article

The Correlation between Islet β Cell Secretion Function and Gallbladder Stone Disease: A Retrospective Study Based on Chinese Patients with Newly Diagnosed Type 2 Diabetes Mellitus

Tiantian Wu *, Qiang Wang, Changsheng Pu and Keming Zhang

Department of Hepatobiliary Surgery, Peking University International Hospital, Beijing 100001, China; wangqiang1@pkuih.edu.cn (Q.W.); puchangsheng@pkuih.edu.cn (C.P.); zhangkeming@pkuih.edu.cn (K.Z.)
* Correspondence: matthewwu1979@163.com

Abstract: Background: This study aimed to analyze the correlation between islet β cell function and gallbladder stone (GBS) in newly diagnosed type 2 diabetes mellitus (T2DM) patients. Methods: A total of 438 newly diagnosed T2DM patients in Peking University International Hospital from January 2017 to August 2022 were retrospectively analyzed and divided into a non-GBS group and a GBS group. Results: (1) The homeostasis model assessment of the insulin resistance (HOMA-IR) of the GBS group was higher than that of the non-GBS group ($p < 0.05$), while the homeostasis model assessment of β cell (HOMA-β), disposition index (DI0), and Matsuda index of the GBS group were lower than those of the non-GBS group (all $p < 0.05$). (2) For male patients, HOMA-IR is an independent risk factor for GBS (OR = 2.00, 95% CI:1.03, 3.88, $p < 0.05$), and the Matsuda index value is a protective factor for GBS (OR = 0.76, 95% CI:0.60, 0.96, $p < 0.05$). For female patients, HOMA-IR is an independent risk factor for GBS (OR = 2.80, 95% CI:1.03, 7.58, $p < 0.05$) and the Matsuda index value is a protective factor for GBS (OR = 0.59, 95% CI:0.39, 0.90, $p < 0.05$). (3) For male patients, the area under curve (AUC) for predicting GBS was 0.77 (95% CI 0.67, 0.87), with a specificity of 75.26%, a sensitivity of 80.00%, and an accuracy of 75.64%. For female patients, the AUC for predicting GBS was 0.77 (95% CI 0.63, 0.88), with a specificity of 79.63%, a sensitivity of 71.43%, and an accuracy of 78.69%. Conclusions: Insulin resistance may be an independent risk factor for the incidence of GBS in patients with newly diagnosed T2DM, both male or female, which provides a new clinical basis and research direction for the prevention and treatment of GBS in patients with T2DM. This study has established a predictive model of GBS in T2DM and found it to be accurate, thus representing an effective tool for the early prediction of GBS in patients with T2DM.

Keywords: insulin resistance; islet β cell; type 2 diabetes mellitus; gallbladder stone; HbA1c

1. Introduction

Gallbladder stone (GBS) is one of the most common diseases requiring surgery in health care systems. In recent years, with the improvement in people's living standards and the change in eating habits, the incidence of this disease has increased year by year [1,2]. Results have shown that the prevalence of diabetes mellitus (DM) with GBS is about two times that of normal people, and about 1/3 of GBS patients are found to have DM when biliary tract surgery is performed [3,4]. Elmehdawi et al. [5] found that obese and elderly patients with DM were more likely to suffer from GBS and believed that weight, age, and gender were risk factors for diabetes associated with GBS. Early studies believed that diabetes fat metabolism disorder, insulin resistance, and autonomic neuropathy were high-risk factors for the formation of gallstones associated with diabetes. In recent years, there has been some research progress, such as studies on adiponectin, leptin, metabolic syndrome, cholecystokinin (CCK), and so on. The dyslipidemia in patients with DM is characterized by hypertriglyceridemia, lower levels of high-density lipoprotein cholesterol (HDL-C), and higher levels of low-density lipoprotein cholesterol (LDL-C) [6]. DM is complicated with GBS, and its symptoms are closely related to the decline in HDL and the rise in LDL. In addition, due to insulin resistance or insufficient insulin secretion, DM cannot effectively inhibit fat decomposition, and type 2 diabetes mellitus (T2DM) is often accompanied by obesity, hyperinsulinemia, and dyslipidemia, which ultimately leads to an increase in cholesterol synthesized in the liver, an imbalance in the proportion of cholesterol, bile acid and phospholipid in bile, a saturated cholesterol, and poor water solubility, which increases the risk of forming GBS significantly [7].

The clinical manifestations of GBS are severe pain in the upper abdomen or right upper abdomen and radiation to the right shoulder or back, accompanied by nausea and vomiting. If complicated with acute cholecystitis or pancreatitis, there may even be chills and fever. However, most patients with DM have neuropathy, and their sensitivity to pain is reduced. When they have GBS, they always have no obvious symptoms, and once they get sick, they may suffer from gangrene and perforation of gallbladder, or even severe cholangitis and severe pancreatitis. Therefore, exploring the risk factors of GBS in T2DM patients is of great clinical significance to prevent serious complications of GBS in patients with T2DM.

It has been shown that dyslipidemia and diabetic autonomic neuropathy are the highest risk factors of GBS in T2DM patients. At the same time, some studies have shown that the changes in adiponectin, leptin, and cholecystokinin levels in T2DM patients are also closely related to the incidence of GBS. Recent studies have found that [8] the insulin levels of patients with T2DM and GBS are also significantly higher than in those without GBS. However, due to the limitation of sample size and the fact that the islet β cell secretion levels of newly diagnosed patients will be affected by the duration of DM, previous studies cannot truly reflect the relationship between islet β cell secretion function and GBS in T2DM patients. Therefore, the innovation in our study was to explore the relationship between islet β cell secretion function and GBS in newly diagnosed T2DM patients, in order to minimize the bias caused by medication and the duration of T2DM.

In our study, the relationship between insulin resistance and islet β cell secretion function and the incidence of GBS in patients with newly diagnosed T2DM were analyzed to further clarify the influence of islet β cell function on the incidence of GBS and to provide clinical evidence for the prevention and progression of GBS.

2. Materials and Methods

2.1. Ethics Statement

This study was approved by the Ethics Committee of Peking University International Hospital, and all methods were performed in accordance with the relevant guidelines and regulations. Due to the retrospective nature of the study, the Ethics Committee of Peking University International Hospital waived the need to obtain informed consent.

2.2. Research Subjects

This study retrospectively analyzed 438 newly diagnosed T2DM patients from January 2017 to August 2022 in Peking University International Hospital, including 315 males and 123 females, with an average age of 55.49 $\pm$ 13.65 years. All patients met the diagnostic criteria for diabetes issued by the World Health Organization (WHO) in 1999 [9], including: ① typical symptoms of diabetes and random blood glucose $\geq$ 11.1 mmol/L; ② fasting blood glucose $\geq$ 7.0 mmol/L; ③ in the oral glucose tolerance test (OGTT), blood glucose $\geq$ 11.1 mmol/L after taking 75 g glucose for 2 h. If there are no symptoms of diabetes, the above examination should be repeated on another day. If one of the three criteria is then met, the patient is diagnosed as suffering from diabetes and meets the diagnostic criteria for type 2 diabetes according to the clinical classification.

The exclusion criteria of this study were ① patients with type 1 diabetes, gestational diabetes, and other special types of diabetes; ② acute complications of diabetes; ③ patients with severe liver and kidney function diseases; ④ patients who have been diagnosed with GBS in the past; and ⑤ patients with hematological diseases and malignant tumors.

The graphical scheme of the study design is shown below.

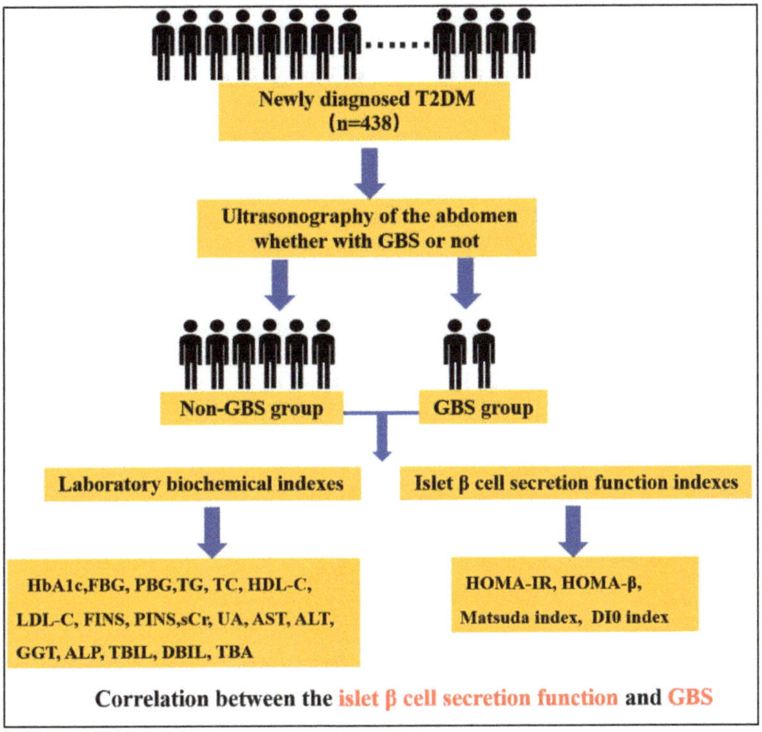

2.3. General Conditions and Clinical Data

The data of 438 patients were retrospectively analyzed, and the general conditions of the patients, including sex, age, height, weight, systolic blood pressure (SBP), and diastolic blood pressure (DBP) were recorded. The body mass index (BMI) was calculated and recorded for the patients: BMI (kg/m^2) = height (kg)/body weight^2 (m^2).

2.4. Laboratory Biochemical Indexes

All subjects were patients with T2DM diagnosed in the outpatient department or in the hospital for the first time. All subjects had had an empty stomach for more than 8 h, and the OGTT was performed in the morning of the next day; the fasting biochemical indexes include glycosylated hemoglobin (HbA1c), fasting blood glucose (FBG), triglyceride (TG), total cholesterol (TC), high-density lipoprotein cholesterol (HDL-C), low-density lipoprotein cholesterol (LDL-C), fasting insulin (FINS), serum creatinine (sCr), uric acid (UA), aspartate aminotransferase (AST), alanine aminotransferase (ALT), gamma-glutamyl transpeptidase (GGT), alkaline phosphatase (ALP), total bilirubin (TBIL), direct bilirubin (DBIL), and total bile acid (TBA). A total of 75 g of glucose powder was then dissolved in 300 mL of warm boiled water and this was drunk within 5 min. Starting from the first sip of glucose, postprandial blood glucose (PBG) and postprandial insulin (PINS) were measured after 2 h. Glomerular filtration rates (eGFR) were calculated based on the sCr of the study subjects. All blood tests were performed at the central laboratory of Peking University International Hospital. FBG, UA, sCr, AST, ALT, GGT, ALP, TBIL, DBIL, and TBA were measured using enzyme-based techniques. HbA1c was determined through high-performance liquid chromatography, and the detection instrument model was Japan Dongcao G8 glycosylated hemoglobin analyzer.

2.5. Islet β Cell Secretion Function Index Evaluation

According to the measurement results, homeostasis model assessment (HOMA) was used to assess insulin sensitivity and insulin resistance, and the homeostasis model assessment of β cell (HOMA–β) was used to evaluate islet β cell secretion function, using the following calculation formula: HOMA-β = FINS × 20/(FBG − 3.5).

The Matsuda index [10] was used to evaluate insulin sensitivity after glucose load, and the following calculation formula was used: Matsuda index = $10{,}000/\sqrt{FINS * FBG * MeanBG * MeanINS}$).

The homeostasis model assessment of insulin resistance (HOMA-IR) was used to evaluate the degree of insulin resistance, and the calculation formula used was as follows: HOMA-IR = FINS × FBG/22.5.

The disposition index (DI0) [11] was used to evaluate the basic islet β cell secretion function after adjustment of HOMA-IR, and the calculation formula was as follows: DI0 = HOMA-β/HOMA-IR.

2.6. Ultrasonography of the Abdomen

All patients were required to fast for more than 12 h before testing. The following morning, a qualified ultrasound physician used an Echolaser X4 (Esaote SpA, Genoa, Italy) color Doppler ultrasound instrument and performed an abdominal ultrasound on each patient. The status of the gallbladder and bile duct were recorded in detail.

The patients were divided into two groups according to the presence of GBS: the GBS group (n = 39) and the normal group (n = 399).

2.7. Statistical Methods

SPSS 22.0 software (IBM, Chicago, IL, USA) was used for statistical analysis. The measurement data of the normal distribution is expressed by mean ± standard deviation (x ± s). The data of non-normal distribution is converted to normal distribution via square root (SQRT) and then analyzed, and t-test was used to compare the normal distribution data between the two groups. The ratio was used to describe counting data, and this study uses the χ2 test to compare counting data between two groups. This study used an unconditional linear regression model to conduct univariate and multivariate analysis of the risk factors for GBS occurrence, as well as calculated odds ratios (OR) and 95% confidence intervals (CI). This study evaluated the predictive and diagnostic abilities of the models by drawing the receiver operating characteristic curve (ROC). All statistical tests were performed as two-sided tests, and a p-value < 0.05 was considered statistically significant.

3. Results

3.1. Comparison of General Conditions and Biochemical Indexes between the Two Groups

Compared with the normal group, the GBS group was older ($p < 0.05$). The GGT of the GBS group was higher than that of the normal group ($p < 0.05$), while the FINS was higher in the GBS group ($p < 0.05$). The SQRTHOMA-IR of the GBS group was higher than that of the normal group ($p < 0.05$), while the SQRTHOMA-β, SQRTDI0, and SQRTMatsuda of the GBS group were lower than that of the normal group ($p < 0.05$, respectively).There were no significant differences in sex, BMI, SBP, DBP, FBG, PBG, HbA1c, AST, ALT, ALP, TC, TG, LDL-C, HDL-C, TBIL, DBIL, TBA, PINS, eGFR, and UA levels between the two groups ($p > 0.05$, respectively) (Table 1).

Table 1. Comparison of general conditions and biochemical indexes between the two groups.

Index	Non-GBS Group	GBS Group	t(χ2)	*p*
	(*n* = 399)	(*n* = 39)		
Age (years)	47.66 ± 14.83	57.13 ± 15.60	−3.83	<0.05
Sex (female%)	109 (27.32%)	14 (35.90%)	1.29	0.26
BMI (kg/m^2)	26.45 ± 4.37	27.29 ± 4.70	−1.12	0.26
SBP (mmHg)	131.28 ± 17.51	133.90 ± 14.10	−0.91	0.37
DBP (mmHg)	81.05 ± 11.87	80.23 ± 10.38	0.42	0.68
AST (U/L)	26.73 ± 9.66	23.72 ± 17.48	1.94	0.08
ALT (U/L)	27.50 ± 10.04	28.96 ± 16.84	−0.99	0.45
GGT (U/L)	32.06 ± 21.48	39.35 ± 32.17	−2.15	<0.05
ALP (U/L)	55.58 ± 14.96	50.85 ± 13.96	1.46	0.41
TBIL (umol/L)	19.35 ± 7.09	23.03 ± 6.54	−1.28	0.65
DBIL (umol/L)	4.39 ± 0.43	4.40 ± 0.54	−0.43	0.85
TBA (umol/L)	4.86 ± 1.09	4.07 ± 1.15	0.78	0.34
TC (mmol/L)	4.60 ± 1.29	4.53 ± 1.57	0.29	0.77
TG (mmol/L)	2.32 ± 1.71	2.15 ± 2.71	1.48	0.14
LDL-C (mmol/L)	2.83 ± 0.92	2.71 ± 1.35	0.69	0.49
HDL-C (mmol/L)	0.94 ± 0.22	0.93 ± 0.22	0.15	0.88
UA (umol/L)	335.90 ± 89.21	324.76 ± 80.23	0.96	0.65
eGFR	103.27 ± 18.69	108.54 ± 18.87	−1.88	0.07
HbA1c (%)	9.47 ± 2.43	10.01 ± 2.32	−1.06	0.29
FBG (mmol/L)	9.26 ± 3.80	9.79 ± 3.83	−0.78	0.44
PBG (mmol/L)	12.23 ± 5.59	11.98 ± 4.18	0.26	0.79
FINS (uU/mL)	14.65 ± 16.06	19.75 ± 7.27	−2.02	<0.05
PINS (uU/mL)	42.76 ± 40.79	46.02 ± 63.28	−1.20	0.24
SQRTHOMA-IR	2.15 ± 0.64	2.50 ± 0.83	−3.23	<0.05
SQRTHOMA-β	8.23 ± 3.81	7.00 ± 3.08	2.33	<0.05
SQRTDI0	4.15 ± 2.36	3.20 ± 1.86	2.45	<0.05
SQRTMatsuda	8.57 ± 2.83	7.00 ± 1.40	3.42	<0.05

Note: BMI is the abbreviation for body mass index, SBP is the abbreviation for systolic blood pressure, DBP is the abbreviation for diastolic blood pressure, FBG is the abbreviation for fasting blood glucose, PBG is the abbreviation for postprandial blood glucose, FINS is the abbreviation for fasting insulin, PINS is the abbreviation for postprandial insulin, HbA1c is the abbreviation for glycosylated hemoglobin, eGFR is the abbreviation for glomerular filtration rates, UA is the abbreviation for uric acid, UACR is the abbreviation for urinary albuminuria creatinine ratio, TC is the abbreviation for total cholesterol, TG is the abbreviation for triglycerides, LDL-C is the abbreviation for low-density lipoprotein cholesterol, HDL-C is the abbreviation for high-density lipoprotein cholesterol, AST is the abbreviation for aspartate aminotransferase, ALT is the abbreviation for alanine aminotransferase, GGT is the abbreviation for gamma-glutamyl transpeptidase, ALP is the abbreviation for alkaline phosphatase, TBIL is the abbreviation for total bilirubin, DBIL is the abbreviation for direct bilirubin, TBA is the abbreviation for total bile acid, SQRTHOMA-IR is the abbreviation for square root of homeostasis model assessment insulin resistance, SQRTHOMA-β is the abbreviation for square root of homeostasis model assessment β, SQRTDI0 is the abbreviation for square root of disposition index, SQRTMatsuda is the abbreviation for square root of Matsuda.

3.2. Comparison of Islet β Cell Function Index Evaluation between the Two Groups

In male patients, the SQRTHOMA-IR of the GBS group was higher than that of the normal group ($p < 0.05$), while the SQRTHOMA-β, SQRTDI0, and SQRTMatsuda of the GBS group were lower than those of the normal group ($p < 0.05$, respectively).

In female patients, the SQRTHOMA-IR of the GBS group was higher than that of the normal group ($p < 0.05$), while the SQRTHOMA-β, SQRTDI0, and SQRTMatsuda of the GBS group were lower than those of the normal group ($p < 0.05$, respectively) (Figure 1).

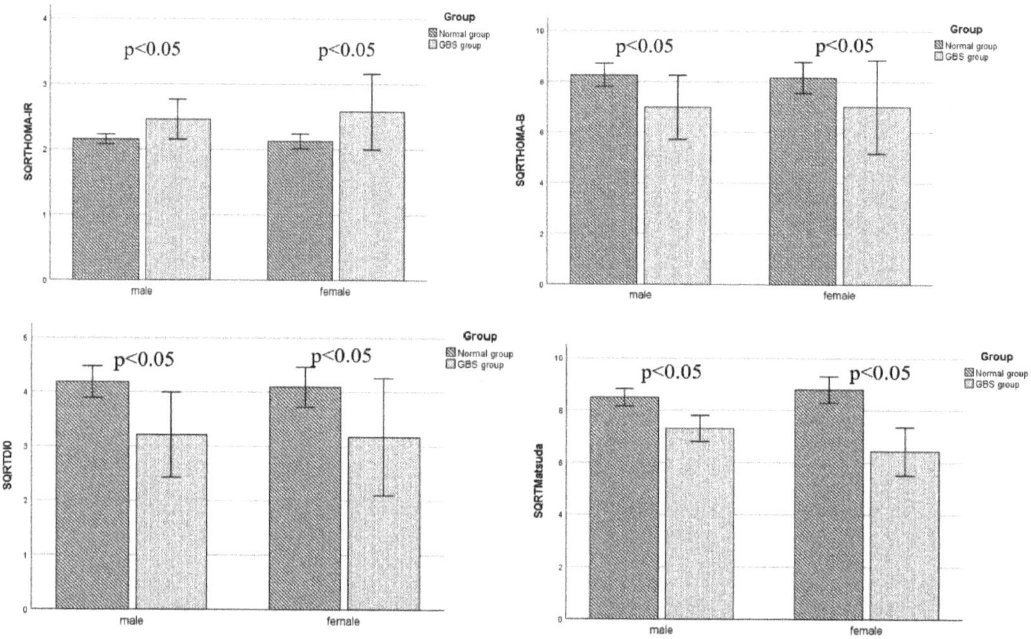

Figure 1. Comparison of islet β cell function index evaluation between the two groups. In both male and female patients, the SQRTHOMA-IR of the GBS group was higher than that of the normal group (all $p < 0.05$), while the SQRTHOMA-β, SQRTDI0, and SQRTMatsuda of the GBS group were lower than those of the normal group (all $p < 0.05$).

3.3. Univariate Logistic Regression Analysis of GBS

Taking GBS as the dependent variable, a univariate logistic regression model was established. For male patients, after adjustment for age, BMI, ALT, and eGFR, HOMA-IR is an independent risk factor for GBS (OR = 2.00, 95% CI:1.03, 3.88, $p < 0.05$). The Matsuda index value is a protective factor for GBS (OR = 0.76, 95% CI:0.60, 0.96, $p < 0.05$). For female patients, after adjustment for age, BMI, ALT, and eGFR, HOMA-IR is an independent risk factor for GBS (OR = 2.80, 95% CI:1.03, 7.58, $p < 0.05$). The Matsuda index value is a protective factor for GBS (OR = 0.59, 95% CI:0.39, 0.90, $p < 0.05$) (Figure 2).

3.4. Multivariate Predictive Model for Predicting GBS

For male patients, multivariate predictive model for predicting the occurrence of GBS was established with GBS as the dependent variable and sex, age, BMI, HOMA-IR, HOMA-β, DI0, and Matsuda as independent variables. The logistic regression model for predicting the GBS was $-3.73510 + 0.06236\times\text{age} + 0.02119\times\text{BMI} + 0.37235\times\text{HOMA-IR} - 0.26797\times\text{HOMA-}\beta + 0.33766\times\text{DI0-}0.32066\times\text{Matsuda}$. The area under curve (AUC) of the model for predicting GBS was 0.77 (95% CI 0.67, 0.87), with the specificity of the model being 75.26%, the sensitivity of the model being 80.00%, and the accuracy of the model being 75.64%.

For female patients, a multivariate predictive model for predicting the occurrence of GBS was established with GBS as the dependent variable and sex, age, BMI, HOMA-IR, HOMA-β, DI0, and Matsuda as independent variables. The logistic regression model for predicting the GBS was $1.62159 + 0.01908\times\text{age} - 0.15143\times\text{HOMA-IR} - 0.09614\times\text{DI0} - 0.54718\times\text{Matsuda}$. The area under curve (AUC) of the model for predicting GBS was 0.77 (95% CI 0.63, 0.88), with the specificity of the model being 79.63%, the sensitivity of the model being 71.43%, and the accuracy of the model being 78.69% (Figure 3).

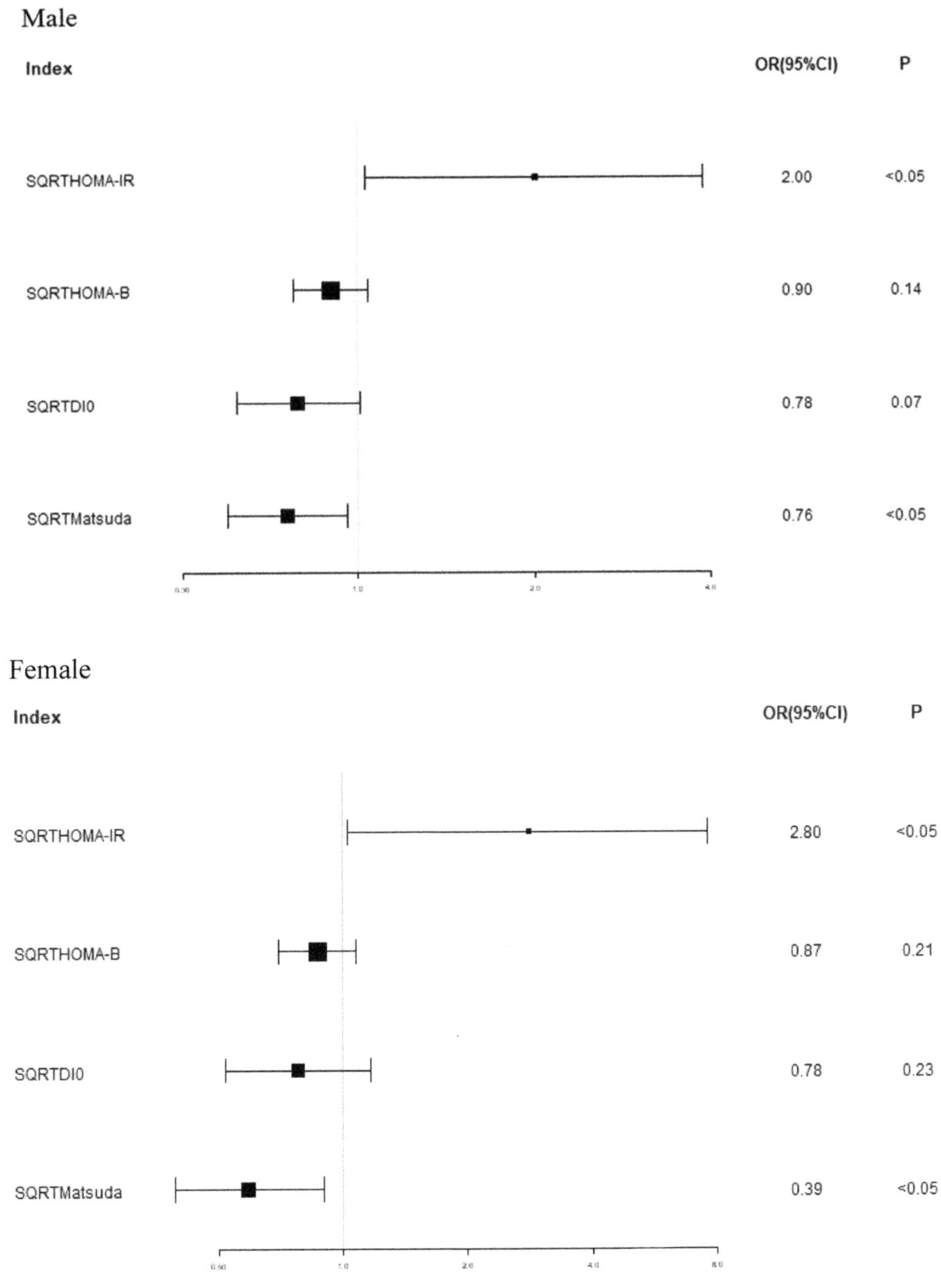

Figure 2. Univariate logistic regression analysis of GBS. In both male and female patients, HOMA-IR is an independent risk factor for GBS (male: OR = 2.00, 95% CI:1.03, 3.88, $p < 0.05$; female: OR = 2.80, 95% CI:1.03, 7.58, $p < 0.05$), and Matsuda index value is a protective factor for GBS (male: OR = 0.76, 95% CI:0.60, 0.96, $p < 0.05$; female: OR = 0.59, 95% CI:0.39, 0.90, $p < 0.05$).

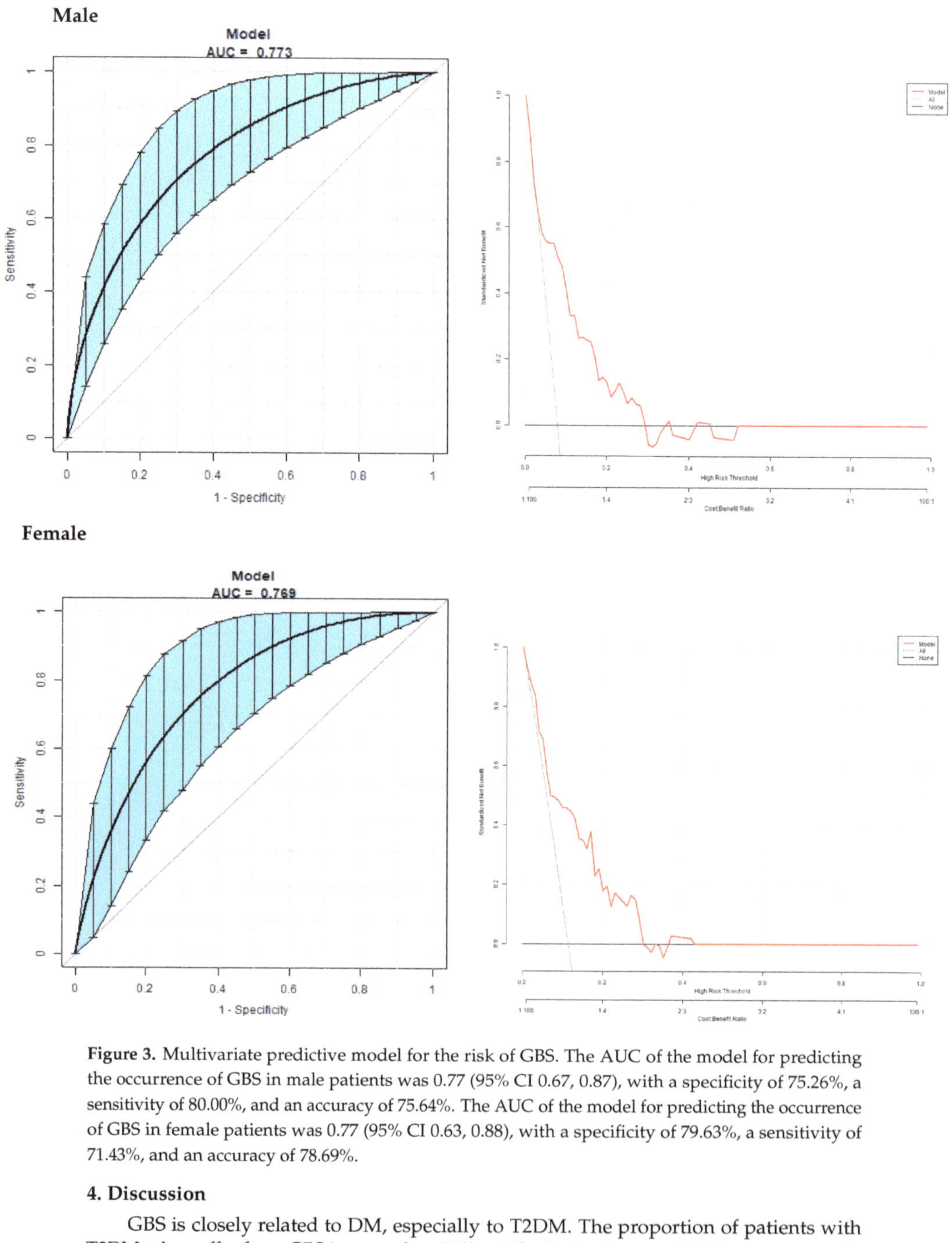

Figure 3. Multivariate predictive model for the risk of GBS. The AUC of the model for predicting the occurrence of GBS in male patients was 0.77 (95% CI 0.67, 0.87), with a specificity of 75.26%, a sensitivity of 80.00%, and an accuracy of 75.64%. The AUC of the model for predicting the occurrence of GBS in female patients was 0.77 (95% CI 0.63, 0.88), with a specificity of 79.63%, a sensitivity of 71.43%, and an accuracy of 78.69%.

4. Discussion

GBS is closely related to DM, especially to T2DM. The proportion of patients with T2DM who suffer from GBS is more than 30%; while the incidence of GBS in patients without DM is only 10%, the incidence of GBS with DM is three times that without DM [12,13]. Therefore, the study of the relationship between GBS and T2DM has important clinical significance for the diagnosis and treatment of patients with both GBS and T2DM.

As early as more than 50 years ago, Sampler et al. found in epidemiological studies that the incidence of GBS in Indians with hyperinsulinemia and significant insulin resistance was extremely high. This study suggests that insulin resistance may be related to the incidence of GBS [14]. Scragg et al. also found that the plasma insulin level was closely related to the risk of GBS [15]. In patients with GBS, fasting insulin levels were higher than those in controls, and the insulin level was a risk factor independent of age, BMI, and TG. A study has found that the incidence of GBS is related to metabolic syndrome and the key factor is hyperinsulinemia [16]. Kboi Q et al. found that hyperglycemia, hyperinsulinemia, and hyperlipidemia can reduce the contractility of gallbladder smooth muscle because of various neurotransmitters in the study of mouse gallbladders in vitro [17].

The clinical features of patients with T2DM are mainly hyperinsulinemia and insulin resistance. The mechanism of GBS induced by increasing insulin level is still unclear and may include the following aspects: (1) Insulin may increase the activity of hydroxymethylglutaryl-coenzyme A reductase, which leads to increased cholesterol synthesis and increased hepatic cholesterol secretion [18] to saturate the cholesterol in the bile. And it may promote the formation of GBS. (2) Insulin inhibits the rate-limiting enzyme-7α of bile salt synthesis. The activity of hydroxylase can reduce the bile acid secretion in the bile duct, increase the calcium ion content in the bile, and induce the gallbladder to secrete more mucopolysaccharide substances, which are known as nucleating factors in the bile, breaking the dynamic balance between pro-nucleation and anti-nucleation factors in bile and accelerating the crystallization rate of cholesterol in bile, thereby promoting the formation of GBS [19]. (3) The elevation of insulin can increase the number of LDL receptors, thereby improving the activity of LDL receptors and increasing the amount of LDL-C transferred from the blood circulation to the liver, which may prompt the liver to excrete more cholesterol into the bile and further increase the saturation of cholesterol in the bile [20]. (4) Insulin regulates the contraction of smooth muscle cells by regulating the ion concentration of the intracellular Na^+ -K^+ pump, thereby reducing the activity of the gallbladder and causing the formation of GBS. (5) Patients with DM often exhibit abnormal symptoms of autonomic nervous function, which lead to impaired gallbladder contraction function, thickening, and deposition of bile secretion concentration, which is conducive to the formation of GBS [21]. (6) Diabetes causes endocrine disorders, especially the regulation of the lipid metabolism, which is closely related to the incidence of hyperlipidemia and cholesterolemia, especially affecting the secretion of cholesterol, leading to an increase in free cholesterol and fatty acids, thus promoting the formation of stones [22].

Studies have shown that there are many methods currently used clinically to evaluate the islet β cell function and insulin resistance in patients with T2DM, including direct detection of insulin sensitivity and indirect detection of insulin sensitivity. Hyperinsulinemic euglycemic clamp (HEC) technology and the insulin suppression test (IST) were used in the pathogenesis research and new drug evaluation of various metabolic diseases. For population research, it is still appropriate to use indirect detection methods of insulin sensitivity in the fasting state, such as HOMA-IR and HOMA-β. However, for T2DM patients with a long duration and those who have previously used hypoglycemic drugs, such as sulfonylureas and other insulin secretagogue, insulin levels cannot truly reflect the islet β-cell function, and a homeostasis model evaluation may not reflect the degree of insulin resistance in T2DM patients. However, in this study, all the subjects were patients diagnosed with T2DM for the first time, who had not used hypoglycemic therapy before, so that the insulin levels of the subjects, and especially the insulin resistance index calculated by the homeostasis model, can better reflect the islet β-cell secretion function and the degree of insulin resistance.

The results of this study showed that after sex stratification, the HOMA-IR of the GBS group was higher than that of the normal group ($p < 0.05$), while the HOMA-β, DI0, and Matsuda of the GBS group were lower than those of the normal group ($p < 0.05$, respectively). And in univariate regression analysis, for male patients, after adjustment for age, BMI, ALT, and eGFR, HOMA-IR is an independent risk factor for GBS (OR = 2.00,

95% CI:1.03, 3.88, $p < 0.05$). The Matsuda index value is a protective factor for GBS (OR = 0.76, 95% CI:0.60, 0.96, $p < 0.05$). For female patients, after adjustment for age, BMI, ALT, and eGFR, HOMA-IR is an independent risk factor for GBS (OR = 2.80, 95% CI:1.03, 7.58, $p < 0.05$). The Matsuda index value is a protective factor for GBS (OR = 0.59, 95% CI:0.39, 0.90, $p < 0.05$). This result is consistent with previous research results [23,24]. In a study that included 4125 Korean postmenopausal women [24], the results showed that in a multiple logistic regression analysis, LDL-C was an independent factor of GBS in premenopausal women and HOMA-IR was significantly associated with the occurrence of the GBS. However, previous studies only analyzed the correlation between insulin levels and GBS, while we further adopted more accurate indicators that reflect islet β cell secretion levels and insulin resistance indexes, which can better verify that the severity of insulin resistance in T2DM patients is an independent risk factor for the incidence of GBS, and that the degree of islet β cell secretion is closely related to the incidence of GBS.

In recent studies, there are also many reports about the related risk factors for GBS in T2DM patients [25]. Physiological factors, especially sex and age, have a great influence on the incidence of GBS in patients with T2DM. With the increase in age, the function of various organs in the human body exhibits an aging failure trend, which directly leads to the decrease in cholesterol transformation into bile acid. The decrease in cholesterol decomposition increases the concentration of cholesterol in the total cholesterol pool and thus increases the cholesterol excretion in the biliary tract. The results of this study also confirm this point, as the average age in the GBS group was higher than that in the normal group ($p < 0.05$).

Estrogen is the main factor responsible for the different incidence rates of GBS between men and women. Studies have shown that the level of estrogen in women can affect the secretion of bile acids. The higher the estrogen level, the lower the amount of bile acids secretion, which results in an increase in the incidence of GBS. However, the results of this study have shown that compared with the normal group, the proportion of female patients in the GBS group was a little higher, without a significant difference. This difference between studies may be the result of the limited sample size. Also, the effect of sex difference on GBS is mainly due to the difference in estrogen levels. The women included in a previous study [26] were young, so there was a significant correlation between being female and GBS. However, the average age of the women in our study was more than 50 years old, most of them were postmenopausal women, and the estrogen levels in postmenopausal women are significantly lower than in younger women. Therefore, our results could not reflect the effect of estrogen levels on GBS in patients with T2DM.

Our results showed that the levels of GGT in the GBS group were slightly higher than those in the non-GBS group ($p < 0.05$), but there were no significant differences in the levels of TBIL, DBIL, ALP, and TBA between the two groups (all $p > 0.05$). In the further univariate logistic regression analysis, none of the above indexes reflecting liver and gallbladder functions were risk factors for GBS in T2DM patients ($p > 0.05$), which may be because these indexes only reflect the physiological functions of the liver and gallbladder and do not directly affect cholesterol excretion, so there is no apparent correlation between them and the incidence of GBS.

In this study, a multivariate logistic regression model was established for predicting the incidence of GBS. For male patients, the multivariate predictive model was established with GBS as the dependent variable and sex, age, BMI, SQRTHOMA-IR, SQRTHOMA-β, SQRTDI0, and SQRTMatsuda as independent variables. The equation of the logistic regression model was logit (GBS) = −3.73510 + 0.06236*age + 0.02119*BMI + 0.37235*HOMA-IR − 0.26797*HOMA-β + 0.33766*DI0-0.32066*Matsuda. And the AUC of the model for male patients is 0.77 (95% CI 0.67, 0.87), with a specificity of 75.26%, a sensitivity of 80.00%, and an accuracy of 75.64%. For female patients, the multivariate predictive model was established with GBS as the dependent variable and sex, age, BMI, SQRTHOMA-IR, SQRTHOMA-β, SQRTDI0, and SQRTMatsuda as independent variables. The logistic regression equation of the model was logit (GBS) = 1.62159 + 0.01908*age − 0.15143* HOMA-IR − 0.09614*DI0 −

0.54718* Matsuda. The AUC of the model for female patients is 0.77 (95% CI 0.63, 0.88), with a specificity of 79.63%, a sensitivity of 71.43%, and an accuracy of 78.69%.

This study not only identified the risk factors for GBS in T2DM patients, but also further established a predictive model for GBS in T2DM patients, which has a certain predictive value. This model has not been investigated in previous studies. Through the establishment of this model, we can evaluate the risk of GBS occurrence in newly diagnosed T2DM patients. For T2DM patients with a higher risk, further diagnosis and evaluation of the necessity of surgery for GBS should be actively carried out to prevent the deterioration of GBS.

There are still some limitations to this study. First, one of the limitations of our research is that it is a retrospective study, and we had limited control over the quality of the data used for analysis. Secondly, some biochemical indexes were tested only once, which may lead to variation. In the future, studies with larger samples need to be carried out. In addition, this study did not reveal the pathophysiological mechanism of the close relationship between islet β cell secretion and GBS. In the future, more animal studies are needed to better understand the pathophysiological basis for the close relationship between islet β cell secretion and GBS. Finally, the sample size of this study was small, especially the sample size of the GBS group, which was only 39 cases. In order to avoid the influence of hypoglycemic treatment and the diabetes duration on insulin function and insulin resistance as much as possible, the subjects of this study were newly diagnosed T2DM patients. Although the sample size was limited, the sample size ratio of the non-GBS group and GBS group was 10:1, which was in line with statistical requirements. At the time of writing, there were not many studies on the correlation between insulin function, insulin resistance indexes, and GBS in newly diagnosed T2DM patients. At that point, our study had the largest sample size, but this was only a preliminary exploration. In future research, we will further expand the sample size to better reveal the correlation between pancreatic function, insulin resistance indicators, and GBS.

5. Conclusions

Insulin resistance may be an independent risk factor for the incidence of GBS in patients with newly diagnosed T2DM, both male and female, which provides a new clinical basis and research direction for the prevention and treatment of GBS in patients with T2DM. This study has established a predictive model of GBS in T2DM and found it to be accurate, thus representing an effective tool for the early prediction of GBS in patients with T2DM.

Author Contributions: T.W. and Q.W. conceived and designed the study; T.W. and C.P. collected the data and conducted the research; C.P. analyzed and interpreted the data; T.W. and Q.W. wrote the initial draft; K.Z. revised the manuscript; T.W. and K.Z. had primary responsibility for the final content. All authors have read and agreed to the published version of the manuscript.

Funding: This research received no external funding.

Institutional Review Board Statement: This study was approved by the Ethics Committee of Peking University International Hospital. The number of the ethics approval is 2022-KY-0030-01.

Informed Consent Statement: Due to the retrospective nature of the study, the Ethics Committee of Peking University International Hospital waived the need for obtaining informed consent.

Data Availability Statement: The datasets generated and analyzed during the current study are not publicly available due to limitations of ethical approval involving patient data and anonymity but are available from the corresponding author on reasonable request.

Conflicts of Interest: The authors declare no conflict of interest.

References

1. Kratzer, W.; Klysik, M.; Binzberger, A.; Schmidberger, J. Gallbladder stone incidence and prevalence in Germany: A population-based study. *Z. Gastroenterol.* **2021**, *59*, 859–864. [CrossRef] [PubMed]

2. Portincasa, P.; Di Ciaula, A.; de Bari, O.; Garruti, G.; Palmieri, V.O.; Wang, D.Q. Management of gallstones and its related complications. *Expert. Rev. Gastroenterol. Hepatol.* **2016**, *10*, 93–112. [CrossRef] [PubMed]
3. Aune, D.; Vatten, L.J. Diabetes mellitus and the risk of gallbladder disease: A systematic review and meta-analysis of prospective studies. *J. Diabetes Complicat.* **2016**, *30*, 368–373. [CrossRef]
4. Almobarak, A.O.; Jervase, A.; Fadl, A.A.; Garelnabi, N.I.A.; Hakem, S.A.; Hussein, T.M.; Ahmad, A.A.A.; Ahmed, I.S.E.-D.; Badi, S.; Ahmed, M.H. The prevalence of diabetes and metabolic syndrome and associated risk factors in Sudanese individuals with gallstones: A cross sectional survey. *Transl. Gastroenterol. Hepatol.* **2020**, *5*, 14. [CrossRef]
5. Elmehdawi, R.; Elmajberi, S.; Behieh, A.; Elramli, A. Prevalence of Gall Bladder Stones among Type 2 Diabetic Patients in Benghazi Libya: A Case-control Study. *Libyan J. Med.* **2009**, *4*, 27–30. [CrossRef]
6. Rana, J.S.; Visser, M.E.; Arsenault, B.J.; Després, J.-P.; Stroes, E.S.; Kastelein, J.J.; Wareham, N.J.; Boekholdt, S.M.; Khaw, K.-T. Metabolic dyslipidemia and risk of future coronary heart disease in apparently healthy men and women: The EPIC-Norfolk prospective population study. *Int. J. Cardiol.* **2010**, *143*, 399–404. [CrossRef]
7. Ding, X.; Gong, J.-P.; Lu, C.-Y.; Liu, C.-A.; Shi, Y.-J.; Gao, G.-W. Relation of abnormal gallbladder arterioles to gallbladder emptying in patients with gallstone and diabetes mellitus. *Hepatobiliary Pancreat. Dis. Int.* **2004**, *3*, 275–278.
8. Cortés, V.A.; Barrera, F.; Nervi, F. Pathophysiological connections between gallstone disease, insulin resistance, and obesity. *Obes. Rev.* **2020**, *21*, e12983. [CrossRef]
9. World Health Organization. Definition, diagnosis and classification of diabetes mellitus and its complications. Report of a WHO consultation. In *Part 1: Diagnosis and Classification of Diabetes Mellitus*; WHO: Geneva, Switzerland, 1999; pp. 4–7.
10. Lechner, K.; Lechner, B.; Crispin, A.; Schwarz, P.E.H.; von Bibra, H. Waist-to-height ratio and metabolic phenotype compared to the Matsuda index for the prediction of insulin resistance. *Sci. Rep.* **2021**, *11*, 8224. [CrossRef]
11. Retnakaran, R.; Qi, Y.; Goran, M.I.; Hamilton, J.K. Evaluation of proposed oral disposition index measures in relation to the actual disposition index. *Diabet. Med.* **2009**, *26*, 1198–1203. [CrossRef]
12. Microvascular complications group of diabetes credit association of Chinese Medical Association. Guidelines for the prevention and treatment of diabetes and kidney disease in China. *Chin. J. Diabetes Mellitus* **2021**, *13*, 762–784.
13. Tereshchenko, I.V.; Kamenskikh, Y.A.; Kayushev, P.E. The concurrence of diabetes mellitus and gallstone disease. *Ter. Arkh.* **2015**, *87*, 105–109. [CrossRef] [PubMed]
14. Sampliner, R.E.; Bennett, P.H.; Comess, L.J.; Rose, F.A.; Burch, T.A. Gallbladder disease in pima indians. Demonstration of high prevalence and early onset by cholecystography. *N. Engl. J. Med.* **1970**, *283*, 1358–1364. [CrossRef]
15. Scragg, R.K.; Calvert, G.D.; Oliver, J.R. Plasma lipids and insulin in gall stone disease: A case-control study. *Br. Med. J.* **1984**, *289*, 521–525. [CrossRef]
16. Méndez-Sánchez, N.; Chavez-Tapia, N.C.; Motola-Kuba, D.; Sanchez-Lara, K.; Ponciano-Rodríguez, G.; Baptista, H.; Ramos, M.H.; Uribe, M. Metabolic syndrome as a risk factor for gallstone disease. *World J. Gastroenterol.* **2005**, *11*, 1653–1657. [CrossRef]
17. Tran, K.Q.; Goldblatt, M.I.; Swartz-Basile, D.A.; Svatek, C.; Nakeeb, A.; Pitt, H.A. Diabetes and hyperlipidemia correlate with gallbladder contractility in leptin-related murine obesity. *J. Gastrointest. Surg.* **2003**, *7*, 857–862; discussion 63. [CrossRef]
18. Kharroubi, I.; Rasschaert, J.; Eizirik, D.L.; Cnop, M. Expression of adiponectin receptors in pancreatic beta cells. *Biochem. Biophys. Res. Commun.* **2003**, *312*, 1118–1122. [CrossRef]
19. Stinton, L.M.; Shaffer, E.A. Epidemiology of gallbladder disease: Cholelithiasis and cancer. *Gut Liver.* **2012**, *6*, 172–187. [CrossRef] [PubMed]
20. Chinetti, G.; Zawadski, C.; Fruchart, J.C.; Staels, B. Expression of adiponectin receptors in human macrophages and regulation by agonists of the nuclear receptors PPARalpha, PPARgamma, and LXR. *Biochem. Biophys. Res. Commun.* **2004**, *314*, 151–158. [CrossRef]
21. Reshetnyak, V.I. Concept of the pathogenesis and treatment of cholelithiasis. *World J. Hepatol.* **2012**, *4*, 18–34. [CrossRef]
22. Erichsen, R.; Froslev, T.; Lash, T.L. Long-term statin use and the risk of GBS disease: A population-based case control study. *Am. J. Epidemi.* **2011**, *173*, 162–170. [CrossRef]
23. Cojocaru, C.; Pandele, G.I. Clinical and paraclinical features in diabetic patients cholecystectomized for gallstones. *Rev. Med. Chir. Soc. Med. Nat. Iasi.* **2010**, *114*, 998–1004. [PubMed]
24. Wang, H.; So, H.; Ko, S.W.; Jung, S.W.; Bang, S.J.; Park, E.J. Gallstone Is Associated with Metabolic Factors and Exercise in Korea. *Healthcare* **2022**, *10*, 1372. [CrossRef] [PubMed]
25. Liao, K.F.; Lai, S.W.; Li, C.I.; Chen, W.C. Diabetes mellitus correlates with increased risk of pancreatic cancer: A population-based cohort study in Taiwan. *J. Gastroenterol. Hepatol.* **2012**, *27*, 709–713. [CrossRef] [PubMed]
26. A1-Bayati, S.; Kodayer, S. GBS in a group of Iraqi patients with type 2 diabetes mellitus. *Sandi Med.* **2012**, *33*, 412–417.

biomedicines

MDPI

Article

Progression of Diabetic Kidney Disease and Gastrointestinal Symptoms in Patients with Type I Diabetes

Aleksejs Fedulovs [1], Lilian Tzivian [1], Polina Zalizko [1,2], Santa Ivanova [1], Renāte Bumane [1], Jana Janeviča [1,2], Lelde Krūzmane [1], Eduards Krustins [2] and Jelizaveta Sokolovska [1,*]

1 Faculty of Medicine, University of Latvia, Jelgavas Street 3, LV 1004 Riga, Latvia; aleksejs.fedulovs@lu.lv (A.F.); liliana.civjane@lu.lv (L.T.); polinazalizko@inbox.lv (P.Z.); ivanova63@inbox.lv (S.I.); renate.bumane@gmail.com (R.B.); janevica.jana@gmail.com (J.J.); lelde.kruzmane@gmail.com (L.K.)

2 Pauls Stradins Clinical University Hospital, Pilsoņu Street 13, LV 1002 Riga, Latvia; eduards.krustins@gmail.com

* Correspondence: jelizaveta.sokolovska@lu.lv

Abstract: (1) Background: Little research is conducted on the link between diabetic kidney disease (DKD) progression and diabetic gastroenteropathy in type 1 diabetes (T1D). (2) Methods. We performed a cross-sectional study with 100 T1D patients; 27 of them had progressive DKD, defined as an estimated glomerular filtration rate (eGFR) decline $\geq$3 mL/min/year or increased albuminuria stage, over a mean follow-up time of 5.89 $\pm$ 1.73 years. A newly developed score with 17 questions on gastrointestinal (GI) symptoms was used. Faecal calprotectin was measured by ELISA. Lower GI endoscopies were performed in 21 patients. (3) Results: The gastrointestinal symptom score demonstrated high reliability (Cronbach's α = 0.78). Patients with progressive DKD had higher GI symptom scores compared to those with stable DKD (p = 0.019). The former group demonstrated more frequent bowel movement disorders (p < 0.01). The scores correlated negatively with eGFR (r = −0.335; p = 0.001), positively with albuminuria (r = 0.245; p = 0.015), Hba1c (r = 0.305; p = 0.002), and diabetes duration (r = 0.251; p = 0.012). Faecal calprotectin levels did not differ between DKD groups significantly. The most commonly reported histopathological findings of enteric mucosa were infiltration with eosinophils, lymphocytes, plasmacytes, the presence of lymphoid follicles, and lymphoid aggregates. Conclusion: The progression of DKD is positively correlated with gastrointestinal symptoms; however, more research is needed to clarify the causal relationships of the gut-kidney axis in T1D.

Keywords: type 1 diabetes; diabetic kidney disease; gastrointestinal symptoms; calprotectin; gastrointestinal endoscopy

1. Introduction

The prevalence of type 1 diabetes (T1D) is constantly rising throughout the world. T1D is associated with increased morbidity and mortality, mainly due to its vascular complications, including diabetic kidney disease (DKD), which is the main reason for end-stage renal disease (ESRD) in the developed world [1]. Despite the progress in the understanding of the pathophysiology of DKD [2]., and constantly improving diabetes care to control for the main clinical risk factors of the disease, it is still largely unclear which patients are at increased risk of rapidly progressing DKD (estimated glomerular filtration (eGFR) loss of $\geq$3 mL/min/1.73^2 per year [1].

Diabetic gastroenteropathy is a condition characterized by various oesophageal, gastric, intestinal, and anorectal symptoms caused by diabetes [3,4]. Gastrointestinal symptoms in T1D are twice as common as in the general population and were associated with worse glycaemic control and lower quality of life in studies [5,6]. A hypothesis was proposed that diabetic gastroenteropathy might predispose affected individuals to augmented intestinal inflammation and permeability and higher levels of systemic inflammation [7]. Low-grade systemic inflammation is in turn associated with the progression of complications of diabetes, including DKD [8,9]. To support the concept of this so-called gut-kidney axis, it was described that patients with T1D and macroalbuminuria have a higher level of the faecal inflammatory marker calprotectin compared to normoalbuminuric patients [10,11]. Unfortunately, the latter studies did not report symptoms of gastroenteropathy. Existing data on possible associations between DKD and gastrointestinal symptoms in T1D is currently limited to ESRD patients [12]. In the latter case, severe electrolyte imbalance, uraemia, oedema of the mucosa, medications, and generally very poor health might potentiate the symptoms. That is why data obtained in ESRD can hardly be extrapolated to patients with initial DKD stages.

Gastrointestinal symptoms are insufficiently recognised and investigated, both in clinical practise and research. Specifically, endoscopic examination of the gastrointestinal tract might be avoided by T1D patients despite indications due to the increased risk of hypoglycemia and other complications [13]. Indirectly supporting the latter statement, we found only two papers reporting data on histological and immunohistochemical examination of intestinal mucosal biopsies of patients with T1D [12,14].

To summarize, diabetic gastroenteropathy as assessed by gastrointestinal symptom scores, instrumental examinations, and biomarkers (such as calprotectin) remains a little studied factor predisposing to or potentiating the progression of DKD. However, such data are of extreme importance for clinical practice, as they could promote the development of novel treatment and prevention options for DKD [15].

To fill this gap, the aim of this work was to analyse the prevalence of gastrointestinal symptoms, history of previous gastrointestinal conditions, data from endoscopic gastrointestinal investigations, levels of faecal calprotectin in patients with T1D, and different velocities of DKD progression in a cross-sectional study.

2. Materials and Methods

2.1. Patients and Ethics

This study is a part of the longitudinal LatDiane study, initiated in 2013 (and participating in the international InterDiane consortium). LatDiane recruits adult patients with T1D diagnosed before the age of 40 with insulin treatment initiated within one year of diagnosis and C-peptide levels below 0.3 nmol/L. Patients with a history of chronic kidney disease apart from DKD are excluded from LatDiane. Follow-up visits and re-assessments of the status of complications of diabetes take place every three years. Currently, more than 400 patients have been recruited, with approximately 150 having attended one or more follow-up visits. Study protocol includes recording diabetes and other disease histories, basic clinical and anthropometric investigation, collection of blood samples for preparation of serum and plasma and DNA extraction, collection of urine, as well as assessment of dietary and physical activity habits, socioeconomic factors, and psychologic condition with the help of questionnaires [16–24]. The protocol of the general LatDiane and sub-study devoted to gut health described here were approved by the Latvian Central Ethics Committee and received permissions No 01-29.1/3 (dated 10 July 2013), Nr. A-17/19-10-17 (dated 17 October 2019), and Nr. 01-29.1/2226 (dated 30 April 2020).

Recruitment of this study participants, biobanking, and sample storage were performed in accordance with the procedures of the Genome Database of the Latvian population [25] and are described in detail in [22]. This study is in line with the 1964 Declaration of Helsinki and its later amendments. Written informed consent was obtained from all study participants prior to inclusion in this study.

Recruitment for this study took place between 15 January 2021 and 31 August 2022 in Latvia, Riga, Pilsoņu 13 str., building 10 (in the rooms of the Laboratory for Personalized Medicine of the University of Latvia). Information about this study was disseminated via the webpage and social media of the University of Latvia.

Inclusion criteria for this study were: T1D duration of at least 8 years and available data on progression of DKD (at least three yearly serum creatinine measurements and albuminuria measurements available between the baseline visit of the LatDiane study in 2013–2019 and this study) (Figure 1).

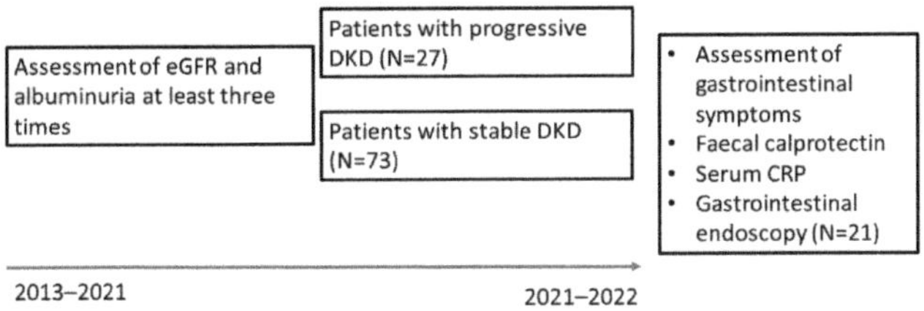

Figure 1. Recruitment scheme. eGFR—estimated glomerular filtration rate; DKD—diabetic kidney disease; CRP—C-reactive protein.

As for exclusion criteria, they were: pregnancy, subjects with a history of inflammatory bowel disease (Crohn disease or Ulcerative colitis), coeliac disease, acute intestinal infection within 2 months of the planned faecal collection, asymptomatic coeliac disease (detected via screening of serum transglutaminase IgA antibodies), clinical signs of acute inflammation, and fever.

On the study day, patients were investigated for the collection of anthropometric measures, questionnaires were filled out, blood samples were collected, and subjects received instructions and vials for the collection of the faecal sample.

2.2. Clinical Investigation and Monitoring of Diabetic Complications and Co-Morbidities

Clinical investigation included assessment of weight and height to calculate the body mass index (BMI, weight (kg)/height (m)^2). We also measured blood pressure. Patients with systolic blood pressure $\geq$ 140 mmHg (18.7 kPa) or diastolic blood pressure $\geq$ 90 mmHg (12.0 kPa) or a history of antihypertensive drug usage were defined as having arterial hypertension.

Smoking was self-reported in the questionnaire; the "smokers" group referred to patients currently smoking at least one cigarette per day.

Assessment of cardiovascular disease (CVD) and complications of diabetes, such as retinopathy, neuropathy, and DKD, was based on medical files. We defined CVD as a history of acute myocardial infarction, coronary bypass/percutaneous transluminal coronary angioplasty stroke, amputation, or peripheral vascular disease.

The albumin-to-creatinine ratio in morning spot urine samples was used for the definition of albuminuria at each study visit during the follow-up. The estimated glomerular filtration rate (eGFR) was calculated according to the Chronic Kidney Disease Epidemiology Collaboration (CKD-EPI).

ESRD was defined as eGFR < 15 mL/min/1.73 m^2, dialysis, or kidney transplantation.

Progressive DKD was defined as an eGFR decline exceeding 3 mL/min/1.73 m^2/year [2] and/or increase in albuminuria stage over the follow-up period. At least three yearly serum creatinine measurements were used for the calculation of at least three eGFR values during the follow-up period. These data were used for eGFR slope plotting. The number of serum creatinine measurements ranged from three to fifteen during the follow-up for each patient.

2.3. Blood Samples and Faecal Collection

The blood samples were collected via venous puncture. Blood samples and morning spot urine samples were sent for assessment of clinical markers (blood count, clinical chemistry, and albuminuria) to a certified clinical lab.

Except for several patients who could collect the stool sample during the recruitment visit, stool samples were collected within two weeks after blood collection and assessment of gastrointestinal symptoms. Participants collected their faecal samples at home using sterile collection tubes without buffer (the collection date and time were marked). Within 24 h samples were delivered to the laboratory for calprotectin measurement in unfrozen samples.

Faecal calprotectin was measured by the Alegria® Calprotectin Elisa kit (Organotech Diagnostika GmbH, Budapest, Hungary, REF ORG280) in a certified clinical lab.

2.4. Monitoring of Gastrointestinal Disease and Symptoms

The history of gastrointestinal disease was self-reported via an assisted study questionnaire in the majority of cases, and this information was supported by medical files. For reporting in this paper, we defined upper gastrointestinal disease as gastritis/duodenitis, peptic ulcer, gastroesophageal reflux disease, gastroparesis, diaphragmal hernia, and *Haelicobacter pylori* infection; lower gastrointestinal disease was defined as hemorrhoids, appendicitis, coeliac disease, irritable bowel syndrome, and lactose intolerance; and liver and pancreas disease were defined as histories of fatty liver, pancreatitis, viral hepatitis, gallstones, diverticulitis, and irritable bowel syndrome.

A newly developed scale questionnaire for assessment of gastrointestinal symptoms was filled out during this study visit. It was elaborated on the basis of the diabetes and bowel symptom questionnaire [26], which previously demonstrated good test-retest reliability and concurrent validity (median kappa: 0.63 and 0.47, respectively) for the gastrointestinal items. Our newly developed scale questionnaire included 17 questions about pain, discomfort, impaired bowel movement such as diarrhoea, and constipation (Supplement S1).

2.5. Endoscopy in Patients with Indications and "Red Flag" Symptoms

Patients who had increased calprotectin levels and persistent symptoms of gastrointestinal disorders in the last 2 months were referred to a gastroenterologist for evaluation of indications for endoscopic examination (colonoscopy and/or endoscopy according to indications). As indications for endoscopy, the following criteria were used: unexplained weight loss, clinical suspicion of inflammatory bowel disease, unclear abdominal pain, unclear anaemia (especially iron deficiency anaemia), unclear diarrhoea, constipation or changing bowel movements, bowel movements with mucus admixture, family history of inflammatory bowel disease or colorectal cancer, history of polyps, elevated faecal calprotectin >50 μg/g, or as a screening colonoscopy for subjects over the age of 50 [27–29]. Out of 100 T1D patients, 47 were selected to undergo endoscopic examination, and 21 of them accepted the invitation and went through the procedure. Endoscopic biopsy specimens were examined by a histopathologist. *H. pylori* was identified by rapid urease testing (RUT) and histological staining (Giemsa).

Patients who consented to lower endoscopy received recommendations from endocrinologists for preparation for the procedure based on international recommendations [13,30–32]. It included advice for food choices in the week preceding colonoscopy ("white foods", avoidance of fibre-containing and red foods, etc.), frequent blood glucose monitoring during the reduced nutritional intake period, fasting to avoid hypoglycemia, and an approach to correction of hyper- and hypoglycemia during the preparation (Supplement S2). Patients were prescribed a polyethylene glycol (PEG)-based osmotic laxative (PEG-3350, Sodium Sulfate, Sodium Chloride, Potassium Chloride, Sodium Ascorbate, and Ascorbic Acid for Oral Solution) for bowel cleaning.

2.6. Statistical Analysis

Descriptive statistics were performed for all study variables. For group variables, we presented numbers and percentages from the whole study sample. We used a one-sample Kolmogorov-Smirnov test and the graphical presentation of data by the histogram to check the normality of this study variables. As all the continuous variables were distributed differently than normal, we presented medians and interquartile ranges (IQR).

We performed the univariate analysis to assess the difference in socio-demographic variables between this study groups (we used the Chi-square test for the group variables and the Mann-Whitney test for continuous variables).

We calculated the mean value from the 17 questions of the gastrointestinal symptom score to assess the mean frequency and intensity of all investigated gastrointestinal symptoms, as well as the mean value of the frequency of use of medications. The Cronbach Alpha test was applied to check the reliability of this scale.

In addition, we evaluated the answers to questions about upper and lower gastrointestinal disease, history of liver and pancreatic diseases, history of gastrointestinal malignancy, and history of abdominal surgery.

We investigated the difference between those with stable and progressive DKD in gastrointestinal symptoms (Cramer's V test), symptom intensity (Mann-Whitney test), use of medications (Mann-Whitney test), and presence and history of diseases (Chi-square test).

A Spearman correlation was performed to identify the relationship between markers of kidney disease and demographic and blood/urine parameters. The p values < 0.05 were considered statistically significant.

We built multiple logistic regression models to assess the association between the progression of DKD and gastrointestinal symptoms. We adjusted the model for the variables that displayed statistical significance in the univariate analysis or had clinical relevance. The full adjustment set included sex, diabetes duration, HbA1c, and BMI.

3. Results

3.1. Description of this Study Groups and Inflammatory Markers

This study sample consists of 100 patients with T1D, mostly women (62%) with a mean age of 42.59 ± 13.18 and a mean BMI of 25.98 ± 4.69 1 kg/m^2. The mean follow-up time in the cohort is 5.89 ± 1.73 years. Most of the participants were non-smokers (63%), and they had hypertension (53%). The mean duration of diabetes was 24.38 ± 11.92 years, and the mean HbA1c was 8.28 ± 1.74%. 52 (52%) of subjects had retinopathy, 27 (27%) had autoimmune thyroid disease, and 16 (16%) had CVD. Study groups (with stable DKD disease and with progressive DKD) differed by smoking (more smokers among those with progressive DKD), hypertension (more patients with hypertension among those with progressive DKD), length of diabetes (longer history of diabetes for patients with progressive DKD), retinopathy, HbA1c, CVD, eGFR, albuminuria, serum bilirubin, blood haemoglobin concentration, and erythrocyte counts. The level of calprotectin in faeces and serum CRP did not differ between the groups of patients with progressive DKD and patients with stable DKD statistically significantly (Table 1). Moreover, of the 100 patients in this study, only 10 had faecal calprotectin ≥50 µg/g.

3.2. Gastrointestinal Diseases and Symptoms

The gastrointestinal symptom score demonstrated high reliability (Cronbach's $\alpha = 0.78$). Patients with progressive DKD had higher gastro-intestinal symptoms scores (Supplement S1) compared to those with stable DKD ($p = 0.019$). In addition, 14 (52%) of patients with progressive DKD had bowel movement disorders, versus 16 (22%) in patients with stable DKD ($p < 0.01$) (Table 2.)

There was no statistically significant difference between the patients with progressive DKD and patients with stable DKD on previous upper and lower gastrointestinal disease ($p = 0.50$ and $p = 0.35$, respectively). There was no difference between groups in the history of liver and pancreatic diseases ($p = 0.74$) or in the history of gastrointestinal malignancy ($p = 0.10$). The history of abdominal surgery was more frequent in patients with progressive DKD at the significance level of $p = 0.07$. There were no statistically significant differences between DKD patients with progressive DKD and patients with stable DKD in their use of medications for gastrointestinal disorders ($p = 0.54$).

Table 1. Differences in socio-demographic and disease-related data among study groups.

	DKD Stable, N = 73	DKD Progressive, N = 27	*p* Value
Male gender, N (%)	31 (42.5%)	7 (25.9%)	0.99
Age, years,	44.0 (31.5–52.0)	39.0 (34.0–50.0)	0.86
BMI, kg/m^2	24.85 (22.63–28.15)	25.40 (22.60–28.40)	0.95
Smokers, N (%)	13 (17.8%)	6 (22.2%)	<0.01
Hypertension, N (%)	32 (43.8%)	21 (77.8%)	<0.01
Length of diabetes, years	21 (13–31)	27 (24–37)	<0.01
Mean follow-up, years	7.00 (5.50–7.00)	7.00 (3.00–7.00)	0.72
Retinopathy, N (%)	30 (41.1%)	22 (81.5%)	<0.01
Cardiovascular disease, N (%)	7 (9.6%)	9 (33.3%)	<0.01
On ACEI/ARB, N (%)	12 (16.4%)	8 (29.6%)	0.14
On lipid lowering medication, N (%)	17 (23.3%)	10 (37.0%)	0.16
Autoimmune thyroid disease, N (%)	18 (24.7%)	9 (33.3%)	0.27
Other autoimmune disease, N (%)	11 (15.1%)	5 (18.5%)	0.67
Haemoglobin A1C, %	7.60 (7.00–8.70)	8.90 (07.54–10.30)	0.02
Haemoglobin A1C, mmol/mol	59.56 (53.00–71.58)	73.77 (58.90–89.07)	0.02
Estimated glomerular filtration rate, mL/min/1.73 m^2	107.98(92.52–117.63)	72.81(40.72–105.27)	<0.01
End stage renal disease, N (%)	0 (0%)	4 (14.8%)	<0.01
Albumin/creatinine ratio in urine, mg/mmol	0.45(0.19–0.99)	19.65 (4.98–112.50)	<0.01
C-reactive protein, mg/L	0.9 (0.5–2.8)	1.5 (0.5–3.48)	0.72
Faecal calprotectin, μg/g	7.60 (2.75–23.20)	16.20 (5.80–22.00)	0.21
Faecal calprotectin > 50 μg/g, N (%)	8 (11.0%)	2 (7.4%)	0.59
Total cholesterol, mmol/L	5.02(4.30–5.79)	4.96(4.12–5.88)	0.95
Low density lipoproteins, mmol/L	2.87(2.10–3.40)	3.04(2.10–3.46)	0.41
Triglycerides, mmol/L	1.14(0.85–1.45)	1.31(0.86–2.11)	0.14
Alanine transaminase, U/L	19.00(15.50–29.00)	21.00(17.00–24.00)	0.64
Gamma-glutamyl Transferase, U/L	16.00(13.00–25.50)	17.00(15.00–26.00)	0.41
Bilirubin, μmol/L	9.30(7.80–12.40)	6.51(5.10–9.20)	0.001
Haemoglobin, g/L	140.00(132.00–150.00)	129.00(120.00–141.00)	0.001
Erythrocytes, 10 × 12/L	4.70(4.40–5.00)	4.40(4.00–4.73)	0.002
Leukocytes, 10 × 9/L	6.13(5.01–7.22)	6.53(5.71–7.64)	0.14
Thrombocytes, 10 × 9/L	259.00(228.00–284.00)	231.00(200.00–299.00)	0.21

Continuous variables are presented as medians (IQR). DKD—diabetic kidney disease. eGFR—estimated glomerular filtration rate. Diabetic retinopathy—history of any stage of retinopathy based on medical recordings. Arterial hypertension—systolic blood pressure ≥ 140 mmHg (18.7 kPa) or diastolic blood pressure ≥ 90 mmHg (12.0 kPa), or a history of antihypertensive drug treatment. Autoimmune thyroid disease—Hashimoto's thyroiditis or Graves' disease Other autoimmune diseases—history of autoimmune rheumatologic diseases such as rheumatoid arthritis, sacroiliitis, psoriasis, asthma, etc. CVD—cardiovascular disease, defined as a history of acute myocardial infarction, coronary bypass/percutaneous transluminal coronary angioplasty stroke, amputation, or peripheral vascular disease.

Table 2. Gastrointestinal conditions and symptoms in this study groups.

	DKD Stable, N = 73	DKD Progressive, N = 27	*p* Value
History of upper gastrointestinal disease, N (%)	29 (39.7%)	13 (48.1%)	0.50
History of lower gastrointestinal disease, N (%)	24 (32.9%)	12 (44.4%)	0.28
History of gastrointestinal malignancy, N (%)	0 (0.0%)	1 (3.7%)	0.10
History of liver and pancreas disease, N (%)	27 (37.0%)	9 (33.3%)	0.74
History of abdominal surgery, N (%)	21 (28.8%)	13 (48.1%)	0.07
Mean value of gastrointestinal symptom score	1.05 (0.73–1.35)	1.27 (1.00–1.82)	0.019
Bowel movement disorders, N (%)	16 (21.9%)	14 (51.9%)	<0.01
Usage of medications for gastrointestinal disorders	0.16 (0.00–0.50)	0.33 (0.00–0.66)	0.54

Continuous variables are presented as medians (IQR). Bowel movement disorders—constipation, diarrhoea, intermittent constipation, and diarrhoea. DKD—diabetic kidney disease.

3.3. Correlation between Gastrointestinal Symptom Scores with Clinical Markers and Regression Analysis

We investigated correlations between the gastrointestinal symptom score and several clinical markers in this study sample. The scores correlated negatively with eGFR (r = −0.335; p = 0.001), weight (r = −0.236, p = 0.018), blood erythrocyte counts (r = −0.313, p = 0.002), and blood haemoglobin (r = −0.321, p = 0.001) and positively with albuminuria (r = 0.245; p = 0.015), Hba1c (r = 0.305, p = 0.002), and diabetes duration (r = 0.251, p = 0.012).

Faecal calprotectin did not correlate with the gastrointestinal symptom score, eGFR, or albuminuria.

In univariate regression analysis, higher scores in gastrointestinal symptoms were associated with higher odds of DKD progression (3.086 (1.209, 7.879), p = 0.018). The association remained significant when the model was adjusted for sex and BMI. However, the association was no longer significant when the model was adjusted for sex, BMI, diabetes duration, and HbA1c, with diabetes duration remaining the only significant predictor of DKD (odds ratio 1.058 (1.011, 1.106), p = 0.014) in the model and HbA1c demonstrating association at a significance level of 0.075 (odds ratio 1.302 (0.978, 1.734). The results of the logistic regression analysis are summarised in Table 3.

Table 3. Association between the progression of diabetic kidney disease and gastrointestinal symptoms.

Variable	Model	Odds Ratio, OR	95% Confidence Interval (CI)	*p* Value
Mean Symptoms	1	3.086	1.20; 7.87	0.02
Mean Symptoms	2	2.77	1.06; 7.24	0.04
Mean symptoms	3	2.394	0.886; 6.467	0.085
Mean Symptoms	4	1.99	0.71; 5.54	0.18

Results of the logistic regression analysis with the presence of progressive diabetic kidney disease as the response variable. Data are presented as odds ratios with 95% CI and *p*-values. Model 1—univariate. Model 2 was adjusted for sex and BMI. Model 3 was adjusted for sex, BMI, and diabetes duration. Model 4 was adjusted for sex, BMI, diabetes duration, and HbA1c.

3.4. Endoscopy

Prevalence of indications for colonoscopy did not differ between the patients with and without DKD progression.

From the 47 patients who were selected to undergo colonoscopy, 13 had progressive DKD and 34 did not (48.1% and 46.5% of the progressive DKD and non-progressive DKD groups, respectively). Only 21 patients (4 patients with progressive DKD and 17 patients with stable DKD) accepted the invitation and went through the procedure. The reasons for non-acceptance of the invitation included a complicated preparation procedure for the colonoscopy with the necessity of fasting and intensive glucose control, a fear of hypoglycemia, and a fear of complications during anaesthesia. Many patients refused to undergo the investigation because of their poor health status due to complications of diabetes and co-morbidities.

Among patients who underwent the endoscopic examination, the most frequent indications for endoscopic examination were abdominal pain (n = 17; 81%), bowel movement disorders (n = 9; 43%), and elevated faecal calprotectin (>50 μg/g) (n = 5; 24%).

Of the 10 individuals who underwent upper GI endoscopy, 7 (70%) had abnormal macroscopic findings and were analysed for H. pylori infection by rapid urease tests (RUT). None of the patients had a positive RUT; however, histopathology identified two patients with *H. pylori*, visible on special staining. Most of the gastric lesions were minor endoscopic findings (Table 4). Of the five endoscopically reported hyperaemic gastropathy and duodenopathy patients, two had active gastritis and two had chronic atrophic gastritis. Of the three patients with macroscopically normal upper GI endoscopy, one had chronic atrophic gastritis and one had active gastritis with erosive gastropathy.

Table 4. Summary of macroscopic and microscopic lesions identified during gastrointestinal endoscopic examination.

Procedure	Macroscopic Lesions	Histopathologic Lesions
Upper endoscopy, N = 10	(1) Hyperaemic gastropathy (n = 4) (2) Hyperaemic duodenopathy (n = 1) (3) oesophageal candidiasis (n = 1) (4) gastric intestinal metaplasia (n = 1)	(1) active gastritis (N = 3) (2) chronic atrophic gastritis (N = 3)
Colonoscopy, N = 21	(1) polyps (n = 2) (2) diverticulosis (n = 1) (3) erosion of sigmoid colon (n = 1) (4) perianal papilloma (n = 1)	(1) eosinophilic infiltration (n = 8, 38%) (2) lymphoid follicles/lymphoid aggregates (n = 7, 33%) (3) lymphoplasmacytic infiltration (n = 5, 24%). (4) lymphocyte and macrophage infiltration (n = 3, 14%) (5) stromal fibrosis (n = 3, 14%) (6) mononuclear cell infiltration (n = 2, 9.5%) (7) tubular adenomas (n = 2, 9.5%). (8) Active inflammation 6 (29%) (9) active colitis 1 (4.76%)

In total, 21 colonoscopies were performed. Five (24%) of the colonoscopies performed showed abnormal macroscopic findings (Tables 4, S1 and S2). The most commonly reported histopathological findings were infiltration with eosinophils, lymphocytes, plasmacytes, the presence of lymphoid follicles, and lymphoid aggregates. We also observed stromal fibrosis, mononuclear cell and macrophage infiltration, and tubular adenomas in several patients. Active inflammation was found in six patients, and one patient had active colitis on histopathological examination. No malignancies were found.

4. Discussion

The main finding of our study is that in patients with T1D and progressive DKD, the frequency and severity of gastrointestinal symptoms are higher compared to patients with stable kidney markers, as assessed by the gastrointestinal symptom score. The link between progressive DKD and diabetic gastroenteropathy was additionally confirmed by statistically significant correlations between gastrointestinal symptom scores, eGFR, and albuminuria, as well as in the logistic regression models.

We demonstrate in our work that gastrointestinal disorders start to manifest already in the initial stages of DKD progression, as the median eGFR is 72.81(40.72–105.27) mL/min/1.73 m^2 in the group of progressive DKD in our study. Our findings cannot be directly compared to previous data due to the deficiency of studies on the association of diabetic gastroenteropathy with progressive DKD in T1D. We only found one paper by D'Addio and colleagues reporting higher scores of gastrointestinal symptoms in patients with T1D and DKD. However, that paper investigated diabetic gastroenteropathy only in patients with ESRD compared to healthy individuals and did not cover subjects with DKD or the initial stages of chronic kidney disease [12]. More pronounced gastrointestinal symptoms in ESRD from any cause were already reported and might result from metabolic disorders and treatment of ESRD [27]. D'Addio and colleagues also report that the gastrointestinal symptoms of patients subsided significantly several years after successful treatment with kidney-pancreas transplantation. However, this was not the case in patients who only received kidney transplants, indicating hyperglycemia per se as the main factor in diabetic gastroenteropathy. Although we think that immunosuppressive treatment after transplantation might be one of the factors alleviating the gastrointestinal derangements in the above study, our results of the regression analysis with a fully adjusted model agree with the latter finding. Specifically, after adjustment of the regression model for diabetes duration, gastrointestinal symptom scores were no longer significant predictors of progressive DKD. We suggest that a larger longitudinal study is needed to obtain more conclusive results about mutual associations between gastrointestinal derangements and DKD progression in T1D. Such a study is necessary for the development of future approaches to DKD prevention and treatment. Indeed, gastrointestinal symptoms are usually a sign of dysfunction in the gastrointestinal tract. Therefore, they might be associated with impaired nutritional balance and increased gut permeability, resulting in augmented low-grade inflammation, which has been shown to be associated with DKD progression [7–10,33,34].

In contrast to some previous studies in T1D reporting higher calprotectin levels in patients with DKD [10,11,35], we did not observe higher faecal calprotectin levels in patients with progressive DKD compared to subjects with stable kidney markers. Moreover, faecal calprotectin did not exhibit any correlations with gastrointestinal symptom scores, eGFR, or albuminuria in our study. Our findings might mean that gastrointestinal symptoms in our patients were not associated with neutrophil-mediated inflammation, resulting in an increase in calprotectin and a severe inflammatory reaction, which is observed in inflammatory bowel disease [36]. Indeed, in the histological investigation of the colon biopsies of patients who underwent endoscopic examination, eosinophilic infiltration, lymphoid follicles/lymphoid aggregates, and lymphoplasmacytic infiltration were the most frequent findings. In 21 subjects who underwent colonoscopy, infiltration with polymorphonuclear neutrophils was not registered, mononuclear cell infiltration was observed only in two patients, and active inflammation was reported only in six subjects (only one of them with progressive DKD). Thus, histologic changes observed by us indicate increased reactivity of the mucosa and chronic pathology [37], when increased calprotectin levels are unlikely. On the other hand, lymphoplasmacytic infiltration is a predictor of more severe colitis in the future [37], and a study in T1D with ESRD reports more severe histologic changes of the mucosa as compared to our findings [12]. Thus, it is possible that an increase in calprotectin is observed in more advanced DKD stages.

Our study's limitations include a relatively low number of subjects, especially in the group of progressive DKD, which might have influenced the results. Further, the cross-sectional nature of this study does not allow us to evaluate the causal relationship between symptoms of diabetic gastroenteropathy and DKD. Other limitations include the self-evaluation of gastrointestinal symptoms in this study and the self-reporting of previous gastrointestinal diseases in a subset of patients due to unavailable central medical records in Latvia. We also did not perform an evaluation of autonomic neuropathy, which might have influenced the gastrointestinal symptoms; however, to our opinion, these data would not alter our conclusions or the clinical value of our study due to the availability of treatment for autonomic neuropathy nowadays. Lack of endoscopic evaluation in all study participants is another limitation. However, all study participants did not have indications for endoscopy. In addition, not all of the invited patients responded to the invitation due to complicated preparation procedures, fear of hypoglycemia, fear of complications during anaesthesia, or generally poor health status.

The major strength of this study is the analysis of gastrointestinal symptoms in patients with different rates of progression of DKD, in contrast to previous studies addressing either patients with T1D generally or patients with T1D and ESRD in comparison to healthy subjects. In addition, we have demonstrated results on histological colon biopsies in 21 patients with T1D, previously described only in one study [12].

5. Conclusions

To conclude, in patients with T1D and progressive DKD, the frequency and severity of gastrointestinal symptoms are higher compared to patients with stable kidney markers, as assessed by gastrointestinal symptom scores. Moreover, gastrointestinal symptom scores correlate with kidney markers. Further research is needed to clarify the causal relationships of the gut-kidney axis in T1D.

Supplementary Materials: The following supporting information can be downloaded at: https://www.mdpi.com/article/10.3390/biomedicines11102679/s1, Supplement S1: Gastrointestinal symptom score, Supplement S2: Instructions for patients with type 1 diabetes for preparation for lower endoscopy, Table S1: Histopathology findings of upper endoscopy in the study groups, Table S2: Histopathology findings of lower endoscopy in the study groups.

Author Contributions: A.F. recruited subjects, analysed data, wrote the paper; L.T. consulted on study design, analysed data, edited the paper; P.Z. participated in this study design, development of questionnaires and instructions, recruited the patients, edited the paper; S.I. worked with data and recruited patients, edited the paper; R.B. worked with data and recruited patients, edited the paper; J.J. participated inpatients' surveillance, participated in study design, edited the paper; L.K. participated inpatients' surveillance, participated in study design, edited the paper; E.K. performed endoscopic examinations, edited the paper; J.S. designed this study and wrote this paper. All authors have read and agreed to the published version of the manuscript.

Funding: European Regional Development Fund, project Nr. 1.1.1.2/VIAA/3/19/525 "Intestinal inflammation as a potentially modifiable risk factor for complications in type 1 diabetes".

Institutional Review Board Statement: This study protocol of the general LatDiane and sub-study devoted to gut health described here were approved by the Latvian Central Ethics Committee and received permissions No. 01-29.1/3 (dated 10 July 2013), Nr. A-17/19-10-17 (dated 17 October 2019), and Nr. 01-29.1/2226 (dated 30 April 2020).

Informed Consent Statement: All study participants provided written informed consent for their participation.

Data Availability Statement: All data are not available publicly due to privacy restrictions. The data are available from the corresponding author on request.

Acknowledgments: We thank Irēna Puzirevska for the coordination of patient recruitment. We acknowledge Latvian Biomedical Research and Study centre and Latvian National Biobank—Genome Database of Latvian population -for providing materials for recruitment and sample processing.

Conflicts of Interest: The authors declare no conflict of interest.

References

1. Bikbov, B.; Purcell, C.A.; Levey, A.S.; Smith, M.; Abdoli, A.; Abebe, M.; Adebayo, O.M.; Afarideh, M.; Agarwal, S.K.; Agudelo-Botero, M.; et al. Global, regional, and national burden of chronic kidney disease, 1990–2017: A systematic analysis for the Global Burden of Disease Study 2017. *Lancet* **2020**, *395*, 709–733. [CrossRef] [PubMed]
2. Colombo, M.; Valo, E.; McGurnaghan, S.J.; Sandholm, N.; Blackbourn, L.A.K.; Dalton, R.N.; Dunger, D.; Groop, P.H.; McKeigue, P.M.; Forsblom, C.; et al. Biomarker panels associated with progression of renal disease in type 1 diabetes. *Diabetologia* **2019**, *62*, 1616–1627. [CrossRef] [PubMed]
3. Du, Y.T.; Rayner, C.K.; Jones, K.L.; Talley, N.J.; Horowitz, M. Gastrointestinal Symptoms in Diabetes: Prevalence, Assessment, Pathogenesis, and Management. *Diabetes Care* **2018**, *41*, 627–637. [CrossRef] [PubMed]
4. Lomer, M.C. Review article: The aetiology, diagnosis, mechanisms and clinical evidence for food intolerance. *Aliment. Pharmacol. Ther.* **2015**, *41*, 262–275. [CrossRef] [PubMed]
5. Leeds, J.S.; Hadjivassiliou, M.; Tesfaye, S.; Sanders, D.S. Lower gastrointestinal symptoms are associated with worse glycemic control and quality of life in type 1 diabetes mellitus. *BMJ Open Diabetes Res. Care* **2018**, *6*, e000514. [CrossRef]
6. Porter, J.A.; MacKenzie, K.E.; Darlow, B.A.; Pearson, J.F.; Day, A.S. A questionnaire-based assessment of gastrointestinal symptoms in children with type 1 diabetes mellitus. *Transl. Pediatr.* **2020**, *9*, 743–749. [CrossRef]

7. Lehto, M.; Groop, P.H. The Gut-Kidney Axis: Putative Interconnections Between Gastrointestinal and Renal Disorders. *Front. Endocrinol.* **2018**, *9*, 553. [CrossRef]
8. Ni, Y.; Zheng, L.; Nan, S.; Ke, L.; Fu, Z.; Jin, J. Enterorenal crosstalks in diabetic nephropathy and novel therapeutics targeting the gut microbiota. *Acta Biochim. Biophys. Sin.* **2022**, *54*, 1406–1420. [CrossRef]
9. Guo, W.; Song, Y.; Sun, Y.; Du, H.; Cai, Y.; You, Q.; Fu, H.; Shao, L. Systemic immune-inflammation index is associated with diabetic kidney disease in Type 2 diabetes mellitus patients: Evidence from NHANES 2011–2018. *Front. Endocrinol.* **2022**, *13*, 1071465. [CrossRef]
10. Winther, S.A.; Mannerla, M.M.; Frimodt-Møller, M.; Persson, F.; Hansen, T.W.; Lehto, M.; Hörkkö, S.; Blaut, M.; Forsblom, C.; Groop, P.H.; et al. Faecal biomarkers in type 1 diabetes with and without diabetic nephropathy. *Sci. Rep.* **2021**, *11*, 15208. [CrossRef]
11. Lassenius, M.I.; Fogarty, C.L.; Blaut, M.; Haimila, K.; Riittinen, L.; Paju, A.; Kirveskari, J.; Järvelä, J.; Ahola, A.J.; Gordin, D.; et al. Intestinal alkaline phosphatase at the crossroad of intestinal health and disease—A putative role in type 1 diabetes. *J. Intern. Med.* **2017**, *281*, 586–600. [CrossRef] [PubMed]
12. D'Addio, F.; La Rosa, S.; Maestroni, A.; Jung, P.; Orsenigo, E.; Ben Nasr, M.; Tezza, S.; Bassi, R.; Finzi, G.; Marando, A.; et al. Circulating IGF-I and IGFBP3 Levels Control Human Colonic Stem Cell Function and Are Disrupted in Diabetic Enteropathy. *Cell Stem Cell* **2015**, *17*, 486–498. [CrossRef] [PubMed]
13. Hochberg, I.; Segol, O.; Shental, R.; Shimoni, P.; Eldor, R. Antihyperglycemic therapy during colonoscopy preparation: A review and suggestions for practical recommendations. *United Eur. Gastroenterol. J.* **2019**, *7*, 735–740. [CrossRef] [PubMed]
14. Pellegrini, S.; Sordi, V.; Bolla, A.M.; Saita, D.; Ferrarese, R.; Canducci, F.; Clementi, M.; Invernizzi, F.; Mariani, A.; Bonfanti, R.; et al. Duodenal Mucosa of Patients with Type 1 Diabetes Shows Distinctive Inflammatory Profile and Microbiota. *J. Clin. Endocrinol. Metab.* **2017**, *102*, 1468–1477. [CrossRef]
15. Paul, P.; Kaul, R.; Chaari, A. Renal Health Improvement in Diabetes through Microbiome Modulation of the Gut-Kidney Axis with Biotics: A Systematic and Narrative Review of Randomized Controlled Trials. *Int. J. Mol. Sci.* **2022**, *23*, 14838. [CrossRef]
16. Ahola, A.J.; Radzeviciene, L.; Zaharenko, L.; Bulum, T.; Skrebinska, S.; Prakapiene, E.; Blaslov, K.; Roso, V.; Rovite, V.; Pirags, V.; et al. Association between symptoms of depression, diabetes complications and vascular risk factors in four European cohorts of individuals with type 1 diabetes—InterDiane Consortium. *Diabetes Res. Clin. Pract.* **2020**, *170*, 108495. [CrossRef]
17. Tzivian, L.; Sokolovska, J.; Grike, A.E.; Kalcenaua, A.; Seidmann, A.; Benis, A.; Mednis, M.; Danovska, I.; Berzins, U.; Bogdanovs, A.; et al. Quantitative and qualitative analysis of the quality of life of Type 1 diabetes patients using insulin pumps and of those receiving multiple daily insulin injections. *Health Qual. Life Outcomes* **2022**, *20*, 120. [CrossRef]
18. Svikle, Z.; Pahirko, L.; Zariņa, L.; Baumane, K.; Kardonaite, D.; Radzeviciene, L.; Daugintyte-Petrusiene, L.; Balciuniene, V.J.; Verkauskiene, R.; Tiščuka, A.; et al. Telomere Lengths and Serum Proteasome Concentrations in Patients with Type 1 Diabetes and Different Severities of Diabetic Retinopathy in Latvia and Lithuania. *J. Clin. Med.* **2022**, *11*, 2768. [CrossRef]
19. Salna, I.; Salna, E.; Pahirko, L.; Skrebinska, S.; Krikova, R.; Folkmane, I.; Pīrāgs, V.; Sokolovska, J. Achievement of treatment targets predicts progression of vascular complications in type 1 diabetes. *J. Diabetes Complicat.* **2021**, *35*, 108072. [CrossRef]
20. Rostoka, E.; Salna, I.; Dekante, A.; Pahirko, L.; Borisovs, V.; Celma, L.; Valeinis, J.; Sjakste, N.; Sokolovska, J. DNA damage in leukocytes and serum nitrite concentration are negatively associated in type 1 diabetes. *Mutagenesis* **2021**, *36*, 213–222. [CrossRef]
21. Sokolovska, J.; Stefanovics, J.; Gersone, G.; Pahirko, L.; Valeinis, J.; Kalva-Vaivode, S.; Rovite, V.; Blumfelds, L.; Pirags, V.; Tretjakovs, P. Angiopoietin 2 and Neuropeptide Y are Associated with Diabetic Kidney Disease in Type 1 Diabetes Mellitus. *Exp. Clin. Endocrinol. Diabetes* **2020**, *128*, 654–662. [CrossRef] [PubMed]
22. Sokolovska, J.; Dekante, A.; Baumane, L.; Pahirko, L.; Valeinis, J.; Dislere, K.; Rovite, V.; Pirags, V.; Sjakste, N. Nitric oxide metabolism is impaired by type 1 diabetes and diabetic nephropathy. *Biomed. Rep.* **2020**, *12*, 251–258. [CrossRef] [PubMed]
23. Salem, R.M.; Todd, J.N.; Sandholm, N.; Cole, J.B.; Chen, W.M.; Andrews, D.; Pezzolesi, M.G.; McKeigue, P.M.; Hiraki, L.T.; Qiu, C.; et al. Genome-Wide Association Study of Diabetic Kidney Disease Highlights Biology Involved in Glomerular Basement Membrane Collagen. *J. Am. Soc. Nephrol.* **2019**, *30*, 2000–2016. [CrossRef] [PubMed]
24. Sviklāne, L.; Olmane, E.; Dzērve, Z.; Kupčs, K.; Pīrāgs, V.; Sokolovska, J. Fatty liver index and hepatic steatosis index for prediction of non-alcoholic fatty liver disease in type 1 diabetes. *J. Gastroenterol. Hepatol.* **2018**, *33*, 270–276. [CrossRef]
25. Rovite, V.; Wolff-Sagi, Y.; Zaharenko, L.; Nikitina-Zake, L.; Grens, E.; Klovins, J. Genome Database of the Latvian Population (LGDB): Design, Goals, and Primary Results. *J. Epidemiol.* **2018**, *28*, 353–360. [CrossRef] [PubMed]
26. Quan, C.; Talley, N.J.; Cross, S.; Jones, M.; Hammer, J.; Giles, N.; Horowitz, M. Development and validation of the Diabetes Bowel Symptom Questionnaire. *Aliment. Pharmacol. Ther.* **2003**, *17*, 1179–1187. [CrossRef]
27. Karahan, D.; Şahin, İ. Comparison of gastrointestinal symptoms and findings in renal replacement therapy modalities. *BMC Nephrol.* **2022**, *23*, 261. [CrossRef]
28. Bouri, S.; Martin, J. Investigation of iron deficiency anaemia. *Clin. Med.* **2018**, *18*, 242–244. [CrossRef]
29. Lewandowski, K.; Rydzewska, G.; Ledwoń, T.K. Preparation for endoscopic examinations in patients with diabetes and hypoglycaemia. *Przegląd Gastroenterol.* **2021**, *16*, 297–305. [CrossRef]
30. Hassan, C.; Bretthauer, M.; Kaminski, M.F.; Polkowski, M.; Rembacken, B.; Saunders, B.; Benamouzig, R.; Holme, O.; Green, S.; Kuiper, T.; et al. Bowel preparation for colonoscopy: European Society of Gastrointestinal Endoscopy (ESGE) guideline. *Endoscopy* **2013**, *45*, 142–150. [CrossRef]

31. Hinkelbein, J.; Lamperti, M.; Akeson, J.; Santos, J.; Costa, J.; De Robertis, E.; Longrois, D.; Novak-Jankovic, V.; Petrini, F.; Struys, M.; et al. European Society of Anaesthesiology and European Board of Anaesthesiology guidelines for procedural sedation and analgesia in adults. *Eur. J. Anaesthesiol.* **2018**, *35*, 6–24. [CrossRef] [PubMed]
32. Saltzman, J.R.; Cash, B.D.; Pasha, S.F.; Early, D.S.; Muthusamy, V.R.; Khashab, M.A.; Chathadi, K.V.; Fanelli, R.D.; Chandrasekhara, V.; Lightdale, J.R.; et al. Bowel preparation before colonoscopy. *Gastrointest. Endosc.* **2015**, *81*, 781–794. [CrossRef] [PubMed]
33. Zhang, J.; Chen, Y.; Zou, L.; Gong, R. Prognostic nutritional index as a risk factor for diabetic kidney disease and mortality in patients with type 2 diabetes mellitus. *Acta Diabetol.* **2023**, *60*, 235–245. [CrossRef] [PubMed]
34. Aktas, G.; Yilmaz, S.; Kantarci, D.B.; Duman, T.T.; Bilgin, S.; Balci, S.B.; Atak Tel, B.M. Is serum uric acid-to-HDL cholesterol ratio elevation associated with diabetic kidney injury? *Postgrad. Med.* **2023**, *135*, 519–523. [CrossRef]
35. Schön, E.-M.; Winter, D.; Escalona, M.J.; Thomaschewski, J. *Key Challenges in Agile Requirements Engineering*; Springer: Cham, Switzerland, 2017; pp. 37–51.
36. Shi, J.T.; Chen, N.; Xu, J.; Goyal, H.; Wu, Z.Q.; Zhang, J.X.; Xu, H.G. Diagnostic Accuracy of Fecal Calprotectin for Predicting Relapse in Inflammatory Bowel Disease: A Meta-Analysis. *J. Clin. Med.* **2023**, *12*, 1206. [CrossRef]
37. Rezazadeh Ardabili, A.; Goudkade, D.; Wintjens, D.; Romberg-Camps, M.; Winkens, B.; Pierik, M.; Grabsch, H.I.; Jonkers, D. Histopathological Features in Colonic Biopsies at Diagnosis Predict Long-term Disease Course in Patients with Crohn's Disease. *J. Crohn's Colitis* **2021**, *15*, 1885–1897. [CrossRef]

biomedicines

MDPI

Article

Relationship between β-Cell Autoantibodies and Their Combination with Anthropometric and Metabolic Components and Microvascular Complications in Latent Autoimmune Diabetes in Adults

Tomislav Bulum [1,2,*], Marijana Vučić Lovrenčić [3,4], Jadranka Knežević Ćuća [3], Martina Tomić [5], Sandra Vučković-Rebrina [6] and Lea Duvnjak [1,2]

1 Department of Diabetes and Endocrinology, Vuk Vrhovac University Clinic for Diabetes, Endocrinology and Metabolic Diseases, Merkur University Hospital, 10000 Zagreb, Croatia
2 Medical School, University of Zagreb, 10000 Zagreb, Croatia
3 Clinical Department of Medical Biochemistry and Laboratory Medicine, Merkur University Hospital, 10000 Zagreb, Croatia
4 Scientific Research Unit, Merkur University Hospital, 10000 Zagreb, Croatia
5 Department of Ophthalmology, Vuk Vrhovac University Clinic for Diabetes, Endocrinology and Metabolic Diseases, Merkur University Hospital, 10000 Zagreb, Croatia
6 Department of Neurology, Vuk Vrhovac University Clinic for Diabetes, Endocrinology and Metabolic Diseases, Merkur University Hospital, 10000 Zagreb, Croatia
* Correspondence: tomobulum@gmail.com

Abstract: Aims: Our study aimed to investigate the relationship between three autoantibodies and their combination with anthropometric and metabolic components and microvascular complications in patients with latent autoimmune diabetes in adults (LADA). Methods: Our study included 189 LADA patients divided into four subgroups according to the autoantibodies present: glutamic acid decarboxylase autoantibodies (GADA) only; zinc transporter-8 autoantibodies (ZnT8A)+GADA; insulinoma-associated-2 autoantibodies (IA-2)+GADA; and ZnT8+IA-2+GADA. Results: Compared to GADA positivity only, patients with ZnT8+GADA positivity and ZnT8+IA-2+GADA positivity had a shorter diabetes duration and lower body mass index (BMI); patients with ZnT8+GADA positivity were younger and showed an increase in glomerular filtration rate, while those with ZnT8+IA-2+GADA positivity had lower C-peptide and lower insulin resistance measured with HOMA2-IR. In a multiple regression analysis, ZnT8 positivity was associated with lower BMI ($p = 0.0024$), female sex ($p = 0.0005$), and shorter duration of disease ($p = 0.0034$), while IA-2 positivity was associated with lower C-peptide levels ($p = 0.0034$) and shorter diabetes duration ($p = 0.02$). No association between antibody positivity and microvascular complications of diabetes, including retinopathy, neuropathy, and microalbuminuria, as well as with variables of glucose control and β-cell function were found. Conclusion: The results of our study suggest that ZnT8 and IA-2 autoantibodies are present in a significant number of LADA patients and associated with clinical and metabolic characteristics resembling classic type 1 diabetes. Due to increased LADA prevalence, earlier identification of patients requiring frequent monitoring with the earlier intensification of insulin therapy might be of special clinical interest.

Keywords: autoimmune diabetes in adults; autoimmunity; glutamic acid decarboxylase autoantibodies

1. Introduction

Type 1 diabetes mellitus (T1DM) and latent autoimmune diabetes in adults (LADA) are autoimmune conditions associated with circulating autoantibodies which indicate the destruction of pancreatic islet β-cells, leading to insulin deficiency and hyperglycemia [1]. Compared to classic type 1 diabetes, which develops in childhood and progresses rapidly,

LADA is characterized by a slow progression of the disease and slower pancreatic β-cell dysfunction and usually manifests itself in later adulthood [2,3]. Such patients were previously diagnosed with type 2 diabetes, although most did not have the clinical features of metabolic syndrome. Due to the slow progression of the disease, patients with LADA can achieve optimal glucose control with oral antihyperglycemic agents only for years with preserved β-cell function measured with C-peptide [4]. Diagnosis of LADA is confirmed with a positive test for circulating specific β-cell autoantibodies (glutamic acid decarboxylase enzyme autoantibodies (GADA), zinc transporter-8 autoantibodies (ZnT8), and tyrosine phosphatase-like transmembrane glycoprotein autoantibodies (IA2)) [5–8]. GADA autoantibodies are predominant in the definition of LADA, although detectable GADA does not always confirm autoimmune diabetes etiology [9]. After verifying the diagnosis of LADA, the main goal of treatment, as in patients with type 1 diabetes and type 2 diabetes, is to achieve optimal glucoregulation to prevent the development and progression of micro- and macrovascular complications.

It is suggested that LADA is not a unique subtype of diabetes but instead represents a combination of two heterogeneous populations with very different phenotypes. One phenotype represents type 1 diabetes and the other represents type 2 diabetes [10]. Single autoantibody positivity and lower titer are more closely related to the type 2 diabetes phenotype, whereas the high titer of GADA as well as simultaneous positivity for ZnT8 and IA2 autoantibodies are more closely associated with the type 1 diabetes phenotype [9,11]. Generally, metabolic syndrome and its component disorders (obesity, blood pressure, and triglycerides) and cardiovascular disease are more common in patients with LADA than in classic type 1 diabetes but less common than in those with classic type 2 diabetes [12,13]. Also, the GADA titer is negatively associated with the age of onset, total cholesterol and triglycerides, obesity, and C-peptide concentrations and positively associated with the hemoglobin A_1c and high-density lipoprotein cholesterol (HDL-C) concentrations [14]. GADA titer negatively correlates with the C-peptide concentration, and LADA patients with higher GADA titers show more insulin deficiency [15,16]. Different autoantibody titers and their positivity affect LADA patients' different phenotypes and clinical characteristics [17]. In addition, up to 10% of all patients with type 2 diabetes meet the criteria for LADA [18].

Diabetes-related comorbidities of patients with LADA and positivity for single or simultaneous autoantibodies are not fully understood. Some patients develop micro- and macrovascular complications despite improved glycemic control and independently of metabolic syndrome features [15,19]. Our study aimed to investigate the relationship between three specific β-cell autoantibodies, GADA, IA-2, and ZnT8, and their combination with anthropometric and metabolic components and with microvascular complications in adult patients with autoimmune diabetes.

2. Methods

2.1. Study Design and Ethics Statement

This cross-sectional study was performed at the Department of Diabetes and Endocrinology and Clinical Department of Medical Biochemistry and Laboratory Medicine at Merkur University Hospital in Zagreb, Croatia. A total of 189 LADA patients aged over 35 years with a minimum of 1 year since being diagnosed with diabetes and GADA-positive autoantibodies were included in the study. The study was conducted following the Declaration of Helsinki and approved by the hospital's ethics committee (protocol number 05/01-850, approval date: 16 September 2020). All study participants received written and oral information about the study and signed the written informed consent form.

2.2. Demographic Data, Medical Records, and Clinical Characteristics

Demographic data of patients included age, gender, and diabetes duration. Body mass index (BMI) was calculated by dividing weight and height squared (kg/m^2). Weight and height were measured using a balance-beam scale and a wall-mounted stadiometer.

Systolic/diastolic blood pressure (SBP/DBP) were measured with an ambulatory digital sphygmomanometer after a 10-min resting period using a cuff appropriate to the length and circumference of the arm and expressed in mmHg.

2.3. Measure of β-Cell Function

Fasting venous blood samples were collected to determine the biochemistry panel, including glucose, C-peptide, and HbA_1c. HbA_1c was measured in EDTA-anticoagulated whole blood samples using an automated turbidimetric inhibition immunoassay (HbA_1c Gen 3, Cobas Integra 400 Plus, Roche Diagnostic, Basel, Switzerland), traceable to the International Federation of Clinical Chemistry and Laboratory Medicine (IFCC) reference system and reported in National Glycohemoglobin Standardization Program (NGSP) units (%). Fasting serum C-peptide concentration was determined using an automated chemiluminescent immunoassay (Advia Centaur XP, Siemens Healthineers, Tarrytown, NY, USA). HOMA2-%B and HOMA2-IR were determined using the HOMA2 Calculator (available at https://www.dtu.ox.ac.uk/homacalculator/download.php, accessed on 14 September 2023; Oxford Centre for Diabetes, Endocrinology and Metabolism, Oxford, UK). We used fasting blood glucose and serum C-peptide levels to calculate the HOMA2 score. The secretory capacity of the pancreatic islet β-cells is expressed using the HOMA2 calculator as HOMA2-%B, where the higher the value, the more insulin the β-cells can secrete to respond to blood glucose levels. Higher HOMA2-%B and HOMA2-IR scores indicate increased insulin sensitivity and insulin resistance, respectively.

2.4. Detection of Autoantibodies

GAD and IA-2 antibodies were analyzed using their respective bridge ELISA immunoassays (Euroimmun, Lübeck, Germany) calibrated to international units (IU) with the 1st WHO reference reagent for islet cell antibodies (WHO, 1999, reagent 97/550, National Institute for Biological Standards and Control, Hertfordshire, UK). By definition, the NIBSC 97/550 reference reagent contains 100 IU of anti-GAD or anti-IA2 per ampoule. Human recombinant glutamic acid decarboxylase, isoform GAD65, and human recombinant tyrosine phosphatase (IA2) were used as antigens in the respective immunoassays. The lower detection limits for GAD and anti-IA2 are 0.59 IU/mL and 1.04 IU/mL, respectively, and the cut-off values are set at 10 IU/mL for both assays.

ZnT8 autoantibodies were detected using a bridge ELISA (RSR Limited, Cardiff, United Kingdom) capable of detecting and quantifying autoantibodies specific to R 325 (Arg) to W 325 (Trp) or residue 325 non-specific variants. In this assay, ZnT8 Ab in patients' sera, calibrators, and controls react with ZnT8 coated onto ELISA plate wells. After a 16–20-h incubation, the samples are discarded, ZnT8-Biotin conjugate is added, and ZnT8 Ab in the samples forms a bridge between ZnT8 bound to the wells and ZnT8-Biotin via polyvalent binding. Unbound ZnT8-Biotin is removed by washing, and the amount of bound ZnT8-Biotin is determined by adding streptavidin peroxidase (S-P), which binds specifically to biotin. After washing the unbound S-P, the peroxidase substrate 3,3′, 5,5′ tetramethyl-benzidine (TMB) is added, which results in a chromogenic reaction. After stopping the reaction with acidification, the absorbance of the reaction mixture is read (405/450 nm) using an ELISA plate reader. The absorbance is proportional to the ZnT8 antibody positivity in the sample.

The assay is calibrated against proprietary calibrators manufactured from rabbit serum positive for ZnT8 Ab and values assigned to the RSR arbitrary units. The assay range is 10–2000 U/mL, with a lower detection limit of 1.2 U/mL and the recommended cut-off for positivity at 15 U/mL.

The cut-off limit was 5 IU/mL for GADA, 10 IU/mL for IA2 autoantibodies, and 10 U/mL for ZnT8 autoantibodies, respectively [20]. The patients with autoantibody titers over the established cut-off were considered seropositive [21].

2.5. Chronic Complications of Diabetes

Renal function was determined using serum creatinine, glomerular filtration rate (GFR), and albumin/creatinine (A/C) ratio. Serum creatinine was determined using a compensated Jaffe spectrophotometric method traceable to Standard Reference Material 967 provided by the US National Institute of Standards and Technology (NIST). GFR was estimated using the Chronic Kidney Disease Epidemiology Collaboration (CKD-EPI) formula [22], and a random urine sample was collected to determine the A/C ratio using a turbidimetric immunoassay and photometric assay, respectively. Normoalbuminuria was defined as an A/C ratio < 3 mg/mmol and microalbuminuria as an A/C ratio $\geq 3 < 30$ mg/mmol. Those with chronic kidney disease, defined as macroalbuminuria (A/C ratio $\geq$ 30 mg/mmol) and/or estimated GFR < 60 mL/min^{-1}1.73 m^{-2}, were excluded from the study.

Diabetic retinopathy was diagnosed via binocular indirect slit lamp fundoscopy and color fundus photographs of two fields of both eyes were taken with a suitable 45° fundus camera (VISUCAM, Zeiss, Germany) according to the EURODIAB retinal photography methodology [23]. Evaluation of peripheral sensorimotor neuropathy was based on clinical symptoms (neuropathy symptom score), signs (neuropathy disability score), quantitative sensory testing (vibration perception threshold), and electroneuromyography testing.

2.6. Statistical Analysis

The normality of distribution was tested using the Shapiro–Wilk test. Data are expressed as mean ± SD for normally distributed variables and median with range for non-normally distributed variables. Pearson's and Spearman's rank correlations were used to assess the relationship between normally and non-normally distributed variables, respectively. Depending on the data distribution, differences between the groups were examined using parametric (*t*-test) or non-parametric tests (Mann–Whitney). A *p*-value of less than 0.05 was considered statistically significant in all analyses. Statistical analysis was performed using Stata/IC ver. 14.2, StataCorp LLC, and MedCalc Statistical Software version 18.11.6 (MedCalc Software bvba, Ostend, Belgium; https://www.medcalc.org; accessed on 1 January 2019).

3. Results

Among 189 adult subjects (91 males (M) and 98 females (F)) with diabetes and GAD-positive autoantibodies included in the study, ZnT8 autoantibodies were detected in 81 subjects (M/F = 38/53) and IA-2 autoantibodies in 67 subjects (M/F = 27/40) while 91 subjects (M/F = 53/38) had only GADA positivity. Regarding autoantibody combinations, 31/17 GADA-positive subjects had ZnT8/IA-2 autoantibody positivity, whereas, in 50 subjects, all three antibodies were detected (Figure 1).

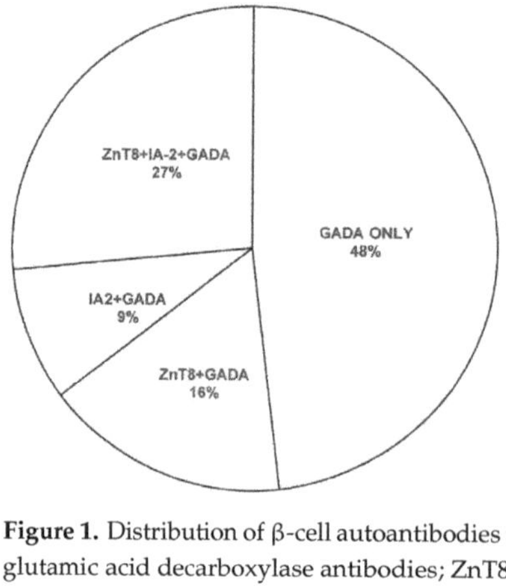

Figure 1. Distribution of β-cell autoantibodies in GADA-positive adult patients with diabetes. GADA: glutamic acid decarboxylase antibodies; ZnT8: zinc transporter-8; IA-2: anti-islet-2 antibodies.

3.1. Autoantibodies and Clinical Phenotype

There were significant differences in age, BMI, diabetes duration, C-peptide levels, HOMA2-IR, and eGFR between four subgroups of patients with various antibody patterns (GADA only, ZnT8+GADA; IA-2+GADA; and ZnT8+IA-2+GADA). Patients with a combination of either ZnT8+GADA or ZnT8+IA-2+GADA positivity had a shorter diabetes duration and lower BMI than patients who had GADA only. Compared to the GADA-only positive subgroup, patients with the ZnT8+GADA combination were younger and had a higher eGFR, while those with a combination of all three autoantibodies had lower C-peptide and HOMA2-IR values. Also, various antibody patterns were unevenly distributed according to sex, with predominately males in the subgroups of GADA only and IA-2+GADA positivity, while there were more females in the subgroups of ZnT8-positive patients, either combined with GADA alone or IA-2+GADA ($\chi^2 = 10.49$, df = 3, $p = 0.0148$).

Males had significantly higher GADA titers than females ($p = 0.034$; Mann–Whitney test), whereas no sex-related differences were observed in other parameters except for BMI in the entire study cohort.

No significant differences in the variables of fasting plasma glucose, HbA_1c, HOMA2-estimated β-cell function, TSH, and albuminuria between the subgroups of patients with various antibody patterns were observed (Table 1).

Table 1. Clinical characteristics of the GAD-positive adult diabetic patients according to the diabetes-specific autoantibody patterns.

Variable	Entire Cohort	Antibody-Positivity-Related Subgroup				p-Value
		GADA Only	ZnT8+GADA	IA-2+GADA	ZnT8+IA-2+GADA	
N	189	91	31	17	50	
% of the total	100	48	16	9	27	
Sex (M/F)	91/98	53/38	11/20	10/7	17/33	**0.0148**
Age (years)	53 (39–63)	56 (42–66)	**47 (37–56) ***	49 (38–62)	50 (36–60)	**0.0261**
Diabetes duration (years)	4 (2–11)	6 (2–15)	**3 (1–7) ***	4 (2–8)	**2 (1–7) ***	**<0.001**
BMI (kg/m^2)	25.6 (22.0–29.0)	28.0 ± 5.5	**24.7 ± 5.6 ***	25 (22–27)	**24.0 ± 3.7 ***	**<0.001**
C-peptide (nmol/L)	0.28 (0.18–0.47)	0.33 (0.22–0.54)	0.3 (0.22–0.43)	0.21 (0.12–0.36)	**0.22 (0.15–0.35) ***	**0.0038**
HOMA2-B (%)	25.9 (13.4–39.6)	29.4 (15.7–44.4)	18.6 (13.5–33.5)	22.1 (9.4–35.4)	23.9 (9.6–36.7)	0.1228
HOMA2-IRI (1/1)	0.84 (0.51–1.39)	0.98 (0.55–1.71)	0.83 (0.65–1.08)	0.82 (0.32–1.00)	**0.64 (0.44–1.20) ***	0.0327
FPG (mmol/L)	8.7 (7.0–12.0)	8.5 (6.9–11.3)	9.6 (7.5–13.3)	8.9 (7.2–13.1)	8.5 (6.9–11.5)	0.8432
HbA_1c (%)	7.4 (6.5–8.7)	7.4 (6.4–8.8)	7.1 (6.6–9.8)	7.1 (6.0–8.3)	7.4 (6.6–8.4)	0.7247
eGFR (mL/min/1.72 m^2)	97 (85–107)	93 (80–101)	**106 (94–118) ***	100 (91–109)	100 (87–110)	**0.0011**
U-ACR (mg/mmol)	1.3 (0.6–3.7)	1.5 (0.8–4.9)	1.5 (0.6–4.2)	0.9 (0.63–1.98)	0.8 (0.5–2.4)	0.0548
TSH (mIU/L)	1.80 (1.20–2.77)	1.87 (1.19–2.90)	1.93 (1.20–2.82)	1.52 (1.32–2.05)	1.70 (1.18–2.65)	0.6608

Values are presented as median (interquartile range) or mean ± SD, depending on the data distribution. Chi-square test for categorical variables; Kruskal–Wallis ANOVA for continuous variables. * $p < 0.05$ compared to GADA only subgroup (Dunn's post-hoc test) (bold values). GADA: glutamic acid decarboxylase antibodies; ZnT8: zinc transporter-8; IA-2: anti-islet-2 antibodies; HOMA2-B: homeostatic model assessment 2 β-cell function; HOMA2-IRI: homeostatic model assessment 2 insulin resistance index; eGFR: estimated glomerular filtration rate; U-ACR: urinary albumin to creatinine ratio.

GADA titers were significantly higher in the ZnT8+GADA subgroup but not in the IA-2+GADA and ZnT8+IA-2+GADA-positive subgroup when compared to GADA-only positive patients (Figure 2). There were no significant differences in the titers of ZnT8 and IA-2 autoantibodies between the subgroups of ZnT8+GADA and ZnT8+IA-2+GADA-positivity ($p = 0.1423$) and IA-2+GADA and ZnT8+IA-2+GADA-positivity ($p = 0.0576$), respectively (Mann–Whitney U test).

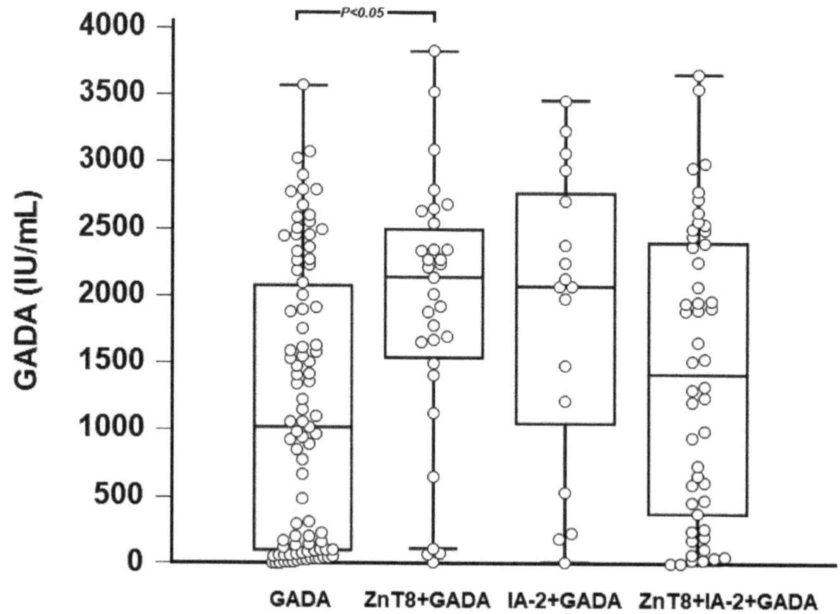

Figure 2. GADA titers in subgroups of patients with various diabetes-specific autoantibody patterns. GADA-only autoantibodies were present in 91 patients, ZnT8+GADA in 31 patients, IA-2+GADA in 17 patients, and ZnT8+IA-2+GADA in 50 patients. The results are medians/IQR (Kruskal–Wallis ANOVA followed by Dunn's post-hoc test). GADA: glutamic acid decarboxylase antibodies; ZnT8: zinc transporter-8; IA-2: anti-islet-2 antibodies.

ZnT8 positivity was associated with lower BMI (OR/C.I. = 0.8788/0.8086 to 0.9551, $p = 0.0024$), female sex (OR/C.I. = 4.0371/1.8325 to 8.8960, $p = 0.0005$), and shorter duration of disease (OR/C.I = 0.8933/0.8284 to 0.9633, $p = 0.0034$). On the other hand, IA-2 positivity could be predicted with lower C-peptide levels (OR/C.I. = 0.0675/0.0111 to 0.4102, $p = 0.0034$) and shorter duration of disease (OR/C.I. = 0.9347/0.8829 to 0.9896, $p = 0.02025$). Other variables included in the logistic regression model, including GADA titer, HOMA2-B, HOMA2-IR, eGFR, and HbA_1c, could not predict ZnT8 and IA-2 antibody positivity, respectively. Thirty-four patients (17%) had hypothyroidism, assessed as either TSH level > 4.5 mIU/L, levothyroxine replacement therapy, or both. GADA titer and HOMA2-B were significant predictors of hypothyroidism (OR/C.I. = 1.0011/1.0006 to 1.0016, $p = 0.0001$ and 1.0228/1.0042 to 1.0417, $p = 0.0160$, respectively). There were no associations between thyroid status and age, sex, duration of diabetes, BMI, and ZnT8/IA-2 positivity in the logistic regression model used.

3.2. *Associations with Glucose Control and Complications*

A multiple logistic regression analysis revealed that GADA titer, duration of diabetes, and HOMA2-estimated β-cell function significantly predicted glucose control, set at an HbA_1c cut-off of 7.0%, while age, sex, BMI, HOMA2-IR, and positivity for IA-2 and ZnT8 antibodies did not influence glucose control (Table 2). The model was significant ($\chi^2 = 37.6$, $p < 0.0001$) and correctly classified 71.3% of the cases (AUC = 0.783, SE = 0.038; C.I. = 0.7007 to 0.847).

Table 2. Predictors of glucose control ($HbA_1c \leq 7.0\%$/N = 100—good control;$HbA_1c > 7.0\%$/ N = 89—poor control) in GADA-positive adult diabetic patients.

Variable	Odds Ratio	95% Conf. Interval	*p*-Value
GADA (U/mL)	1.0008	1.0004–1.0011	<0.0001
HOMA2-B (%)	0.9670	0.9478–0.9865	0.0010
Duration of diabetes (years)	1.0804	1.0200–1.1444	0.0084

Multiple logistic regression analysis. Variables not retained in the model: age, sex, BMI, IRI, IA-2 positivity, ZnT8 positivity. GADA: glutamic acid decarboxylase antibodies; HOMA2-B: homeostatic model assessment 2 β-cell function.

No association between antibody positivity and microvascular complications of diabetes including retinopathy, neuropathy, and microalbuminuria were found. Also, neither BMI nor β-cell function, insulin resistance, HbA_1c, sex, and eGFR were significant determinants of microvascular complications in the multiple logistic regression model. However, the duration of diabetes had a remarkable effect, significantly predicting retinopathy, neuropathy, and microalbuminuria (OR/C.I. = 1.1499/1.0713 to 1.2344, p = 0.0001; 1.1169/1.0321 to 1.2087, p = 0.0060 and 1.0846/1.0257 to 1.1468, p = 0.0044, respectively). Furthermore, hypertension was positively associated with microalbuminuria (OR/C.I. = 4.7287/1.8996 to 11.7713, p = 0.008), and age was positively associated with neuropathy (OR/C.I. = 1.0639/1.0252 to 1.1041, p = 0.0011).

4. Discussion

This cross-sectional study included GADA-positive adult diabetic patients classified according to the presence of other β-cell autoimmune markers (ZnT8 and IA2) into groups with single, double, and triple antibody positivity. Our study included only GADA-positive adult diabetic patients because it is questionable whether positivity for a single low-titer islet autoantibody other than GADA is a reliable indicator of autoimmune disease. GADA titers were significantly higher in the ZnT8+GADA subgroup but not in the IA-2+GADA and ZnT8+IA-2+GADA-positive subgroups when compared to GADA-only positive patients. Although ZnT8 is an autoantibody antigen used to diagnose type 1 diabetes, ZnT8 autoantibodies are also detected in many patients with LADA. Unlike GADA and IA-2, the ZnT8 autoantibody is exclusively expressed in pancreatic β-cells and targets the autoimmune process in adult-onset diabetes [24]. In addition, the prevalence of ZnT8 autoantibodies is low in younger individuals but increases dramatically from 3 years onward, peaking at 80% in late adolescence and tending to decline after that [25]. We also observed more females in the subgroups of ZnT8-positive patients combined with GADA alone or IA-2+GADA. It is well known that females have an increased incidence of autoimmune diseases generally, although no gender difference in the incidence of type 1 diabetes was found [26]. ZnT8 autoantibodies were detected in a significant proportion of our patients and thus seem to be a valuable marker of patients with adult-onset autoimmune diabetes. On the contrary, it is suggested that GADA and/or IA-2 antibody positivity in middle-aged individuals at risk for diabetes is not a clinically relevant risk factor for progression to diabetes [27].

Patients with a combination of either ZnT8+GADA or ZnT8+IA-2+GADA positivity had a shorter diabetes duration, lower C-peptide and HOMA2-IR values, and younger age with lower BMI than patients who had GADA only. Compared to only GADA-positive adult diabetic patients, those with multiple antibodies exhibited characteristics more similar to those of type 1 diabetes, with a younger age at disease onset, lower BMI, lower C-peptide level, and higher insulin sensitivity [24,28]. Multiple autoantibody positivity can identify patients with a more severe form of β-cell exhaustion in whom early insulinization might be needed to preserve β-cell function [29]. Those with a single GADA positivity exhibited characteristics similar to those with classic type 2 diabetes. In a clinical setting, it is essential to differentiate these two clinical phenotypes within the adult patient population because the prevalence of LADA has reached a high level in some countries. Nowadays, there is an increased prevalence of LADA in up to 5.9% of newly diagnosed patients with type 2 diabetes over the age of 30 and in almost 65% of patients with newly diagnosed T1DM in China [30].

A multiple logistic regression analysis revealed that GADA titer, along with the duration of diabetes and HOMA2-estimated β-cell function, significantly predicted glucose control, set at an HbA_1c cut-off of 7.0%, while IA-2 and ZnT8 antibodies did not influence glucose control. Patients with a high GADA titer have an accelerated loss of β-cell function early in the development of the disease, and those with a high GADA titer have worse glycemic control despite higher insulin requirements [31]. In contrast, in patients with type 1 diabetes at diabetes diagnosis, there were no differences in the ZnT8 autoantibody status according to HbA_1c, and during diabetes follow-up, there were no statistically significant differences in glycemic control and vascular complications related to ZnT8 autoantibody positivity [32]. In addition, in patients with type 2 diabetes, although ZnT8-positive participants experienced a loss of glycemic control during treatment, they exhibited lower rates of diabetic complications than other groups [33].

No association between autoantibody positivity and microvascular complications of diabetes including retinopathy, neuropathy, and microalbuminuria were found in our study. The apparent explanation is that our cohort had a short duration of diabetes (4 years) with reasonably controlled glycemia (median HbA_1c 7.4%). However, as previously mentioned, ZnT8 antibody positivity in patients with type 2 diabetes was associated with a lower rate of diabetic complications despite a loss of glycemic control on treatment [33]. Also, GAD-positive patients with recent onset of type 1 diabetes reported worse glycemic control but without clinical neuropathy and slightly decreased somatosensory and autonomic nerve function [34]. In our study, patients with single GADA and ZnT8+GADA positivity had a marginally higher (non-significant) risk of microalbuminuria. However, it was documented that in LADA patients, compared with the GADA-negative patients, microalbuminuria was less frequent both at baseline and during follow-up [35]. In another study, patients with GADA had a significantly lower prevalence of diabetic retinopathy compared with patients without GADA (19.2 vs. 47.9%; $p < 0.05$), with a similar prevalence of nephropathy and neuropathy [36]. In patients with a long duration of type 1 diabetes, higher GADA levels were shown to be more common in patients with peripheral neuropathy and less likely in patients with severe retinopathy [37]. In support of that data, we previously observed in a sample of 461 LADA patients that GADA is associated with peripheral neuropathy; however, that cohort has a significantly longer duration of diabetes compared to this study [38]. There is no consensus, and the majority of cross-sectional studies did not reveal significant associations between specific β-cell autoantibodies and the risk of development of microvascular complications in diabetes [39,40]. It seems that the assessment of diabetes-associated autoantibodies at diagnosis does not help predict the development of future microvascular complications, although higher GADA levels have been associated with subsequent nerve damage [41].

Due to increased LADA prevalence in clinical settings, earlier identification of patients requiring frequent monitoring with the earlier intensification of insulin therapy might be of particular clinical interest. Those with simultaneous GADA, ZnT8, and IA-2 positivity have a more severe form of β-cell autoimmunity, and their residual β-cell function might be preserved by early introduction of insulin therapy [42]. A high GADA titer with ZnT8 and IA-2 positivity in the first year after diagnosis significantly increases the progression toward insulin requirement in patients with LADA [43]. Although a high titer of GADA is generally connected with a shorter insulin-free period, results from the significant and essential United Kingdom Prospective Diabetes Study (UKPDS) suggest that GADA autoantibodies persist for six years after diagnosis of LADA but are not associated with disease progression [44]. Several autoantibodies, more so than high titers of GADA, predict insulin dependence, and the presence of multiple β-cell autoantibodies is highly correlated with a faster decline of islet function in patients with LADA [45,46].

The present study has several potential limitations. First, this was a single hospital-based cross-sectional study with a limited number of study participants that most probably are not representative of the population of LADA. Therefore, the data must be confirmed in prospective studies with more patients. Second, our analyses were based on a single measurement of autoantibodies, which might not reflect the dynamic nature of autoimmunity over time. Third, clinical methods used to diagnose diabetic retinopathy and neuropathy may influence the results, making it difficult to compare findings between studies. Fourth, since our study only included patients from the white European population, there was no racial/ethnic diversity.

In conclusion, our study, which included 189 adult LADA patients, revealed diverse associations between individual-specific β-cell autoantibodies and their combination with clinical and metabolic phenotypes. The patients with a single GADA positivity exhibited characteristics more similar to those with classic type 2 diabetes, while those with positivity to all three autoantibodies had clinical and metabolic characteristics of classic type 1 diabetes. In a clinical setting, it is essential to differentiate these two clinical phenotypes within the adult patient population because the prevalence of LADA nowadays is increasing significantly due to the growing awareness of this subtype of diabetes. A diagnostic approach using multiple specific β-cell antibodies may help identify subpopulations of adult patients with diabetes requiring more frequent monitoring to improve patient outcomes. No association between antibody positivity and microvascular complications of diabetes was found in our study, probably because of the short duration of diabetes and relatively satisfactorily controlled disease. However, the relationship between β-cell autoimmunity and chronic complications of diabetes merits further investigation in long-term prospective studies.

Author Contributions: Conceptualization, T.B. and M.V.L.; data curation, L.D.; formal analysis, T.B., M.T. and M.V.L.; methodology, M.V.L., J.K.Ć., T.B. and L.D.; project administration, M.V.L.; resources, M.V.L.; supervision, L.D.; writing—original draft, T.B. and M.V.L.; writing—review and editing, T.B., M.V.L., M.T., S.V.-R. and L.D. All authors have read and agreed to the published version of the manuscript.

Funding: This research received no external funding.

Institutional Review Board Statement: This study was conducted following the Declaration of Helsinki and approved by the hospital's ethics committee (protocol number 05/01-849, approval date: 16 September 2020).

Informed Consent Statement: All patients included in this study received both written and oral information about the study and signed the written informed consent form.

Data Availability Statement: The data presented in this study are available on request from the corresponding author.

Conflicts of Interest: The authors declare no conflict of interest.

References

1. Alberti, K.G.; Zimmet, P.Z. Definition, diagnosis and classification of diabetes mellitus and its complications. Part 1: Diagnosis and classification of diabetes mellitus: Provisional report of a WHO consultation. *Diabet. Med.* **1998**, *15*, 539–553. [CrossRef]
2. WHO/ADA, Report of the Expert Committee on the diagnosis and classification of diabetes mellitus. *Diabetes Care* **1997**, *20*, 1183–1197. [CrossRef]
3. Redondo, M.J. LADA: Time for a new definition. *Diabetes* **2013**, *62*, 339–340. [CrossRef] [PubMed]
4. Buzzetti, R.; Tuomi, T.; Mauricio, D.; Pietropaolo, M.; Zhou, Z.; Pozzilli, P.; Leslie, R.D. Management of Latent Autoimmune Diabetes in Adults: A Consensus Statement From an International Expert Panel. *Diabetes* **2020**, *69*, 2037–2047. [CrossRef] [PubMed]
5. Botazzo, G.F.; Floorin-Christensen, A.; Doniach, D. Islet cell antibodies in diabetes mellitus with autoimmune polyendocrine deficiencies. *Lancet* **1974**, *304*, 1279–1283. [CrossRef]
6. Palmer, J.P.; Asplin, C.M.; Clemons, P.; Lyen, K.; Tatpati, O.; Raghu, P.K.; Paquetteet, T.L. Insulin antibodies in insulin-dependent diabetes before insulin treatment. *Science* **1983**, *222*, 1337–1339. [CrossRef] [PubMed]

7. Baekkeskov, S.; Anastoot, H.J.; Chirstgau, S.; Reetz, A.; Solimena, M.; Cascalho, M.; Folli, F.; Richter-Olesen, H.; De Camilliet, P. Identification of the 64K autoantigen in insulin-dependent diabetes as the GABA synthesizing enzyme glutamic acid decarboxylase. *Nature* **1990**, *347*, 151–156. [CrossRef]
8. Lan, M.S.; Lu, J.; Goto, Y.; Notkins, A.L. Molecular cloning and identification of a receptor-type protein tyrosine phosphatase, IA2, from human insulinoma. *DNA Cell Biol.* **1994**, *13*, 505–514. [CrossRef] [PubMed]
9. Jones, A.G.; McDonald, T.J.; Shields, B.M.; Hagopian, W.; Hattersley, A.T. Latent Autoimmune Diabetes of Adults (LADA) Is Likely to Represent a Mixed Population of Autoimmune (Type 1) and Nonautoimmune (Type 2) Diabetes. *Diabetes Care* **2021**, *44*, 1243–1251. [CrossRef]
10. Blaslov, K.; Bulum, T.; Knežević-Ćuća, J.; Duvnjak, L. Relationship between autoantibodies combination, metabolic syndrome components and diabetic complications in autoimmune diabetes in adults. *Endocrine* **2015**, *48*, 551–556. [CrossRef]
11. Brophy, S.; Yderstraede, K.; Mauricio, D.; Hunter, S.; Hawa, M.; Pozzilli, P.; Schernthaner, G.; Schloot, N.; Buzzetti, R.; Davies, H.; et al. Time to insulin initiation cannot be used in defining latent autoimmune diabetes in adults. *Diabetes Care* **2008**, *31*, 439–441. [CrossRef] [PubMed]
12. Tuomi, T.; Carlsson, A.; Li, H.; Isomaa, B.; Miettinen, A.; Nilsson, A.; Nissén, M.; Ehrnström, B.O.; Forsén, B.; Snickars, B.; et al. Clinical and genetic characteristics of type 2 diabetes with and without GAD antibodies. *Diabetes* **1999**, *48*, 150–157. [CrossRef] [PubMed]
13. Mollo, A.; Hernandez, M.; Marsal, J.R.; Esquerda, A.; Rius, F.; Blanco-Vaca, F.; Verdaguer, J.; Pozzilli, P.; de Leiva, A.; Mauricio, D. Latent autoimmune diabetes in adults is perched between type 1 and type 2: Evidence from adults in one region of Spain. *Diabetes Metab. Res. Rev.* **2013**, *29*, 446–451. [CrossRef]
14. Roh, M.O.; Jung, C.H.; Kim, B.Y.; Mok, J.O.; Kim, C.H. The prevalence and characteristics of latent autoimmune diabetes in adults (LADA) and its relation with chronic complications in a clinical department of a university hospital in Korea. *Acta Diabetol.* **2013**, *50*, 129–134. [CrossRef]
15. Buzzetti, R.; Di Pietro, S.; Giaccari, A.; Petrone, A.; Locatelli, M.; Suraci, C.; Capizzi, M.; Arpi, M.L.; Bazzigaluppi, E.; Dotta, F.; et al. High titer of autoantibodies to GAD identifies a specific phenotype of adult-onset autoimmune diabetes. *Diabetes Care* **2007**, *30*, 932–938. [CrossRef]
16. Genovese, S.; Bazzigaluppi, E.; Goncalves, D.; Ciucci, A.; Cavallo, M.G.; Purrello, F.; Anello, M.; Rotella, C.M.; Bardini, G.; Vaccaro, O.; et al. Clinical phenotype and beta-cell autoimmunity in Italian patients with adult-onset diabetes. *Eur. J. Endocrinol.* **2006**, *154*, 441–447. [CrossRef]
17. Zhang, Y.; Yin, T.; Wang, X.; Zhang, R.; Yuan, J.; Sun, Y.; Zong, J.; Cui, S.; Gu, Y. Relationships between Islet-Specific Autoantibody Titers and the Clinical Characteristics of Patients with Diabetes Mellitus. *Diabetes Metab. J.* **2021**, *45*, 404–416. [CrossRef]
18. Tuomi, T.; Santoro, N.; Caprio, S.; Cai, M.; Weng, J.; Groop, L. The many faces of diabetes: A disease with increasing heterogeneity. *Lancet* **2014**, *383*, 1084–1094. [CrossRef]
19. Katsarou, A.; Gudbjornsdottir, S.; Rawshani, A.; Dabelea, D.; Bonifacio, E.; Anderson, B.J.; Jacobsen, L.M.; Schatz, D.A.; Lernmark, A. Type 1 diabetes mellitus. *Nat. Rev. Dis. Primers* **2017**, *3*, 17016. [CrossRef]
20. Schlosser, M.; Mueller, P.W.; Torn, C.; Bonifacio, E.; Bingley, P.J. Participating Laboratories, Diabetes antibody standardization program: Evaluation of assays for insulin autoantibodies. *Diabetologia* **2010**, *53*, 2611–2620. [CrossRef]
21. Li, X.; Zhou, Z.G.; Huang, G.; Yan, X.; Yang, L.; Chen, X.Y.; Wang, J.P. Optimal cutoff point of glutamate decarboxylase antibody titers in differentiating two subtypes of adult-onset latent autoimmune diabetes. *Ann. N. Y. Acad. Sci.* **2004**, *1037*, 122–126. [CrossRef] [PubMed]
22. Levey, A.S.; Stevens, L.A. Estimating GFR using the CKD Epidemiology Collaboration (CKD-EPI) creatinine equation: More accurate GFR estimates, lower CKD prevalence estimates, and better risk predictions. *Am. J. Kidney Dis.* **2010**, *55*, 622–627. [CrossRef] [PubMed]
23. Aldington, S.J.; Kohner, E.M.; Meuer, S.; Klein, R.; Sjølie, A.K. Methodology for retinal photography and assessment of diabetic retinopathy: The EURODIAB IDDM complications study. *Diabetologia* **1995**, *38*, 437–4344. [CrossRef] [PubMed]
24. Lampasona, V.; Petrone, A.; Tiberti, C.; Capizzi, M.; Spoletini, M.; di Pietro, S.; Songini, M.; Bonicchio, S.; Giorgino, F.; Bonifacio, E.; et al. Zinc Transporter 8 Antibodies Complement GAD and IA-2 Antibodies in the Identification and Characterization of Adult-Onset Autoimmune Diabetes. *Diabetes Care* **2010**, *33*, 104–108. [CrossRef]
25. Wenzlau, J.M.; Juhl, K.; Yu, L.; Moua, O.; Sarkar, S.A.; Gottlieb, P.; Rewers, M.; Eisenbarth, G.S.; Jensen, J.; Davidson, H.W.; et al. The cation efflux transporter ZnT8 (Slc30A8) is a major autoantigen in human type 1 diabetes. *Proc. Natl. Acad. Sci. USA* **2007**, *104*, 17040–17045. [CrossRef] [PubMed]
26. Lindholm, E.; Hallengren, B.; Agardh, C.D. Gender differences in GAD antibody-positive diabetes mellitus in relation to age at onset, C-peptide and other endocrine autoimmune diseases. *Diabetes Metab. Res. Rev.* **2004**, *20*, 158–164. [CrossRef]
27. The Diabetes Prevention Program Research Group; Dabelea, D.; Ma, Y.; Knowler, W.C.; Marcovina, S.; Saudek, C.D.; Arakaki, R.; White, N.H.; Kahn, S.E.; Orchard, T.J.; et al. Diabetes autoantibodies do not predict progression to diabetes in adults: The Diabetes Prevention Program. *Diabet. Med.* **2014**, *9*, 1064–1068. [CrossRef]
28. Lohmann, T.; Kellner, K.; Verlohren, H.J.; Krug, J.; Steindorf, J.; Scherbaum, W.A.; Seissler, J. Titre and combination of ICA and autoantibodies to glutamic acid decarboxylase discriminate two clinically distinct types of latent autoimmune diabetes in adults (LADA). *Diabetologia* **2001**, *44*, 1005–1010. [CrossRef]

29. O'Neal, K.S.; Johnson, J.L.; Panak, R.L. Recognizing and appropriately treating latent autoimmune diabetes in adults. *Diabetes Spectr.* **2016**, *29*, 249–252. [CrossRef]
30. Qiu, J.; Xiao, Z.; Zhang, Z.; Luo, S.; Zhou, Z. Latent autoimmune diabetes in adults in China. *Front. Immunol.* **2022**, *13*, 977413. [CrossRef]
31. Hoeldtke, R.D.; Bryner, K.D.; Horvath, G.G.; Byerly, M.R.; Hobbs, G.R.; Marcovina, S.M.; Lernmark, A. Antibodies to GAD and glycemic control in recent-onset IDDM. *Diabetes Care* **1997**, *20*, 1900–1904. [CrossRef] [PubMed]
32. Dahl, A.R.; Jenkins, S.M.; Pittock, S.J.; Pittock, S.T. Clinical Utility and Outcome Prediction of Early ZnT8-IgG Testing and Titer in Type 1 Diabetes. *J. Clin. Res. Pediatr. Endocrinol.* **2023**, *15*, 35–41. [CrossRef] [PubMed]
33. Higgins, J.; Zeitler, P.; Drews, K.L.; Arslanian, S.; Copeland, K.; Goland, R.; Klingensmith, G.; Lipman, T.H.; Tollefsen, S.; TODAY Study Group. ZnT8 autoantibody prevalence is low in youth with type 2 diabetes and associated with higher insulin sensitivity, lower insulin secretion, and lower disposition index. *J. Clin. Transl. Endocrinol.* **2022**, *29*, 100300. [CrossRef]
34. Hoeldtke, R.D.; Bryner, K.D.; Hobbs, G.R.; Horvath, G.G.; Riggs, J.E.; Christie, I.; Ganser, G.; Marcovina, S.M.; Lernmark, A. Antibodies to glutamic acid decarboxylase and peripheral nerve function in type 1 diabetes. *J. Clin. Endocrinol. Metab.* **2000**, *85*, 3297–3308. [CrossRef]
35. Myhill, P.; Davis, W.A.; Bruce, D.G.; Mackay, I.R.; Zimmet, P.; Davis, T.M.E. Chronic complications and mortality in community-based patients with latent autoimmune diabetes in adults: The Fremantle Diabetes Study. *Diabet. Med.* **2008**, *25*, 1245–1250. [CrossRef] [PubMed]
36. Chung, J.O.; Cho, D.H.; Chung, D.J.; Chung, M.Y. Chronic Complications in Adult Diabetic Patients with and without GAD Antibody. *Korean Diabetes J.* **2009**, *33*, 124–133. [CrossRef]
37. Kaufman, D.L.; Erlander, M.G.; Clare-Salzler, M.; Atkinson, M.A.; Maclaren, N.K.; Tobin, A.J. Autoimmunity to two forms of glutamate decarboxylase in insulin-dependent diabetes mellitus. *J. Clin. Investig.* **1992**, *89*, 283–292. [CrossRef]
38. Duvnjak, L.; Blaslov, K.; Bulum, T.; Vučković-Rebrina, S.; Knežević Ćuća, J. Glutamic acid decarboxylase autoantibody is associated with peripheral neuropathy in autoimmune diabetes in adults. *Diabetes* **2017**, *66* (Suppl. S1), A32.
39. Roll, U.; Number, A.; Schroder, A.; Gerlach, E.; Janka, H.U.; Ziegler, A.G. No association of antibodies to glutamic acid decarboxylase and diabetic complications in patients with IDDM. *Diabetes Care* **1995**, *18*, 210–215. [CrossRef]
40. Zanone, M.M.; Burchio, S.; Quadri, R.; Pietropaolo, M.; Sacchetti, C.; Rabbone, I.; Chiandussi, L.; Cerutti, F.; Peakman, M. Autonomic function and autoantibodies to autonomic nervous structures, glutamic acid decarboxylase and islet tyrosine phosphatase in adolescent patients with IDDM. *J. Neuroimmunol.* **1998**, *87*, 1–10. [CrossRef]
41. Glastras, S.J.; Craig, M.E.; Verge, C.F.; Chan, A.K.; Cusumano, J.M.; Donaghue, K.C. The role of autoimmunity at diagnosis of type 1 diabetes in the development of thyroid and celiac disease and microvascular complications. *Diabetes Care* **2005**, *28*, 2170–2175. [CrossRef]
42. Gottsäter, A.; Landin-Olsson, M.; Lernmark, A.; Fernlund, P.; Sundkvist, G. Islet cell antibodies are associated with beta-cell failure also in obese adult-onset diabetic patients. *Acta. Diabetol.* **1994**, *31*, 226–231. [CrossRef]
43. Zampetti, S.; Campagna, G.; Tiberti, C.; Songini, M.; Arpi, M.L.; De Simone, G.; Cossu, E.; Cocco, L.; Osborn, J.; Bosi, E.; et al. High GADA titer increases the risk of insulin requirement in LADA patients: A 7-year follow-up (NIRAD study 7). *Eur. J. Endocrinol.* **2014**, *171*, 697–704. [CrossRef] [PubMed]
44. Desai, M.; Cull, C.A.; Horton, V.A.; Christie, M.R.; Bonifacio, E.; Lampasona, V.; Bingley, P.J.; Levy, J.C.; Mackay, I.R.; Zimmet, P.; et al. GAD autoantibodies and epitope reactivities persist after diagnosis in latent autoimmune diabetes in adults but do not predict disease progression: UKPDS 77. *Diabetologia* **2007**, *50*, 2052–2060. [CrossRef] [PubMed]
45. Maioli, M.; Pes, G.M.; Delitala, G.; Puddu, L.; Falorni, A.; Tolu, F.; Lampis, R.; Orrù, V.; Secchi, G.; Cicalò, A.M.; et al. Number of autoantibodies and HLA genotype, more than high titers of glutamic acid decarboxylase autoantibodies, predict insulin dependence in latent autoimmune diabetes of adults. *Eur. J. Endocrinol.* **2010**, *163*, 541–549. [CrossRef] [PubMed]
46. Yang, L.; Zhou, Z.G.; Huang, G.; Ouyang, L.L.; Li, X.; Yan, X. Six-year follow-up of pancreatic beta cell function in adults with latent autoimmune diabetes. *World J. Gastroenterol.* **2005**, *11*, 2900–2905. [CrossRef]

biomedicines

MDPI

Article

Identifying Aging-Related Biomarkers and Immune Infiltration Features in Diabetic Nephropathy Using Integrative Bioinformatics Approaches and Machine-Learning Strategies

Tao Liu [1,2,†], Xing-Xing Zhuang [3,†] and Jia-Rong Gao [1,2,*]

1 Department of Pharmacy, The First Affiliated Hospital of Anhui University of Chinese Medicine, Hefei 230012, China; 2020205219007@stu.ahtcm.edu.cn
2 College of Pharmacy, Anhui University of Chinese Medicine, Hefei 230011, China
3 Department of Pharmacy, Chaohu Hospital of Anhui Medical University, Chaohu 238000, China; zxx900913@126.com
* Correspondence: zyfygjr2006@163.com; Tel.: +86-0554-62838556
† These authors contributed equally to this work.

Abstract: Background: Aging plays an essential role in the development of diabetic nephropathy (DN). This study aimed to identify and verify potential aging-related genes associated with DN using bioinformatics analysis. Methods: To begin with, we combined the datasets from GEO microarrays (GSE104954 and GSE30528) to find the genes that were differentially expressed (DEGs) across samples from DN and healthy patient populations. By overlapping DEGs, weighted co-expression network analysis (WGCNA), and 1357 aging-related genes (ARGs), differentially expressed ARGs (DEARGs) were discovered. We next performed functional analysis to determine DEARGs' possible roles. Moreover, protein–protein interactions were examined using STRING. The hub DEARGs were identified using the CytoHubba, MCODE, and LASSO algorithms. We next used two validation datasets and Receiver Operating Characteristic (ROC) curves to determine the diagnostic significance of the hub DEARGs. RT-qPCR, meanwhile, was used to confirm the hub DEARGs' expression levels in vitro. In addition, we investigated the relationships between immune cells and hub DEARGs. Next, Gene Set Enrichment Analysis (GSEA) was used to identify each biomarker's biological role. The hub DEARGs' subcellular location and cell subpopulations were both identified and predicted using the HPA and COMPARTMENTS databases, respectively. Finally, drug–protein interactions were predicted and validated using STITCH and AutoDock Vina. Results: A total of 57 DEARGs were identified, and functional analysis reveals that they play a major role in inflammatory processes and immunomodulation in DN. In particular, aging and the AGE-RAGE signaling pathway in diabetic complications are significantly enriched. Four hub DEARGs (CCR2, VCAM1, CSF1R, and ITGAM) were further screened using the interaction network, CytoHubba, MCODE, and LASSO algorithms. The results above were further supported by validation sets, ROC curves, and RT-qPCR. According to an evaluation of immune infiltration, DN had significantly more resting mast cells and delta gamma T cells but fewer regulatory T cells and active mast cells. Four DEARGs have statistical correlations with them as well. Further investigation revealed that four DEARGs were implicated in immune cell abnormalities and regulated a wide range of immunological and inflammatory responses. Furthermore, the drug–protein interactions included four possible therapeutic medicines that target four DEARGs, and molecular docking could make this association practical. Conclusions: This study identified four DEARGs (CCR2, VCAM1, CSF1R, and ITGAM) associated with DN, which might play a key role in the development of DN and could be potential biomarkers in DN.

Keywords: diabetic nephropathy; aging; diagnostic biomarker; immune cell infiltration; molecular docking

1. Introduction

Diabetic kidney disease (DN), one of the most common microvascular effects of diabetes, is the leading cause of end-stage renal disease (ESRD) worldwide [1]. The major lesion of DN, visible in the glomeruli, is characterized by extracellular matrix deposition and basement membrane thickening [2]. There is still much to learn about the pathogenesis and etiology of DN. Historically, the presence of microalbuminuria (MA) and the progression of diabetes mellitus (DM) have been used to make an early diagnosis of DN [3]. This approach is ineffective, though, as only 30% of cases had pathology confirm them, and the remaining cases were DM with primary glomerular illnesses present [4]. The lack of complete and efficient therapy for DN makes it the main contributor to renal dysfunction and ESRD development [5]. Even though there are several potential causes of DN, including obesity, heredity, and environment, the general pathophysiological pathways remain unknown. Consequently, understanding the causes of DN is essential for discovering and identifying diagnostic biomarkers for the incidence and progression of DN.

Recent research shows that DN is highly associated with accelerated aging in various cell types, including endothelial, tubular, and podocyte cells [6–8]. Increased cortical surface roughness, the number of cysts, and reduced cortical volume are just a few of the macrostructural changes that the aging kidneys experience [9]. These changes correspond to the typical microstructural features of glomerulosclerosis, tubular atrophy, interstitial fibrosis, and nephron loss [10]. Notably, mesangial and tubular cells were susceptible to direct cellular senescence induction by hyperglycemia [11–14]. Low-grade inflammation and cellular aging could be promoted by excessive glucose, which is also capable of making macrophages release SASP components [15]. Along with hyperglycemia, AGE generation, oxidative stress induction, chronic persistent inflammation, glucose toxicity, and lipid metabolism problems could all work in concert to foster the development of a favorable milieu for aging cells [16]. Aging is also accompanied by dysregulation of the immune system, which is characterized as immune aging and involves impaired immune responses and overwhelming inflammation [17]. Immune dysregulation and inflammation linked with immune aging have been identified as risk factors for a wide range of age-related illnesses [18,19]. Immune aging can eventually lead to increased vulnerability to age-related comorbidities such as cancer, autoimmune illnesses, and infectious diseases [20].

In this investigation, we employed gene expression profiles specific to DN, combined with aging-related databases, bioinformatic analyses, and validation tests, to identify aging-associated genes that serve as potential biomarkers for DN development. Furthermore, we elucidated the immune mechanisms underlying DN by conducting an immune infiltration analysis, thereby uncovering the immunological basis of these biomarkers. Our study aimed to provide novel insights into the intricate relationship between aging, immune responses, and the progression of DN.

2. Material and Methods

This study's objective was to investigate DN-related gene sets via the lens of ARGs. The study flowchart is depicted in Figure 1.

2.1. Data Preprocessing and Differentially Expressed Genes (DEGs) and Aging-Related Genes (ARGs) Identifying in DN

First, to investigate the DEGs in DN patients compared to healthy individuals, we obtained the gene expression profiles of DN patients from the publicly available GEO database. The NCBI GEO GSE104954 and GSE30528 datasets provided datasets with clinical details on DN and healthy kidney samples. The 7 DN kidney tissues and 18 normal tissues in the GSE104954 data set were based on the Affymetrix Human Genome U133 Plus 2.0 Array of the GPL22945 platform. The 9 DN kidney tissues and 13 normal tissues in the GSE30528 data set were based on the Affymetrix Human Genome U133A 2.0 Array of the GPL571 platform. We processed the datasets using the inSilicoMerging [21] R program to combine the various datasets. In order to exclude group effects, we also applied the

Johnson et al. technique [22]. The follow-up analysis of this study includes a total of 16 DN samples and 31 normal tissue samples. The limma R tool was then used in differential analysis to find the genes that differ between the DN group and the control group [23]. The |fold-change (FC)| > 1.5 and p-value < 0.05 were the statistical thresholds for screening RNA expression. Subsequently, in order to obtain ARGs, we retrieved 1357 ARGs from the GeneCards database (Supplementary Table S1) with a relevance score of greater than 5 [24].

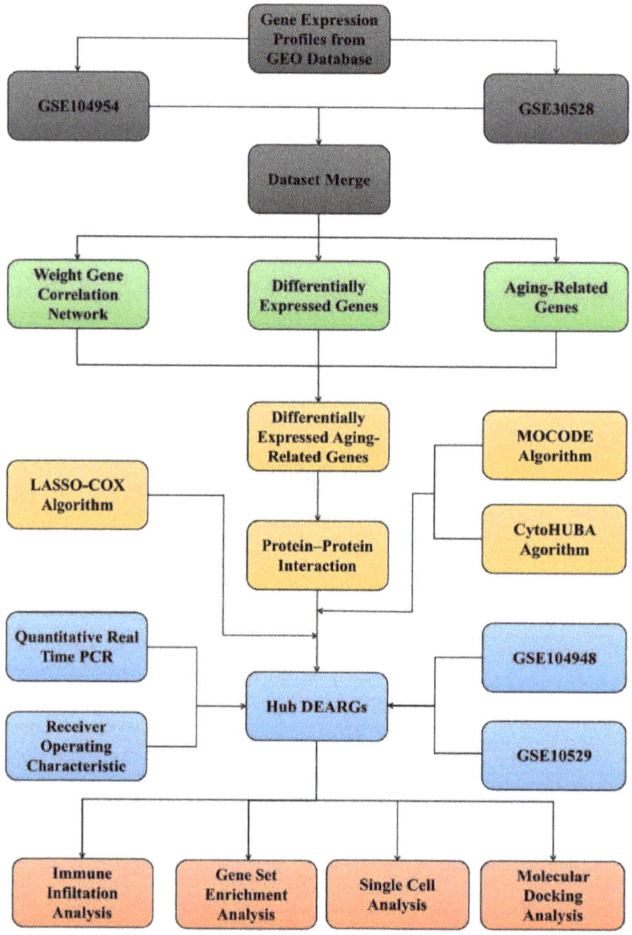

Figure 1. The study flowchart for DN based on integrative bioinformatics approaches and machine-learning strategies.

2.2. *Identification of Clinically Significant Modules Based on Weight Gene Correlation Network Analysis (WGCNA)*

Next, we employed the WGCNA to further identify gene clusters that play crucial roles in the onset and progression of DN. In order to create the scale-free co-expression network, we removed outlier DEGs and probes using the R program WGCNA. To be more precise, all pair-wise genes were first subjected to the average linkage approach and Pearson's correlation matrices. A soft-thresholding parameter, β, emphasized strong gene connections and penalized weak ones. In order to measure the network connectivity of a gene, which is defined as the sum of its adjacency with all other genes for network gene ratio, the adjacency was transformed into a topological overlap matrix (TOM) after selecting the power of 6, and the corresponding dissimilarity (1-TOM) was calculated. Average linkage hierarchical clustering was carried out using the TOM-based dissimilarity measure with a minimum size (gene group) of 10 for the gene dendrogram in order to arrange genes with comparable expression profiles into gene modules. We determined the dissimilarity of the module eigengenes, selected a cut line for the module dendrogram, and combined several modules in order to further investigate the module.

2.3. Functional Enrichment Analysis of DEGs and DEARGs

Furthermore, we performed functional enrichment analysis to explore the biological roles of DEGs and DEARGs in DN. Based on the Molecular Signatures Database (MSigDB) and the DAVID database, we obtained gene annotations for the Human Phenotype Ontology (HPO), Gene Ontology (GO), and Kyoto Encyclopedia of Genes and Genomes (KEGG), respectively. We used the ClusterProfiler R package and DAVID database to perform HPO, GO, and KEGG function analysis to acquire the results of the DEGs enrichment. Statistical significance was defined as p-value < 0.05. The maximum and minimum gene sets are 5000 and 5, respectively.

2.4. Identification of Hub Biomarkers Based on Protein–Protein Interaction (PPI) and Machine Learning Algorithm

Moreover, we employed PPI analysis and a machine learning algorithm to identify hub biomarkers that play pivotal roles among DEARGs. The STRING database was utilized to examine the interactions of different module genes with filtering criteria (score > 0.4). The network was displayed using Cytoscape 3.8.1. The Molecular Complex Detection (MCODE) plug-in for Cytoscape was used to examine the primary functional modules. These criteria for selection are defined as follows: K Core = 2, Cut Grade = 2, Maximum Depth = 100, Cut Node Score = 0.3. Each node gene is scored using the Maximum Clique Centrality (MCC) by the cytoHubba plug-in for Cytoscape. The top 10 nodal genes of each algorithm's MCC score were used to screen for the pivot genes. Then, the hub biomarkers were found using Cox regression with the Least Absolute Shrinkage and Selection Operator (LASSO). Based on the 3-fold cross-validation method, we calculated the penalty parameter, selected the best value corresponding to the lowest cross-validation error, and listed the gene names matching that value utilizing the "glmnet" software package. The GeneMANIA database (http://genemania.org/ (accessed on 1 May 2023)) is a website for building PPI networks. Using GeneMANIA, we identified PPI networks of hub biomarkers in this study.

2.5. Diagnostic Value of Characteristic Biomarkers and Data Validation in DN

To validate the diagnostic value of the selected hub genes, we built a logistics model and visualized the results with the ggplot2 package. The area under the ROC curve was used to evaluate the biomarkers' diagnostic value (AUC, which was between 0.5 and 1). The diagnosis is more accurate when the AUC is near 1. Additionally, we also utilized the RNA expression datasets GSE104948 (which included 7 DN samples and 18 control samples) and GSE30529 (which included 10 DN samples and 12 control samples) as validation sets to conduct a controlled reliability study.

2.6. RT-qPCR

The SV40-MES-13 mouse mesangial cell line was obtained from BNCC Biological Technology (Beijing, China) and cultured in DMEM medium (Solarbio, Beijing, China) supplemented with 10% fetal bovine serum (FBS; BI) and 1% penicillin/streptomycin. The cells were incubated at 37 °C in a 5% CO2-humidified atmosphere. Control cells were cultured in a normal medium containing 5.5 mM glucose, while the model cells were treated with 40 mM high glucose for 24 h. Total RNA was isolated from the cells using the TRIzol kit (Thermo Fisher Scientific, Waltham, MA, USA) following the manufacturer's protocol. The isolated RNA was then reverse-transcribed into cDNA using the M-MuLV

First Strand cDNA Synthesis Kit (Sangon Biotech, Shanghai, China). Quantitative real-time PCR was performed using the SYBR Premix EX Taq™ II (Tli RNaseH Plus) kit (Takara Bio, Inc., Kusatsu, Japan) and an ABI Stepone plus PCR system (ABI, Oakland, CA, USA). The expression levels of the hub genes were normalized to GAPDH and analyzed using the $2^{-\Delta\Delta Ct}$ method. The primer sequences can be found in Supplementary Table S17.

2.7. Evaluation of Immune Cell Infiltration and Correlation Analysis between Diagnostic Markers and Infiltrating Immune Cells

The expression of immune cells plays a crucial role in the development of kidney diseases. In order to estimate the frequency of immunological invasion, the 1000 permutation deconvolution method CIBERSORT [25] converts the expression matrix into different immune cell types. Then, generate a histogram to illustrate the different cell components. A correlation heatmap of different cell components was created to show associations between different subtypes. A box plot was also used to show the differential analysis between immune cells from DN and healthy tissue. A correlation analysis of Spearman's rank was utilized to examine and illustrate relationships between the detected biomarkers and the quantity of invading immune cells using dot-bar graphs.

2.8. Gene Set Enrichment Analysis (GSEA) of Biomarkers

In order to explore the possible roles of the chosen biomarkers in DN, we used the GSEA analysis [26] to explore Human Phenotypic Ontology, GO items, and KEGG pathways. Based on the biomarker expression levels, all samples were split into low-expression groups (50%) and high-expression groups (50%). Reference gene sets included the Molecular Signatures Database datasets c5.go.bp.v7.4.symbols.gmt, c2.cp.kegg.v7.4.symbols.gmt, and c5.hpo.v7.4.symbols.gmt. For GSEA analysis with default settings, $p < 0.05$ was regarded as statistically significant.

2.9. Single-Cell Expression Analysis and Subcellular Localization of Biomarkers

On the basis of the HPA database [27,28] (https://www.proteinatlas.org/ (accessed on 1 May 2023)), single-cell data and transcriptional data were utilized to assess the expression of biomarkers in kidney cells. Based on the COMPARTMENTS database (https://compartments.jensenlab.org/ (accessed on 1 May 2023)), we also predicted biomarker protein subcellular localization. This website serves as a prediction tool for proteins' subcellular locations.

2.10. Drug–Protein Interaction and Molecular Docking Analysis of Biomarkers

The Drugbank database (https://go.drugbank.com/ (accessed on 1 May 2023)) was used to identify existing or possibly relevant drug compounds in order to investigate drug–protein interactions. The 3D structures of target proteins and ligands were found using the AlphaFold Protein Structure database (https://alphafold.ebi.ac.uk/ (accessed on 1 May 2023)) and the PubChem database (https://pubchem.ncbi.nlm.nih.gov/ (accessed on 1 May 2023)). Docking simulations and visualizations were performed and presented using PyMOL software 2.3.0 and AutoDock Vina 1.2.0 [29,30].

2.11. Statistical Analysis

Statistical analyses were conducted using GraphPad Prism 8.0.2 and R (version 4.2.1). For comparing data between two groups, either Student's *t*-test or Mann–Whitney U-test was applied, depending on the normality of the data. A significance level of $p < 0.05$ was considered statistically significant. The level of significance was denoted as follows: * $p < 0.05$, ** $p < 0.01$, *** $p < 0.001$, and **** $p < 0.0001$.

3. Results

3.1. Data Preprocessing

Firstly, to obtain gene expression profiles of DN patients, we downloaded two large-scale clinical datasets, GSE104954 and GSE30528, from the GEO database. We eliminated batch impact from the gene expression matrix after merging the GSE104954 and GSE30528 datasets (Supplementary Tables S2 and S3). The box diagram in Figure 2A,B demonstrated that the datasets' sample distributions differed significantly before batch impact was eliminated, implying batch variance's existence. After batch impact removal, the datasets' sample median distributions tend to be the same. In addition, UMAP findings in Figure 2C,D indicated that the two datasets were independent of one another and did not intersect before batch impact was removed. After batch variance was removed, the sample distributions tended to be similar. Moreover, density curves in Figure 2E,F revealed a substantial variation between the two datasets' sample distributions prior to batch impact exclusion. After it was removed, the sample distributions between the datasets were almost consistent.

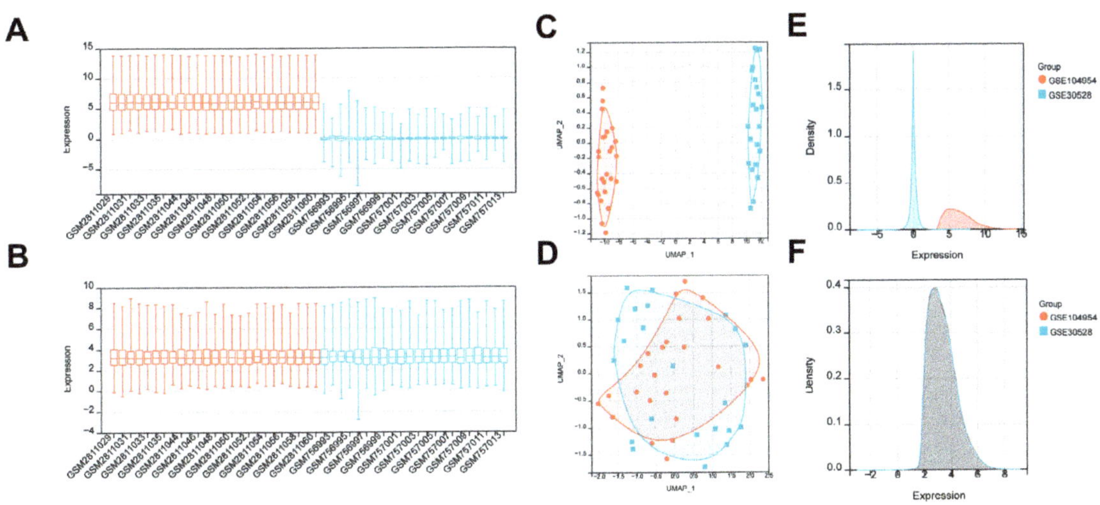

Figure 2. Data preprocessing. (**A**,**B**) Box diagram shows the dataset sample distributions before and after batch removal. (**C**,**D**) UMAP shows the dataset sample distributions before and after batch removal. (**E**,**F**) Density map shows the dataset sample distributions before and after batch removal.

3.2. Identification and Function Enrichment of DEGs for DN

We obtained the DEGs from the gene expression matrix after merging the datasets. A total of 559 genes were screened as DEGs under the conditions of p-value > 0.05 and |fold-change (FC)| > 1.5, with 270 genes up-regulated and 289 genes down-regulated (Figure 3A,B) (Supplementary Table S4). The biological functions and pathways related to 559 DEGs were then examined using HPO, GO, and KEGG enrichment analyses (Supplementary Tables S5–S7). The top 10 HPO results showed that abnormal renal glomerulus morphology, abnormal renal cortex morphology, nephrotic syndrome, glomerulonephritis, and abnormal urine protein levels were significantly enriched (Figure 3C), which confirmed our data's dependability. More importantly, the top 10 GO analysis showed that a large number of biological processes related to immune and inflammatory responses were significantly enriched, including inflammatory response, immune response, antigen processing, and presentation of exogenous peptide antigen via MHC class II, positive regulation of T cell activation, positive regulation of ERK1 and ERK2 cascade, and cellular response to interleukin-1 (Figure 3D). In addition, cell adhesion, angiogenesis, and positive regulation of cell migration were also enriched. In terms of the KEGG pathway, complement and coagulation cascades, cytokine-cytokine receptor interaction, the AGE-RAGE signaling pathway in diabetic complications, and the NF-kappa B signaling pathway were significantly enriched (Figure 3E). The findings above clearly imply that inflammation and autoimmunity are crucial components of DN development.

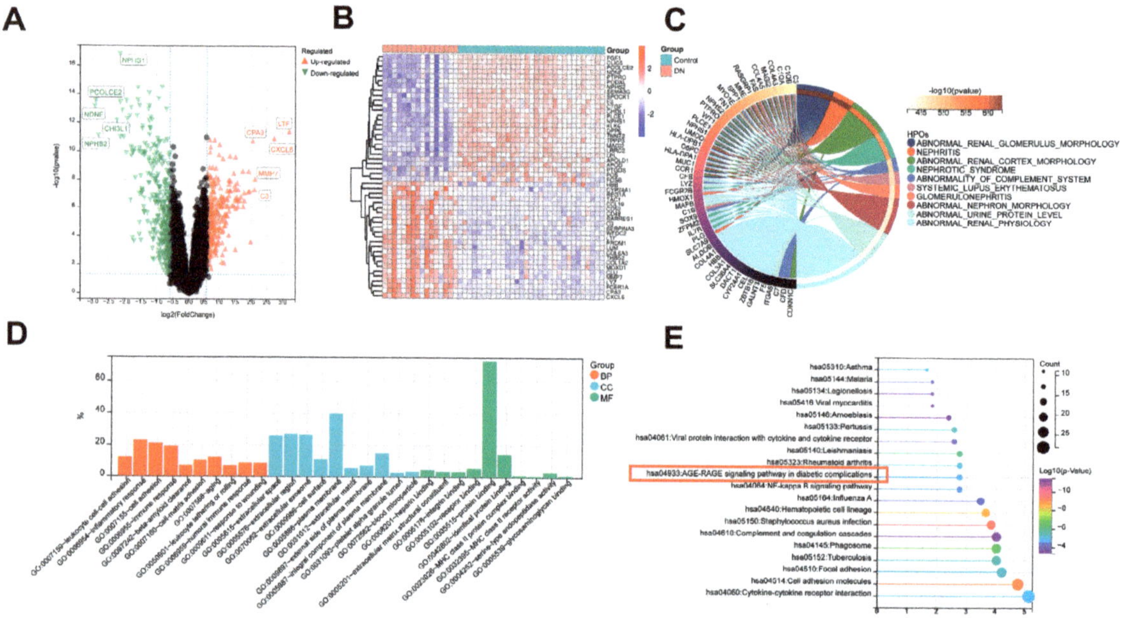

Figure 3. Identification and function enrichment of DEGs for DN. (**A**,**B**) Volcano plot and cluster heatmap show DEGs between the DN and control group. (**C**) Human phenotype ontology analysis for DEGs. (**D**) GO biological processes analysis for DEGs. (**E**) KEGG pathway analysis for DEGs.

3.3. *Weighted Gene Co-Expression Network Construction and Identification of Clinically Significant Modules*

In order to determine the critical modules most closely related to DN, WGCNA was carried out using the combined gene expression profile (Supplementary Table S8). Then, when R2 = 0.86 and the average connectivity is high, we set the soft threshold to 10 (Figure 4A,B). After combining strong association modules with a cluster height limit of 0.25, a total of 19 modules were found (Figure 4C). Then, the clustering of module feature vectors was explored, and the results showed the distance between them (Figure 4D). The relationships between modules and clinical symptoms were also investigated. The top 4 results demonstrated the strongest correlation between the "group" attribute (i.e., DN and Control) and the brown module, the royal blue module, the salmon module, and the green module, especially the green module (Figure 4E,F).

To comprehend the biological roles that the green module's genes perform, we carried out functional enrichment (Supplementary Tables S9–S11). The top 10 HPO results demonstrated that abnormal inflammatory response, abnormal lymphocyte morphology, immunodeficiency, abnormal immune system morphology, abnormality of the lymph nodes, and lymphopenia were significantly enriched (Figure 4G). According to the results of GO and KEGG analysis, DEGs in the green module were related to numerous biological processes and pathways that were linked to infection, inflammation, and autoimmunity. GO enrichment analysis showed that the green module's genes have immune response, inflammatory response, antigen processing and presentation, innate immune response, antigen processing and presentation of exogenous peptide antigen via MHC class II, positive regulation of T cell activation, and cellular response to interleukin-1 (Figure 4H). In addition, cell adhesion, positive regulation of apoptotic process, and defense response were also enriched, showing their potential pathogenesis in DN. More importantly, KEGG analysis was associated with cell adhesion molecules, Type I diabetes mellitus, complement and coagulation cascades, and NF-kappa B signaling pathway (Figure 4I).

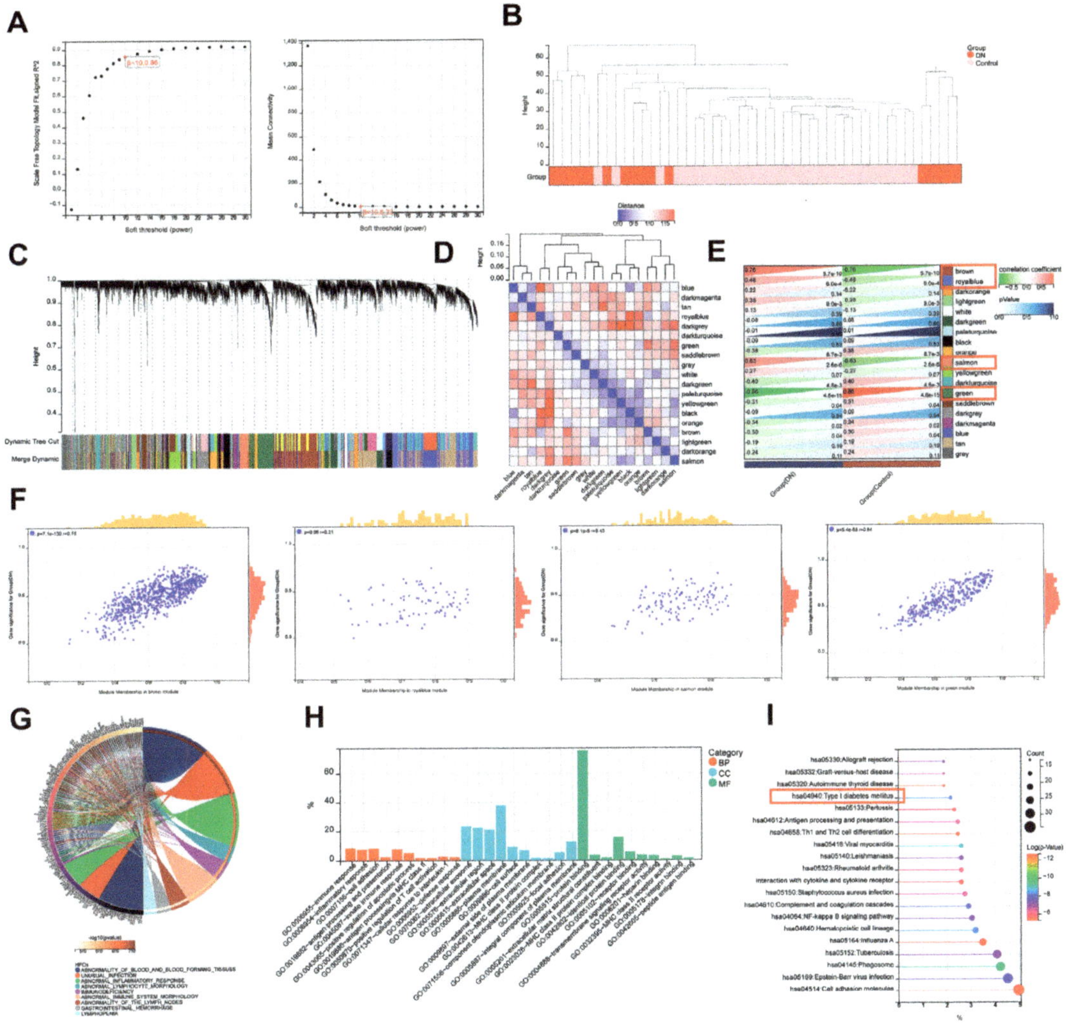

Figure 4. Identification of DN-associated key modules based on WGCNA analysis. (**A**) Scale-free fitting index analysis and mean connectivity of soft threshold power from 1 to 30. (**B**) Clustering dendrogram with tree leaves corresponding to individual samples. (**C**) Clustering dendrogram of all expressed genes based on a dissimilarity measure (1-TOM). (**D**) Correlation heatmap of the module feature vector. (**E**) Correlation heatmap between module eigengene and DN clinical trait. (**F**) Correlation scatter plot between DN gene significance and green module membership. (**G**) Human phenotype ontology analysis for green module genes. (**H**) GO biological processes analysis for green module genes. (**I**) KEGG pathway analysis for green module genes.

3.4. Identification and Function Enrichment of DEARGs for DN

Then, the DEGs, the WGCNA green module genes, and aging-related genes were overlapping. We intersected 57 genes (DEARGs) in total (Figure 5A). The heat map displayed the expression features for 57 DEARGs in DN individuals as well as controls (Figure 5B). In addition, a functional analysis was performed on the 57 DEARGs (Supplementary Tables S12–S14). In HPO results, abnormal circulating creatinine concentration, abnormal circulating nitrogen compound concentration, hyperuricemia, severe infection, and renal corticomedullary cysts were enriched (Figure 5C). In BP results, the leukocyte cell-cell adhesion, inflammatory response, immune response, aging, and humoral immune response were enriched (Figure 5D). The KEGG results indicated that complement and coagulation cascades, cell adhesion molecules, AGE-RAGE signaling pathway in diabetic complications, and cytokine-cytokine receptor interaction might participate in the pathogenesis of DN (Figure 5E).

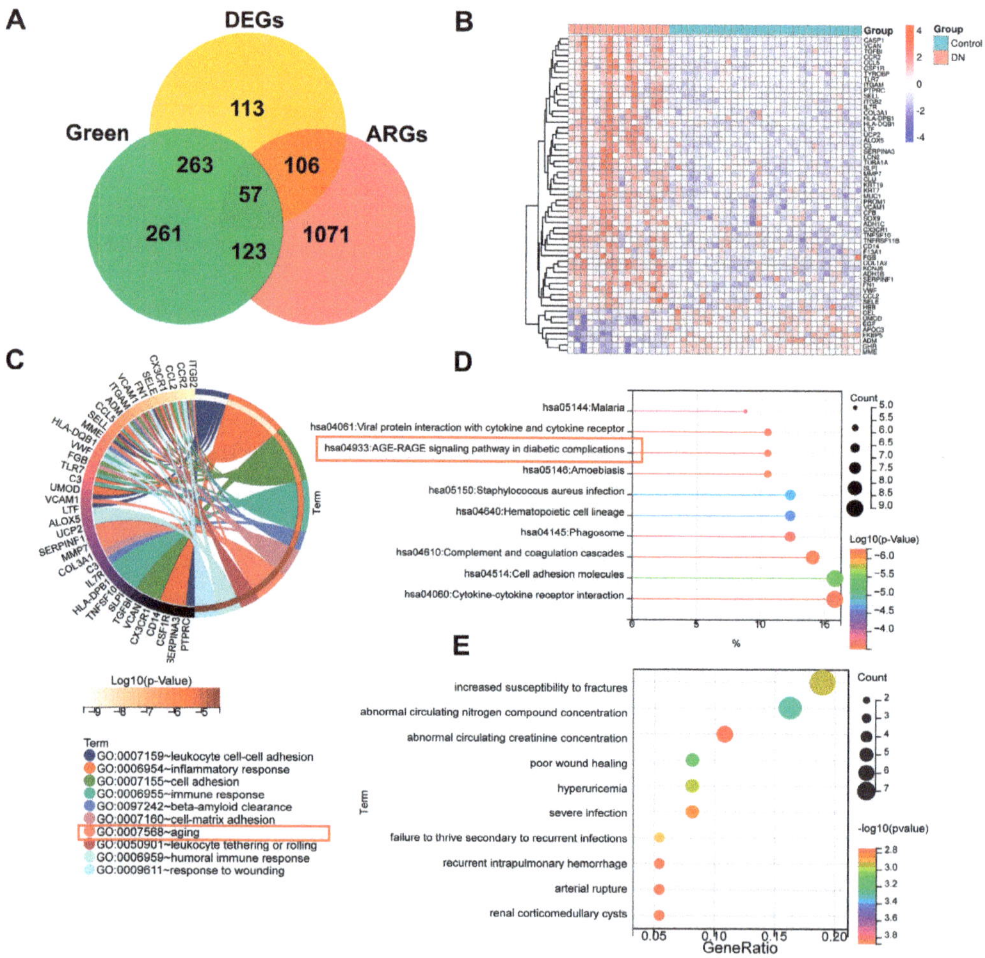

Figure 5. Identification and function enrichment of DEARGs for DN. (**A**) Identification of DEARGs with a Venn diagram. (**B**) Heat map showing differences in DEARGs between the DN and control group. (**C**) Human phenotype ontology analysis for DEARGs. (**D**) GO biological processes analysis for DEARGs. (**E**) KEGG pathway analysis for DEARGs.

3.5. Identification of Hub DEARGs with a Least Absolute Shrinkage and Selection Operator (LASSO) Algorithm

To further explore DN-associated hub DEARGs and relative mechanisms, we uploaded the aforementioned 57 DEARGs to the STRING website and built a PPI network consisting of 51 nodes and 297 edges (Figure 6A) (Supplementary Table S15). The top 10 genes among the 51 nodes with a high binding degree were identified using the MCODE and MCC calculation algorithms in Cytoscape (Figure 6B). We selected the candidate genes for feature gene screening through LASSO regression. The results of the LASSO regression identified four hub DEARGs (CCR2, VCAM1, CSF1R, and ITGAM) with non-zero regression coefficients and the optimal lambda value of lambda. min = 0.16 (Figure 6C,D).

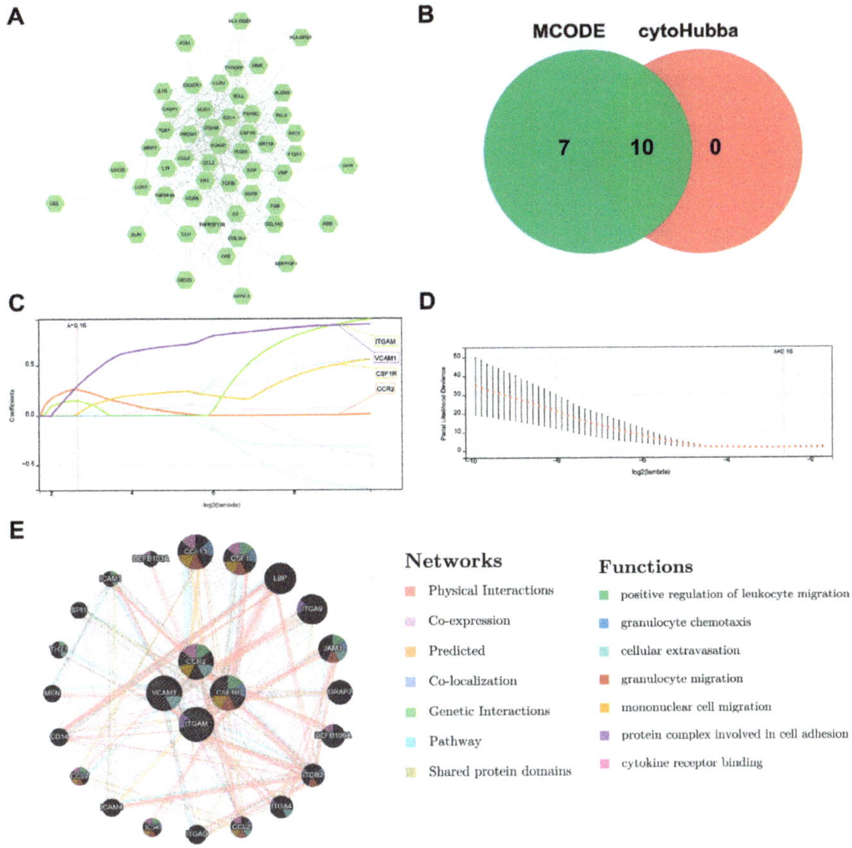

Figure 6. Identification of hub DEARGs of DN. (**A**) PPI network of DEARGs. (**B**) Venn diagram showing the intersections of the DEARGs by cytoHubba and MCODE. (**C**,**D**) Four feature genes with non-zero coefficients were selected by optimal lambda based on the LASSO regression model. (**E**) GeneMANIA database showing DEARGs and their co-expression gene networks.

The GeneMANIA database was then used to study the hub DEARGs co-expression networks and probable roles (Figure 6E) (Supplementary Table S16). We discovered a complex PPI network with 0.60% protein domain, 1.88% pathway, 2.87% genetic relationships, 3.64% co-localization, 5.37% predicted interactions, 8.01% co-expression, and 77.64% physical interactions. According to a function study, they were mostly linked to various immunological and inflammatory processes, including positive regulation of leukocyte migration, granulocyte chemotaxis, cellular extravasation, granulocyte migration, mononuclear cell migration, a protein complex involved in cell adhesion, and cytokine receptor binding, indicating their critical involvement in the etiology of DN.

3.6. RT-qPCR and Datasets Validation and Diagnostic Value of Hub DEARGs for DN

In order to confirm the expression of CCR2, VCAM1, CSF1R, and ITGAM in DN, we created an in vitro high glucose-induced human mesangial cell model. We discovered that, compared to control subjects, these proteins were all substantially expressed in the cells of the model group, revealing the accuracy of our bioinformatics predictions (Figure 7A) (Supplementary Table S17). Further analysis was done on the other two new DN-related datasets, GSE104948 and GSE30529 (Figure 7B,C). Verification revealed that hub biomarker expressions were all higher in DN groups than in control groups (Supplementary Table S18). The results fully validated the presumption that CCR2, VCAM1, CSF1R, and ITGAM may serve as DN diagnostic biomarkers.

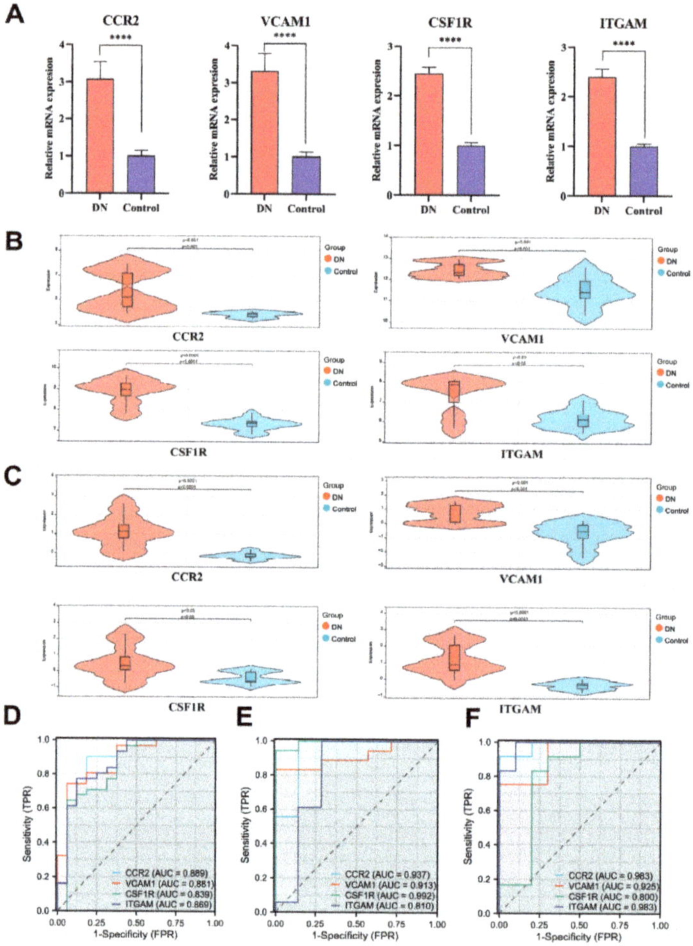

Figure 7. RT-qPCR and datasets validation, and diagnostic value of hub DEARGs for DN. (**A**) RT-qPCR validation of hub DEARGs. (**B**) Dataset validation of hub DEARGs by GSE104948. (**C**) Dataset validation of hub DEARGs by GSE30529. (**D**) ROC curves estimate the diagnostic values of DEARGs in merged datasets. (**E**) ROC curves estimate the diagnostic values of DEARGs in GSE104948. (**F**) ROC curves estimate the diagnostic values of DEARGs in GSE30529. (Note: **** $p < 0.0001$).

Next, we used ROC curves to investigate the association between hub DEARG expressions and DN patient prognosis in order to evaluate the potential predictive usefulness of four hub markers in DN (Supplementary Table S19). High diagnostic specificity and sensitivity for DN were regarded as having an AUC greater than 0.800. According to Figure 7D, CCR2 is 0.889 (95% CI: 0.775–1.000), VCAM1 is 0.881 (95% CI: 0.777–0.986), CSF1R is 0.839 (95% CI: 0.700–0.978), and ITGAM is 0.869 (95% CI: 0.749–0.989). Moreover, the AUC values of two new DN-related datasets also showed excellent diagnostic utility (Figure 7E,F). The findings demonstrated the high DN diagnostic value of CCR2, VCAM1, CSF1R, and ITGAM.

3.7. Immune Cell Infiltration Analysis

To analyze immunological patterns in DN and normal tissues, we used CIBERSORT to compute the proportion of 22 immune cells in each sample through the matrix of gene expression (Supplementary Table S20). Each sample's 22 different categories of immune cells were represented by a histogram (Figure 8A). Each histogram's colors showed the immune cell percentages, with a sum of 1 for each sample. The findings showed that the most prevalently infiltrated immune cells in all 47 samples were resting dendritic cells (47), plasma cells (46), regulatory T cells (46), and M2 macrophages (46). Eosinophils (2), CD4 memory resting T cells (2), and CD4 naive T cells (7) were infiltrating less, though. In the subsequent study, the correlation between 22 categories of immuno-infiltrated cells in two groups was investigated (Figure 8B). Delta gamma T cells were strongly positively correlated with activated CD4 memory T cells and negatively correlated with regulatory T cells and activated mast cells, according to the correlation heat map of different immune cells. Violin plots of the differential in immune cell infiltration revealed that compared to the normal control sample, memory B cells, naive CD4 T cells, delta gamma T cells, and resting mast cells infiltrated more, whereas naive B cells, regulatory T cells, and activated mast cells infiltrated less (Figure 8C).

3.8. Correlation between Hub DEARGs and Immune Cells

We next investigated the relationship between hub DEARG expression and immune cell abundance (Supplementary Table S21). The results of Pearson's correlation showed that a total of four types of immune cells were associated with all four DEARGs. As shown in Figure 9A–D, regulatory T cells and active mast cells were statistically negatively correlated with CCR2, VCAM1, CSF1R, and ITGAM, but delta gamma T cells and resting mast cells were positively correlated with them, suggesting they may play crucial roles in DN formation.

A

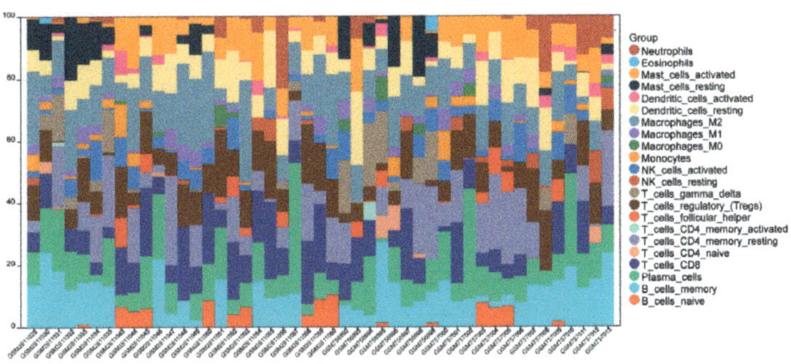

Figure 8. *Cont.*

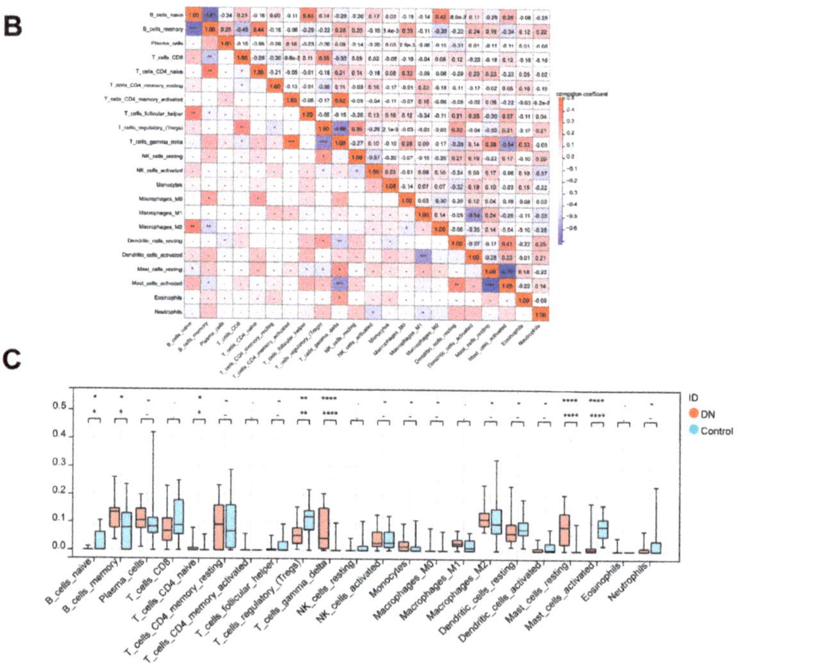

Figure 8. Immune infiltration analysis of DN. (**A**) Each sample's proportion of different immune cells. (**B**) Correlation between different immune cells. (**C**) Expression abundance of different immune cells in DN and control. (Note: * $p < 0.05$, ** $p < 0.01$, *** $p < 0.001$ and **** $p < 0.0001$).

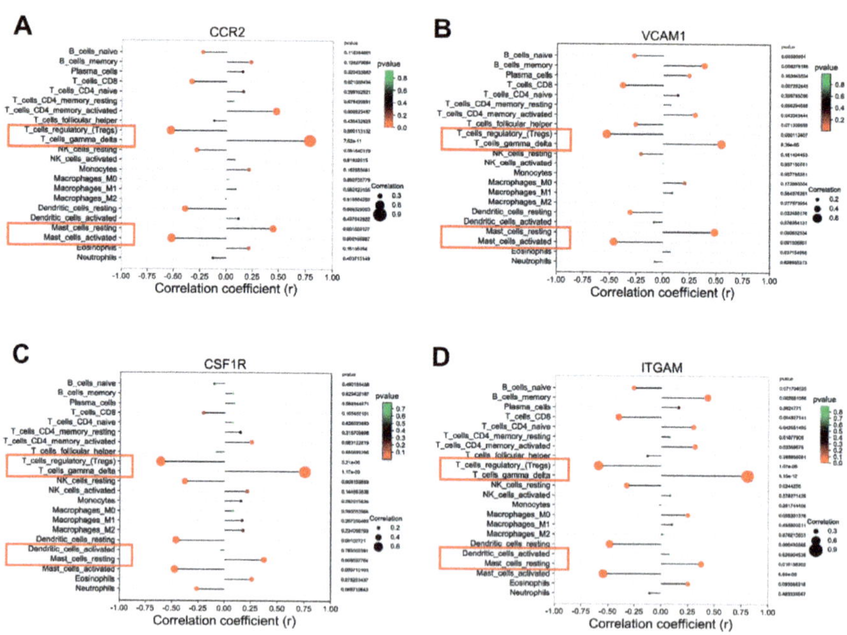

Figure 9. Correlation between the hub DEARGs and different immune cells. (**A**) CCR2; (**B**) VCAM1; (**C**) CSF1R; (**D**) ITGAM.

3.9. GSEA of Hub DEARGs

Furthermore, we investigated the precise signaling pathways and the probable biological processes of the hub DEARGs that regulated DN development (Supplementary Tables S22–S25). The top 10 GSEA HPO results revealed that CCR2 was mostly relevant for abnormalities in a variety of immune cells, including abnormal granulocyte count, B lymphocytopenia, vasculitis, abnormal lymphocyte morphology, and abnormal immune system morphology (Figure 10A). The main enriched items for VCAM1 were recurrent pneumonia, meningitis, and basal cell carcinoma (Figure 10B). The main enriched items for CSF1R were recurrent lower respiratory tract infections, viral hepatitis, and abnormal lymphocyte physiology (Figure 10C). As for ITGAM, the main enriched items were autoimmunity, leukocytosis, and B lymphocytopenia (Figure 10D).

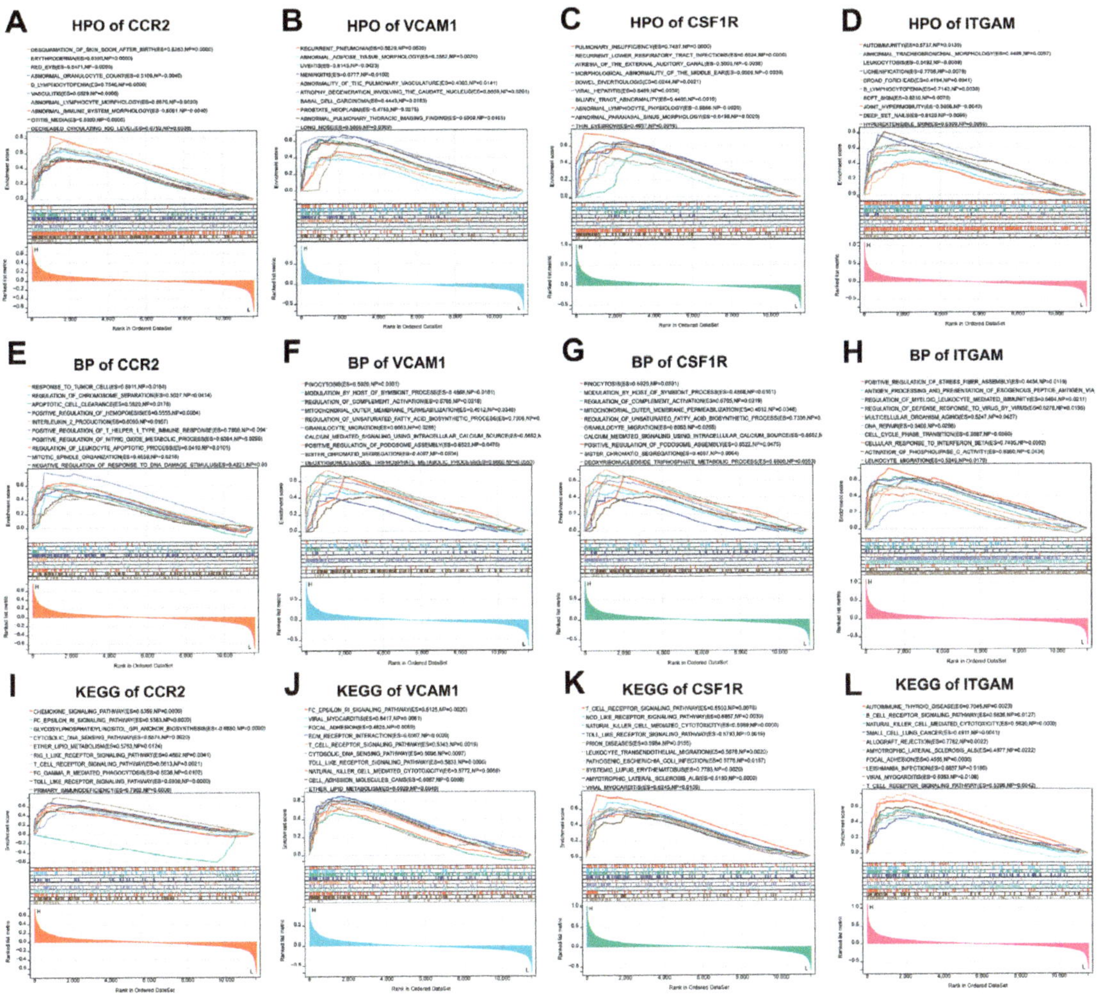

Figure 10. GSEA of hub DEARGs. (**A–D**) Human phenotype ontology analysis for (**A**) CCR2, (**B**) VCAM1, (**C**) CSF1R, and (**D**) ITGAM. (**E–H**) GO biological processes analysis for (**E**) CCR2, (**F**) VCAM1, (**G**) CSF1R, and (**H**) ITGAM. (**I–L**) KEGG pathway analysis for (**I**) CCR2, (**J**) VCAM1, (**K**) CSF1R, and (**L**) ITGAM.

What is more, the top 10 GO BP results revealed that CCR2 regulated a variety of immunological responses, including regulation of chromosome separation, apoptotic cell clearance, interleukin-2 production, positive regulation of T helper 1 type immune response, and regulation of leukocyte apoptotic process (Figure 10E). The main enriched terms for VCAM1 were regulation of complement activation, mitochondrial outer membrane permeabilization, regulation of unsaturated fatty acid synthetic processes, granulocyte migration, and calcium-mediated signaling using intracellular calcium (Figure 10F). The main enriched terms for CSF1R expression were leukocyte differentiation, lymphocyte activation, leukocyte migration, apoptotic cell clearance, and regulation of lymphocyte activation (Figure 10G). As for ITGAM, the main enriched terms were antigen processing and presentation of exogenous peptide antigen via MHC class I, regulation of myeloid leukocyte-mediated immunity, regulation of defense response to virus by virus, and multicellular organism aging (Figure 10H).

Meanwhile, KEGG gene sets found that CCR2 was primarily enriched in the chemokine signaling pathway, the T cell receptor signaling pathway, Fc gamma R mediated phagocytosis, the Toll-like receptor signaling pathway, and primary immunodeficiency (Figure 10I). The main enriched pathways for VCAM1 were the Fc epsilon ri signaling pathway, ECM receptor interaction, T cell receptor signaling pathway, Toll-like receptor signaling pathway, and natural killer cell-mediated cytotoxicity (Figure 10J). The main enriched pathways for CSF1R were the T cell receptor signaling pathway, the Nod-like receptor signaling pathway, natural killer cell-mediated cytotoxicity, the Toll-like receptor signaling pathway, and leukocyte transendothelial migration (Figure 10K). As for ITGAM, the main enriched pathways were the B cell receptor signaling pathway, natural killer cell-mediated cytotoxicity, allograft rejection, focal adhesion, and the T cell receptor signaling pathway (Figure 10L). The above results suggest that all of these hub DEARGs might play essential roles in the regulation of immunity and inflammation in DN.

3.10. Single Cell Analysis and Subcellular Localization of Hub DEARGs

To more precisely delineate the expression of hub DEARGs in human kidney tissues, we interrogated a scRNA-seq based on the HPA database to identify the cell populations expressing in DN. Clustering identified 15 kidney cell subpopulations, as shown in the UMAP plot. The outcomes further revealed the major expression of CCR2 in macrophages and T cells (Figure 11A), VCAM1 in proximal tubular cells (Figure 11B), CSF1R in macrophages, T cells, and B cells (Figure 11C), and ITGAM in macrophages (Figure 11D). Proteins have different biological functions depending on where they are in the cell. Based on the COMPARTMENTS database (Supplementary Table S26), we further predicted the protein subcellular localization of hub DEARGs. CCR2 is primarily distributed in the nucleus and plasma membrane (Figure 11E), VCAM1 is primarily distributed in the Golgi apparatus, endosome, endoplasmic reticulum, cytoskeleton, extracellular, and plasma membrane (Figure 11F), CSF1R is primarily distributed in the nucleus and plasma membrane (Figure 11G), and ITGAM is primarily distributed in extracellular and plasma membrane (Figure 11H).

3.11. Drug–Gene Interaction and Molecular Docking Analysis of Hub DEARGs

Developing possible therapeutic medicines that target CCR2, VCAM1, CSF1R, and ITGAM offers a unique therapy strategy. Four small molecular medicines, including cenicriviroc, carvedilol, sunitinib, and atorvastatin, were ultimately obtained based on the GeneCards database (Table 1). The potential for binding was then assessed by docking the aforementioned four bioactive chemical ligands with the proteins CCR2, VCAM1, CSF1R, and ITGAM. The docking 3D and 2D models of the proteins CCR2, VCAM1, CSF1R, and ITGAM, as well as four small-molecule medications with the firmest binding, were shown in Figure 12A–D, demonstrating their ability to lessen or even reverse the development of DN (Supplementary Table S27).

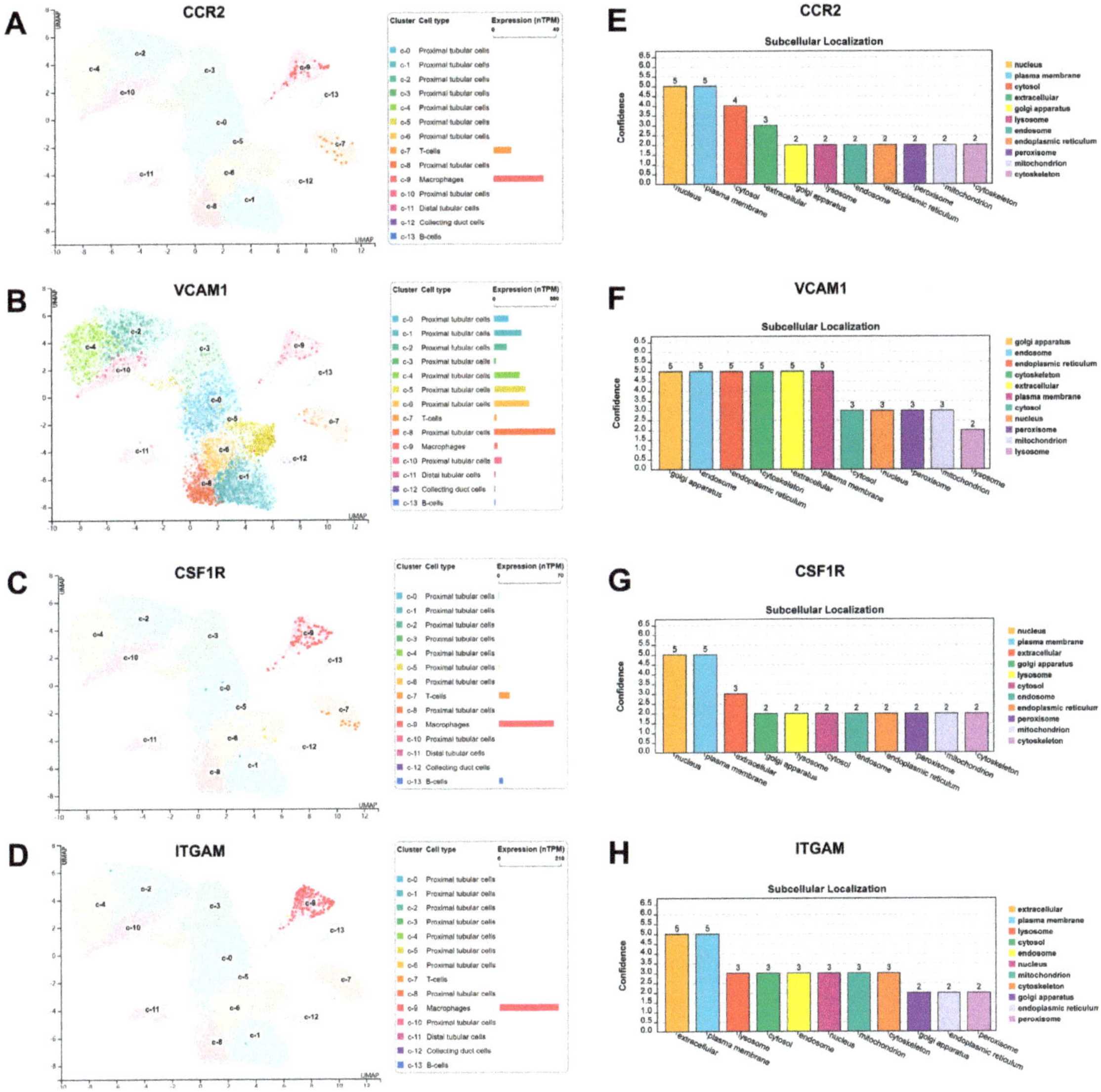

Figure 11. Single-cell expression analysis and subcellular localization of hub DEARGs. (**A–D**) Single-cell expression analysis for (**A**) CCR2, (**B**) VCAM1, (**C**) CSF1R, and (**D**) ITGAM. (**E–H**) Subcellular localization of (**E**) CCR2, (**F**) VCAM1, (**G**) CSF1R, and (**H**) ITGAM.

Table 1. The details of the candidate small molecular drugs targeting hub DEARGs.

DRUGBANK ID	NAME	TYPE	Chemical Formula	DRUG GROUP	ACTIONS
DB11758	Cenicriviroc	Small Molecule	$C_{41}H_{52}N_4O_4S$	investigational	inhibitor
DB01136	Carvedilol	Small Molecule	$C_{24}H_{26}N_2O_4$	approved, investigational	inhibitor
DB01268	Sunitinib	Small Molecule	$C_{22}H_{27}FN_4O_2$	approved, investigational	inhibitor
DB01076	Atorvastatin	Small Molecule	$C_{33}H_{35}FN_2O_5$	approved	inhibitor

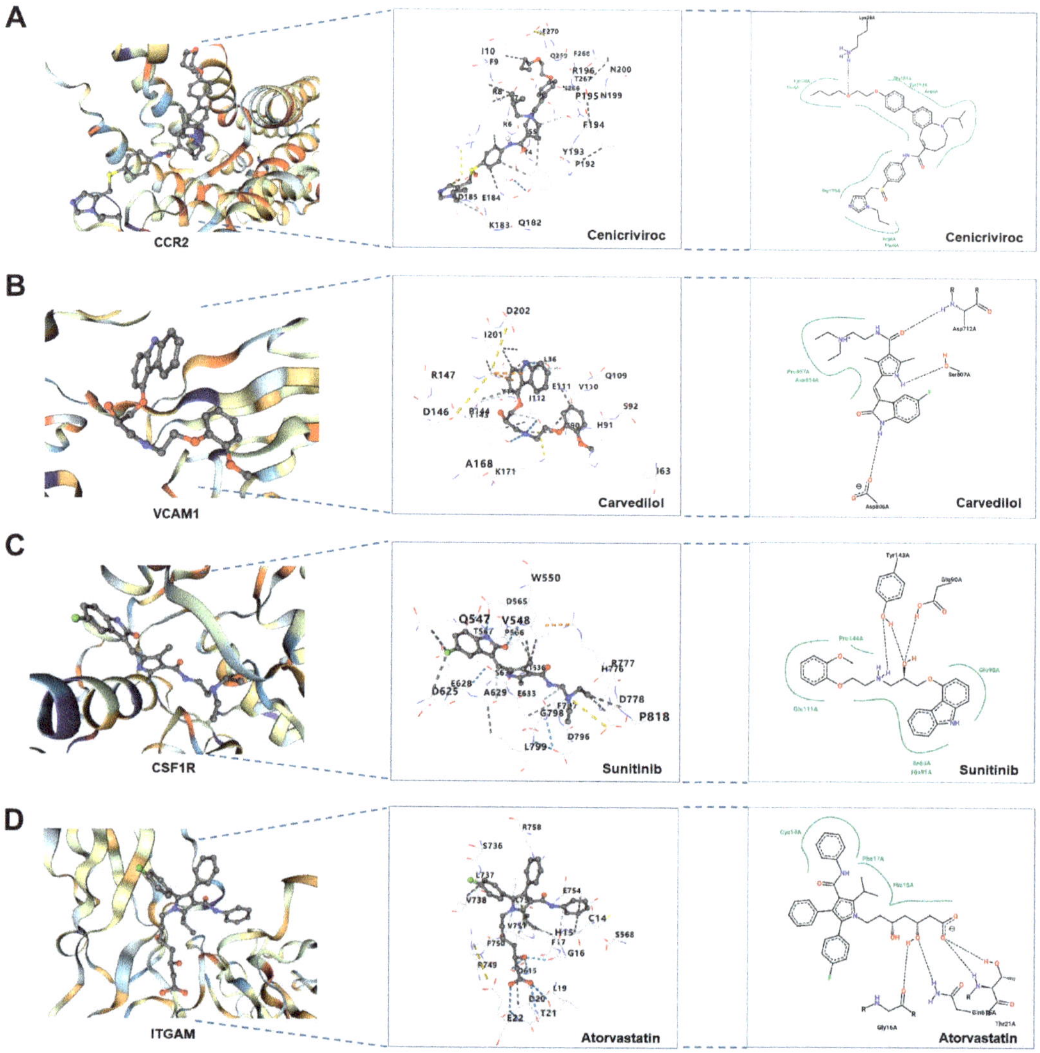

Figure 12. Drug–protein interactions based on molecular docking. (**A**) Molecular docking of CCR2 and cenicriviroc. (**B**) Molecular docking of VCAM1 and carvedilol. (**C**) Molecular docking of CSF1R and sunitinib. (**D**) Molecular docking of ITGAM and atorvastatin.

4. Discussion

The aging of the kidneys is a complicated process that interacts with a variety of disorders, particularly those that are more common in the elderly. Glomerular filtration rate (GFR) decline, a physiological feature of DN, is a manifestation of kidney aging [31,32]. Beyond age 35, the GFR declines by roughly 5–10% per decade, while those between the ages of 18 and 29 had 48% more intact nephrons than those between the ages of 70 and 75 [33,34]. The increase in senescent cells leads to two main effects. First, as one might anticipate, the senescence of cells may result in a lack of self-repair and regeneration potential due to persistent cell cycle arrest [35–38]. This might cause other progenitor or stem cells, in addition to renal cells, to run out. According to a study, people with chronic renal disease have 30–50% fewer endothelial progenitor cells than healthy subjects [39]. In kidneys with DN, there is a small reservoir, a diminished population, and a low rate of stem cell renewal [40,41], all of which would inevitably hasten the disease's course. Second, the aging process also affects the immune system, including immune-cell function and biomolecules that act as effectors, which results in immunosenescence, immunoactivation, and inflammatory processes [42,43]. Cytokines that promote inflammation and matrix synthesis, such as IL-6 and TGF-β, can be produced by senescent cells. These SASP-associated compounds may have a paracrine and autocrine role in stem and kidney cell renewal, as well as persistent inflammation and fibrosis [44,45]. In summary, cellular senescence engages in various pathogenic processes collectively to promote the development of DN.

In this work, we screened 559 DEGs and discovered 289 down-regulated genes and 270 up-regulated genes. Further GO enrichment analysis revealed that a large number of biological processes associated with immunological and inflammatory responses (inflammatory response, immune response, positive regulation of T cell activation, and cellular response to interleukin-1) are considerably enriched, whereas a KEGG enrichment study revealed some correlation with complement and coagulation cascades, cytokine-cytokine receptor interaction, the AGE-RAGE signaling pathway in diabetic complications, and the NF-kB signaling pathway. Also, the results above are further supported by Human Phenotype Ontology analysis. The primary enriched terms were abnormal renal glomerulus morphology, abnormal renal cortex morphology, nephrotic syndrome, glomerulonephritis, and abnormal urine protein level. As a result, it is possible that the DEGs have a role in DN pathogenesis.

Then, based on WGCNA analysis, we discovered 19 DN-related modules. Many biological functions and pathways associated with inflammation and the immune system have been revealed to involve DEGs in the green module. We got a total of 57 DEARGs by overlapping the DEGs, the green module genes, and the ARGs. To further identify DN-related hub DEARGs, we estimated the expression of the aforementioned 57 DEARGs using MCODE, MCC, and LASSO methods and then identified four DEARGs (CCR2, VCAM1, CSF1R, and ITGAM). Fewer of them have been reported in the development of DN, but many of them have been linked to immunological and inflammatory responses in other disorders.

C-C chemokine receptor type 2 (CCR2) modulates the immune response by causing the migration of macrophages and monocytes to areas of inflammation [46,47]. In fact, it has been demonstrated that CCR2 is engaged in the DN process. According to research, macrophages play a direct role in the renal injury of diabetic nephropathy, and genetic CCR2 deletion provides kidney protection in renal injury [48]. The 90-kDa glycoprotein known as Vascular Cell Adhesion Molecule 1 (VCAM-1) is mostly expressed in endothelial cells. The first identification of VCAM-1 as an endothelial cell surface glycoprotein occurred in 1989 [49,50]. Inflammatory cytokines, including TNF, ROS, oxidized LDL, elevated blood sugar levels, toll-like receptor agonists, and shear stress, all stimulate the production of VCAM-1 [51]. A class of tyrosine/serine kinases known as colony-stimulating factor 1 receptor (CSF1R) are primarily in charge of controlling the proliferation and differentiation of microglia and macrophages [52]. In both human and rat RA models, CSF1R blockade lowers inflammation [53]. CSF1R is bound by CSF, which increases cell survival and proliferation [54]. In RA, synovial endothelial cells generate CSF [55] and IL-1β and TNF [56] in vitro. Integrin Subunit Alpha M (ITGAM) encodes the CD11b-subunit of the Mac1 or CD11b/CD18 integrin, which has been repeatedly linked to susceptibility to systemic lupus erythematosus (SLE) [57]. In diabetic nephropathy, ITGAM may contribute to kidney injury by increasing macrophage recruitment in the kidneys and causing histological abnormalities in the glomeruli [58].

For a comprehensive understanding of the dysregulated immune cells in DN, an immune infiltration investigation was conducted. We discovered that DN tissue had higher levels of resting mast cells and delta gamma T cells but lower levels of regulatory T cells and activated mast cells. Moreover, our investigation demonstrated that several main immune cells were statistically correlated to all four DEARGs (CCR2, VCAM1, CSF1R, and ITGAM).

For instance, delta gamma T cells and resting mast cells showed a positive correlation with all hub genes, but regulatory T cells and activated mast cells showed a negative correlation with them. They might, therefore, be extremely important in the immunomodulation of DN and be linked to the malfunctioning of inflammatory cells in DN. The immunological response of effector T cells, B cells, and innate immune cells is suppressed by CD4+ T cells known as Tregs (regulatory T cells). Tregs limit inflammatory immunity in numerous ways, including through the renal and systemic systems [59]. Current research indicates that kidney disease may cause a decline in the proportion of Tregs and an impairment of their regulatory capabilities [60]. Delta gamma T cells are the primary warriors of both the innate and adaptive immune systems, making up an average of 3.7% of CD3+ T cells in peripheral blood [61,62]. The fact that delta gamma T cells are classified as T lymphocytes have TCR rearrangement, have the capacity to create immunological memory, and can lyse target cells all point to them being an important component of the adaptive immune system [63]. Studies have shown that T lymphocytes control renal operational processes. Mast cells are mononuclear, non-dividing cells that are a component of the innate immune system [64]. The two phenotypes of mast cells that are typically distinguished are those that secrete tryptase and chymase and those that exclusively secrete tryptase. Tryptase-secreting mast cells may perform many functions in the immunological response, whereas chymase-secreting mast cells may also participate in revascularization and tissue repair [65,66]. The release of mediators by mast cells during inflammation may result in the loss of kidney structure, and mast cells have also been recognized as significant effector cells in renal inflammation [67]. Despite this, there are not many researches that investigate how hub DEARGs relate to resting memory CD4 T cells, gamma delta T cells, and mast cells in the DN, which could be a fascinating discovery.

Following that, we looked into the particular signal pathways that the four hub DEARGs enriched and investigated how the hub DEARGs might affect the development of DN. Four DEARGs were implicated in immune cell abnormalities, and GSEA analysis revealed that they controlled a great deal of immune system responses and inflammatory pathways, including apoptosis, interleukin-2 production, complement activation, Nod-like receptor signal pathways, and Toll-like receptor signal pathways, indicating that hub DEARGs may be a potential biomarker for DN diagnosis and prognosis. Apoptosis, a sort of active, programmed cell death, maintains the stability of the body's environment [68]. Apoptosis and proliferation of cells are directly controlled by genes, ensuring the equilibrium state of the body's cells [69]. It has been discovered that apoptosis has a significant impact on glomerular remodeling and regulates glomerular cell regression during CGN recovery [70,71]. Interleukin 2 (IL-2) is a multipotent cytokine with a 15.5 kDa four-helix bundle that plays a crucial role in immune control. Antigen-stimulated CD4+ T cells are the predominant producers, but NK T cells, CD8+ T cells, mast cells, and dendritic cells can also generate it [72–76]. Long-term IL-2 treatment decreased the activity and proliferation of intrarenal conventional CD4+ T cells, which was accompanied by a clinical and histological improvement of lupus nephritis, according to research, while short-term IL-2 treatment increased the intrarenal Treg population in mice with active lupus nephritis [77]. Moreover, IL-2 often protects against caspase-8-mediated apoptotic injury, making it a potentially new and practical method to avoid tubular injury in autoimmune kidney diseases [78]. Complement and coagulation cascades perform significant functions in inflammatory-related events and the immune system's protection and regulation [79]. Coagulation, complement, the fibrinolysis system, and platelets all work together to build a tight network in the blood circulation. Systemic lupus erythematosus, C3 glomerulonephritis, and ischemia-reperfusion damage are just a few examples of illnesses that can advance clinically as a result of dysregulation of any cascade system [80]. A family of pattern recognition receptors (PRRs) known as the NOD-like receptor (NLR) family of proteins is known to mediate the early innate immune response to cellular injury and stress. Its activation occurs not only in immune cells but also in resident cells, including endothelial cells and podocytes in the glomeruli [81,82]. Inflammation and other cellular damage are the results of NLRP3 inflammasome activation, which has been linked to ESRD and glomerular injury in studies [83]. Similar to this, the toll-like receptor family (TLRs) plays a crucial manipulative function in the innate immune system. According to a current study, the transduction of TLR signals affects how the kidney responds to various external and internal stimuli by triggering its inflammatory response [84]. Besides, TLRs also play new roles in addition to their well-known ones in host defense, such as regulating body homeostasis and healing wounds [85].

Moreover, we explored cell subpopulations and the subcellular localization of hub DEARGs in the kidney. The results identified 15 kidney cell subpopulations and predicted various organelles, such as the Golgi apparatus, endosome, endoplasmic reticulum, cytoskeleton, extracellular, and plasma membrane. However, hub DEARGs are mostly expressed in macrophages as well as on the cell membrane in the kidney. Lastly, we discovered four prospective therapeutic medicines that target hub DEARGs, suggesting a potential therapeutic strategy for DN. According to molecular docking, precise molecule binding strengthens the reliability of this association.

Our investigation was subject to certain limitations. Specifically, we quantified gene expression levels exclusively in high glucose-induced mesangial cells rather than in actual tissue samples. Although this approach provided a representative model, it may not fully capture the intricacies of the in vivo setting. To address this, we intend to conduct future experiments utilizing clinical samples, thereby offering a more direct validation of our findings. By doing so, we aim to enhance the robustness and clinical relevance of our results.

5. Conclusions

In conclusion, four potential aging-related genes (CCR2, VCAM1, CSF1R, and ITGAM) associated with DN were identified in this study using bioinformatic analysis and machine learning methods. By controlling senescence, these genes may influence the development and prognosis of DN, and they may also aid in the development of future therapeutic approaches.

Supplementary Materials: The following supporting information can be downloaded at https://www.mdpi.com/article/10.3390/biomedicines11092454/s1, Table S1: Aging-related genes from GeneCards. Table S2: The merged datasets before batch removal. Table S3: The merged datasets after batch removal. Table S4: Differentially expressed mRNAs in DN. Table S5: The results of Human phenotype ontology enrichment analyses. Table S6: The results of GO enrichment analyses. Table S7: The results of KEGG enrichment analyses. Table S8: The results of differential mRNAs in 19 modules based on WGCNA analysis. Table S9: The results of Human phenotype ontology enrichment analyses. Table S10: The results of GO enrichment analyses. Table S11: The results of KEGG enrichment analyses. Table S12: The results of Human phenotype ontology enrichment analyses. Table S13: The results of GO enrichment analyses. Table S14: The results of KEGG enrichment analyses. Table S15: PPI interactions based on STRING database. Table S16: The results of GeneMANIA database. Table S17: The results of RT-qPCR. Table S18: Hub DEARGs expression data of GSE104948 and GSE30529. Table S19: Hub DEARGs expression data for ROC analysis. Table S20: Calculation of 22 types of immune cells in each sample based on CIBERSORT. Table S21: Correlation analysis between hub genes and immune cells. Table S22: The results of functional enrichment analyses for CCR2. Table S23: The results of functional enrichment analyses for VCAM1. Table S24: The results of functional enrichment analyses for CSF1R. Table S25: The results of functional enrichment analyses for ITGAM. Table S26: The subcellular localization of hub DEARGs. Table S27: The details of molecular docking for hub DEARGs.

Author Contributions: Conceptualization, T.L. and X.-X.Z.; data curation, T.L. and X.-X.Z.; formal analysis, T.L. and X.-X.Z.; funding acquisition, J.-R.G.; investigation, T.L. and X.-X.Z.; methodology, T.L. and X.-X.Z.; project administration, J.-R.G.; resources, T.L. and X.-X.Z.; software, T.L. and X.-X.Z.; supervision, J.-R.G.; validation, T.L. and X.-X.Z.; visualization, T.L. and X.-X.Z.; writing—original draft, T.L. and X.-X.Z.; writing—review and editing, J.-R.G. All authors have read and agreed to the published version of the manuscript.

Funding: This study was financially supported by the Key Research and Development Plan Projects of Anhui Province (No. 2022e07020024) and the National Natural Science Foundation of China (No. 81973546).

Institutional Review Board Statement: Not applicable.

Informed Consent Statement: Not applicable.

Data Availability Statement: The data used and analyzed to support the findings of this study are available from the corresponding author upon request.

Conflicts of Interest: We declare that we do not have any commercial or associative interest that represents a conflict of interest in connection with the work submitted.

References

1. Alicic, R.Z.; Rooney, M.T.; Tuttle, K.R. Diabetic Kidney Disease: Challenges, Progress, and Possibilities. *Clin. J. Am. Soc. Nephrol* **2017**, *12*, 2032–2045. [CrossRef] [PubMed]
2. Wada, J.; Makino, H. Inflammation and the pathogenesis of diabetic nephropathy. *Clin. Sci.* **2013**, *124*, 139–152. [CrossRef] [PubMed]
3. Papadopoulou-Marketou, N.; Kanaka-Gantenbein, C.; Marketos, N.; Chrousos, G.P.; Papassotiriou, I. Biomarkers of diabetic nephropathy: A 2017 update. *Crit. Rev. Clin. Lab. Sci.* **2017**, *54*, 326–342. [CrossRef] [PubMed]
4. Oh, S.W.; Kim, S.; Na, K.Y.; Chae, D.-W.; Kim, S.; Jin, D.C.; Chin, H.J. Clinical implications of pathologic diagnosis and classification for diabetic nephropathy. *Diabetes Res. Clin. Pract.* **2012**, *97*, 418–424. [CrossRef]
5. Quan, K.Y.; Yap, C.G.; Jahan, N.K.; Pillai, N. Review of early circulating biomolecules associated with diabetes nephropathy—Ideal candidates for early biomarker array test for DN. *Diabetes Res. Clin. Pract.* **2021**, *182*, 109122. [CrossRef] [PubMed]
6. D'onofrio, N.; Servillo, L.; Giovane, A.; Casale, R.; Vitiello, M.; Marfella, R.; Paolisso, G.; Balestrieri, M.L. Ergothioneine oxidation in the protection against high-glucose induced endothelial senescence: Involvement of SIRT1 and SIRT6. *Free. Radic. Biol. Med.* **2016**, *96*, 211–222. [CrossRef]
7. Kitada, K.; Nakano, D.; Ohsaki, H.; Hitomi, H.; Minamino, T.; Yatabe, J.; Felder, R.A.; Mori, H.; Masaki, T.; Kobori, H.; et al. Hyperglycemia causes cellular senescence via a SGLT2- and p21-dependent pathway in proximal tubules in the early stage of diabetic nephropathy. *J. Diabetes Its Complicat.* **2014**, *28*, 604–611. [CrossRef]
8. Van Deursen, J.M. The role of senescent cells in ageing. *Nature* **2014**, *509*, 439–446. [CrossRef]
9. Hommos, M.S.; Glassock, R.J.; Rule, A.D. Structural and Functional Changes in Human Kidneys with Healthy Aging. *J. Am. Soc. Nephrol.* **2017**, *28*, 2838–2844. [CrossRef]
10. Rule, A.D.; Amer, H.; Cornell, L.D.; Taler, S.J.; Cosio, F.G.; Kremers, W.K.; Textor, S.C.; Stegall, M.D. The Association between Age and Nephrosclerosis on Renal Biopsy Among Healthy Adults. *Ann. Intern. Med.* **2010**, *152*, 561–567. [CrossRef]
11. Zhang, X.; Chen, X.; Wu, D.; Liu, W.; Wang, J.; Feng, Z.; Cai, G.; Fu, B.; Hong, Q.; Du, J. Downregulation of Connexin 43 Expression by High Glucose Induces Senescence in Glomerular Mesangial Cells. *J. Am. Soc. Nephrol.* **2006**, *17*, 1532–1542. [CrossRef] [PubMed]
12. Liu, J.; Yang, J.R.; Chen, X.M.; Cai, G.Y.; Lin, L.R.; He, Y.N. Impact of ER stress-regulated ATF4/p16 signaling on the premature senescence of renal tubular epithelial cells in diabetic nephropathy. *Am. J. Physiol.-Cell Physiol.* **2015**, *308*, C621–C630. [CrossRef] [PubMed]
13. Chen, K.; Dai, H.; Yuan, J.; Chen, J.; Lin, L.; Zhang, W.; Wang, L.; Zhang, J.; Li, K.; He, Y. Optineurin-mediated mitophagy protects renal tubular epithelial cells against accelerated senescence in diabetic nephropathy. *Cell Death Dis.* **2018**, *9*, 105. [CrossRef] [PubMed]
14. Fu, B.; Yang, J.; Chen, J.; Lin, L.; Chen, K.; Zhang, W.; Zhang, J.; He, Y. Preventive effect of Shenkang injection against high glucose-induced senescence of renal tubular cells. *Front. Med.* **2018**, *13*, 267–276. [CrossRef]
15. Prattichizzo, F.; De Nigris, V.; Mancuso, E.; Spiga, R.; Giuliani, A.; Matacchione, G.; Lazzarini, R.; Marcheselli, F.; Recchioni, R.; Testa, R.; et al. Short-term sustained hyperglycaemia fosters an archetypal senescence-associated secretory phenotype in endothelial cells and macrophages. *Redox Biol.* **2017**, *15*, 170–181. [CrossRef]
16. Tamura, Y.; Takubo, K.; Aida, J.; Araki, A.; Ito, H. Telomere attrition and diabetes mellitus. *Geriatr. Gerontol. Int.* **2016**, *16*, 66–74. [CrossRef]
17. Linton, P.J.; Dorshkind, K. Age-related changes in lymphocyte development and function. *Nat. Immunol.* **2004**, *5*, 133–139. [CrossRef]
18. Pawelec, G.; Goldeck, D.; Derhovanessian, E. Inflammation, ageing and chronic disease. *Curr. Opin. Immunol.* **2014**, *29*, 23–28. [CrossRef]
19. Franceschi, C.; Campisi, J. Chronic Inflammation (Inflammaging) and Its Potential Contribution to Age-Associated Diseases. *J. Gerontol. A Ser. Biol. Sci. Med. Sci.* **2014**, *69*, S4–S9. [CrossRef]
20. Chou, J.P.; Effros, R.B. T cell replicative senescence in human aging. *Curr. Pharm. Des.* **2013**, *19*, 1680–1698.

21. Taminau, J.; Meganck, S.; Lazar, C.; Steenhoff, D.; Coletta, A.; Molter, C.; Duque, R.; de Schaetzen, V.; Solís, D.Y.W.; Bersini, H.; et al. Unlocking the potential of publicly available microarray data using inSilicoDb and inSilicoMerging R/Bioconductor packages. *BMC Bioinform.* **2012**, *13*, 335. [CrossRef] [PubMed]
22. Johnson, W.E.; Li, C.; Rabinovic, A. Adjusting batch effects in microarray expression data using empirical Bayes methods. *Biostatistics* **2006**, *8*, 118–127. [CrossRef] [PubMed]
23. Ritchie, M.E.; Phipson, B.; Wu, D.; Hu, Y.; Law, C.W.; Shi, W.; Smyth, G.K. Limma powers differential expression analyses for RNA-sequencing and microarray studies. *Nucleic Acids Res.* **2015**, *43*, e47. [CrossRef]
24. Stelzer, G.; Rosen, N.; Plaschkes, I.; Zimmerman, S.; Twik, M.; Fishilevich, S.; Stein, T.I.; Nudel, R.; Lieder, I.; Mazor, Y.; et al. The GeneCards Suite: From Gene Data Mining to Disease Genome Sequence Analyses. *Curr. Protoc. Bioinform.* **2016**, *54*, 1.30.1–1.30.33. [CrossRef]
25. Chen, B.; Khodadoust, M.S.; Liu, C.L.; Newman, A.M.; Alizadeh, A.A. Profiling Tumor Infiltrating Immune Cells with CIBERSORT. *Cancer Syst. Biol. Methods Protoc.* **2018**, *1711*, 243–259.
26. Subramanian, A.; Tamayo, P.; Mootha, V.K.; Mukherjee, S.; Ebert, B.L.; Gillette, M.A.; Paulovich, A.; Pomeroy, S.L.; Golub, T.R.; Lander, E.S.; et al. Gene set enrichment analysis: A knowledge-based approach for interpreting genome-wide expression profiles. *Proc. Natl. Acad. Sci. USA* **2005**, *102*, 15545–15550. [CrossRef]
27. Uhlen, M.; Karlsson, M.J.; Zhong, W.; Tebani, A.; Pou, C.; Mikes, J.; Lakshmikanth, T.; Forsström, B.; Edfors, F.; Odeberg, J.; et al. A genome-wide transcriptomic analysis of protein-coding genes in human blood cells. *Science* **2019**, *366*, eaax9198. [CrossRef]
28. Karlsson, M.; Zhang, C.; Méar, L.; Zhong, W.; Digre, A.; Katona, B.; Sjöstedt, E.; Butler, L.; Odeberg, J.; Dusart, P.; et al. A single–cell type transcriptomics map of human tissues. *Sci. Adv.* **2021**, *7*, eabh2169. [CrossRef]
29. Nguyen, N.T.; Nguyen, T.H.; Pham, T.N.H.; Huy, N.T.; Van Bay, M.; Pham, M.Q.; Nam, P.C.; Vu, V.V.; Ngo, S.T. Autodock Vina Adopts More Accurate Binding Poses but Autodock4 Forms Better Binding Affinity. *J. Chem. Inf. Model.* **2019**, *60*, 204–211. [CrossRef]
30. Lam, W.W.T.; Siu, S.W.I. PyMOL mControl: Manipulating molecular visualization with mobile devices. *Biochem. Mol. Biol. Educ.* **2016**, *45*, 76–83. [CrossRef]
31. Schmitt, R.; Melk, A. Molecular mechanisms of renal aging. *Kidney Int.* **2017**, *92*, 569–579. [CrossRef] [PubMed]
32. Musso, C.G.; Oreopoulos, D.G. Aging and Physiological Changes of the Kidneys Including Changes in Glomerular Filtration Rate. *Nephron Physiol.* **2011**, *119*, 1–5. [CrossRef] [PubMed]
33. Denic, A.; Lieske, J.C.; Chakkera, H.A.; Poggio, E.D.; Alexander, M.P.; Singh, P.; Kremers, W.K.; Lerman, L.O.; Rule, A.D. The Substantial Loss of Nephrons in Healthy Human Kidneys with Aging. *J. Am. Soc. Nephrol.* **2016**, *28*, 313–320. [CrossRef] [PubMed]
34. Glassock, R.J.; Rule, A.D. Aging and the Kidneys: Anatomy, Physiology and Consequences for Defining Chronic Kidney Disease. *Nephron* **2016**, *134*, 25–29. [CrossRef]
35. Bernet, J.D.; Doles, J.D.; Hall, J.K.; Tanaka, K.K.; Carter, T.A.; Olwin, B.B. p38 MAPK signaling underlies a cell-autonomous loss of stem cell self-renewal in skeletal muscle of aged mice. *Nat. Med.* **2014**, *20*, 265–271. [CrossRef]
36. Cosgrove, B.D.; Gilbert, P.M.; Porpiglia, E.; Mourkioti, F.; Lee, S.P.; Corbel, S.Y.; Llewellyn, M.E.; Delp, S.L.; Blau, H.M. Rejuvenation of the muscle stem cell population restores strength to injured aged muscles. *Nat. Med.* **2014**, *20*, 255–264. [CrossRef]
37. García-Prat, L.; Martínez-Vicente, M.; Perdiguero, E.; Ortet, L.; Rodríguez-Ubreva, J.; Rebollo, E.; Ruiz-Bonilla, V.; Gutarra, S.; Ballestar, E.; Serrano, A.L.; et al. Autophagy maintains stemness by preventing senescence. *Nature* **2016**, *529*, 37–42. [CrossRef]
38. Choudhury, A.R.; Ju, Z.; Djojosubroto, M.W.; Schienke, A.; Lechel, A.; Schaetzlein, S.; Jiang, H.; Stepczynska, A.; Wang, C.; Buer, J.; et al. Cdkn1a deletion improves stem cell function and lifespan of mice with dysfunctional telomeres without accelerating cancer formation. *Nat. Genet.* **2006**, *39*, 99–105. [CrossRef]
39. Chade, A.R.; Zhu, X.-Y.; Krier, J.D.; Jordan, K.L.; Textor, S.C.; Grande, J.P.; Lerman, A.; Lerman, L.O. Endothelial Progenitor Cells Homing and Renal Repair in Experimental Renovascular Disease. *Stem Cells* **2010**, *28*, 1039–1047. [CrossRef]
40. Bartek, J.; Hodny, Z. Ageing: Old blood stem cells feel the stress. *Nature* **2014**, *512*, 140–141. [CrossRef]
41. Niccoli, T.; Partridge, L. Ageing as a Risk Factor for Disease. *Curr. Biol.* **2012**, *22*, R741–R752. [CrossRef] [PubMed]
42. O'Connor, J.E.; Herrera, G.; Martinez-Romero, A.; de Oyanguren, F.S.; Diaz, L.; Gomes, A.; Balaguer, S.; Callaghan, R.C. Systems Biology and immune aging. *Immunol. Lett.* **2014**, *162*, 334–345. [CrossRef] [PubMed]
43. Flynn, M.G.; Markofski, M.M.; Carrillo, A.E. Elevated Inflammatory Status and Increased Risk of Chronic Disease in Chronological Aging: Inflamm-aging or Inflamm-inactivity? *Aging Dis.* **2019**, *10*, 147–156. [CrossRef] [PubMed]
44. Tchkonia, T.; Zhu, Y.; van Deursen, J.; Campisi, J.; Kirkland, J.L. Cellular senescence and the senescent secretory phenotype: Therapeutic opportunities. *J. Clin. Investig.* **2013**, *123*, 966–972. [CrossRef] [PubMed]
45. Ovadya, Y.; Krizhanovsky, V. Senescent cells: SASPected drivers of age-related pathologies. *Biogerontology* **2014**, *15*, 627–642. [CrossRef]
46. Amano, H.; Morimoto, K.; Senba, M.; Wang, H.; Ishida, Y.; Kumatori, A.; Yoshimine, H.; Oishi, K.; Mukaida, N.; Nagatake, T. Essential contribution of monocyte chemoattractant protein-1/C-C chemokine ligand-2 to resolution and repair processes in acute bacterial pneumonia. *J Immunol.* **2004**, *172*, 398–409. [CrossRef]
47. França, C.N.; Izar, M.C.; Hortêncio, M.N.; Amaral, J.B.D.; Ferreira, C.E.; Tuleta, I.D.; Fonseca, F.A. Monocyte subtypes and the CCR2 chemokine receptor in cardiovascular disease. *Clin. Sci.* **2017**, *131*, 1215–1224. [CrossRef]
48. You, H.; Gao, T.; Raup-Konsavage, W.M.; Cooper, T.K.; Bronson, S.K.; Reeves, W.B.; Awad, A.S. Podocyte-specific chemokine (C-C motif) receptor 2 overexpression mediates diabetic renal injury in mice. *Kidney Int.* **2016**, *91*, 671–682. [CrossRef]

49. Rice, G.E.; Bevilacqua, M.P. An Inducible Endothelial Cell Surface Glycoprotein Mediates Melanoma Adhesion. *Science* **1989**, *246*, 1303–1306. [CrossRef]
50. Osborn, L.; Hession, C.; Tizard, R.; Vassallo, C.; Luhowskyj, S.; Chi-Rosso, G.; Lobb, R. Direct expression cloning of vascular cell adhesion molecule 1, a cytokine-induced endothelial protein that binds to lymphocytes. *Cell* **1989**, *59*, 1203–1211. [CrossRef]
51. Cook-Mills, J.M.; Marchese, M.E.; Abdala-Valencia, H. Vascular Cell Adhesion Molecule-1 Expression and Signaling During Disease: Regulation by Reactive Oxygen Species and Antioxidants. *Antioxid. Redox Signal.* **2011**, *15*, 1607–1638. [CrossRef]
52. Oosterhof, N.; Kuil, L.E.; van der Linde, H.C.; Burm, S.M.; Berdowski, W.; van Ijcken, W.F.; van Swieten, J.C.; Hol, E.M.; Verheijen, M.H.; van Ham, T.J. Colony-Stimulating Factor 1 Receptor (CSF1R) Regulates Microglia Density and Distribution, but Not Microglia Differentiation In Vivo. *Cell Rep.* **2018**, *24*, 1203–1217. [CrossRef] [PubMed]
53. Garcia, S.; Hartkamp, L.M.; Malvar-Fernandez, B.; van Es, I.E.; Lin, H.; Wong, J.; Long, L.; Zanghi, J.A.; Rankin, A.L.; Masteller, E.L.; et al. Colony-stimulating factor (CSF) 1 receptor blockade reduces inflammation in human and murine models of rheumatoid arthritis. *Thromb. Haemost.* **2016**, *18*, 75. [CrossRef] [PubMed]
54. Hume, D.A.; MacDonald, K.P.A. Therapeutic applications of macrophage colony-stimulating factor-1 (CSF-1) and antagonists of CSF-1 receptor (CSF-1R) signaling. *Blood* **2012**, *119*, 1810–1820. [CrossRef] [PubMed]
55. Nakano, K.; Okada, Y.; Saito, K.; Tanikawa, R.; Sawamukai, N.; Sasaguri, Y.; Kohro, T.; Wada, Y.; Kodama, T.; Tanaka, Y. Rheumatoid synovial endothelial cells produce macrophage colony-stimulating factor leading to osteoclastogenesis in rheumatoid arthritis. *Rheumatology* **2007**, *46*, 597–603. [CrossRef] [PubMed]
56. Campbell, I.K.; Ianches, G.; Hamilton, J.A. Production of macrophage colony-stimulating factor (M-CSF) by human articular cartilage and chondrocytes. Modulation by interleukin-1 and tumor necrosis factor α. *Biochim. Biophys. Acta Mol. Basis Dis.* **1993**, *1182*, 57–63. [CrossRef]
57. Ramírez-Bello, J.; Sun, C.; Valencia-Pacheco, G.; Singh, B.; Barbosa-Cobos, R.E.; Saavedra, M.A.; López-Villanueva, R.F.; Nath, S.K. ITGAM is a risk factor to systemic lupus erythematosus and possibly a protection factor to rheumatoid arthritis in patients from Mexico. *PLoS ONE* **2019**, *14*, e0224543. [CrossRef]
58. You, H.; Gao, T.; Cooper, T.K.; Reeves, W.B.; Awad, A.S.; Morris, S.M.; Vacher, J.; Kashyap, S.; Warner, G.M.; Hartono, S.P.; et al. Macrophages directly mediate diabetic renal injury. *Am. J. Physiol.-Ren. Physiol.* **2013**, *305*, F1719–F1727. [CrossRef]
59. Ghali, J.R.; Wang, Y.M.; Holdsworth, S.R.; Kitching, A.R. Regulatory T cells in immune-mediated renal disease. *Nephrol.* **2016**, *21*, 86–96. [CrossRef]
60. Hu, M.; Wang, Y.M.; Wang, Y.; Zhang, G.Y.; Zheng, G.; Yi, S.; O'Connell, P.J.; Harris, D.C.; Alexander, S.I. Regulatory T cells in kidney disease and transplantation. *Kidney Int.* **2016**, *90*, 502–514. [CrossRef]
61. Pauza, C.D.; Poonia, B.; Li, H.; Cairo, C.; Chaudhry, S. γδ T Cells in HIV Disease: Past, Present, and Future. *Front. Immunol.* **2015**, *5*, 687. [CrossRef] [PubMed]
62. Lawand, M.; Déchanet-Merville, J.; Dieu-Nosjean, M.-C. Key Features of Gamma-Delta T-Cell Subsets in Human Diseases and Their Immunotherapeutic Implications. *Front. Immunol.* **2017**, *8*, 761. [CrossRef] [PubMed]
63. Betjes, M.G.H. Immune cell dysfunction and inflammation in end-stage renal disease. *Nat. Rev. Nephrol.* **2013**, *9*, 255–265. [CrossRef]
64. Wilcock, A.; Bahri, R.; Bulfone-Paus, S.; Arkwright, P.D. Mast cell disorders: From infancy to maturity. *Allergy* **2018**, *74*, 53–63. [CrossRef]
65. Tomino, Y. Predictors of prognosis in IgA nephropathy. *Kaohsiung J. Med. Sci.* **2012**, *28*, 517–520. [CrossRef] [PubMed]
66. Bradding, P.; Pejler, G. The controversial role of mast cells in fibrosis. *Immunol. Rev.* **2018**, *282*, 198–231. [CrossRef] [PubMed]
67. Blank, U.; Essig, M.; Scandiuzzi, L.; Benhamou, M.; Kanamaru, Y. Mast cells and inflammatory kidney disease. *Immunol. Rev.* **2007**, *217*, 79–95. [CrossRef] [PubMed]
68. Zhao, S.-Y.; Liao, L.-X.; Tu, P.-F.; Li, W.-W.; Zeng, K.-W. Icariin Inhibits AGE-Induced Injury in PC12 Cells by Directly Targeting Apoptosis Regulator Bax. *Oxidative Med. Cell. Longev.* **2019**, *2019*, 7940808. [CrossRef]
69. Guan, X.; Lu, J.; Sun, F.; Li, Q.; Pang, Y. The Molecular Evolution and Functional Divergence of Lamprey Programmed Cell Death Genes. *Front. Immunol.* **2019**, *10*, 1382. [CrossRef]
70. Hughes, J.; Savill, J.S. Apoptosis in glomerulonephritis. *Curr. Opin. Nephrol. Hypertens.* **2005**, *14*, 389–395. [CrossRef]
71. Shimizu, A.; Masuda, Y.; Kitamura, H.; Ishizaki, M.; Sugisaki, Y.; Yamanaka, N. Apoptosis in progressive crescentic glomerulonephritis. *Lab. Investig.* **1996**, *74*, 941–951. [PubMed]
72. Choudhry, H.; Helmi, N.; Abdulaal, W.H.; Zeyadi, M.; Zamzami, M.A.; Wu, W.; Mahmoud, M.M.; Warsi, M.K.; Rasool, M.; Jamal, M.S. Prospects of IL-2 in Cancer Immunotherapy. *BioMed Res. Int.* **2018**, *2018*, 9056173. [CrossRef] [PubMed]
73. Paliard, X.; Malefijt, R.d.W.; Yssel, H.; Blanchard, D.; Chrétien, I.; Abrams, J.; de Vries, J.; Spits, H. Simultaneous production of IL-2, IL-4, and IFN-gamma by activated human CD4+ and CD8+ T cell clones. *J. Immunol.* **1988**, *141*, 849–855. [CrossRef]
74. Granucci, F.; Vizzardelli, C.; Pavelka, N.; Feau, S.; Persico, M.; Virzi, E.; Rescigno, M.; Moro, G.; Ricciardi-Castagnoli, P. Inducible IL-2 production by dendritic cells revealed by global gene expression analysis. *Nat. Immunol.* **2001**, *2*, 882–888. [CrossRef]
75. Yui, M.A.; Sharp, L.L.; Havran, W.L.; Rothenberg, E.V. Preferential activation of an IL-2 regulatory sequence transgene in TCR gamma delta and NKT cells: Subset-specific differences in IL-2 regulation. *J. Immunol.* **2004**, *172*, 4691–4699. [CrossRef] [PubMed]
76. Hershko, A.Y.; Suzuki, R.; Charles, N.; Alvarez-Errico, D.; Sargent, J.L.; Laurence, A.; Rivera, J. Mast Cell Interleukin-2 Production Contributes to Suppression of Chronic Allergic Dermatitis. *Immunity* **2011**, *35*, 562–571. [CrossRef]

77. Rose, A.; von Spee-Mayer, C.; Kloke, L.; Wu, K.; Kühl, A.; Enghard, P.; Burmester, G.-R.; Riemekasten, G.; Humrich, J.Y. IL-2 Therapy Diminishes Renal Inflammation and the Activity of Kidney-Infiltrating CD4+ T Cells in Murine Lupus Nephritis. *Cells* **2019**, *8*, 1234. [CrossRef]
78. Du, C.; Guan, Q.; Yin, Z.; Zhong, R.; Jevnikar, A.M. IL-2–mediated apoptosis of kidney tubular epithelial cells is regulated by the caspase-8 inhibitor c-FLIP. *Kidney Int.* **2005**, *67*, 1397–1409. [CrossRef]
79. Wiegner, R.; Chakraborty, S.; Huber-Lang, M. Complement-coagulation crosstalk on cellular and artificial surfaces. *Immunobiology* **2016**, *221*, 1073–1079. [CrossRef]
80. Luo, S.; Hu, D.; Wang, M.; Zipfel, P.F.; Hu, Y. Complement in Hemolysis- and Thrombosis- Related Diseases. *Front. Immunol.* **2020**, *11*, 1212. [CrossRef]
81. Platnich, J.M.; Muruve, D.A. NOD-like receptors and inflammasomes: A review of their canonical and non-canonical signaling pathways. *Arch. Biochem. Biophys.* **2019**, *670*, 4–14. [CrossRef] [PubMed]
82. Conley, S.M.; Abais, J.M.; Boini, K.M.; Li, P.-L. Inflammasome Activation in Chronic Glomerular Diseases. *Curr. Drug Targets* **2017**, *18*, 1019–1029. [CrossRef] [PubMed]
83. Komada, T.; Muruve, D.A. The role of inflammasomes in kidney disease. *Nat. Rev. Nephrol.* **2019**, *15*, 501–520. [CrossRef]
84. Garibotto, G.; Carta, A.; Picciotto, D.; Viazzi, F.; Verzola, D. Toll-like receptor-4 signaling mediates inflammation and tissue injury in diabetic nephropathy. *J. Nephrol.* **2017**, *30*, 719–727. [CrossRef] [PubMed]
85. Ramnath, D.; Powell, E.E.; Scholz, G.M.; Sweet, M.J. The toll-like receptor 3 pathway in homeostasis, responses to injury and wound repair. *Semin. Cell Dev. Biol.* **2017**, *61*, 22–30. [CrossRef]

biomedicines

MDPI

Article

The Impact of GLP-1 RAs and DPP-4is on Hospitalisation and Mortality in the COVID-19 Era: A Two-Year Observational Study

Salvatore Greco [1,2,†], Vincenzo M. Monda [3,†], Giorgia Valpiani [4], Nicola Napoli [5], Carlo Crespini [6], Fabio Pieraccini [7], Anna Marra [6] and Angelina Passaro [1,4,8,*]

1 Department of Translational Medicine, University of Ferrara, Via Luigi Borsari, 46, I-44121 Ferrara, FE, Italy; grcsvt@unife.it
2 Department of Internal Medicine, Ospedale del Delta, Via Valle Oppio, 2, I-44023 Lagosanto, FE, Italy
3 Primary Care Department, Diabetes Unit of "SS. Annunziata" Hospital, Via Giovanni Vicini 2, I-44042 Cento, FE, Italy; v.monda@ausl.fe.it
4 Research and Innovation Section, University Hospital of Ferrara Arcispedale Sant'Anna, Via Aldo Moro 8, I-44124 Cona, FE, Italy; giorgia.valpiani@unife.it
5 Programming and Management Control Unit, University Hospital of Ferrara Arcispedale Sant'Anna, Via Aldo Moro 8, I-44124 Cona, FE, Italy; n.napoli@ospfe.it
6 Pharmaceutical Department, University Hospital of Ferrara Arcispedale Sant'Anna, Via Aldo Moro 8, I-44124 Cona, FE, Italy; c.crespini@ospfe.it (C.C.); a.marra@ospfe.it (A.M.)
7 Pharmaceutical Care Department, Azienda Unità Sanitaria Locale della Romagna, Via Carlo Forlanini 34, I-47121 Forlì, FC, Italy; farmaciainterna.fo@auslromagna.it
8 Department of Internal Medicine, University Hospital of Ferrara Arcispedale Sant'Anna, Via Aldo Moro 8, I-44124 Cona, FE, Italy
* Correspondence: angelina.passaro@unife.it
† These authors contributed equally to this work.

Abstract: Novel antidiabetic drugs have the ability to produce anti-inflammatory effects regardless of their glucose-lowering action. For this reason, these molecules (including GLP-1 RAs and DPP-4is) were hypothesized to be effective against COVID-19, which is characterized by cytokines hyperactivity and multiorgan inflammation. The aim of our work is to explore the potential protective role of GLP-1 RAs and DPP-4is in COVID-19 (with the disease intended to be a model of an acute stressor) and non-COVID-19 patients over a two-year observation period. Retrospective and one-versus-one analyses were conducted to assess the impact of antidiabetic drugs on the need for hospitalization (in both COVID-19- and non-COVID-19-related cases), in-hospital mortality, and two-year mortality. Logistic regression analyses were conducted to identify the variables associated with these outcomes. Additionally, log-rank tests were used to plot survival curves for each group of subjects, based on their antidiabetic treatment. The performed analyses revealed that despite similar hospitalization rates, subjects undergoing home therapy with GLP-1 RAs exhibited significantly lower mortality rates, even over a two-year period. These individuals demonstrated improved survival estimates both within hospital and non-hospital settings, even during a longer observation period.

Keywords: diabetes; GLP-1 RAs; DPP-4is; cardiovascular risk; inflammation

1. Introduction

Type 2 diabetes mellitus (T2DM) is known for being one of the most significant cardiovascular risk factors and has experienced a substantial increase in recent decades due to the rising burden of overweight and obesity [1]. Furthermore, in the past year, it has been strongly linked to the severe form of COVID-19 (coronavirus disease 19) [2], a genuine acute stressor for the diabetic population, resulting in generally high mortality rates [3,4]. Given that, according to various studies, the prevalence of diabetes in COVID-19 patients ranges from 5% to 36% [5], it is reasonable to assume that any additional cardiovascular risk factor can predispose individuals with both diabetes and COVID-19 to even worse clinical outcomes [6].

COVID-19 is characterized by a hyperinflammatory acute state [7–9], while also featuring low-grade inflammation that leads to chronic complications. The simultaneous presence of these two conditions likely explains why patients with T2DM suffer from higher mortality rates compared to other subjects. Another point connecting diabetes with coronaviruses is that both SARS-CoV (severe acute respiratory syndrome coronavirus) and SARS-CoV-2 (the causative agent of COVID-19) can enter respiratory tract cells by exploiting the angiotensin-converting enzyme 2 (ACE2) and binding to the spike protein on the virion surface [10]; the effects of this enzyme are multifold, and it also has a major role in micro and macrovascular complications in subjects with diabetes [11].

In contrast, MERS-CoV (Middle East respiratory syndrome), the second member of the coronaviruses family, uses a different receptor for cell penetration, known as dipeptidyl-peptidase-4 (DPP-4) [12]. This receptor can degrade glucagon-like peptide-1 (GLP-1), a hormone produced by L cells in the distal ileum in response to glucose passing through the intestines, a phenomenon called the "incretin effect" [13]. The expression of GLP-1 receptors is not limited to the gastrointestinal tract; they have been found in other systems such as the central nervous system, respiratory system, and cardiovascular system. These receptors also regulate glucose homeostasis in non-diabetic patients, promoting insulin secretion and inhibiting glucagon production [14]. When these mechanisms malfunction, as is the case in T2DM, uncontrolled glucose homeostasis leads to chronic inflammation [15].

Diabetes and inflammation are closely intertwined regardless of other diagnoses, and some antidiabetic drugs have been developed to provide enhanced cardiovascular protection through their anti-inflammatory effects, independent of their glucose-lowering actions [16]. This effect of the novel classes of diabetes medications is one potential mechanism to consider when examining their cardiovascular benefits, even though evidence on this matter is still limited, necessitating further clinical trials to explore this aspect of diabetes.

COVID-19 shares with diabetes the ability to intensely stimulate the immune system. However, the infection caused by SARS-CoV-2 can exploit this function more rapidly compared to diabetes, which requires more time. Based on this, COVID-19 can be considered, in all respects, an acute stressor for the body, like a major adverse cardiovascular event (MACE). Other anti-inflammatory drugs have previously been suggested to be protective against COVID-19. Orally delivered DPP-4 inhibitors (DPP-4is) (such as sitagliptin, vildagliptin, saxagliptin with mimetic inhibition mechanisms, alogliptin, and linagliptin with non-mimetic inhibition) and GLP-1 receptor agonists (GLP-1 RAs) with daily (exenatide, lixisenatide, liraglutide) or weekly (semaglutide, exenatide LAR, dulaglutide) subcutaneous administration [17,18] or once-daily oral administration (semaglutide) are among these potential treatments [19].

In this article, we delve into the role of antidiabetic drugs in relation to SARS-CoV-2 infection as an acute stressor, with a particular focus on individuals chronically treated with GLP-1 RAs or DPP4-is. Our work has three main objectives: (a) comparing, in a "real-world" setting, the hospitalization rates of various medical conditions in T2DM patients on home therapy with GLP-1 RAs or DPP-4is (either alone or in combination with other antidiabetic drugs) versus those on home therapy with different antidiabetic agents and/or insulin; (b) comparing the length of hospital stays between the two groups; and (c) calculating the mortality rates (all-cause and COVID-19-related mortality) of subjects with diabetes in the different groups. The observation period was extended to a second year following the initial observation.

2. Materials and Methods

2.1. Study Design

This is a retrospective, multi-center, non-interventional, observational cohort study. We enrolled a total of 76,764 patients from hospitals in the districts of Ferrara and Romagna (the University Hospital of Ferrara (Coordinating Centre), as well as the Ferrara and Romagna Local Health Units (LHUs)). Additional details about the participating centers can be found in Supplementary Table S1.

The databases used for analysis included the demographic database, pharmaceutical database (containing data related to dispensed drugs, categorized by the Anatomical–Therapeutic Chemical [ATC] codes FED for "Farmaci a erogazione diretta" and AFT for "Assistenza Farmaceutica Territoriale"), and hospitalization database. Hospital discharge cards (HDCs) were used to track internal transfers between operating units, providing information such as admission, transfer, and discharge dates and times, admission diagnoses, and previous history of major adverse cardiovascular events (MACEs), including non-fatal myocardial infarction (MI), non-fatal cerebrovascular accident (CVA), heart failure (HF), malignant dysrhythmias (MD), and cardiac shock (CS).

Clinical diagnoses were classified using the International Classification of Diseases, 9th Revision, Clinical Modification (ICD-9-CM), while mortality data were collected daily from the ReM (Relevation of Mortality) service for the Emilia Romagna Region. Information about individuals with diabetes in each region was gathered in collaboration with local diabetology units.

SARS-CoV-2 infection was confirmed through nasopharyngeal swabs with virus-specific RNA detection and amplification using real-time polymerase chain reaction assays (RT-PCR). Hospitalization was categorized as "COVID-19-associated" or "-related" based on diagnoses listed on the hospital discharge card for coronavirus infections, as communicated by the hospital assistance service of the Emilia Romagna region in March 2020.

The inclusion criteria consisted of two factors: (a) age, individuals aged 18 or older; and (b) diabetes-specific drugs used directly for diabetes treatment following the Anatomical Therapeutic Chemical (ATC) classification, A10. The observation period spanned two years, from January 2020 to December 2021.

The use of an anonymous unique numeric code ensured full compliance with the European General Data Protection Regulation (GDPR) (2016/679). The analysis was performed exclusively on anonymized data, thereby adhering to privacy regulations. Results were presented only in aggregated form, preventing attribution to any single institution, department, doctor, or individual prescribing behavior. The study was conducted in accordance with current legislation for retrospective studies. According to the Data Privacy Guarantor Authority (the General Authorization for personal data treatment for scientific research purposes—n.9/2014); informed consent was not required due to organizational constraints. The study adhered to Italian law on observational studies, with notification to and approval from the ethics committee of each participating entity.

2.2. Demographic Data

The University Hospital of Ferrara (UHF) and Ferrara Local Health Units (LHUs) collectively cover an area inhabited by 345,503 people (45,387 of whom are under 18 years old, and 300,116 of whom are older), while the region served by the Romagna LHUs has a population of 1,125,574 individuals (174,618 under 18 years old and 950,956 older), making a total of 1,471,077 residents.

Regarding adult T2DM patients, the Ferrara district reported 17,797 individuals (constituting 5.2% of the population), and the Romagna area had 59,327 cases (equivalent to 6.2%). This resulted in a combined diabetic population of 76,764 patients, accounting for 6.1% of the adult population. It is worth noting that these figures align closely with the national average, considering the prevalence of diabetes in Italy (which stood at 5.9% for both female and male subjects in 2020; source: www.istat.it, accessed on 1 January 2023). This demonstrates the significant consistency of our region's data with the country's overall statistics. Additional details concerning the demographic breakdown of subjects can be found in Supplementary Figure S1.

We divided the overall population with T2DM into several subgroups based on their respective home antidiabetic therapies. Additionally, the cohort of patients who were hospitalized was further divided into two subgroups, categorized by the reason for their hospital admission (COVID-19-related or other reasons).

The term "non-COVID-19-associated-related hospitalization" refers to admissions prompted by various causes requiring hospital treatment, excluding SARS-CoV-2 infection. Examples of such causes include cardiovascular events, routine or emergency surgeries, infections, respiratory insufficiency, and more.

The hospitalized population with T2DM was further characterized and classified based on their home antidiabetic therapy and their history of major adverse cardiovascular events (MACEs). We sought to identify differences between groups in terms of individual MACEs (such as non-fatal myocardial infarction, MI; non-fatal cerebrovascular accident, CVA; heart failure, HF; malignant dysrhythmias, MD; cardiac shock, CS), 2-point MACEs (non-fatal MI and non-fatal CVA), 3-point MACEs (non-fatal MI, non-fatal CVA, and HF with or without CS), and 4-point MACEs (non-fatal MI, non-fatal CVA, HF with or without CS, and MD).

2.3. Statistical Analysis

Data analyses were carried out using IBM SPSS Statistics version 26.0 (IBM Corporation). The normality of the distribution of continuous variables was assessed using the Shapiro–Wilk test. In case of normal distribution of data, continuous variables were presented with their mean and standard deviation (SD), while in case of non-normal distribution, with their median value and interquartile range [1Q 3Q]. Categorical data were presented as total numbers and percentages (%).

Differences between groups were examined in terms of age, sex distribution, length of stay, mortality (both in-hospital and cumulative deaths within the two-year observation period), and antidiabetic treatment. Percentages were compared using the chi-square test, Fisher's exact test, or Yates' correction if necessary. Continuous data were assessed using Student's *t*-test or the Mann–Whitney test as appropriate.

Box plots were employed to compare the lengths of stay among different groups of inpatients. Additionally, chi-square tests were conducted for risk estimates, and one-versus-one analyses among the primary antidiabetic treatments, with computation of relative odds ratios (ORs) and 95% confidence intervals (CIs). These ORs and 95% CIs were calculated using an unadjusted logistic regression model, with the need for hospitalization, in-hospital deaths, and cumulative deaths as dependent variables, and age, sex, 4-point MACE events, and antidiabetic treatments as independent variables. Survival curves were generated using the Kaplan–Meier method and compared between various subgroups using the log-rank test. A significance level of $p < 0.05$ was considered statistically significant.

Throughout the development of this article, STROBE (Strengthening the Reporting of Observational Studies in Epidemiology) guidelines were adhered to in each phase.

3. Results

3.1. Antidiabetic Prescriptions

We categorized the population with T2DM based on their respective home antidiabetic treatments. As anticipated, a significant proportion of the population (30,238 individuals, accounting for 39.4% of the total) were undergoing therapy exclusively with metformin. Furthermore, 14,739 individuals (19.2%) were treated with either insulin or insulin secretagogues. An additional breakdown of the population included 2037 individuals (2.4%) utilizing a combination of DPP-4 inhibitors (DPP-4is) and metformin; 1169 individuals (1.5%) on DPP-4is alone; 1095 individuals (1.4%) taking DPP-4is along with insulin or insulin secretagogues like glimepiride, glyburide, or glipizide; 910 individuals (1.2%) using GLP-1 receptor agonists (GLP-1 RAs) alongside metformin; 190 individuals (0.2%) on a regimen of GLP-1 RAs in combination with insulin or insulin secretagogues; and 127 individuals (0.2%) solely on GLP-1 RAs. Moreover, 26,259 individuals (34.2%) were on various other drug combinations or alternative medications such as SGLT-2 inhibitors, acarbose, or thiazolidinediones (refer to Table 1).

Table 1. Population characteristics.

Variables		Total	Non-Hospitalized Subjects	Hospitalized Subjects (n = 2910)		p Value
				Non-COVID-19 Hospitalization	COVID-19 Hospitalization	
Subjects, n (%)		76,764	73,854 (96.2)	988 (34.0)	1922 (66.0)	<0.001
Age (years), mean ± SD		70 ± 13	70 ± 13	74 ± 13	73 ± 13	0.05
Age < 60 years, n (%)		14,861 (19.4)	14,435 (19.5)	135 (13.7)	291 (15.1)	0.36
Age 60–69 years, n (%)		18,291 (23.8)	17,789 (24.1)	164 (16.6)	338 (17.6)	0.57
Age 70–79 years, n (%)		24,278 (31.6)	23,372 (31.6)	288 (29.1)	618 (32.2)	0.23
Age ≥ 80 years, n (%)		19,334 (25.2)	18,258 (24.7)	401 (40.6)	675 (35.1)	0.05
Sex, n (%)	Female	35,418 (46.1)	34,231 (46.5)	410 (41.5)	777 (40.4)	<0.001
	Male	41,251 (53.9)	39,528 (53.5)	578 (58.5)	1145 (59.6)	
Days of hospital stay, mean ± SD		-	-	18.5 ± 16.3	18.2 ± 17.7	0.73
In-hospital death, n (%)		739 (1.0)	-	318 (32.2)	421 (21.9)	<0.001
Cumulative death, n (%)		6926 (9.0)	5947 (8.1)	423 (42.8)	556 (28.9)	<0.001
Cardiovascular events						
Non-fatal MI, n (%)		573 (0.7)	524 (0.7)	22 (2.2)	27 (1.4)	0.11
Non-fatal CVA, n (%)		1470 (1.9)	1277 (1.7)	81 (8.2)	112 (5.8)	0.023
Heart failure (HF), n (%)		1898 (2.5)	1589 (2.2)	125 (12.7)	184 (9.6)	0.022
Malignant dysrhythmia (MD), n (%)		323 (0.4)	287 (0.4)	14 (1.4)	22 (1.1)	0.53
Cardiac shock (CS), n (%)		50 (0.1)	40 (0.1)	0 (0.0)	10 (0.5)	0.019
4-point MACE, n (%)		3794 (4.9)	3263 (4.4)	215 (21.8)	316 (16.4)	0.004
Antidiabetic drugs						
Metformin, n (%)		30,238 (39.4)	29,455 (39.9)	239 (24.2)	544 (28.3)	0.07
Insulin or insulin secretagogues, n (%)		14,739 (19.2)	13,976 (18.9)	284 (28.7)	479 (24.9)	0.09
GLP-1 RAs, n (%)		1227 (1.6)	1175 (1.6)	18 (1.8)	34 (1.8)	0.92
GLP-1 RAs + metformin, n (%)		910 (1.2)	875 (1.2)	9 (0.9)	26 (1.4)	0.31
GLP-1 RA alone, n (%)		127 (0.2)	122 (0.2)	2 (0.2)	3 (0.2)	0.78
GLP-1 RAs + insulin or insulin secretagogues, n (%)		190 (0.2)	178 (0.2)	7 (0.7)	5 (0.3)	0.08
DPP-4is, n (%)		4301 (5.6)	4060 (5.5)	87 (8.8)	154 (8.0)	0.50
DPP-4i alone, n (%)		1169 (1.5)	1078 (1.5)	38 (3.8)	53 (2.8)	0.12
DPP-4is + metformin, n (%)		2037 (2.7)	1972 (2.7)	16 (1.6)	49 (2.5)	0.12
DPP-4is + insulin or insulin secretagogues, n (%)		1095 (1.4)	1010 (1.4)	33 (3.3)	52 (2.7)	0.35
Other drug combinations or other drugs, n (%)		26,259 (34.2)	25,188 (34.1)	360 (36.4)	711 (37.0)	0.84

Non-COVID-19 hospitalization, non-COVID-19-related/associated hospitalization but for other reasons; COVID-19 hospitalization, COVID-19-related/associated hospitalization; MI = myocardial infarction; CVA = cardiovascular accidents; HF = heart failure; CS = cardiac shock; MD = malignant dysrhythmia; 4-point MACE = 4-point major adverse cardiovascular events (non-fatal MI, non-fatal CVA, HF with or without CS, and MD); GLP-1 RAs = GLP-1 receptor agonists; DPP-4is = DPP-4 inhibitors. Data are presented as number (%), and if not are appropriately specified.

3.2. Population Characteristics

Within the primary cohort of individuals with T2DM, a total of 2910 required hospitalization, representing 3.8% of the cohort. Among these hospitalizations, 1922 cases (66.0%) were attributed to COVID-19, while the remaining 988 cases (34.0%) were due to other reasons. Table 1 provides a comprehensive overview of the distinctions between the two groups of subjects who were hospitalized for COVID-19 or alternative reasons. The p-values resulting from the comparison of COVID-19 and non-COVID-19 inpatients are presented.

Substantial differences were observed in terms of age; COVID-19 patients were relatively younger, with an average age of 73 ± 13 years compared to 74 ± 13 years for non-COVID-19 inpatients (p = 0.05). This age difference was particularly pronounced within the subgroup of individuals aged over 80, where those hospitalized for non-COVID-19 reasons were generally older (p = 0.05). Regarding sex distribution, males were more prevalent in both subgroups of inpatients.

In-hospital mortality rates demonstrated significant variation; COVID-19 patients experienced notably lower mortality, with rates of 21.9% compared to 32.2% for those hospitalized for other reasons ($p < 0.001$). Cumulative mortality data further supported this trend, with COVID-19-related mortality at a lower level of 28.9% in contrast to 42.8% for non-COVID-19-related reasons ($p < 0.001$).

The same categorization (subjects with T2DM hospitalized for COVID-19 versus those hospitalized for other reasons) was maintained in the second section of Table 1, wherein we assessed the differences in terms of individual MACEs and subsequently, 2-point, 3-point, and 4-point MACEs, as elaborated above. Noteworthy differences between the two groups emerged for non-fatal cerebrovascular accidents (CVA) (8.2% vs. 5.8%, $p = 0.023$), heart failure (HF) (12.7% vs. 9.6%, $p = 0.022$), and cardiac shock (CS) (0% vs. 0.5%, $p = 0.019$). COVID-19 inpatients presented generally lower rates of 4-point MACE (16.4% vs. 21.8%, $p = 0.004$). Aside from CS, where subjects admitted for other reasons did not experience this outcome, those admitted due to COVID-19 generally exhibited a lower occurrence of MACEs. This trend persisted across 2-point, 3-point, and 4-point MACE analyses.

Regarding antidiabetic treatments, no substantial differences were encountered in the comparisons between groups.

In Supplementary Table S2, we have presented the prevalence of each individual MACE, categorized based on patients' antidiabetic home treatment. Given the notably low percentage of occurrences for each MACE within all subgroups, no statistical analysis or intergroup comparison was deemed relevant.

3.3. Antidiabetic Drugs and Outcomes

In Figure 1, we direct our attention to the primary treatment groups discussed earlier, excluding the subgroup treated with other drugs or combinations of drugs. For each treatment group, we calculated the respective percentages of hospitalizations (attributed to COVID-19 or other reasons), in-hospital deaths (separating COVID-19-related and other reasons), and cumulative deaths (encompassing both hospitalized and non-hospitalized subjects).

Regarding the need for hospitalization (Figure 1A), the breakdown is as follows: among subjects treated with metformin, 1.8% required hospitalization due to COVID-19, and 0.8% for other reasons; within the group receiving insulin/insulin secretagogues, 3.2% were hospitalized for COVID-19, and 1.9% for other reasons. For those treated with GLP-1 Ras, 2.8% were admitted due to COVID-19, and 1.5% for other reasons, while among the subjects treated with DPP-4 inhibitors (DPP-4is), the respective percentages were 3.6% for COVID-19-related hospitalization and 2.0% for other reasons.

The analysis pertaining to mortality yielded different results; among all treatment groups, patients with the lowest in-hospital mortality rates were those treated with GLP-1 RAs (0.4% due to COVID-19, and 0.2% for other reasons). Similar findings were observed for cumulative death over the two-year observation period. This trend persisted across all subjects, including those who did not require hospitalization within the two-year span, as well as those who experienced at least one hospitalization (Figure 1B,C).

Assessment of the length of stay, defined as the number of days spent during the primary hospitalization, revealed minimal disparities between the various subject groups. This observation held true even when comparing lengths of stay between COVID-19 and non-COVID-19 inpatients (refer to Supplementary Figure S2).

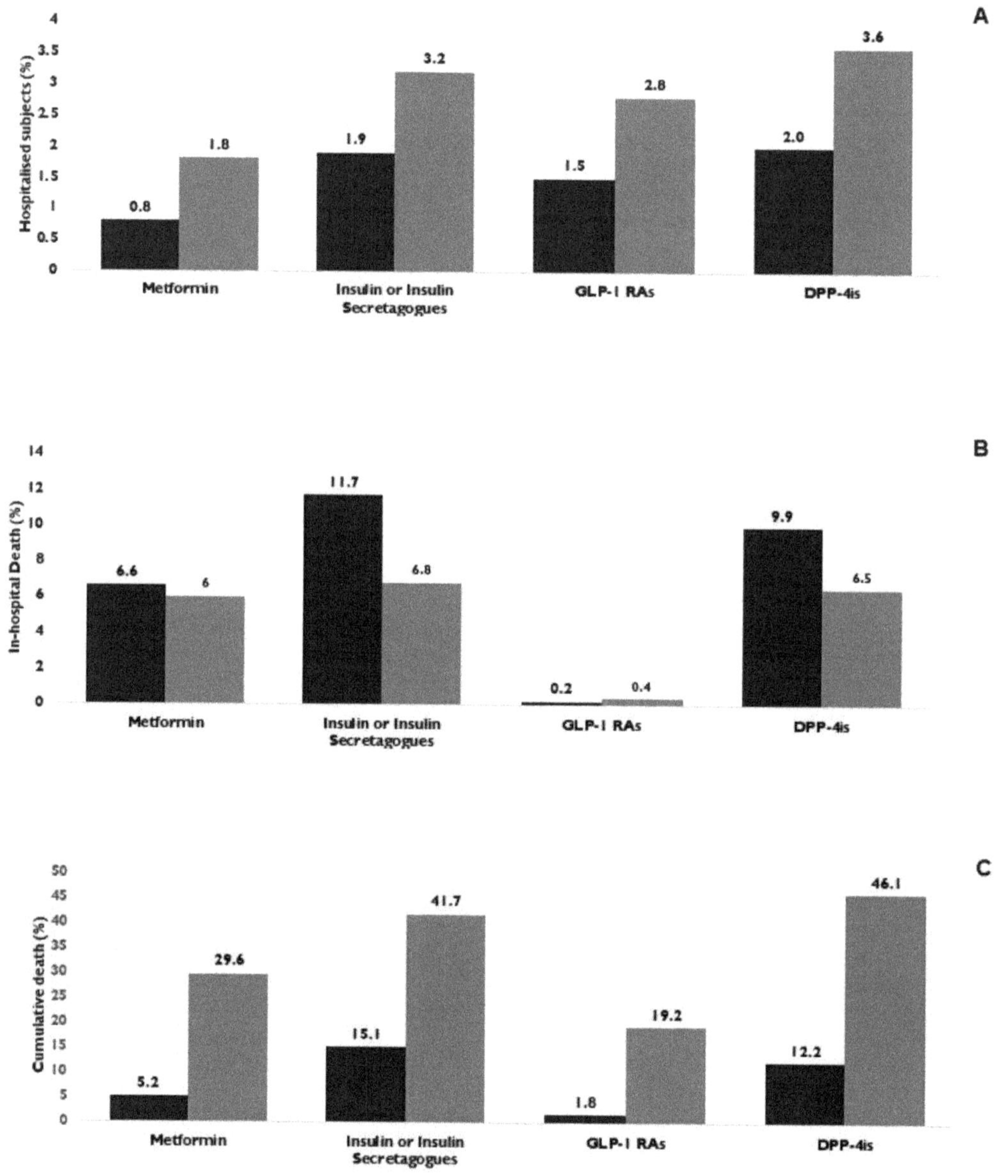

Figure 1. Comparison between the main four subgroups of diabetic inpatients in terms of hospital admission (admitted for COVID-19, right column, and for other reasons, left column) (**A**); Metformin vs. all drugs $p < 0.001$. Differences between groups in terms of in-hospital death (admitted for COVID-19, right column, and for other reasons, left column) (**B**); Metformin versus insulin/insulin secretagogues and versus DPP-4is. $p < 0.001$, GLP-1RAs vs. other drugs $p < 0.001$. Differences between groups in terms of cumulative death within the period of observation (admitted to hospital, right column, and not admitted to hospital, left column) (**C**). GLP-1 RAs vs. metformin and insulin/insulin secretagogues $p < 0.001$. DPP-4is vs. metformin and insulin/insulin secretagogues $p < 0.005$.

3.4. One-versus-One Comparisons

One-versus-one analyses revealed notable differences when considering the risks associated with hospital admission, COVID-19-related hospitalization, in-hospital death, and cumulative death (refer to Figure 2). In terms of hospital admission, insulin/insulin secretagogues, GLP-1 RAs, and DPP-4 inhibitors (DPP-4is) exhibited higher risks when each category was compared to metformin (with ORs of 2.05 [95% CI 1.86–2.27], 1.67 [95% CI 1.25–2.22], and 2.23 [1.93–2.59], respectively). Moreover, DPP-4is displayed a significantly higher risk than GLP-1 RAs (with an OR of 1.34) in terms of hospital admission.

Outcome	Drug 1	Drug 2	OR	Lower 95% CI	Upper 95% CI	p value
Hospital Admission	Insulin or Insulin secretagogues	Metformin	2.05	1.86	2.27	0.001
	GLP-1 RAs	Metformin	1.67	1.25	2.22	0.001
	DPP-4is	Metformin	2.23	1.93	2.59	0.001
	DPP-4is	GLP-1 RAs	1.34	0.99	1.82	0.06
COVID-19 related/associated hospitalisation	Insulin or Insulin secretagogues	Metformin	0.74	0.60	0.92	0.006
	GLP-1 RAs	Metformin	0.83	0.46	1.50	0.54
	DPP-4is	Metformin	0.78	0.57	1.05	0.11
	DPP-4is	GLP-1 RAs	0.94	0.50	1.76	0.88
In hospital Death	Insulin or Insulin secretagogues	Metformin	2.82	2.32	3.42	0.001
	GLP-1 RAs	Metformin	1.23	0.63	2.40	0.07
	DPP-4is	Metformin	3.19	2.45	4.15	0.001
	DPP-4is	GLP-1 RAs	2.60	1.30	5.19	0.002
Cumulative death	Insulin or Insulin secretagogues	Metformin	3.19	2.99	3.41	0.001
	GLP-1 RAs	Metformin	0.42	0.29	0.60	0.001
	DPP-4is	Metformin	2.65	2.40	2.92	0.001
	DPP-4is	GLP-1 RAs	6.33	4.39	9.13	0.001

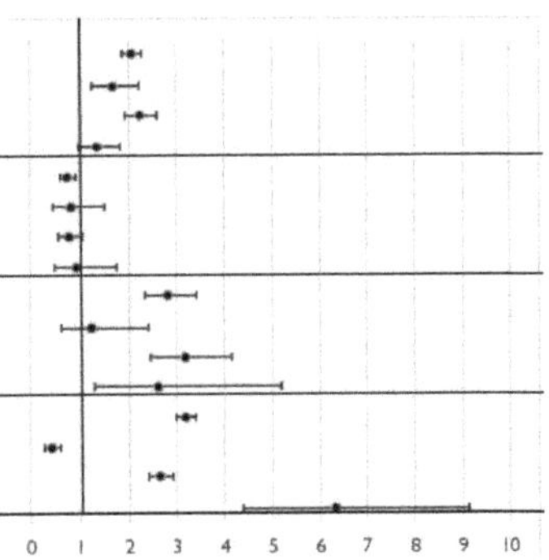

Figure 2. One-versus-one analyses evaluating the risk for worse outcomes (hospital admission, COVID-19-related/associated hospitalization, in-hospital death, and cumulative death). OR = odds ratio; 95% CI = 95% confidence interval; GLP-1 RAs = GLP-1 receptor agonists; DPP-4is = DPP-4 inhibitors.

Regarding COVID-19-related hospitalization, the most significant comparison was between insulin/insulin secretagogues and metformin (with an OR of 0.74 [95% CI 0.60–0.92]), indicating a lower risk associated with metformin use.

The most substantial findings emerged from the one-versus-one analyses related to mortality; concerning in-hospital death, both insulin/insulin secretagogues and DPP-4is demonstrated lower levels of protection compared to metformin (with ORs of 2.82 [95% CI 2.32–3.42] and 3.19 [95% CI 2.45–4.15], respectively). Furthermore, DPP-4is exhibited a higher risk of mortality than GLP-1 RAs (with an OR of 2.60 [95% CI 1.30–5.19]). However, the comparison between GLP-1 RAs and metformin did not yield statistically significant results in terms of in-hospital death.

These analyses provide important insights into the relative risks associated with different antidiabetic treatments in the context of hospitalization and mortality outcomes.

Indeed, the analyses pertaining to cumulative death provide some of the most compelling insights. These analyses reaffirm what was presented in Figure 1, highlighting that insulin/insulin secretagogues and DPP-4 inhibitors (DPP-4is) continue to exhibit worse outcomes compared to metformin (with ORs of 3.19 [95% CI 2.99–3.41] and 2.65 [95% CI 2.40–2.92], respectively). Furthermore, DPP-4is, when compared to GLP-1 receptor agonists (GLP-1 RAs), continue to display an elevated risk of cumulative death (with an OR of 6.33 [95% CI 4.39–9.13]).

However, a distinct finding emerges from the one-versus-one analysis between GLP-1 RAs and metformin. This analysis yields an OR of 0.42 (95% CI 0.29–0.60, $p < 0.001$). This substantial OR signifies the powerful protective effect exerted by GLP-1 RAs against mortality over a two-year period.

3.5. Logistic Regression Analyses

Logistic regression analyses were conducted to assess the individual contribution of each variable in influencing the three selected outcomes: hospital admission, in-hospital death, and cumulative death. The reference categories chosen for comparison were as follows: female sex, age below 60 years for age categories, and metformin for antidiabetic treatments. Notably, female sex was found to be independently associated with lower ORs across all considered outcomes, indicating a lower risk. Conversely, higher ORs were observed for the variable "4-point MACE" in relation to all outcomes (as detailed in Table 2).

Table 2. Logistic regression analyses.

	B	S.E.	Wald	df	*p* Value	OR	95% CI (Upper-Lower)
Hospital admission							
Sex (F/M)	−0.27	0.05	29.63	1	<0.001	0.77	0.70–0.84
Age < 60 years	-	-	82.01	3	<0.001	-	-
Age 60–69 years	−0.01	0.09	0.01	1	0.99	1.00	0.84–1.18
Age 70–79 years	0.23	0.08	8.87	1	0.003	1.26	1.08–1.46
Age ≥ 80 years	0.55	0.08	51.96	1	<0.001	1.73	1.49–2.01
4-point MACE	1.31	0.07	396.51	1	<0.001	3.72	3.27–4.24
Metformin	-	-	115.75	3	<0.001	-	-
Insulin or insulin secretagogues	0.51	0.05	88.79	1	<0.001	1.66	1.50–1.85
GLP-1 RAs	0.64	0.15	18.37	1	<0.001	1.69	1.41–2.52
DPP-4is	0.58	0.08	55.97	1	<0.001	1.78	1.53–2.08
In-hospital death							
Sex (F/M)	−0.50	0.09	29.09	1	<0.001	0.61	0.51–0.72
Age < 60 years			179.07	3	<0.001	-	-
Age 60–69 years	0.67	0.30	4.88	1	0.03	1.95	1.08–3.53
Age 70–79 years	1.74	0.27	43.04	1	<0.001	5.68	3.38–9.53
Age ≥ 80 years	2.45	0.26	88.65	1	<0.001	11.62	6.97–19.35
4-point MACE	1.55	0.10	229.20	1	<0.001	4.71	3.85–5.75
Metformin			42.07	3	<0.001	-	-
Insulin or insulin secretagogues	0.59	0.10	33.33	1	<0.001	1.81	1.48–2.20
GLP-1 RAs	0.80	0.35	5.33	1	0.021	1.84	1.13–4.42
DPP-4is	0.67	0.14	23.59	1	<0.001	1.96	1.49–2.56
Cumulative death							
Sex (F/M)	−0.24	0.03	53.59	1	<0.001	0.79	0.74–0.84
Age < 60 years	-	-	2269.81	3	<0.001	-	-
Age 60–69 years	1.02	0.10	107.46	1	<0.001	2.76	2.28–3.35
Age 70–79 years	1.72	0.09	368.67	1	<0.001	5.57	4.67–6.64
Age ≥ 80 years	2.84	0.09	1066.26	1	<0.001	17.14	14.45–20.33
4-point MACE	1.16	0.05	578.85	1	<0.001	3.20	2.91–3.51
Metformin	-	-	565.10	3	<0.001	-	-
Insulin or insulin secretagogues	0.82	0.04	545.72	1	<0.001	2.28	2.13–2.44
GLP-1 RAs	−0.20	0.19	1.12	1	0.29	0.82	0.57–1.18
DPP-4is	0.60	0.05	124.76	1	<0.001	1.81	1.63–2.01

Logistic regression modelling for identifying the variables associated with outcomes (hospital admission, in-hospital death, and cumulative death). OR = odds ratio; 95% CI = 95% confidence interval; 4-point MACE = 4-point major adverse cardiovascular events (non-fatal MI, non-fatal CVA, HF with or without CS, and MD); GLP-1 RAs = GLP-1 receptor agonists; DPP-4is = DPP-4 inhibitors.

Insulin/insulin secretagogues and DPP-4 inhibitors (DPP-4is) displayed notably elevated and statistically significant ORs for all three outcomes examined. In contrast,

GLP-1 receptor agonists (GLP-1 RAs) demonstrated comparable results only in relation to hospital admission and in-hospital death, with ORs of 1.69 (95% CI 1.41–2.52) and 1.84 (95% CI 1.13–4.42), respectively. However, no significant differences were observed concerning cumulative death when GLP-1 RAs were compared to metformin as the reference treatment.

3.6. Survival Estimates

The Mantel–Cox log-rank tests conducted over the course of the two-year observation period (Figure 3) revealed significant differences ($p < 0.001$) in terms of cumulative survival between subjects who were hospitalized and those who were not. As anticipated, non-hospitalized subjects exhibited markedly higher survival rates (Figure 3A). This initial observation prompted us to delve deeper into our investigation, wherein we sought differences among both the hospitalized and non-hospitalized subjects, while stratifying for different antidiabetic drugs.

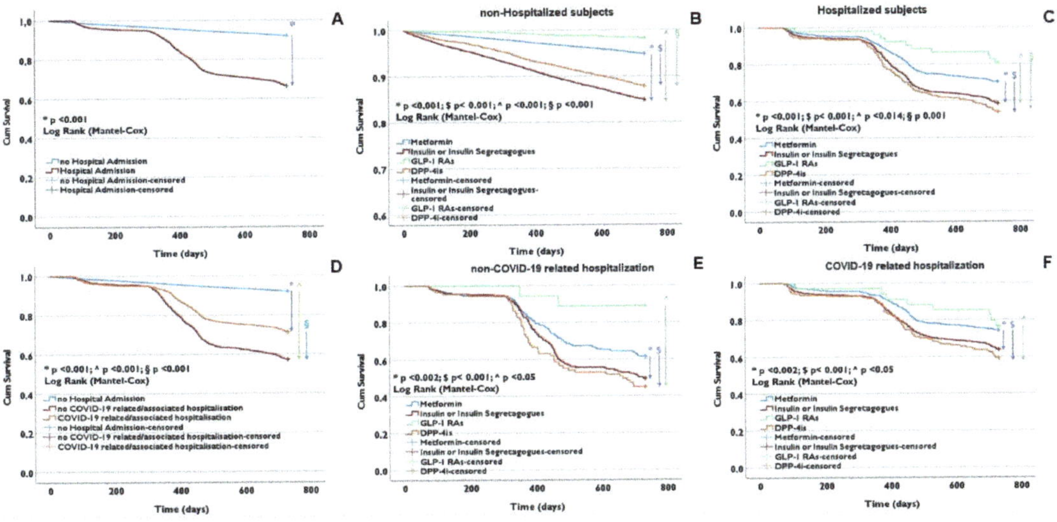

Figure 3. Mantel–Cox log-rank tests. Analysis of two-year survival among diabetic subjects subcohorts. Differences in terms of cumulative survival between hospitalised and non-hospitalised subjects (**A**); cumulative survival among non-hospitalised subjects based on antidiabetic treatment (**B**); cumulative survival among hospitalised subjects based on antidiabetic treatment (**C**); differences in terms of cumulative survival among non-hospitalised, hospitalised for COVID-19 and hospitalised for other reasons (**D**); cumulative survival among subjects hospitalised for other reasons based on antidiabetic treatment (**E**); cumulative survival among subjects hospitalised for COVID-19 based on antidiabetic treatment (**F**).

Remarkably, GLP-1 receptor agonists (GLP-1 RAs) exhibited significantly better survival estimates ($p < 0.001$) for both cohorts of subjects throughout the entire observation period (Figure 3B,C). The Kaplan–Meier survival curves among hospitalized subjects displayed a consistent decline over time across all treatment groups. Conversely, for non-hospitalized subjects, the curves maintained a relatively stable trajectory up to around 300 days, after which they experienced a more rapid decrease across all treatment groups. Notably, non-hospitalized subjects treated with GLP-1 RAs demonstrated a higher likelihood of survival compared to those treated with other medications (with $p < 0.05$).

These findings persisted even when variables associated with COVID-19 and non-COVID-19-related hospitalizations were introduced into the analysis. Once again, GLP-1 receptor agonists (GLP-1 RAs) demonstrated significantly improved survival curves when compared to all other antidiabetic drugs (with p-values < 0.05) (Figure 3D–F).

4. Discussion

In addition to their hypoglycemic effects, DPP-4 inhibitors (DPP-4is) and GLP-1 receptor agonists (GLP-1 RAs) exert a broad anti-inflammatory influence. They achieve this by facilitating the transformation of blood and tissue monocyto-macrophagic cells into the anti-inflammatory M2 phenotype. Simultaneously, they decrease the production of inflammatory cytokines [15,20–22].

A recent study conducted on a total of 338 COVID-19 inpatients revealed that the administration of sitagliptin, a DPP-4 inhibitor, upon admission yielded substantial benefits. Among the group of 169 patients treated with sitagliptin, there was a significant reduction in in-hospital mortality when compared to the control group of 169 patients receiving conventional insulin treatment (18% vs. 37%; Hazard Ratio [HR] = 0.44). Notably, the use of sitagliptin was also associated with a reduced risk of mechanical ventilation and admission to intensive care units (ICUs), with Hazard Ratios (HRs) of 0.27 and 0.51, respectively [23]. In addition to these data and always in the context of COVID-19 inpatients, a multination meta-analysis showed that DPP-4is administration was associated with significantly reduced overall mortality rates (OR 0.75) [24].

GLP-1 RAs were considered excellent candidates for treating COVID-19 also in patients without diagnosis of T2DM owing to their multiple beneficial effects on excessive inflammation-induced acute lung injury [8], once again showing that COVID-19 can be considered a model of acute stressor against which molecules with a marked anti-inflammatory role can act.

A plausible explanation for the favorable effect of GLP-1 receptor agonists (GLP-1 RAs) on the clinical course of COVID-19 stems from an experimental study conducted in an animal model using streptozotocin-induced diabetes rats. This study demonstrated that liraglutide, a type of GLP-1 RA, can stimulate the expression of pulmonary ACE2 and Angiotensin (1-7) [A(1-7)], thereby reversing the imbalance within the renin-angiotensin system (RAS) in rats with type 1 diabetes mellitus (T1DM). This imbalance is characterized by a preponderance of the vasoconstrictor component of the RAS. This results in elevated levels of angiotensin II (AII), which subsequently leads to right ventricle hypertrophy. The study's findings revealed that liraglutide effectively counteracted right ventricle hypertrophy and promoted increased production of proteins A and B of the pulmonary surfactant (SP-A and SP-B) in diabetic rats [25].

The role of ACE2 expression in COVID-19 pathogenesis was already hypothesized in many previous studies and its modulation was thought to be one of the keys for modulating the inflammatory response [26,27]. Moreover, it was also theorised that uncontrolled hyperglycemia may cause aberrant glycosylation of ACE2 in lungs, nasal airways, tongue, and oropharynx, thus increasing SARS-CoV-2 viral binding sites and leading to a higher trend of SARS-CoV-2 infections and more severe forms of COVID-19 [28]. For this reason, an efficacy regulation of plasma sugar levels plays a fundamental role in COVID-19 management.

The activation of the ACE2/A(1-7)/MasR axis is also able to determine an important antithrombotic effect [29,30], mediated by the production of prostacyclin and nitric oxide (NO) [31]. Furthermore, the restoration of the renin-angiotensin system (RAS) balance achieved by enhancing the activity of the ACE2/Angiotensin (1-7)/MasR axis has the potential to mitigate the pro-inflammatory state and suppress the excessive activation of the coagulation process. This modulation of the RAS can also help mitigate the development of thrombotic complications commonly associated with COVID-19, which is often referred to as COVID-19 coagulopathy [32,33], which plays a fundamental role in the pathogenesis of ARDS and multi-organ failure during SARS-CoV-2 infection [34] and is often associated with an ominous prognosis of COVID-19 [35]. Therefore, it is conceivable that the previously described effects of GLP-1 RAs on the synthesis of pulmonary surfactants proteins [25], may be able to determine a further protective effect on the COVID-19 clinical outcomes. Additionally, while the elevated expression of ACE2 might be assumed as a potential facilitator for SARS-CoV-2 cell entry, it is plausible that GLP-1 receptor agonists (GLP-1 RAs), through their counteraction of pro-inflammatory cytokine effects and restoration of RAS balance (including the enhancement of the ACE2/Angiotensin(1-7)/MasR axis activity), could potentially exert a protective effect against lung damage and the onset of multi-organ failure. In this context, GLP-1 RAs might contribute to reducing the severity of COVID-19 by mitigating the detrimental impact on lung function and overall organ health [9,36].

In the current state of research, numerous literature reports have emphasized the necessity for conducting clinical and epidemiological studies with the objective of evaluating the effects of GLP-1 receptor agonists (GLP-1 RAs) on the clinical outcomes of COVID-19 in patients with type 2 diabetes (T2DM) [8,9]. A recent retrospective observational clinical study highlighted that the prior use of GLP-1 RAs and SGLT-2 inhibitors (SGLT-2is), when compared to the utilization of DPP-4 inhibitors (DPP-4is), was linked to a substantial 60-day mortality reduction. Additionally, it was associated with noteworthy reductions in overall mortality, Emergency Room (ER) admissions, and hospitalizations [37]. Conversely, another retrospective observational study conducted in Denmark indicated that the utilization of incretin-based therapies was not associated with improved COVID-19 outcomes. However, it is worth noting that statistical power was constrained due to a small sample size [38].

A neutral effect of both incretin-based therapies (and SGLT-2is) on COVID-19-related mortality was also showed by a national retrospective observational study performed in England on a total of 2,851,465 T2DM patients [39].

Researchers from Indonesia conducted a study that revealed a significant association between the pre-admission use of GLP-1 receptor agonists (GLP-1 RAs) and a reduction in mortality rates related to COVID-19 among patients with type 2 diabetes (T2DM). The OR calculated for this association was 0.53, indicating a substantial reduction in the odds of mortality for those who were using GLP-1 RAs prior to their admission due to COVID-19. Importantly, this association held irrespective of other factors such as age, sex, pre-existing diagnosis of hypertension or other cardiovascular diseases, and the administration of other antidiabetic medications like metformin or insulin [40].

Two other recent meta-analyses have delved into the effects of preadmission use of antidiabetic medications on the in-hospital mortality of patients with type 2 diabetes (T2DM) and COVID-19. In the first meta-analysis, which encompassed 61 studies, it was found that preadmission use of certain antidiabetic medications correlated with distinct outcomes in terms of in-hospital mortality. Specifically, the use of metformin (OR 0.54), GLP-1 RAs (OR 0.51), and SGLT-2is (OR 0.60) was associated with lower mortality rates in individuals with diabetes and COVID-19. Conversely, the use of DPP-4is (OR 1.23) and insulin (OR 1.70) was linked to elevated mortality rates. Other antidiabetic medications such as sulfonylureas, thiazolidinediones, and alpha-glucosidase inhibitors exhibited a neutral impact on mortality outcomes [41]. The second meta-analysis showed instead that treatment with metformin (OR 0.74), DPP-4is (OR 0.88), SGLT-2is (OR 0.82), and GLP-1 RAs (OR 0.91) was related to reduced COVID-19 mortality rates in T2DM subjects, while insulin to increased mortality [42]. Additionally, GLP-1 RAs exhibited the most substantial and significant protective effect in reducing mortality rate, followed by SGLT-2is and metformin.

As for comparisons between the use of DPP-4is and GLP-1 RAs towards COVID-19 outcomes, conflicting results have been reported. While some studies have not shown a significant favourable effect on COVID-19 outcomes by DPP-4is [43,44], some others showed a possible protective action [45,46]. Moreover, while a recent meta-analysis performed on a total of 10 studies showed that DPP-4is therapy is not able to determine a significant improvement in COVID-19 outcomes [47], another meta-analysis which included the aforementioned study by Solerte et al. [23], in addition to 2 studies considering the intrahospital use of DPP-4is [46,48], highlighted a significant reduction in terms of mortality among T2DM patients treated with such drugs; the association was weaker in patients who were also taking metformin and/or ACE inhibitors [49]. A second recent meta-analysis by Indian scientists showed that intra-hospital administration of DPP-4is (pre-admission administration was not considered) was associated with significantly lower COVID-19-related mortality [50].

Based on the existing observational studies, it remains challenging to arrive at definitive conclusions regarding the impact of pre-existing DPP-4 inhibitor (DPP-4is) therapy on COVID-19 outcomes [51]. However, there is a plausible hypothesis that the continued use of incretin-based therapies within the hospital setting might have the potential to notably enhance clinical outcomes for COVID-19 patients. Therefore, it is crucial to conduct thorough analyses to investigate the potential effects of pre-admission treatment involving both DPP-4is and GLP-1 RAs on the clinical outcomes of COVID-19.

Even though the study did not specifically discuss treatment with SGLT-2 inhibitors (SGLT-2is), it is worth noting some recent research that highlights the anti-inflammatory effects of SGLT-2is. These medications have been shown to reduce the activity of pro-inflammatory cytokines such as tumor necrosis factor alpha (TNF-α), interleukin-6 (IL-6), and C-reactive protein (CRP) [52–54]. These effects are potentially mediated by SGLT-2is-induced reductions in uric acid, insulin levels [55], and leptin, as well as increases in adiponectin levels [56,57]. Additionally, SGLT-2is have demonstrated the ability to counteract low-grade inflammation and oxidative stress linked to diabetes [58], and they are associated with the polarization of monocyte-macrophage cells into the anti-inflammatory M2 phenotype [59,60].

Regarding sulfonylureas, a retrospective study conducted using the United Health Group Clinical Discovery Database revealed that both sulfonylureas and insulin were associated with increased odds of hospitalization among individuals with T2DM [61]. In contrast, a recent meta-analysis indicated that metformin and sulfonylureas might be linked to a reduced risk of mortality in patients with T2DM and COVID-19 [62]. Moreover, another recent meta-analysis corroborated the protective role of metformin against COVID-19-related deaths [63].

When assessing the effects of various antidiabetic medications on the clinical course of SARS-CoV-2 infection, it is important to note that there is a lack of definitive and conclusive data across the board. However, an exception to this trend appears to be metformin. Existing evidence suggests that metformin generally exerts a favorable effect, both in terms of reducing the risk of hospitalization and lowering mortality rates among individuals with SARS-CoV-2 infection [64–67]. A possible explanation of this phenomenon could involve the population of subjects with T2DM treated with metformin, the first line of treatment for T2DM and usually destinated to subjects with non-complicated forms of T2DM.

Our study demonstrates a favorable effect of GLP-1 RAs home therapy in the cohort of hospitalised and non-hospitalised subjects and also after a subgroups analysis concerning the subjects admitted for COVID-19 or for other reasons. Once again, we could state that GLP-1 RAs are able to offer an additional layer of protection for T2DM patients even under acute stressors like COVID-19, and this is in line with some of the aforementioned studies and meta-analyses [37,40–42]: in our cohort of patients the effects of GLP-1 RAs are evident in each step of the analyses performed, and it is linked to significantly lower percentage of death, even after a period of observation of two years.

The results of the logistic regression analyses performed clearly demonstrate how the burden of major adverse cardiovascular events (MACEs) in subjects with T2DM, coupled with their older age and male sex, directly correlates with a higher likelihood of hospital admission (for various reasons). This observation aligns well with the current literature and does not require further elaboration. Similarly, these same variables contribute to higher mortality rates in T2DM subjects, both during their hospital stay and cumulatively over time, leaving no room for misinterpretation. Simultaneously, the Mantel–Cox log-rank tests unambiguously reveal that both hospitalized and non-hospitalized T2DM subjects who achieve the best survival outcomes are those treated with GLP-1 RAs. This holds true for patients hospitalized due to a clear acute stressor, such as COVID-19, as well as those hospitalized for other medical reasons.

While many of the anti-inflammatory effects of GLP-1 RAs and DPP-4is still require further clarification, the current literature does not offer a consensus on the lasting benefits provided by these two categories of drugs. Additionally, a more extensive body of research dedicated to these antidiabetic agents could shed light on their potential to modulate the course of acute and/or chronic stressors to which patients with diabetes are particularly susceptible.

Our observations are subject to several limitations, primarily stemming from the retrospective nature of the study and variations in sample size among different subject cohorts. The use of current administrative data sources ensures immediate availability but comes with inherent limitations in terms of data variety. Accessing the necessary information would necessitate manual consultation of each patient's electronic health record (EHR), which is both costly and time-consuming, hindering the analysis of comorbidities and the continuity of antidiabetic treatments during hospitalization. Furthermore, we consciously chose not to focus on certain other antidiabetic drugs (e.g., acarbose, SGLT-2is, thiazolidinediones), as their data were grouped under the umbrella category of "other drug combinations or other drugs", a limitation that should also be acknowledged.

Additionally, important information regarding factors that could influence disease severity (such as medical history, level of physical activity, or laboratory results) is lacking due to the aforementioned reasons.

We recognize that drawing definitive conclusions from administrative data requires larger sample sizes and acknowledge the challenges in doing so. Nonetheless, we are confident that this study, akin to those exploring the effects of antidiabetic medications during acute stressors like COVID-19 or other medical conditions, can serve as a foundational step toward arriving at conclusive findings and a deeper understanding of these drugs.

5. Conclusions

In our cohort of individuals with T2DM, those receiving home treatment with GLP-1 RAs exhibit lower mortality rates compared to any other subgroup treated with various antidiabetic medications. Notably, favorable survival trends were consistently observed for both hospitalized individuals (for acute stressors such as COVID-19 or other medical conditions) and those who were not hospitalized. Furthermore, the beneficial impact of GLP-1 RAs appears to be enduring, resulting in enhanced cumulative survival among individuals with diabetes, even over a two-year observation period.

Supplementary Materials: The following supporting information can be downloaded at: https://www.mdpi.com/article/10.3390/biomedicines11082292/s1, Figure S1: Prevalence of diabetes in the overall adult subjects in the districts of Ferrara and Romagna (A), percentage of diabetic subjects in the districts of Ferrara and Romagna and overall average of diabetic subjects (B); Figure S2: Evaluation of the length of stay in terms of days in the subgroup of patients treated with the four main antidiabetic treatments (A); length of stay among the same four subgroups of inpatients and comparison between COVID-19 and non-COVID-19 subjects (B); Table S1: The institutions serving the districts of Ferrara and Romagna participating in the study; Table S2: MACEs and antidiabetic drugs.

Author Contributions: S.G.: acquisition, analysis and interpretation of data, drafting the article; V.M.M.: the conception and design of the study, drafting the article and revising it critically for important intellectual content; G.V. and N.N.: collection and processing of data; C.C., F.P. and A.M.: acquisition of information concerning drug prescriptions and dispensation, processing data relating to local pharmacies; A.P.: conception and design of the study; revising the article critically for important intellectual content; and final approval of the version to be submitted. All authors have read and agreed to the published version of the manuscript.

Funding: This research received no external funding.

Institutional Review Board Statement: The study was reviewed and approved by the local ethics committee and complies with the ethical principles for medical research involving human subjects, as required by the 2013 revision of the Declaration of Helsinki—WMA Declaration of Helsinki—Ethical Principles for Medical Research Involving Human Subjects. The study protocol was approved by the Ethics Committees (Comitato Etico di Area Vasta Emilia Centro—CE- AVEC—and Comitato Etico della Romagna—C.E.ROM.) on 18 March 2021(268/2021/Oss/AOUFe) and 22 July 2022 (Prot. 5415/2022).

Informed Consent Statement: Not applicable.

Data Availability Statement: Data are protected by a research consortium. The corresponding author will share the data upon receipt of a formal proposal from interested researchers.

Acknowledgments: Our sincere thanks to all the patients who decided to participate in the study, to all the members of the medical staff, to all the extremely skillful and valuable nursing staff members, and to our assistance personnel, who work on the front lines for our patients every day. We also thank the personnel employed in the health system and in information management. Special thanks from all the authors and contributors of the study to Paola Bardasi (Azienda Ospedaliero-Universitaria di Ferrara), Monica Calamai (Azienda Unità Sanitaria Locale di Ferrara), and Tiziano Carradori (Azienda Unità Sanitaria Locale della Romagna) for making it possible to share the databases necessary for the development of the study.

Conflicts of Interest: On behalf of all authors, the corresponding author declares no conflict of interest. The authors declare that they have no known competing financial interests or personal relationships that could have appeared to influence the work reported in this paper.

References

1. Dal Canto, E.; Ceriello, A.; Rydén, L.; Ferrini, M.; Hansen, T.B.; Schnell, O.; Standl, E.; Beulens, J.W. Diabetes as a cardiovascular risk factor: An overview of global trends of macro and micro vascular complications. *Eur. J. Prev. Cardiol.* **2019**, *26*, 25–32. [CrossRef] [PubMed]
2. Kim, L.; Garg, S.; O'halloran, A.; Whitaker, M.; Pham, H.; Anderson, E.J.; Armistead, I.; Bennett, N.M.; Billing, L.; Como-Sabetti, K.; et al. Risk Factors for Intensive Care Unit Admission and In-hospital Mortality Among Hospitalized Adults Identified through the US Coronavirus Disease 2019 (COVID-19)-Associated Hospitalization Surveillance Network (COVID-NET). *Clin. Infect. Dis.* **2021**, *72*, e206–e214. [CrossRef]
3. Holman, N.; Knighton, P.; Kar, P.; O'Keefe, J.; Curley, M.; Weaver, A.; Barron, E.; Bakhai, C.; Khunti, K.; Wareham, N.J.; et al. Risk factors for COVID-19-related mortality in people with type 1 and type 2 diabetes in England: A population-based cohort study. *Lancet Diabetes Endocrinol.* **2020**, *8*, 823–833. [CrossRef] [PubMed]
4. Feldman, E.L.; Savelieff, M.G.; Hayek, S.S.; Pennathur, S.; Kretzler, M.; Pop-Busui, R. COVID-19 and Diabetes: A Collision and Collusion of Two Diseases. *Diabetes* **2020**, *69*, 2549–2565. [CrossRef] [PubMed]
5. Corrao, S.; Pinelli, K.; Vacca, M.; Raspanti, M.; Argano, C. Type 2 Diabetes Mellitus and COVID-19: A Narrative Review. *Front. Endocrinol.* **2021**, *12*, 609470. [CrossRef] [PubMed]
6. Williamson, E.J.; Walker, A.J.; Bhaskaran, K.; Bacon, S.; Bates, C.; Morton, C.E.; Curtis, H.J.; Mehrkar, A.; Evans, D.; Inglesby, P.; et al. Factors associated with COVID-19-related death using OpenSAFELY. *Nature* **2020**, *584*, 430–436. [CrossRef]
7. Solerte, S.B.; Di Sabatino, A.; Galli, M.; Fiorina, P. Dipeptidyl peptidase-4 (DPP4) inhibition in COVID-19. *Acta Diabetol.* **2020**, *57*, 779–783. [CrossRef]
8. Mirabelli, M.; Chiefari, E.; Puccio, L.; Foti, D.P.; Brunetti, A. Potential Benefits and Harms of Novel Antidiabetic Drugs During COVID-19 Crisis. *Int. J. Environ. Res. Public Health* **2020**, *17*, 3664. [CrossRef]
9. Monda, V.M.; Porcellati, F.; Strollo, F.; Gentile, S. ACE2 and SARS-CoV-2 Infection: Might GLP-1 Receptor Agonists Play a Role? *Diabetes Ther.* **2020**, *11*, 1909–1914. [CrossRef]
10. Lu, R.; Zhao, X.; Li, J.; Niu, P.; Yang, B.; Wu, H.; Wang, W.; Song, H.; Huang, B.; Zhu, N.; et al. Genomic characterisation and epidemiology of 2019 novel coronavirus: Implications for virus origins and receptor binding. *Lancet* **2020**, *395*, 565–574. [CrossRef]
11. Kuba, K.; Imai, Y.; Rao, S.; Gao, H.; Guo, F.; Guan, B.; Huan, Y.; Yang, P.; Zhang, Y.; Deng, W.; et al. A crucial role of angiotensin converting enzyme 2 (ACE2) in SARS coronavirus–induced lung injury. *Nat. Med.* **2005**, *11*, 875–879. [CrossRef] [PubMed]
12. Raj, V.S.; Mou, H.; Smits, S.L.; Dekkers, D.H.; Müller, M.A.; Dijkman, R.; Muth, D.; Demmers, J.A.; Zaki, A.; Fouchier, R.A.; et al. Dipeptidyl peptidase 4 is a functional receptor for the emerging human coronavirus-EMC. *Nature* **2013**, *495*, 251–254. [CrossRef] [PubMed]
13. Parker, H.E.; Reimann, F.; Gribble, F.M. Molecular mechanisms underlying nutrient-stimulated incretin secretion. *Expert Rev. Mol. Med.* **2010**, *12*, e1. [CrossRef] [PubMed]
14. Rowlands, J.; Heng, J.; Newsholme, P.; Carlessi, R. Pleiotropic Effects of GLP-1 and Analogs on Cell Signaling, Metabolism, and Function. *Front. Endocrinol.* **2018**, *9*, 672. [CrossRef] [PubMed]
15. Lee, Y.-S.; Jun, H.-S. Anti-Inflammatory Effects of GLP-1-Based Therapies beyond Glucose Control. *Mediat. Inflamm.* **2016**, *2016*, 3094642. [CrossRef]

16. Lontchi-Yimagou, E.; Sobngwi, E.; Matsha, T.E.; Kengne, A.P. Diabetes Mellitus and Inflammation. *Curr. Diabetes Rep.* **2013**, *13*, 435–444. [CrossRef]
17. Martin, J.H.; Deacon, C.F.; Gorrell, M.D.; Prins, J.B. Incretin-based therapies—Review of the physiology, pharmacology and emerging clinical experience. *Intern. Med. J.* **2011**, *41*, 299–307. [CrossRef]
18. Hedrington, M.S.; Davis, S.N. Oral semaglutide for the treatment of type 2 diabetes. *Expert Opin. Pharmacother.* **2019**, *20*, 133–141. [CrossRef]
19. Iacobellis, G.; Fricke, A.C.V. Effects of Semaglutide Versus Dulaglutide on Epicardial Fat Thickness in Subjects with Type 2 Diabetes and Obesity. *J. Endocr. Soc.* **2020**, *4*, bvz042. [CrossRef]
20. Lima-Martínez, M.M.; Paoli, M.; Rodney, M.; Balladares, N.; Contreras, M.; D'marco, L.; Iacobellis, G. Effect of sitagliptin on epicardial fat thickness in subjects with type 2 diabetes and obesity: A pilot study. *Endocrine* **2016**, *51*, 448–455. [CrossRef]
21. Ma, X.; Liu, Z.; Ilyas, I.; Little, P.J.; Kamato, D.; Sahebka, A.; Chen, Z.; Luo, S.; Zheng, X.; Weng, J.; et al. GLP-1 receptor agonists (GLP-1RAs): Cardiovascular actions and therapeutic potential. *Int. J. Biol. Sci.* **2021**, *17*, 2050–2068. [CrossRef] [PubMed]
22. He, J.; Yuan, G.; Cheng, F.; Zhang, J.; Guo, X.; Zeman, M.; Vecka, M.; Burda, M.; Tvrzická, E.; Staňková, B.; et al. Mast Cell and M1 Macrophage Infiltration and Local Pro-Inflammatory Factors Were Attenuated with Incretin-Based Therapies in Obesity-Related Glomerulopathy. *Metab. Syndr. Relat. Disord.* **2017**, *15*, 344–353. [CrossRef]
23. Solerte, S.B.; D'addio, F.; Trevisan, R.; Lovati, E.; Rossi, A.; Pastore, I.; Dell'acqua, M.; Ippolito, E.; Scaranna, C.; Bellante, R.; et al. Sitagliptin Treatment at the Time of Hospitalization Was Associated with Reduced Mortality in Patients with Type 2 Diabetes and COVID-19: A Multicenter, Case-Control, Retrospective, Observational Study. *Diabetes Care* **2020**, *43*, 2999–3006. [CrossRef] [PubMed]
24. Zein, A.F.M.Z.; Raffaello, W.M. Dipeptidyl peptidase-4 (DPP-IV) inhibitor was associated with mortality reduction in COVID-19—A systematic review and meta-analysis. *Prim. Care Diabetes* **2022**, *16*, 162–167. [CrossRef]
25. Romaní-Pérez, M.; Outeiriño-Iglesias, V.; Moya, C.M.; Santisteban, P.; González-Matías, L.C.; Vigo, E.; Mallo, F. Activation of the GLP-1 Receptor by Liraglutide Increases ACE2 Expression, Reversing Right Ventricle Hypertrophy, and Improving the Production of SP-A and SP-B in the Lungs of Type 1 Diabetes Rats. *Endocrinology* **2015**, *156*, 3559–3569. [CrossRef]
26. Pal, R.; Bhansali, A. COVID-19, diabetes mellitus and ACE2: The conundrum. *Diabetes Res. Clin. Pract.* **2020**, *162*, 108132. [CrossRef]
27. Chaudhry, F.; Lavandero, S.; Xie, X.; Sabharwal, B.; Zheng, Y.-Y.; Correa, A.; Narula, J.; Levy, P. Manipulation of ACE2 expression in COVID-19. *Open Heart* **2020**, *7*, e001424. [CrossRef]
28. Shajahan, A.; Pepi, L.E.; Rouhani, D.S.; Heiss, C.; Azadi, P. Glycosylation of SARS-CoV-2: Structural and functional insights. *Anal. Bioanal. Chem.* **2021**, *413*, 7179–7193. [CrossRef]
29. Pai, W.-Y.; Lo, W.-Y.; Hsu, T.; Peng, C.-T.; Wang, H.-J. Angiotensin-(1-7) Inhibits Thrombin-Induced Endothelial Phenotypic Changes and Reactive Oxygen Species Production via NADPH Oxidase 5 Downregulation. *Front. Physiol.* **2017**, *8*, 994. [CrossRef]
30. Fraga-Silva, R.A.; Costa-Fraga, F.P.; De Sousa, F.B.; Alenina, N.; Bader, M.; Sinisterra, R.D.; Santos, R.A.S. An orally active formulation of angiotensin-(1-7) produces an antithrombotic effect. *Clinics* **2011**, *66*, 837–841. [CrossRef] [PubMed]
31. Fang, C.; Stavrou, E.; Schmaier, A.A.; Grobe, N.; Morris, M.; Chen, A.; Nieman, M.T.; Adams, G.N.; LaRusch, G.; Zhou, Y.; et al. Angiotensin 1-7 and Mas decrease thrombosis in *Bdkrb2*$^{-/-}$ mice by increasing NO and prostacyclin to reduce platelet spreading and glycoprotein VI activation. *Blood* **2013**, *121*, 3023–3032. [CrossRef] [PubMed]
32. Becker, R.C. COVID-19 update: COVID-19-associated coagulopathy. *J. Thromb. Thrombolysis* **2020**, *50*, 54–67. [CrossRef] [PubMed]
33. Verdecchia, P.; Cavallini, C.; Spanevello, A.; Angeli, F. The pivotal link between ACE2 deficiency and SARS-CoV-2 infection. *Eur. J. Intern. Med.* **2020**, *76*, 14–20. [CrossRef]
34. Asakura, H.; Ogawa, H. COVID-19-associated coagulopathy and disseminated intravascular coagulation. *Int. J. Hematol.* **2021**, *113*, 45–57. [CrossRef] [PubMed]
35. Helms, J.; Tacquard, C.; Severac, F.; Leonard-Lorant, I.; Ohana, M.; Delabranche, X.; Merdji, H.; Clere-Jehl, R.; Schenck, M.; Gandet, F.F.; et al. High risk of thrombosis in patients with severe SARS-CoV-2 infection: A multicenter prospective cohort study. *Intensive Care Med.* **2020**, *46*, 1089–1098. [CrossRef]
36. Shukla, A.K.; Banerjee, M. Angiotensin-Converting-Enzyme 2 and Renin-Angiotensin System Inhibitors in COVID-19: An Update. *High Blood Press. Cardiovasc. Prev.* **2021**, *28*, 129–139. [CrossRef]
37. Kahkoska, A.R.; Abrahamsen, T.J.; Alexander, G.C.; Bennett, T.D.; Chute, C.G.; Haendel, M.A.; Klein, K.R.; Mehta, H.; Miller, J.D.; Moffitt, R.A.; et al. Association Between Glucagon-Like Peptide 1 Receptor Agonist and Sodium–Glucose Cotransporter 2 Inhibitor Use and COVID-19 Outcomes. *Diabetes Care* **2021**, *44*, 1564–1572. [CrossRef]
38. Israelsen, S.B.; Pottegård, A.; Sandholdt, H.; Madsbad, S.; Thomsen, R.W.; Benfield, T. Comparable COVID-19 outcomes with current use of GLP-1 receptor agonists, DPP-4 inhibitors or SGLT-2 inhibitors among patients with diabetes who tested positive for SARS-CoV-2. *Diabetes Obes. Metab.* **2021**, *23*, 1397–1401. [CrossRef]
39. Khunti, K.; Knighton, P.; Zaccardi, F.; Bakhai, C.; Barron, E.; Holman, N.; Kar, P.; Meace, C.; Sattar, N.; Sharp, S.; et al. Prescription of glucose-lowering therapies and risk of COVID-19 mortality in people with type 2 diabetes: A nationwide observational study in England. *Lancet Diabetes Endocrinol.* **2021**, *9*, 293–303. [CrossRef]
40. Hariyanto, T.I.; Intan, D.; Hananto, J.E.; Putri, C.; Kurniawan, A. Pre-admission glucagon-like peptide-1 receptor agonist (GLP-1RA) and mortality from coronavirus disease 2019 (COVID-19): A systematic review, meta-analysis, and meta-regression. *Diabetes Res. Clin. Pract.* **2021**, *179*, 109031. [CrossRef]

41. Nguyen, N.N.; Ho, D.S.; Nguyen, H.S.; Ho, D.K.N.; Li, H.-Y.; Lin, C.-Y.; Chiu, H.-Y.; Chen, Y.-C. Preadmission use of antidiabetic medications and mortality among patients with COVID-19 having type 2 diabetes: A meta-analysis. *Metabolism* **2022**, *131*, 155196. [CrossRef]
42. Chen, Y.; Lv, X.; Lin, S.; Arshad, M.; Dai, M. The Association Between Antidiabetic Agents and Clinical Outcomes of COVID-19 Patients with Diabetes: A Bayesian Network Meta-Analysis. *Front. Endocrinol.* **2022**, *13*, 895458. [CrossRef] [PubMed]
43. Roussel, R.; Darmon, P.; Pichelin, M.; Goronflot, T.; Abouleka, Y.; Bachir, L.A.; Allix, I.; Ancelle, D.; Barraud, S.; Bordier, L.; et al. Use of dipeptidyl peptidase-4 inhibitors and prognosis of COVID-19 in hospitalized patients with type 2 diabetes: A propensity score analysis from the CORONADO study. *Diabetes Obes. Metab.* **2021**, *23*, 1162–1172. [CrossRef]
44. Pérez-Belmonte, L.M.; Torres-Peña, J.D.; López-Carmona, M.D.; Ayala-Gutiérrez, M.M.; Fuentes-Jiménez, F.; Huerta, L.J.; Muñoz, J.A.; Rubio-Rivas, M.; Madrazo, M.; Garcia, M.G.; et al. Mortality and other adverse outcomes in patients with type 2 diabetes mellitus admitted for COVID-19 in association with glucose-lowering drugs: A nationwide cohort study. *BMC Med.* **2020**, *18*, 359. [CrossRef] [PubMed]
45. Rhee, S.Y.; Lee, J.; Nam, H.; Kyoung, D.-S.; Shin, D.W.; Kim, D.J. Effects of a DPP-4 Inhibitor and RAS Blockade on Clinical Outcomes of Patients with Diabetes and COVID-19. *Diabetes Metab. J.* **2021**, *45*, 251–259. [CrossRef]
46. Mirani, M.; Favacchio, G.; Carrone, F.; Betella, N.; Biamonte, E.; Morenghi, E.; Mazziotti, G.; Lania, A.G. Impact of Comorbidities and Glycemia at Admission and Dipeptidyl Peptidase 4 Inhibitors in Patients with Type 2 Diabetes with COVID-19: A Case Series from an Academic Hospital in Lombardy, Italy. *Diabetes Care* **2020**, *43*, 3042–3049. [CrossRef]
47. Hariyanto, T.I.; Kurniawan, A. Dipeptidyl peptidase 4 (DPP4) inhibitor and outcome from coronavirus disease 2019 (COVID-19) in diabetic patients: A systematic review, meta-analysis, and meta-regression. *J. Diabetes Metab. Disord.* **2021**, *20*, 543–550. [CrossRef]
48. Nyland, J.E.; Raja-Khan, N.T.; Bettermann, K.; Haouzi, P.A.; Leslie, D.L.; Kraschnewski, J.L.; Parent, L.J.; Grigson, P.S. Diabetes, Drug Treatment, and Mortality in COVID-19: A Multinational Retrospective Cohort Study. *Diabetes* **2021**, *70*, 2903–2916. [CrossRef]
49. Rakhmat, I.I.; Kusmala, Y.Y.; Handayani, D.R.; Juliastuti, H.; Nawangsih, E.N.; Wibowo, A.; Lim, M.A.; Pranata, R. Dipeptidyl peptidase-4 (DPP-4) inhibitor and mortality in coronavirus disease 2019 (COVID-19)—A systematic review, meta-analysis, and meta-regression. *Diabetes Metab. Syndr. Clin. Res. Rev.* **2021**, *15*, 777–782. [CrossRef] [PubMed]
50. Pal, R.; Banerjee, M.; Mukherjee, S.; Bhogal, R.S.; Kaur, A.; Bhadada, S.K. Dipeptidyl peptidase-4 inhibitor use and mortality in COVID-19 patients with diabetes mellitus: An updated systematic review and meta-analysis. *Ther. Adv. Endocrinol. Metab.* **2021**, *12*, 204201882199648. [CrossRef]
51. Bonora, B.M.; Avogaro, A.; Fadini, G.P. Disentangling conflicting evidence on DPP-4 inhibitors and outcomes of COVID-19: Narrative review and meta-analysis. *J. Endocrinol. Investig.* **2021**, *44*, 1379–1386. [CrossRef] [PubMed]
52. Panchapakesan, U.; Pegg, K.; Gross, S.; Komala, M.G.; Mudaliar, H.; Forbes, J.; Pollock, C.; Mather, A. Effects of SGLT2 Inhibition in Human Kidney Proximal Tubular Cells—Renoprotection in Diabetic Nephropathy? *PLoS ONE* **2013**, *8*, e54442. [CrossRef]
53. Bonnet, F.; Scheen, A.J. Effects of SGLT2 inhibitors on systemic and tissue low-grade inflammation: The potential contribution to diabetes complications and cardiovascular disease. *Diabetes Metab.* **2018**, *44*, 457–464. [CrossRef] [PubMed]
54. Vallon, V.; Gerasimova, M.; Rose, M.A.; Masuda, T.; Satriano, J.; Mayoux, E.; Koepsell, H.; Thomson, S.C.; Rieg, T.; Layton, A.T.; et al. SGLT2 inhibitor empagliflozin reduces renal growth and albuminuria in proportion to hyperglycemia and prevents glomerular hyperfiltration in diabetic Akita mice. *Am. J. Physiol. Physiol.* **2014**, *306*, F194–F204. [CrossRef] [PubMed]
55. La Grotta, R.; de Candia, P.; Olivieri, F.; Matacchione, G.; Giuliani, A.; Rippo, M.R.; Tagliabue, E.; Mancino, M.; Rispoli, F.; Ferroni, S.; et al. Anti-inflammatory effect of SGLT-2 inhibitors via uric acid and insulin. *Cell. Mol. Life Sci.* **2022**, *79*, 273. [CrossRef]
56. Garvey, W.T.; Van Gaal, L.; Leiter, L.A.; Vijapurkar, U.; List, J.; Cuddihy, R.; Ren, J.; Davies, M.J. Effects of canagliflozin versus glimepiride on adipokines and inflammatory biomarkers in type 2 diabetes. *Metabolism* **2018**, *85*, 32–37. [CrossRef] [PubMed]
57. Packer, M. Do sodium-glucose co-transporter-2 inhibitors prevent heart failure with a preserved ejection fraction by counterbalancing the effects of leptin? A novel hypothesis. *Diabetes Obes. Metab.* **2018**, *20*, 1361–1366. [CrossRef]
58. Gager, G.M.; von Lewinski, D.; Sourij, H.; Jilma, B.; Eyileten, C.; Filipiak, K.; Hülsmann, M.; Kubica, J.; Postula, M.; Siller-Matula, J.M. Effects of SGLT2 Inhibitors on Ion Homeostasis and Oxidative Stress associated Mechanisms in Heart Failure. *Biomed. Pharmacother.* **2021**, *143*, 112169. [CrossRef] [PubMed]
59. Xu, L.; Nagata, N.; Nagashimada, M.; Zhuge, F.; Ni, Y.; Chen, G.; Mayoux, E.; Kaneko, S.; Ota, T. SGLT2 Inhibition by Empagliflozin Promotes Fat Utilization and Browning and Attenuates Inflammation and Insulin Resistance by Polarizing M2 Macrophages in Diet-induced Obese Mice. *Ebiomedicine* **2017**, *20*, 137–149. [CrossRef]
60. Xu, L.; Ota, T. Emerging roles of SGLT2 inhibitors in obesity and insulin resistance: Focus on fat browning and macrophage polarization. *Adipocyte* **2017**, *7*, 121–128. [CrossRef]
61. Boye, K.S.; Erdemir, E.T.; Zimmerman, N.; Reddy, A.; Benneyworth, B.D.; Dabora, M.C.; Hankosky, E.R.; Bethel, M.A.; Clark, C.; Lensing, C.J.; et al. Risk Factors Associated with COVID-19 Hospitalization and Mortality: A Large Claims-Based Analysis Among People with Type 2 Diabetes Mellitus in the United States. *Diabetes Ther.* **2021**, *12*, 2223–2239. [CrossRef] [PubMed]
62. Kan, C.; Zhang, Y.; Han, F.; Xu, Q.; Ye, T.; Hou, N.; Sun, X. Mortality Risk of Antidiabetic Agents for Type 2 Diabetes with COVID-19: A Systematic Review and Meta-Analysis. *Front. Endocrinol.* **2021**, *12*, 708494. [CrossRef] [PubMed]
63. Kow, C.S.; Hasan, S.S. Mortality risk with preadmission metformin use in patients with COVID-19 and diabetes: A meta-analysis. *J. Med. Virol.* **2021**, *93*, 695–697. [CrossRef] [PubMed]

64. Li, J.; Wei, Q.; Li, W.X.; McCowen, K.C.; Xiong, W.; Liu, J.; Jiang, W.; Marin, T.; Thomas, R.L.; He, M.; et al. Metformin Use in Diabetes Prior to Hospitalization: Effects on Mortality in COVID-19. *Endocr. Pract.* **2020**, *26*, 1166–1172. [CrossRef] [PubMed]
65. Ghany, R.; Palacio, A.; Dawkins, E.; Chen, G.; McCarter, D.; Forbes, E.; Chung, B.; Tamariz, L. Metformin is associated with lower hospitalizations, mortality and severe coronavirus infection among elderly medicare minority patients in 8 states in USA. *Diabetes Metab. Syndr. Clin. Res. Rev.* **2021**, *15*, 513–518. [CrossRef]
66. Scheen, A. Metformin and COVID-19: From cellular mechanisms to reduced mortality. *Diabetes Metab.* **2020**, *46*, 423–426. [CrossRef] [PubMed]
67. Bramante, C.T.; Ingraham, N.E.; Murray, T.A.; Marmor, S.; Hovertsen, S.; Gronski, J.; McNeil, C.; Feng, R.; Guzman, G.; Abdelwahab, N.; et al. Metformin and risk of mortality in patients hospitalised with COVID-19: A retrospective cohort analysis. *Lancet Healthy Longev.* **2021**, *2*, e34–e41. [CrossRef]

biomedicines

Review

Modern Challenges in Type 2 Diabetes: Balancing New Medications with Multifactorial Care

Alfredo Caturano [1,2,†], Raffaele Galiero [1,†], Maria Rocco [1], Giuseppina Tagliaferri [1], Alessia Piacevole [1], Davide Nilo [1], Giovanni Di Lorenzo [1], Celestino Sardu [1], Erica Vetrano [1], Marcellino Monda [2], Raffaele Marfella [1], Luca Rinaldi [3,*] and Ferdinando Carlo Sasso [1,*]

1 Department of Advanced Medical and Surgical Sciences, University of Campania Luigi Vanvitelli, 80138 Naples, Italy; alfredo.caturano@unicampania.it (A.C.); raffaele.galiero@unicampania.it (R.G.); giuseppina.tagliaferri@gmail.com (G.T.); alessia.piacevole@studenti.unicampania.it (A.P.); nilodavide@gmail.com (D.N.); giuann86@gmail.com (G.D.L.); celestino.sardu@unicampania.it (C.S.); erica.vetrano@unicampania.it (E.V.); raffaele.marfella@unicampania.it (R.M.)

2 Department of Experimental Medicine, University of Campania Luigi Vanvitelli, 80138 Naples, Italy; marcellino.monda@unicampania.it

3 Department of Medicine and Health Sciences "Vincenzo Tiberio", Università degli Studi del Molise, 86100 Campobasso, Italy

* Correspondence: luca.rinaldi@unimol.it (L.R.); ferdinandocarlo.sasso@unicampania.it (F.C.S.)

† These authors contributed equally to this work.

Abstract: Type 2 diabetes mellitus (T2DM) is a prevalent chronic metabolic disorder characterized by insulin resistance and progressive beta cell dysfunction, presenting substantial global health and economic challenges. This review explores recent advancements in diabetes management, emphasizing novel pharmacological therapies and their physiological mechanisms. We highlight the transformative impact of Sodium-Glucose Cotransporter 2 inhibitor (SGLT2i) and Glucagon-Like Peptide 1 Receptor Agonist (GLP-1RA), which target specific physiological pathways to enhance glucose regulation and metabolic health. A key focus of this review is tirzepatide, a dual agonist of the glucose-dependent insulinotropic polypeptide (GIP) and GLP-1 receptors. Tirzepatide illustrates how integrating innovative mechanisms with established physiological pathways can significantly improve glycemic control and support weight management. Additionally, we explore emerging treatments such as glimins and glucokinase activators (GKAs), which offer novel strategies for enhancing insulin secretion and reducing glucose production. We also address future perspectives in diabetes management, including the potential of retatrutide as a triple receptor agonist and evolving guidelines advocating for a comprehensive, multifactorial approach to care. This approach integrates pharmacological advancements with essential lifestyle modifications—such as dietary changes, physical activity, and smoking cessation—to optimize patient outcomes. By focusing on the physiological mechanisms of these new therapies, this review underscores their role in enhancing T2DM management and highlights the importance of personalized care plans to address the complexities of the disease. This holistic perspective aims to improve patient quality of life and long-term health outcomes.

Keywords: insulin resistance; SGLT2i; GLP1-RA; tirzepatide; GIP receptor agonists; diabetes management; comprehensive care approach; pharmacological therapies

1. Introduction

Type 2 diabetes mellitus (T2DM) is a chronic metabolic disorder characterized by insulin resistance and progressive beta cell dysfunction, leading to hyperglycemia. It is the most common form of diabetes, accounting for about 90–95% of all diabetes cases worldwide. The prevalence of T2DM has been rising at an alarming rate, driven by factors such as population aging, urbanization, and lifestyle changes, which include unhealthy diets and physical inactivity. According to the International Diabetes Federation (IDF), as of 2021, approximately 537 million adults (20–79 years) were living with diabetes globally, a figure projected to increase to 643 million by 2030 and 783 million by 2045 [1]. This rapid rise in diabetes cases imposes a substantial burden on individuals and healthcare systems. Diabetes is associated with serious complications such as cardiovascular disease, kidney failure, neuropathy, and retinopathy, which can lead to disability and premature death [2]. In addition to the human cost, diabetes poses significant economic challenges. The global healthcare expenditure on diabetes was estimated to be USD 966 billion in 2021, an increase of 316% over the past 15 years [1]. These statistics underscore the urgent need for effective diabetes management strategies that not only control blood glucose levels but also address the broader health implications and socioeconomic impacts of the disease.

In recent years, the management of diabetes has seen significant advancements with the introduction of innovative medications that offer improved glycemic control and additional health benefits. Medications such as Sodium-Glucose Cotransporter 2 inhibitor (SGLT2i), Glucagon-Like Peptide 1 Receptor Agonist (GLP-1RA), and the novel dual glucose-dependent insulinotropic polypeptide (GIP) and GLP-1 receptor agonist, tirzepatide, have revolutionized diabetes treatment paradigms (Table 1). However, while these pharmacological advancements are crucial, managing diabetes effectively extends beyond medication alone [3–5]. Diabetes management, in fact, requires a multifactorial approach that addresses not only blood glucose control but also the myriad of factors that influence overall health and well-being. Pharmacological treatment alone is insufficient. Multifactorial care integrates dietary modifications, regular physical activity, weight management, and smoking cessation, which are critical in reducing the risk of complications such as cardiovascular disease, nephropathy, and neuropathy. Moreover, continuous patient education and psychological support play vital roles in enhancing treatment adherence, self-management, and quality of life. Personalized care plans must consider individual patient needs, preferences, comorbidities, and control of the entire spectrum of risk factors for cardiovascular disease, not only to prevent the onset of complications but also to enhance overall cardiovascular health. By addressing the diverse aspects of diabetes, a multifactorial care approach aims to achieve comprehensive disease management, improve patient outcomes, and reduce the burden of diabetes on individuals and healthcare systems [6].

Balancing the efficacy and benefits of new medications with comprehensive care strategies ensures that patients receive personalized, effective, and sustainable treatment, ultimately improving their overall quality of life and long-term health outcomes. This review explores the modern challenges in diabetes management by examining the latest therapeutic innovations and their integration into a holistic care framework.

Table 1. Overview of key diabetes medications.

Drug Class	Drug Name	Mechanism of Action	Indications	Drug Formulation	Restrictions	Adverse Effects
SGLT2i	Dapagliflozin Empagliflozin Canagliflozin Sotagliflozin Ertugliflozin	SGLT2 inhibition in the proximal tubule of the kidney, reducing glucose reabsorption	T2DM; T1DM in combination with insulin (Sotagliflozin, Dapagliflozin); HFrEF (Dapagliflozin, Empagliflozin)	Film-coated tablet	Hypersensitivity to the active substance or excipients; caution in patients at high risk of diabetic ketoacidosis	Urogenital infections, diabetic ketoacidosis, diarrhea, increased creatinine, polyuria, pollakiuria, volume depletion
GLP-1RA	Liraglutide Dulaglutide Semaglutide	GLP-1 receptor agonists: enhance insulin secretion, inhibit glucagon release, and slow gastric emptying	T2DM, obesity	Solution for injection in pre-filled pen; tablet (Semaglutide)	Hypersensitivity to the active substance or excipients	Nausea, vomiting, diarrhea, abdominal pain, decreased appetite, fatigue, local injection site reactions, cholelithiasis, gastroesophageal reflux disease, constipation, flatulence

Table 1. *Cont.*

Drug Class	Drug Name	Mechanism of Action	Indications	Drug Formulation	Restrictions	Adverse Effects
GLP-1/GIP Receptor Agonist	Tirzepatide	Dual agonist: acts as both a GIP analogue and GLP-1 receptor agonist, enhancing insulin secretion and reducing glucagon levels	T2DM, obesity	Solution for injection in pre-filled pen	Hypersensitivity to the active substance or excipients	Nausea, vomiting, diarrhea, abdominal pain, fatigue, gastroesophageal reflux disease, constipation, flatulence, local injection site reactions, hypersensitivity reactions
Glimins	Imeglimin	Dual mechanism: improves mitochondrial function, reducing insulin resistance, and enhances insulin secretion from pancreatic beta cells	T2DM	Oral tablets	Restricted in patients with severe renal impairment or hepatic impairment	Nausea, vomiting, diarrhea, possible risk of lactic acidosis
GK Activators	Dorzagliatin	GK activator increases glucose sensitivity and enhances insulin secretion by activating glucokinase	T2DM (investigational)	Oral tablets (investigational)	Limited data available; contraindications pending further clinical trials	Hypoglycemia, gastrointestinal disturbances, potential long-term cardiovascular risks (under investigation)
GLP-1/GIP/ Glucagon Receptor Agonist	Retatrutide	Triple agonist: activates GLP-1, GIP, and glucagon receptors, leading to improved glycemic control, enhanced insulin secretion, weight loss, and lipid control	Obesity, T2DM (under investigation)	Subcutaneous injection (investigational)	Contraindicated in patients with a history of medullary thyroid carcinoma or multiple endocrine neoplasia syndrome	Nausea, vomiting, diarrhea, possible risk of thyroid tumors (under investigation), pancreatitis, and gallbladder issues

2. Research Strategy

In preparing this review, a structured literature search was conducted to identify relevant studies on novel pharmacological therapies and their physiological mechanisms in Type 2 diabetes management. We utilized databases such as PubMed, MEDLINE, Web of Science, and Scopus, focusing on peer-reviewed articles published within the last 10 years. Our search strategy employed key terms such as "Type 2 Diabetes", "SGLT2 inhibitors", "GLP-1 receptor agonists", "tirzepatide", "Glimins", "Glucokinase activators", and "multifactorial care". The inclusion criteria emphasized studies that explored the impact of these novel therapies on glycemic control, weight management, and overall metabolic health. We also prioritized studies that discussed the transition from single drug therapies to their integration within multifactorial care approaches. We included clinical trials, systematic reviews, and meta-analyses to ensure a comprehensive review of the evidence. Exclusion criteria involved studies that lacked clinical relevance and statistical power and where not written in English.

3. SGLT2 Inhibitors: A New Era in Diabetes Treatment

Inhibitors of the SGLT2, also known as gliflozins, are a class of antihyperglycemic drugs crucial in treating T2DM [7]. Healthy kidneys filter approximately 160 g of glucose per day under euglycemic conditions; when blood glucose levels increase to the point that the filtered load exceeds this capacity, the excess is excreted in the urine [8]. Approximately 90% of filtered glucose reabsorption is mediated by SGLT2 located on the apical membrane of the S1 segment of the proximal tubule cells, while SGLT1 reabsorbs the remaining 2–3% under normoglycemic conditions [9]. SGLT2 symporters cotransport glucose and sodium in a 1:1 ratio: glucose is passively transported by GLUT1 and GLUT2 transporters at the anti-luminal site, while sodium is extruded by an active outward movement driven by

ATP [10]. This sodium gradient across the apical membrane is maintained by basolateral Na^+/K^+-adenosine triphosphatase, which pumps out Na+ and pumps in K^+, resulting in low intracellular Na^+ concentration, thereby facilitating glucose reabsorption through the luminal membrane [11]. The capacity for renal glucose reabsorption is enhanced in diabetes due to SGLT2 overexpression in the proximal tubule cells (PTCs), which can be explained by their persistent exposure to high glucose levels [12]. This upregulation has been linked to the activation of angiotensin II (Ang II) AT1 receptors [13] and the transcription factor hepatocyte nuclear factor HNF-1α [14], potentially responding to basolateral hyperglycemia sensed through GLUT2 [15]. Consequently, diabetic patients have a higher threshold for urinary glucose excretion and increased glucose reabsorption compared to healthy individuals [16,17]. Under hyperglycemic conditions, increased reabsorption via SGLT1 and SGLT2 leads to a reduction in sodium concentration in the downstream tubular lumen [18]. This concentration is falsely perceived as effective hypovolemia by the macula densa at the end of the Henle loop, triggering tubulo-glomerular feedback. High sodium levels in the cells inhibit the conversion of ATP into the potent vasoconstrictor adenosine, leading to a reduction in vasodilation of the afferent arteriole, while the intrarenal activation of the renin-angiotensin-aldosterone system constricts the efferent arteriole [19,20]. The resulting increase in intraglomerular pressure induces hyperfiltration and glomerular injury with urinary albumin excretion, potentially leading to kidney damage up to overt diabetic nephropathy. The PTCs also contain the sodium/hydrogen exchanger (NHE) 3, responsible for the reabsorption of approximately two thirds of the total sodium reabsorption. NHE3 exchangers colocalize with SGLT2 symporters, and their activities are linked via the accessory membrane-associated protein 17 [21]. As a result, the increased activity of one may increase the activity of the other, explaining why SGLT2 inhibitors can block NHE3 [22,23]. Indeed, SGLT2 inhibition is associated with a marked inhibition of NHE3, even in the absence of glucose. This result can explain the significant SGLT2 inhibitor-induced natriuresis [24] (Figure 1).

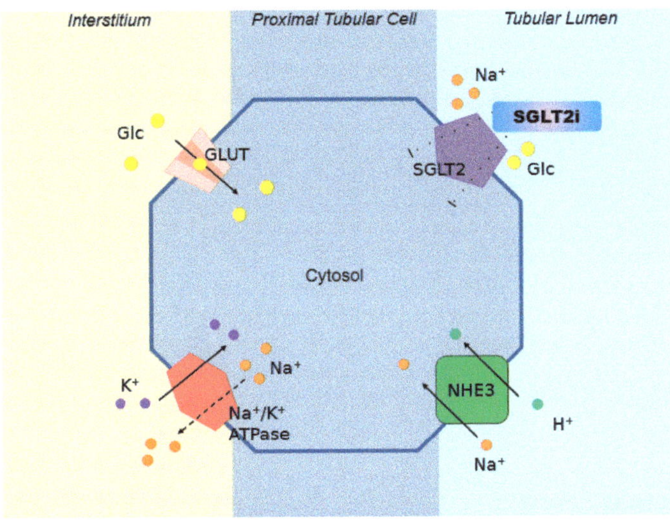

Figure 1. Schematic representation of the mechanism of action of Sodium-Glucose Cotransporter 2 inhibitors (SGLT2is). These inhibitors target SGLT2 transporters in the proximal renal tubules, reducing glucose reabsorption and enhancing glucose excretion in the urine, thereby lowering blood glucose levels. The figure also highlights the roles of the Na^+/H^+ exchanger (NHE3) and the Na+/K+ ATPase pump, which work together to maintain the sodium gradient essential for the operation of SGLT2. Additionally, the glucose transporter (GLUT) is depicted, illustrating its function in facilitating the reabsorption of glucose into the bloodstream.

The induction of glucosuria leads to improved glycemic control in all stages of T2DM, with a low risk of hypoglycemia, because they stop working when the filtered glucose load drops below 80 g per day without interfering with metabolic counter regulation [8]. This antihyperglycemic effect is influenced by specific factors. The efficacy of these drugs decreases progressively as blood glucose concentration falls [25]. Another factor is the glomerular filtration rate (GFR); the lower the GFR, the smaller the glycosuria [26]. These drugs influence glycosylated hemoglobin (HbA1c), which decreases by 7–10 mmol/mol (0.6–0.9%) compared with the placebo [27]. In addition to their main glycosuric effect, this class of drugs is characterized by pleiotropic actions, resulting in benefits for blood pressure, body weight, and particularly cardiovascular and renal protection. SGLT2 inhibition reduces body weight, initially through a diuretic effect, and subsequently by shifting substrate utilization from carbohydrates to lipids, thereby reducing body fat, including visceral and subcutaneous fat. The released free fatty acids are also used for the hepatic formation of ketone bodies, which provide additional energy substrates to improve the performance of cardiac myocytes and kidney epithelia [28,29]. By decreasing blood glucose and body weight, SGLT2 inhibitors cause a sustained improvement in beta cell function and insulin sensitivity [8]. The cardioprotective effect has been analyzed and demonstrated through several clinical trials. The clinical trials EMPAREG OUTCOME, CANVAS, and DECLARE-TIMI 58 showed that this class of drugs improved cardiovascular outcomes in T2DM patients with atherosclerotic cardiovascular disease: they significantly reduced the risk of myocardial infarction (MI), cardiovascular mortality, and all-cause mortality, although they had no effect on strokes [30–32]. In addition to the primary outcomes, several secondary or exploratory endpoints were collected from these trials, including those related to heart failure (HF) and kidney disease [33,34]. All gliflozins significantly reduced the risk of hospitalization for heart failure by approximately 30%, both in newly onset or recurrent HF [35]. Moreover, evidence was also reported by several real-world studies of SGLT2 is having proven to ameliorate cardiac remodeling [36–40]. Regarding kidney disease, several specific trials (CREDENCE, DAPA CKD, EMPA-KIDNEY) demonstrated the ability of SGLT2 inhibitors to reduce a composite of renal outcomes by 40–70%, including the doubling of serum creatinine, development of macroalbuminuria, need for dialysis and/or transplantation, and kidney death, regardless of antihyperglycemic action [41–43] (Table 2).

The primary and well-recognized side effects are euglycemic diabetic ketoacidosis (DKA) and urinary tract infections (UTIs) [44]. DKA has been reported with an incidence rate varying from 0.16 to 0.76 events per 1000 patient-years, with recognized risk factors including malnutrition, infectious diseases, weight loss, vomiting, or imbalanced insulin doses [45]. Moreover, to reduce the risk of euglycemic DKA, the American Diabetes Association Standards of Care recommends that SGLT2 inhibitors be discontinued 3–4 days before surgery [46]. The etiopathogenesis is still not fully clear; some authors suggest that SGLT inhibitors can stimulate lipolysis, liver ketogenesis, and a reduction in insulin production, leading to increased ketone storage and ketonemia. Additionally, it seems that the increased renal reabsorption of ketones and the hypovolemia induced by SGLT inhibitors could increase this risk [47]. The risk of UTIs is associated with glycosuria, which increases the likelihood of glucose accumulation in the urinary tract, thereby promoting bacterial growth [48]. Patients who receive proper training in regular personal hygiene can mitigate this risk. Furthermore, it appears that this effect does not extend to an increased risk of pyelonephritis or upper urinary tract infections [49]. Meta-analyses also confirmed an increased risk of genital infections, particularly among females and those with a prior history of such infections [50–52]. These genital infections, however, are typically non-severe and manageable without necessitating the discontinuation of treatment. An exception is Fournier's gangrene, a rare but life-threatening condition [53,54].

There have been concerns that SGLT2is may affect mineral metabolism, potentially reducing bone density and increasing the risk of fractures [55,56]. Specifically, decreases in total hip bone mineral density (BMD) have been observed after two years of treatment with Canagliflozin. The CANVAS trial indicated a significantly higher risk of fractures overall with Canagliflozin compared to the placebo, though no significant difference in low-trauma fractures was noted. In contrast, the EMPA-REG OUTCOME and DECLARE-TIMI 58 studies did not show a significant difference in fracture risk [30,33]. Additionally, SGLT2is may predispose patients to dehydration and an increased risk of falls, warranting caution when prescribing these drugs, particularly to the elderly population [33].

Table 2. Summary of key clinical trials for cardiovascular and renal outcomes with diabetes medications.

Trial	Drug	Primary Outcome	Secondary Outcomes	Ref.
EMPA-REG OUTCOME	Empagliflozin	Reduced risk of cardiovascular mortality and all-cause mortality in T2DM patients	Improved heart failure outcomes, no significant effect on stroke	[30]
CANVAS	Canagliflozin	Reduced risk of myocardial infarction (MI) and cardiovascular mortality	Increased risk of fractures, reduced hospitalization for heart failure	[31]
DECLARE-TIMI 58	Dapagliflozin	Reduced risk of major cardiovascular events (MACE)	Reduced risk of hospitalization for heart failure	[32]
CREDENCE	Canagliflozin	Reduced risk of renal outcomes (e.g., doubling of serum creatinine)	Reduced progression to dialysis and kidney-related death	[41]
DAPA-CKD	Dapagliflozin	Reduced risk of renal outcomes, regardless of diabetes status	Improved cardiovascular outcomes in CKD patients	[42]
EMPA-KIDNEY	Empagliflozin	Reduced risk of progression to end-stage renal disease (ESRD)	Improved cardiovascular outcomes in kidney disease patients	[43]
LEADER	Liraglutide	Reduced MACE, including cardiovascular death, non-fatal MI, and stroke	Reduced renal mortality and macroalbuminuria	[57]
SUSTAIN-6	Semaglutide	Lowered risk of MACE in T2DM patients	Notable reductions in HbA1c and body weight	[58]
REWIND	Dulaglutide	Reduced MACE in T2DM patients with lower baseline cardiovascular risk	Reduced macroalbuminuria	[59]
HARMONY	Albiglutide	Reduced MACE in T2DM patients	–	[60]
PIONEER-6	Oral Semaglutide	Reduced MACE	–	[61]
AMPLITUDE-O	Efpeglenatide	Cardiovascular benefits similar to other GLP-1Ras	–	[62]
SELECT	Semaglutide	Reduced incidence of cardiovascular death, MI, and stroke in obese patients without T2DM	–	[63]
FLOW	Semaglutide	Nephroprotective effects, including reduced progression to ESRD	–	[64]
STEP HFpEF	Semaglutide	Improved symptoms and physical limitations in HFpEF patients	Greater weight loss, better exercise function	[65]
SURMOUNT-1	Tirzepatide	Significant weight loss in obese patients	Improved cardiovascular outcomes	[66]
SUMMIT	Tirzepatide	Ongoing trial for cardiovascular outcomes in T2DM patients	–	[67]
SURPASS-CVOT	Tirzepatide	Reduced hazard ratio for cardiovascular outcomes in T2DM patients	–	[68]

4. GLP-1 Receptor Agonists: Enhancing Glycemic Control and Beyond

The Glucagon-Like Peptide 1 Receptor (GLP-1R) belongs to the class B family of G protein-coupled receptors [69]. It is primarily expressed in the beta cells of the pancreas but is also found in the neurons of both the central and peripheral nervous systems, as well as various cells in the gastrointestinal tract [70]. The natural ligand for GLP-1R is the incretin hormone GLP-1, which is secreted by enteroendocrine L cells in response to food intake [71]. The binding of GLP-1 to its receptor in the pancreas initiates a signaling cascade that involves cyclic adenosine monophosphate (cAMP) and protein kinase A (PKA), leading to a series of pleiotropic effects crucial for glucose regulation [72].

Endogenous GLP-1 is rapidly degraded by the enzyme dipeptidyl peptidase 4 (DPP-4) into a less active form, which is then quickly eliminated by the kidneys [73]. Due to its short half-life—generally around 1 or 2 min in humans—direct administration of GLP-1 as a drug is limited [74]. This challenge is addressed by GLP-1RAs, which mimic the actions of GLP-1 and have been shown to be a significant advancement in the treatment of T2DM, offering benefits beyond traditional glycemic control [75]. For instance, Coskun et al. developed a GLP-1RA with a half-life of approximately five days, improving patient compliance [76].

GLP-1RAs enhance glycemic control through several mechanisms. Upon binding to GLP-1R on pancreatic beta cells, these agonists activate adenylyl cyclase, converting ATP into cAMP. Elevated cAMP levels activate PKA and exchange protein directly activated by cAMP (EPAC), both of which are pivotal in insulin secretion and glucose regulation [77]. PKA phosphorylates various targets, including those that regulate calcium channels, facilitating calcium entry into the cell, essential for insulin release. Additionally, PKA inhibits ATP-sensitive potassium channels, causing cell membrane depolarization and further increasing calcium influx. This rise in intracellular calcium triggers the exocytosis of insulin granules, releasing insulin into the bloodstream [78] (Figure 2).

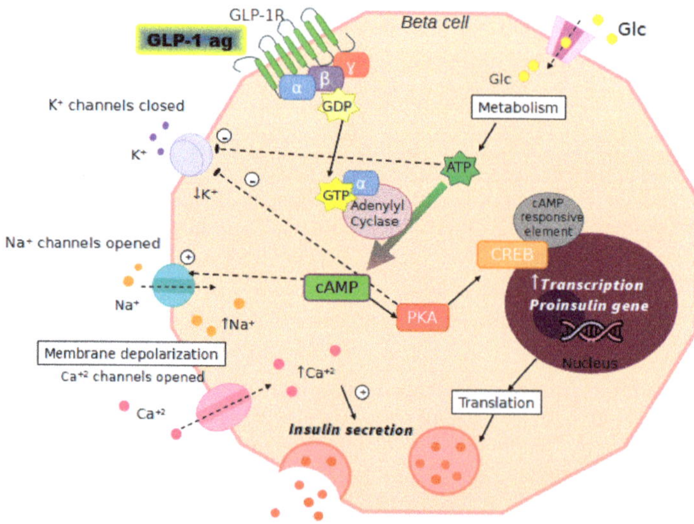

Figure 2. Schematic representation of the molecular pathways involved in the mechanism of action of GLP-1RAs. Upon binding to GLP-1 receptors on pancreatic beta cells, GLP-1RAs activate the cAMP/PKA signaling pathway, leading to the phosphorylation of the cAMP response element-binding protein (CREB). This activation enhances insulin gene transcription and secretion. Additionally, GLP-1RAs inhibit glucagon release from alpha cells via the same signaling pathway, thus decreasing hepatic glucose production. Colored dots represent key molecules in insulin secretion from beta cells. Orange dots (Na^+) and red dots (Ca^{2+}) illustrate ion flow crucial for membrane depolarization, which triggers the release of insulin (dark pink) and amylin (pink), aiding in glucose regulation.

GLP-1RAs also act on pancreatic alpha cells to inhibit glucagon secretion, thereby decreasing hepatic glucose production and contributing to lower blood glucose levels [79]. These agents slow gastric emptying, reducing the rate at which glucose is absorbed into the bloodstream postprandially. This effect is mediated through neural pathways and direct actions on the gastrointestinal tract [80]. Additionally, GLP-1RAs influence the CNS to promote satiety and reduce food intake by activating receptors in the hypothalamus and other brain regions involved in appetite regulation [81].

Beyond the primary cAMP-PKA pathway, GLP-1RAs engage several secondary signaling mechanisms. cAMP activates EPAC2, which activates proteins such as Ras-related protein 1 (RAP1) and phospholipase C (PLC). PLC generates inositol triphosphate (IP3) and diacylglycerol (DAG), promoting calcium release from intracellular stores. PKA also phosphorylates the IP3 receptor, enhancing IP3-mediated calcium release, and modulates enzymes involved in metabolic pathways, increasing glucose uptake and utilization. The combined increase in intracellular calcium and activation of downstream kinases facilitates the docking and fusion of insulin-containing vesicles with the plasma membrane, culminating in insulin release [82].

GLP-1RAs are highly effective in improving glycemic control in T2DM, lowering HbA1c levels by approximately 0.5 to 1.5% depending on the specific drug and patient characteristics [83–85]. Originally developed for diabetes management, GLP-1RAs like semaglutide and liraglutide have also been found to aid in weight reduction [86]. These drugs work by decreasing appetite and hunger while increasing feelings of fullness, which helps reduce overall calorie intake [87–89]. Beyond glycemic control, GLP-1RAs offer significant cardiovascular benefits. Several large-scale cardiovascular outcomes trials (CVOTs) have demonstrated the benefits of GLP-1 receptor agonists in both glycemic control and cardiovascular health. The LEADER trial showed that liraglutide significantly reduced major adverse cardiovascular events (MACEs), including cardiovascular death, non-fatal myocardial infarction, and non-fatal stroke, while also reducing renal mortality and macroalbuminuria in patients with T2DM [57]. Similarly, the SUSTAIN-6 trial confirmed that semaglutide lowered the risk of MACE alongside providing notable reductions in HbA1c and body weight [58]. The REWIND trial, which focused on dulaglutide, demonstrated a reduction in MACEs, even in a population with a lower baseline cardiovascular risk compared to other trials, and also showed reductions in macroalbuminuria. More recent trials continue to highlight the broad benefits of GLP-1Ras [59]. The HARMONY trial [60], with albiglutide, and the PIONEER-6 trial [61], with oral semaglutide, also demonstrated reductions in MACEs. The AMPLITUDE-O trial [62] evaluated efpeglenatide and confirmed similar cardiovascular benefits. The SELECT trial [63] and the ongoing SOUL trial [90] are further exploring the long-term cardiovascular effects of semaglutide, with a continued focus on MACE reduction. The SELECT trial showed that in patients with pre-existing cardiovascular disease and overweight or obesity but without diabetes, weekly subcutaneous semaglutide (2.4 mg) was superior to the placebo in reducing the incidence of death from cardiovascular causes, non-fatal myocardial infarction, or non-fatal stroke [61]. Additionally, newer trials such as the FLOW trial have shown the nephroprotective effects of semaglutide, including reductions in the progression to end-stage renal disease, renal mortality, and creatinine levels [64]. The STEP HFpEF trial demonstrated that in patients with heart failure with preserved ejection fraction and obesity, treatment with semaglutide (2.4 mg) led to larger reductions in symptoms and physical limitations, greater improvements in exercise function, and greater weight loss compared to the placebo [65].

Large-scale cardiovascular outcome trials (CVOTs) have consistently demonstrated that these medications can reduce major adverse cardiovascular events (MACEs), including non-fatal myocardial infarction, non-fatal stroke, and cardiovascular death [91–93] (Table 2). Additionally, they have been observed to lower systolic blood pressure modestly, improve lipid profiles by reducing LDL cholesterol and triglycerides, and potentially offer nephroprotective effects, such as reducing albuminuria and slowing the decline in the estimated glomerular filtration rate (eGFR).

GLP-1RAs are generally well tolerated and are not associated with an increased risk of hypoglycemia, thanks to the glucose-dependent activation of beta cells involving several intracellular mediators, such as EPAC and calcium [94]. However, they do carry some potential risks and side effects. The most common adverse effects are gastrointestinal symptoms, such as nausea, vomiting, and diarrhea, particularly when starting therapy [95]. There have been reports of acute pancreatitis associated with these medications, though a definitive causal relationship has not been established [96]. Additionally, an increased risk of gallbladder-related events, including cholelithiasis and cholecystitis, has been observed. Patients with pre-existing renal impairment should use these medications with caution, as there is potential for worsening renal function. In rodent studies, GLP-1RAs have been linked to an increased risk of thyroid C-cell tumors, but this risk has not been confirmed in humans. Injection site reactions can also occur with these drugs. Despite these potential side effects, the benefits of GLP-1RAs in managing T2DM often outweigh these risks, but healthcare providers should monitor patients closely [97].

5. New Frontiers: The Promise of Tirzepatide

Tirzepatide is a recently developed drug useful in the treatment of T2DM and for weight loss. This molecule shows 80% bioavailability, binds with albumin, undergoes liver metabolism through proteolytic cleavage and fatty acid β-oxidation, and is excreted via the urine and feces, with a half-life of 5 days, allowing for weekly subcutaneous administration. It is considered a long-acting molecule, with its extended activity primarily due to the addition of two residues to its lysine-linked side chain, enabling the drug to exert its benefits longer than its natural homologues [98].

Tirzepatide is a unimolecular dual agonist that acts as an analogue of gastric inhibitory polypeptide (GIP) and as a receptor agonist for glucagon-like peptide 1 (GLP-1). Its structure is a linear synthetic peptide comprising 39 amino acids, 19 of which are similar to those in GIP. Pharmaceutical modifications include a residue in the DPP4-binding site, making this molecule resistant to DPP4 enzymatic action; additionally, a fatty acid side chain linked to a lysine residue promotes a high-affinity bond with albumin, extending its half-life to up to 5 days. GIP and GLP-1 are involved in blood sugar homeostasis; they are secreted by cells in the human gut after food intake and regulate insulin release by pancreatic β-cells. GIP is produced by K cells in the duodenum after nutrient intake, with receptors mainly in the pancreas but also in the heart, adrenal cortex, and fat tissue. GLP-1 is secreted by L cells in the bowel, with receptors predominantly in pancreatic β-cells and, to a lesser degree, in the liver, kidneys, gastric mucosa, and brain (where it regulates satiety and food intake) [98,99] (Figure 3).

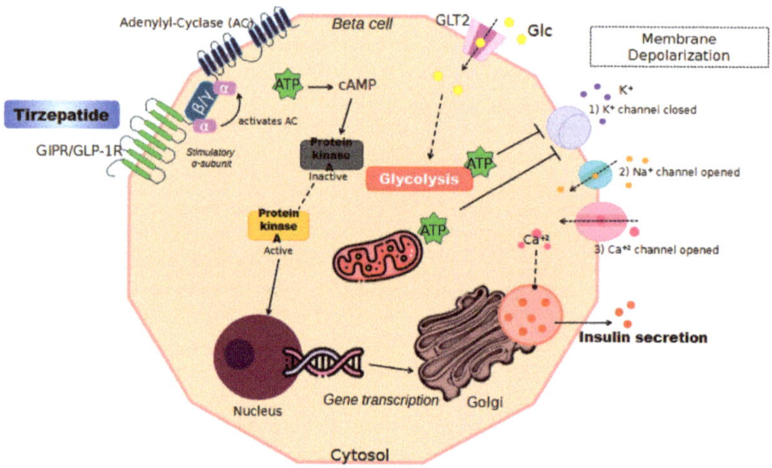

Figure 3. Schematic representation of the molecular pathways involved in the mechanism of action of tirzepatide in pancreatic beta cells. Tirzepatide acts on the GIPR/GLP-1R receptors, leading to the activation of adenylate cyclase (AC) and an increase in cyclic AMP (cAMP) levels. This activates protein kinase A (PKA), which in turn promotes glycolysis, ATP production, and gene transcription. The increase in ATP levels causes membrane depolarization by closing potassium (K^+) channels, and opening sodium (Na^+) and calcium (Ca^{2+}) channels, resulting in Ca^{2+} influx. The elevated intracellular Ca^{2+} concentration stimulates insulin (dark pink) and amylin (pink) secretion.

GIP is the most effective incretin-acting polypeptide in humans, and its action is triggered by increased blood glucose levels, linked with rising levels of cyclic adenosine monophosphate (cAMP). Hyperglycemia stimulates GIP secretion and promotes an increase in GIP receptor expression, enhancing cAMP levels to optimize incretin secretion. Tirzepatide's affinity for both receptors varies; it binds more strongly to GIP receptors compared to GLP-1 receptors. This dual pathway activation significantly increases insulin secretion. Additionally, studies show that this drug improves circulating levels of adiponectin, a protein known for its role in lipid and glucose metabolism [99].

Tirzepatide's health benefits extend to cardiovascular protection and renoprotection. Its cardiovascular benefits are closely related to enhanced GIP effectiveness, promoting anti-atherogenic effects on endothelial cells, activating endothelial nitric oxide synthase (eNOS) for vasodilation, and suppressing advanced glycation end-products (AGEs) and other atherogenic molecules. Furthermore, studies suggest potential therapeutic efficacy in lowering CD36 levels—a membrane protein involved in fatty acid import and acting as a scavenger receptor expressed mostly in abdominal fat, jejunal mucosa, and monocytes—and in suppressing inflammatory responses in macrophage foam cells [100]. A mechanism involving the reduction in triglyceride-rich lipoproteins has been postulated, contributing to the stabilization of atherosclerotic plaques. Three significant studies (SURMOUNT-1, SUMMIT [an ongoing multicentric trial], and SURPASS-CVOT) have evaluated improvements in cardiovascular outcomes in patients with obesity, heart failure, and T2DM, respectively, showing a significant reduction in the hazard ratio [66–68] (Table 2).

In terms of renoprotection, tirzepatide was evaluated in patients with cardiovascular disease, showing a significant reduction in kidney-worsening events, such as renal-related mortality, progression of kidney function decline to end-stage renal disease (ESRD), and new onset of macroalbuminuria, compared with treatment with insulin glargine [68]. Additionally, it is known that increased cAMP levels trigger PKA activation and inhibit oxidative stress-related kidney damage, preventing the progression of diabetic nephropathy [101]. Tirzepatide also appears to stimulate renin-secreting cells in the juxtaglomerular apparatus, enhancing natriuresis and nitric oxide levels (via decreased angiotensin II levels), thereby preventing chronic kidney injury [102].

For these reasons, tirzepatide is a promising therapeutic option for patients with T2DM and those needing significant weight loss, regardless of T2DM status. Comparative studies between standard and innovative T2DM treatments underscore the superiority of this new molecule over both placebo and active comparators (degludec [SURPASS-3], glargine [SURPASS-4], and semaglutide [SURPASS-2]), with significant reductions in HbA1c levels after 40 and 52 weeks, particularly at doses up to 15 mg/week. The same studies, following the same dosage regimen, also reported significant body weight loss [101,103,104].

Tirzepatide is generally well tolerated, with the most adverse effects being gastrointestinal symptoms, such as nausea, vomiting, and diarrhea, occurring within the first month of treatment. More serious adverse events, such as pancreatitis (3%) and cell proliferation in thyroid and pancreatic tissues, which could lead to neoplasms, are rarer [105–107]. The link between tirzepatide administration and endocrine cancers is currently unclear.

In conclusion, this new drug has made significant advancements in therapeutic strategies for T2DM and weight loss. Its potential to treat other metabolic conditions, such as obstructive sleep apnea syndrome (OSAS) and steatohepatitis, highlights its versatility, as demonstrated by recent studies [105,108].

6. Future Perspectives in Diabetes Management

The landscape of diabetes management is rapidly evolving, with promising advancements in therapies and technologies, updated guidelines, and new standards of care.

6.1. Glimins

Among the emerging therapies, glimins represent a new class of oral glucose-lowering drugs with mechanisms distinct from traditional medications. These molecules primarily act within the mitochondria, targeting the mitochondrial respiratory chain complex to reduce the production of reactive oxygen species (ROS) and prevent mitochondrial permeability transition pore opening, thereby protecting cells from death. They achieve this through partial inhibition of Complex I and correction of deficient Complex III activity [109].

Glimins increase glucose-stimulated insulin secretion (GSIS), a defective process in diabetic patients, involving an NAD^+–cyclic ADP-ribose–Ca^{2+} signaling pathway. ATP and NAD^+ production is increased through the "salvage pathway", with an induction of nicotinamide phosphoribosyltransferase (NAMPT) and an increase in the glucose-induced ATP pool [109] (Figure 4).

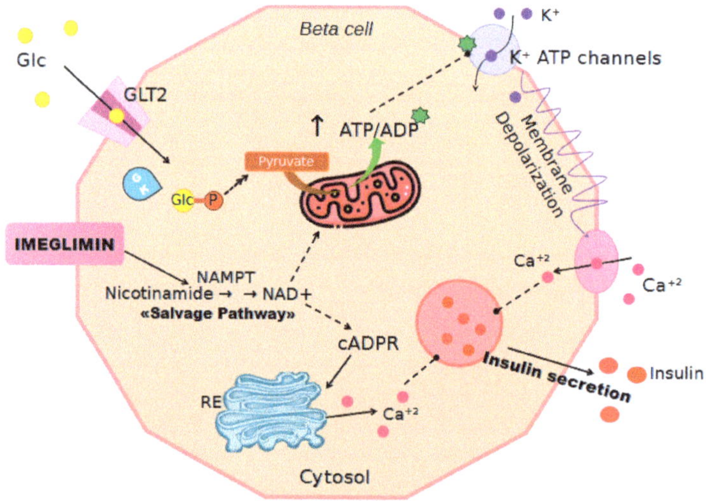

Figure 4. Schematic representation of the mechanism of action of Imeglimin in pancreatic β-cells. Imeglimin acts by inhibiting mitochondrial pyruvate uptake, leading to a reduction in the ATP/ADP ratio. This decrease triggers downstream effects, including the activation of nicotinamide phosphoribosyltransferase (NAMPT), which enhances the salvage pathway, converting nicotinamide into nicotinamide mononucleotide (NMN) and subsequently into nicotinamide adenine dinucleotide (NAD^+) through the action of nicotinamide mononucleotide adenylyltransferase (NMNAT). NAD^+ serves as a substrate for CD38, which catalyzes the formation of cyclic ADP-ribose (cADPR) and nicotinic acid adenine dinucleotide phosphate (NAADP). These molecules facilitate calcium (Ca^{2+}) release from the endoplasmic reticulum (ER) and lysosomes through the ryanodine receptors (RyR) and two-pore channels (TPCs), respectively. The resulting increase in intracellular Ca^{2+} concentration contributes to membrane depolarization and promotes insulin secretion.

Additionally, glimins preserve β-cell mass and increase the number of insulin granules [110], while simultaneously reducing insulin resistance in insulin-sensitive tissues [111]. Glimins also exhibit a protective effect on human endothelial cells by modulating mitochondrial permeability in hyperglycemia-induced oxidative stress environments, without inhibiting mitochondrial respiration, suggesting a potential role in preventing diabetic macrovascular and microvascular complications [112].

Imeglimin, the first molecule of this new class of oral antidiabetic drugs, has shown substantial improvement in glycemic control, safety, and tolerability, even as a monotherapy [113].

6.2. GK Activators

Another promising therapy involves glucokinase activators (GKAs), which address the increased hepatic glucose production fundamental to the pathophysiology of T2DM. Glucokinase (GK) is the key enzyme for gluconeogenesis in hepatocytes, converting glucose into glucose-6-phosphate [114]. GK is also expressed in various other tissues, particularly in the pancreas, where it functions as a glucose sensor in beta cells, regulating insulin secretion [115]. Although there is no established correlation between pancreatic GK function and T2DM [116], GK remains inactive in the liver during fasting, forming a complex with glucokinase regulatory protein (GKRP) in the nucleus. Postprandial increases in glucose levels dissociate this complex, allowing GK to become active in the cytoplasm [117].

While mutations in the GCK gene cause maturity-onset diabetes of the young type 2 (MODY2), no GCK mutations have been clearly identified in the etiology of typical T2DM. However, Haeusler et al. discovered that in diabetic patients with high HbA1c levels (>7.0), GK expression was suppressed by more than 60%, likely due to transcriptional or post-translational effects on the enzyme [118].

In this context, GKAs are a promising class of antidiabetic drugs that regulate glycemia and enhance beta cell function in T2DM patients [119]. Two recent molecules have shown great potential in terms of efficacy and safety. Dorzagliatin, also known as HMS-5552, is a dual-acting GKA that has completed two phase III trials. It targets both the liver and pancreas, working as an allosteric activator to stabilize a high-affinity conformation of the enzyme, thus increasing glucose phosphorylation activity. In the liver, Dorzagliatin activates GK, leading to the dissociation of the GK-GKRP complex. In the pancreas, the drug-activated GK inhibits insulin resistance and increases insulin sensitivity [120] (Figure 5).

TTP399, or Cadisegliatin, is a liver-specific GKA that has completed a phase II trial. Although its structural interaction with GK is still partially unclear, preclinical studies have shown that it binds to the allosteric site of GK, expanding its kinase binding cavity and increasing its catalytic activity without interfering with GK-GKRP interaction [121].

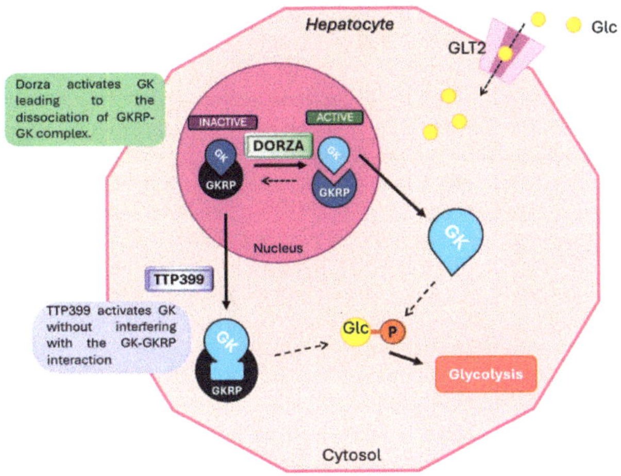

Figure 5. Schematic representation of the mechanism of action of glucokinase (GK) activators. The figure illustrates two distinct mechanisms by which GK activity is modulated in hepatocytes. Dorzagliatin (DORZA) promotes the dissociation of the glucokinase regulatory protein (GKRP)-GK complex within the nucleus, resulting in the release of active GK into the cytosol. This active GK facilitates the phosphorylation of glucose (Glc) to glucose-6-phosphate (Glc-6-P), a key step in glycolysis. In contrast, TTP399 activates GK directly without disrupting the GK-GKRP complex, enhancing the enzyme's catalytic activity. Both mechanisms increase the conversion of glucose to glucose-6-phosphate, thus promoting glycolysis and enhancing glucose utilization. The figure also shows glucose entering the cell through GLUT2 transporters, emphasizing the coordinated regulation of glucose metabolism.

6.3. Retatrutide

Finally, among new drugs for diabetes treatment, retatrutide stands out as a GIP, GLP-1, and glucagon receptor triple agonist. It is a single peptide that interacts with these three different receptors. Compared to the already known tirzepatide (a GLP-1/GIP receptor agonist), retatrutide also acts on the glucagon receptor, increasing energy expenditure in mice [122].

It has been demonstrated that glucagon decreases hunger through the activation of the central nervous system via the vagus nerve. Weight loss induced by glucagon is due to increased energy expenditure, thermogenesis, and fatty acid oxidation, suggesting that this hormone impacts body weight through both feeding-dependent and -independent mechanisms [123]. In 2023, Sanyal et al. studied the effect of a 24-week treatment with retatrutide on liver fat reduction, finding that at least 80% of participants achieved >70% relative reduction in liver fat, and more than 85% achieved resolution of steatosis, defined as <5% total liver fat content. This outcome is superior to that seen with SGLT2is, dulaglutide, tirzepatide, and even semaglutide [124,125].

7. Evolving Guidelines and Standards of Care

In many studies, a decline in diabetes complications has been reported; various factors may be responsible for this change, but one of the most significant reasons is the improved management of risk factors [126]. According to ESC guidelines, it is recommended to screen patients with diabetes for the presence of severe target organ damage (TOD) [127,128] and for symptoms suggestive of atherosclerotic cardiovascular disease (ASCVD) [129,130]. In patients with T2DM without symptomatic ASCVD or severe TOD, it is recommended to estimate cardiovascular (CV) risk [131], considering various factors such as clinical and family history, laboratory tests, and other examinations. The 2023 ESC guidelines introduced the SCORE2-Diabetes tool to calculate the 10-year CV risk in diabetic patients, considering multiple risk factors, including the patient's country of origin. This tool classifies 10-year CV risk into four categories: low risk (<5%), moderate risk (5–10%), high risk (10–20%), and very high risk (>20%) [131].

Once this parameter is calculated, efforts should focus on reducing CV risk through various means. Primarily, improving the patient's lifestyle [2,132] through a balanced low-carb diet and regular exercise can induce weight loss, significantly reducing HbA1c and blood pressure [133]. Smoking cessation is also crucial, as it is associated with a 36% reduction in mortality in cardiovascular disease patients [134–137]. Kim et al. showed that smoking cessation and initiation of exercise after diabetes diagnosis are associated with a 46% reduced risk of cardiovascular disease [136]. Recent research highlights that smoking cessation, rather than reduction, is associated with reduced cardiovascular disease risk [137]. If lifestyle changes are not enough to improve glycemia and other risk factors (such as high blood pressure, lipid abnormalities, and obesity), medication should be used to reduce CV risk [138].

Defining glycemic targets in diabetes management is complex. Tight glycemic control (HbA1c < 7%) decreases the risk of microvascular complications, but there is a U-shaped relationship between HbA1c levels and clinical outcomes, with increased mortality associated with excessively tight control. Hence, lower HbA1c is not always better [139–150]. Individualized glycemic targets should consider life expectancy, comorbidities, and diabetes duration. For patients with a short life expectancy, softer glycemic targets (HbA1c < 8.5%) may be appropriate, whereas tighter targets (HbA1c < 7%) are suitable for those with longer life expectancy, prioritizing agents with proven cardiovascular benefits and low hypoglycemic risk. It is crucial to avoid hypoglycemia, as it is associated with an increased risk of vascular events [151,152]. Figure 6 illustrates the FDA approval timeline for medications used in the treatment of type 2 diabetes. This timeline highlights key milestones in the evolution of therapeutic options, reflecting the continuous advancements in diabetes management [153]. Figure 7 complements this by presenting the chemical structures of these key medications, visually depicting the molecular innovations that underlie their therapeutic effects. As new drugs are developed and approved, they shape clinical guidelines and standards of care, offering healthcare professionals an expanding range of tools to better manage this chronic condition.

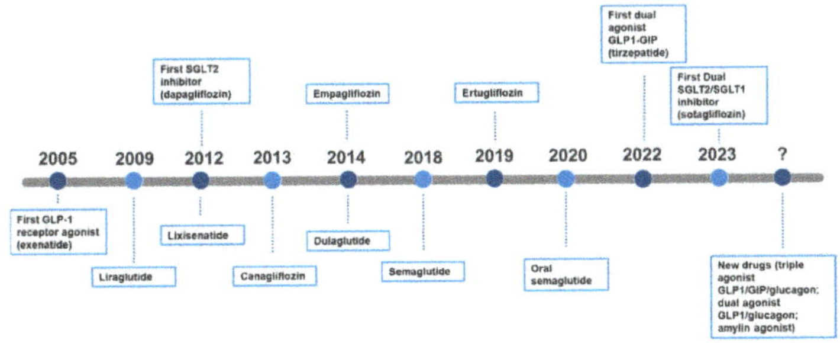

Figure 6. Timeline of FDA-approved drugs for the treatment of type 2 diabetes.

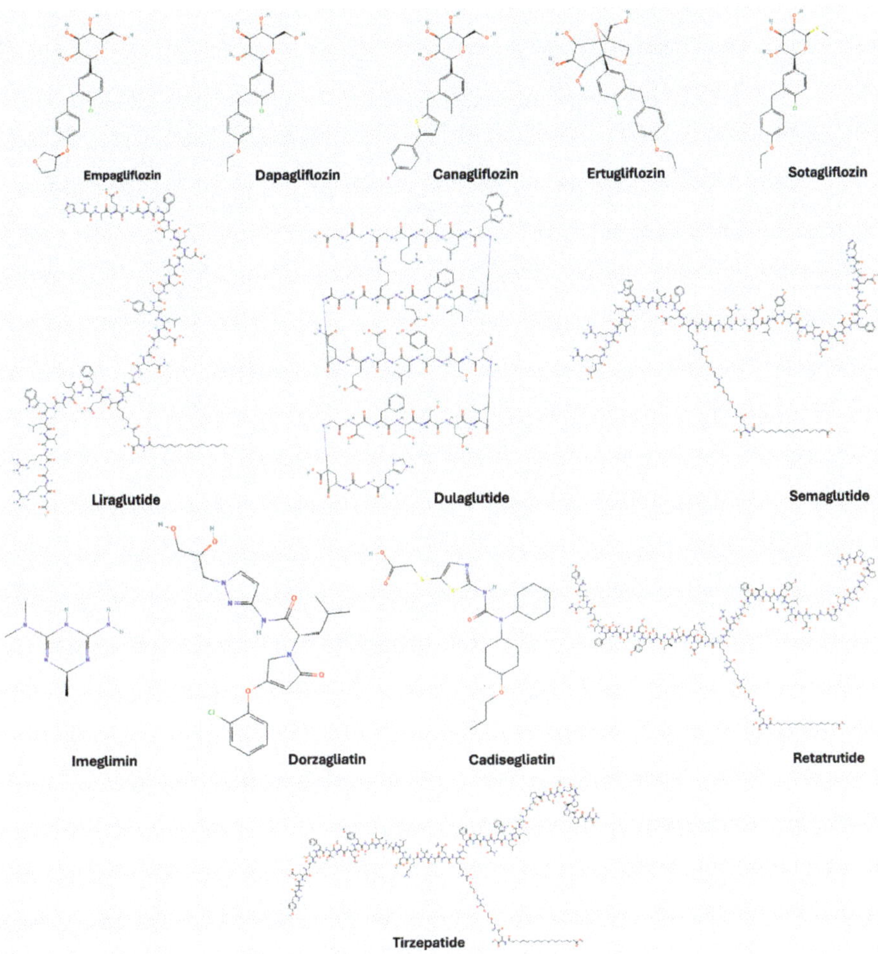

Figure 7. Main chemical structures of key diabetes medications [154–166].

8. Balancing Innovation with Comprehensive Care

8.1. The Importance of Personalized Treatment Plans

In recent decades, scientific evidence, albeit limited, has suggested a shift from a glucocentric therapeutic vision to a multifactorial intervention approach in patients with

T2DM [167]. These findings have shown that in addition to glycemic control, targeting other modifiable cardiovascular risk factors, such as blood pressure, cholesterol, lifestyle, and obesity, can prevent micro- and macrovascular complications [167–169].

Some hypotheses have been proposed to explain the pathophysiological mechanisms underlying the protective effects observed in subjects undergoing multifactorial interventional treatment. According to some studies, an additive protective effect is due to multifactorial intervention on cardiovascular and endothelial inflammatory damage. The effects of blood pressure-lowering treatment with RAS inhibition, the "legacy effect" on AGEs due to glucose-lowering therapy, the impact of statins on LDL and inflammatory cytokines, and the inhibition of platelet adhesion may reduce leukocyte activation and thus atherosclerosis [170,171].

The most up-to-date guidelines have highlighted the fundamental role of "tailored" therapy and the control of cardiovascular risk factors in preventing the development and progression of diabetic disease and its complications [172–174].

8.2. Role in Multifactorial Diabetes Care of New Drug Treatments

For optimal glycemic control, achieving an HbA1c of less than 7% is recommended to reduce the risk of microvascular complications while avoiding hypoglycemic events. For multifactorial intervention, guidelines suggest achieving a target systolic blood pressure of 130 mmHg and LDL-C levels of less than 100 mg/dL for individuals at moderate cardiovascular risk, less than 70 mg/dL for those at high risk, and less than 55 mg/dL for those at very high risk [172].

Currently, no single drug can address and control all cardiovascular risk factors [175]. Metformin, in the absence of contraindications, remains the first-line treatment at the time of diabetes diagnosis [176]. However, recent scientific evidence has shown that new drugs for the treatment of T2DM (GLP1-RAs and SGLT2 inhibitors) may have pleiotropic effects. Besides helping achieve glycemic targets, these drugs can prevent the progression of major cardiovascular risk factors, such as reducing blood pressure, having diuretic effects, lowering body mass index, and reducing heart filling pressures and volumes [125,176,177]. Therefore, the history and clinical characteristics of each patient should guide the best choice of tailored therapy, especially in addition to metformin [174,178–180]. Results from randomized placebo-controlled trials have demonstrated that in subjects with T2DM and atherosclerotic cardiovascular disease, both SGLT2 inhibitors and GLP1-RAs showed proven cardiovascular benefits, including reduced hospitalization and mortality risk. Specifically, in subjects with diabetes and heart failure with reduced ejection fraction, SGLT2 inhibitors are recommended (class I, level A evidence), with specific recommendations for empagliflozin or dapagliflozin in subjects with left ventricular ejection fraction over 40% [6]. Moreover, recent evidence has shown that chronic kidney disease (CKD) is strongly associated with the risk of developing heart failure and major adverse cardiovascular events (MACEs), especially in individuals with T2DM [180,181]. In such conditions, both SGLT2 inhibitors and GLP1-RAs are useful in reducing cardiovascular risk. For subjects with stage IV or V CKD (eGFR < 30 mL/min per 1.73 m^2), GLP1-RAs are primarily recommended [174].

8.3. Addressing Patient Adherence and Lifestyle Modifications

The treatment of T2DM should always begin with lifestyle modifications. The challenge for clinicians often lies in encouraging patients to make lifestyle changes, considering their physical, social, and economic characteristics. Here again, the concept of tailored therapy is crucial in guiding clinicians toward the best choice [6].

In at least 90% of cases, T2DM is associated with overweight or obesity, which in turn often results from an unbalanced lifestyle rich in refined carbohydrates and marked by physical inactivity. Several studies have shown that a lifestyle characterized by moderate weekly physical exercise and a healthy diet can significantly reduce the risk of metabolic diseases and cardiovascular complications (RR: 0.84; 95% CI: 0.77, 0.91) [182,183]. According to guidelines, a Mediterranean diet and 180 min per week of moderate physical activity form the basis of a healthy lifestyle. However, other dietary approaches have also shown promise in reducing cardiovascular risk, though further evidence is needed to confirm these benefits [184–189].

8.4. Coordinating Care among Healthcare Providers

Clinicians, whether working alone or as part of a multidisciplinary team, play a central role in applying the most appropriate therapeutic strategies to address each cardiovascular risk factor. As noted earlier, some trials have demonstrated how multifactorial intervention can reduce the risk of major cardiovascular events (MACEs) and mortality [190].

The Steno-2 study was the first to address this issue. In this trial, subjects with microalbuminuria were randomly assigned to either intensive treatment or conventional therapy. The intensive treatment group aimed for stricter multifactorial treatment targets and, at the end of the study, showed a significant reduction in their risk of nephropathy (HR, 0.39; 95% CI, 0.17 to 0.87), retinopathy (HR, 0.42; 95% CI, 0.21 to 0.86), autonomic neuropathy (HR, 0.37; 95% CI, 0.18 to 0.79), stroke, and mortality (HR, 0.54; 95% CI, 0.32 to 0.89) [191,192]. In another trial, the Japan Diabetes Outcome Intervention Trial (J-DOIT3), individuals with T2DM in the intensive therapy group experienced a significant reduction in their risk of cerebrovascular events (HR, 0.42; 95% CI, 0.24 to 0.74), nephropathic events (HR, 0.68; 95% CI, 0.56 to 0.82), and retinopathic events (HR, 0.86; 95% CI, 0.74 to 1.00) [193]. More recently, the NID-2 study, a trial conducted on subjects with T2DM and high cardiovascular risk, demonstrated the efficacy of multifactorial treatment [170]. The intensive arm showed a 53% lower risk of MACEs (adjusted HR 0.47, 95% CI 0.30–0.74, $p = 0.001$) and a reduced all-cause death risk (adjusted HR 0.53, 95% CI 0.29–0.93, $p = 0.027$). Furthermore, a subsequent post hoc analysis revealed that individuals with a higher number of risk factors at target had better cardiovascular prognoses [155].

9. Limitations and Perspectives

This review provides a comprehensive overview of recent advancements in Type 2 diabetes management, focusing on novel pharmacological therapies. However, several limitations should be acknowledged for proper data interpretation. First, the scope of the literature covered was limited by the availability and selection of published studies, potentially introducing publication bias and restricting the inclusion of emerging but less widely reported treatments. Additionally, the heterogeneity of the included studies—varying in methodology, population, and outcome measures—may challenge the generalizability of the findings. Future research should aim to address these limitations through more systematic, interdisciplinary approaches. Moving forward, the integration of novel treatments into multifactorial care should consider individual patient variability and long-term outcomes [194]. Further exploration of emerging therapies, such as retatrutide, and the development of personalized treatment plans will be critical to advancing Type 2 diabetes care [195]. Incorporating a broader range of studies, including those that evaluate the combination of pharmacological interventions with lifestyle modifications, will be essential to optimizing patient outcomes and addressing the complexities of Type 2 diabetes management [196].

10. Conclusions

The management of T2DM has evolved significantly, with new therapeutic agents and a broader focus on multiple cardiovascular risk factors. This shift from a glucocentric approach has been crucial in reducing both microvascular and macrovascular complications in diabetic patients [197,198].

Medications like GLP-1 receptor agonists, SGLT2 inhibitors, tirzepatide, and glimins not only enhance glycemic control but also provide cardiovascular and renal benefits, underscoring the importance of personalized treatment plans based on individual patient characteristics [197]. Lifestyle modifications, including diet and exercise, remain foundational in T2DM management, highlighting the role of healthcare providers in coordinating comprehensive care [198]. Multidisciplinary approaches, validated in trials such as Steno-2, J-DOIT3, and NID-2, have been effective in reducing major adverse cardiovascular events (MACEs) and improving patient outcomes. These advancements emphasize the need for a holistic treatment strategy that combines emerging therapies with lifestyle interventions and thorough monitoring of cardiovascular and metabolic health [199]. As diabetes management continues to advance, a focus on individualized care and comprehensive risk factor management will be key to optimizing patient outcomes.

Author Contributions: Conceptualization, A.C. and R.G.; writing—original draft preparation, A.C., R.G., M.R., G.T., A.P., D.N., and G.D.L.; writing—review and editing, A.C., R.G., E.V., C.S., L.R., M.M., R.M., and F.C.S.; supervision R.M., M.M., L.R., and F.C.S. All authors have read and agreed to the published version of the manuscript.

Funding: This research received no external funding.

Institutional Review Board Statement: The authors reviewed the literature data and reported the results coming from studies approved by local ethics committees.

Informed Consent Statement: Not applicable.

Data Availability Statement: No dataset was generated for the publication of this article.

Conflicts of Interest: The authors declare no conflicts of interest.

References

1. Diabetes Atlas. Available online: https://diabetesatlas.org/ (accessed on 17 June 2024).
2. Caturano, A.; D'Angelo, M.; Mormone, A.; Russo, V.; Mollica, M.P.; Salvatore, T.; Galiero, R.; Rinaldi, L.; Vetrano, E.; Marfella, R.; et al. Oxidative Stress in Type 2 Diabetes: Impacts from Pathogenesis to Lifestyle Modifications. *Curr. Issues Mol. Biol.* **2023**, *45*, 6651–6666. [CrossRef] [PubMed]
3. Liu, Y.; Nie, D.; Lou, X. The Cardiovascular Benefits of Glucagon-Like Peptide-1 Receptor Agonists as Novel Diabetes Drugs Are Mediated via the Suppression of miR-203a-3p and miR-429 Expression. *DNA Cell Biol.* **2024**, *43*, 387–394. [CrossRef]
4. Nevola, R.; Alfano, M.; Pafundi, P.C.; Brin, C.; Gragnano, F.; Calabrò, P.; Adinolfi, L.E.; Rinaldi, L.; Sasso, F.C.; Caturano, A. Cardiorenal Impact of SGLT-2 Inhibitors: A Conceptual Revolution in The Management of Type 2 Diabetes, Heart Failure and Chronic Kidney Disease. *Rev. Cardiovasc. Med.* **2022**, *23*, 106. [CrossRef] [PubMed]
5. Caturano, A. Cardiovascular and Metabolic Disease: New Treatments and Future Directions 2.0. *Biomedicines.* **2024**, *12*, 1356. [CrossRef]
6. Marx, N.; Federici, M.; Schütt, K.; Müller-Wieland, D.; Ajjan, R.A.; Antunes, M.J.; Christodorescu, R.M.; Crawford, C.; Di Angelantonio, E.; Eliasson, B.; et al. 2023 ESC Guidelines for the management of cardiovascular disease in patients with diabetes. *Eur Heart J.* **2023**, *44*, 4043–4140. [CrossRef]
7. Vallon, V.; Verma, S. Effects of SGLT2 Inhibitors on Kidney and Cardiovascular Function. *Annu. Rev. Physiol.* **2021**, *83*, 503–528. [CrossRef] [PubMed]
8. Vallon, V.; Thomson, S.C. Targeting renal glucose reabsorption to treat hyperglycaemia: The pleiotropic effects of SGLT2 inhibition. *Diabetologia.* **2017**, *60*, 215–225. [CrossRef]
9. Salvatore, T.; Carbonara, O.; Cozzolino, D.; Torella, R.; Nasti, R.; Lascar, N.; Sasso, F.C. Kidney in diabetes: From organ damage target to therapeutic target. *Curr. Drug Metab.* **2011**, *12*, 658. [CrossRef]
10. Wright, E.M.; Loo, D.D.; Hirayama, B.A. Biology of human sodium glucose transporters. *Physiol. Rev.* **2011**, *91*, 733–794. [CrossRef]
11. Ghezzi, C.; Loo, D.D.F.; Wright, E.M. Physiology of renal glucose handling via SGLT1, SGLT2 and GLUT2. *Diabetology.* **2018**, *61*, 2087–2097. [CrossRef]
12. Vallon, V. The proximal tubule in the pathophysiology of the diabetic kidney. *Am. J. Physiol. Integr. Comp. Physiol.* **2011**, *300*, R1009–R1022. [CrossRef]
13. Osorio, H.; Bautista, R.; Rios, A.; Franco, M.; Santamaria, J.; Escalante, B. Sodium-glucose cotransporter inhibition prevents oxidative stress in the kidney of diabetic rats. *Oxid. Med. Cell Longev.* **2012**, *2012*, 542042. [CrossRef] [PubMed]
14. Freitas, H.S.; Anhê, G.F.; Melo, K.F.; Okamoto, M.M.; Oliveira-Souza, M.; Bordin, S.; Machado, U.F. Na^+-glucose transporter-2 messenger ribonucleic acid expression in kidney of diabetic rats correlates with glycemic levels: Involvement of hepatocyte nuclear factor-1alpha expression and activity. *Endocrinology.* **2008**, *149*, 717–724. [CrossRef]
15. Umino, H.; Hasegawa, K.; Minakuchi, H.; Muraoka, H.; Kawaguchi, T.; Kanda, T.; Tokuyama, H.; Wakino, S.; Itoh, H. High Basolateral Glucose Increases Sodium-Glucose Cotransporter 2 and Reduces Sirtuin-1 in Renal Tubules through Glucose Transporter-2 Detection. *Sci. Rep.* **2018**, *8*, 6791. [CrossRef] [PubMed]
16. Rabizadeh, S.; Nakhjavani, M.; Esteghamati, A. Cardiovascular and Renal Benefits of SGLT2 Inhibitors: A Narrative Review. *Int. J. Endocrinol. Metab.* **2019**, *17*, e84353. [CrossRef] [PubMed]

17. Vlotides, G.; Mertens, P.R. Sodium-glucose cotransport inhibitors: Mechanisms, metabolic effects and implications for the treatment of diabetic patients with chronic kidney disease. *Nephrol. Dial. Transplant.* **2015**, *30*, 1272–1276. [CrossRef] [PubMed]
18. Vallon, V.; Rose, M.; Gerasimova, M.; Satriano, J.; Platt, K.A.; Koepsell, H.; Cunard, R.; Sharma, K.; Thomson, S.C.; Rieg, T. Knockout of Na-glucose transporter SGLT2 attenuates hyperglycemia and glomerular hyperfiltration but not kidney growth or injury in diabetes mellitus. *Am. J. Physiol. Physiol.* **2013**, *304*, F156–F167. [CrossRef]
19. Vallon, V.; Schroth, J.; Satriano, J.; Blantz, R.C.; Thomson, S.C.; Rieg, T. Adenosine A1 Receptors Determine Glomerular Hyperfiltration and the Salt Paradox in Early Streptozotocin Diabetes Mellitus. *Nephron Physiol.* **2009**, *111*, 30–38. [CrossRef]
20. Vallon, V.; Thomson, S.C. Renal Function in Diabetic Disease Models: The Tubular System in the Pathophysiology of the Diabetic Kidney. *Annu. Rev. Physiol.* **2012**, *74*, 351–375. [CrossRef]
21. Coady, M.J.; El Tarazi, A.; Santer, R.; Bissonnette, P.; Sasseville, L.J.; Calado, J.; Lussier, Y.; Dumayne, C.; Bichet, D.G.; Lapointe, J.Y. MAP17 Is a Necessary Activator of Renal Na^+/Glucose Cotransporter SGLT2. *J. Am. Soc. Nephrol.* **2017**, *28*, 85–93. [CrossRef]
22. DeFronzo, R.A.; Reeves, W.B.; Awad, A.S. Pathophysiology of diabetic kidney disease: Impact of SGLT2 inhibitors. *Nat. Rev. Nephrol.* **2021**, *17*, 319–334. [CrossRef] [PubMed]
23. Thomson, S.C.; Vallon, V. Renal Effects of Sodium-Glucose Co-Transporter Inhibitors. *Am. J. Cardiol.* **2019**, *124* (Suppl. S1), S28–S35. [CrossRef]
24. Pessoa, T.D.; Campos, L.C.; Carraro-Lacroix, L.; Girardi, A.C.; Malnic, G. Functional role of glucose metabolism, osmotic stress, and sodium-glucose cotransporter isoform-mediated transport on Na^+/H^+ exchanger isoform 3 activity in the renal proximal tubule. *J. Am. Soc. Nephrol.* **2014**, *25*, 2028–2039. [CrossRef]
25. Merovci, A.; Solis-Herrera, C.; Daniele, G.; Eldor, R.; Fiorentino, T.V.; Tripathy, D.; Xiong, J.; Perez, Z.; Norton, L.; Abdul-Ghani, M.A.; et al. Dapagliflozin improves muscle insulinsensitivity but enhances endogenous glucose production. *J. Clin. Investig.* **2014**, *124*, 509–514. [CrossRef]
26. Van Bommel, E.J.; Muskiet, M.H.; Tonneijck, L.; Kramer, M.H.; Nieuwdorp, M.; van Raalte, D.H. SGLT2 Inhibition in the Diabetic Kidney-From Mechanisms to Clinical Outcome. *Clin. J. Am. Soc. Nephrol.* **2017**, *12*, 700–710. [CrossRef]
27. Thomas, M.C.; Cherney, D.Z.I. The actions of SGLT2 inhibitors on metabolism, renal function and blood pressure. *Diabetologia* **2018**, *61*, 2098–2107. [CrossRef] [PubMed]
28. Qiu, H.; Novikov, A.; Vallon, V. Ketosis and diabetic ketoacidosis in response to SGLT2 inhibitors: Basic mechanisms and therapeutic perspectives. *Diabetes Metab. Res. Rev.* **2017**, *33*, e2886. [CrossRef] [PubMed]
29. Tomita, I.; Kume, S.; Sugahara, S.; Osawa, N.; Yamahara, K.; Yasuda-Yamahara, M.; Takeda, N.; Chin-Kanasaki, M.; Kaneko, T.; Mayoux, E.; et al. SGLT2 Inhibition Mediates Protection from Diabetic Kidney Disease by Promoting Ketone Body-Induced mTORC1 Inhibition. *Cell Metab.* **2020**, *32*, 404–419.e6. [CrossRef]
30. Zinman, B.; Wanner, C.; Lachin, J.M.; Fitchett, D.; Bluhmki, E.; Hantel, S.; Mattheus, M.; Devins, T.; Johansen, O.E.; Woerle, H.J.; et al. Empagliflozin, cardiovascular outcomes, and mortality in type 2 diabetes. *N. Engl. J. Med.* **2015**, *373*, 2117–2128. [CrossRef]
31. Wanner, C.; Inzucchi, S.E.; Lachin, J.M.; Fitchett, D.; von Eynatten, M.; Mattheus, M.; Johansen, O.E.; Woerle, H.J.; Broedl, U.C.; Zinman, B. Empagliflozin and progression of kidney disease in type 2 diabetes. *N. Engl. J. Med.* **2016**, *375*, 323–334. [CrossRef]
32. Wiviott, S.D.; Raz, I.; Bonaca, M.P.; Mosenzon, O.; Kato, E.T.; Cahn, A.; Silverman, M.G.; Zelniker, T.A.; Kuder, J.F.; Murphy, S.A.; et al. Dapagliflozin and Cardiovascular Outcomes in Type 2 Diabetes. *N. Engl. J. Med.* **2019**, *380*, 347–357. [CrossRef] [PubMed]
33. Neal, B.; Perkovic, V.; Mahaffey, K.W.; de Zeeuw, D.; Fulcher, G.; Erondu, N.; Shaw, W.; Law, G.; Desai, M.; Matthews, D.R.; et al. Canagliflozin and cardiovascular and renal events in type 2 diabetes. *N. Engl. J. Med.* **2017**, *377*, 644–657. [CrossRef]
34. Mosenzon, O.; Wiviott, S.D.; Cahn, A.; Rozenberg, A.; Yanuv, I.; Goodrich, E.L.; Murphy, S.A.; Heerspink, H.J.L.; Zelniker, T.A.; Dwyer, J.P.; et al. Effects of dapagliflozin on development and progression of kidney disease in patients with type 2 diabetes: An analysis from the DECLARE-TIMI 58 randomised trial. *Lancet Diabetes Endocrinol.* **2019**, *7*, 606–617. [CrossRef]
35. Zelniker, T.A.; Wiviott, S.D.; Raz, I.; Im, K.; Goodrich, E.; Bonaca, M.P.; Mosenzon, O.; Kato, E.; Cahn, A.; Furtado, R.H.M.; et al. SGLT2 inhibitors for primary and secondary prevention of cardiovascular and renal outcomes in type 2 diabetes: A systematic review and meta-analysis of cardiovascular outcome trials. *Lancet* **2019**, *393*, 31–39. [CrossRef]
36. Russo, V.; Malvezzi Caracciolo D'Aquino, M.; Caturano, A.; Scognamiglio, G.; Pezzullo, E.; Fabiani, D.; Del Giudice, C.; Carbone, A.; Bottino, R.; Caso, V.; et al. Improvement of Global Longitudinal Strain and Myocardial Work in Type 2 Diabetes Patients on Sodium-Glucose Cotransporter 2 Inhibitors Therapy. *J. Cardiovasc. Pharmacol.* **2023**, *82*, 196–200. [CrossRef] [PubMed]
37. Palmiero, G.; Cesaro, A.; Galiero, R.; Loffredo, G.; Caturano, A.; Vetrano, E.; Rinaldi, L.; Salvatore, T.; Ruggiero, R.; Rosaria Di Palo, M.; et al. Impact of gliflozins on cardiac remodeling in patients with type 2 diabetes mellitus & reduced ejection fraction heart failure: A pilot prospective study. GLISCAR study. *Diabetes Res. Clin. Pract.* **2023**, *200*, 110686. [CrossRef] [PubMed]
38. Sasso, F.C.; Chiodini, P.; Carbonara, O.; De Nicola, L.; Conte, G.; Salvatore, T.; Nasti, R.; Marfella, R.; Gallo, C.; Signoriello, S.; et al. High cardiovascular risk in patients with Type 2 diabetic nephropathy: The predictive role of albuminuria and glomerular filtration rate. The NID-2 Prospective Cohort Study. *Nephrol. Dial. Transplant.* **2011**, *27*, 2269–2274. [CrossRef]
39. Sasso, F.C.; De Nicola, L.; Carbonara, O.; Nasti, R.; Minutolo, R.; Salvatore, T.; Conte, G.; Torella, R. Cardiovascular Risk Factors and Disease Management in Type 2 Diabetic Patients With Diabetic Nephropathy. *Diabetes Care* **2006**, *29*, 498–503. [CrossRef]
40. Minutolo, R.; Sasso, F.C.; Chiodini, P.; Cianciaruso, B.; Carbonara, O.; Zamboli, P.; Tirino, G.; Pota, A.; Torella, R.; Conte, G.; et al. Management of cardiovascular risk factors in advanced type 2 diabetic nephropathy: A comparative analysis in nephrology, diabetology and primary care settings. *J. Hypertens.* **2006**, *24*, 1655–1661. [CrossRef]

41. Perkovic, V.; Jardine, M.J.; Neal, B.; Bompoint, S.; Heerspink, H.J.L.; Charytan, D.M.; Edwards, R.; Agarwal, R.; Bakris, G.; Bull, S.; et al. Canagliflozin and Renal Outcomes in Type 2 Diabetes and Nephropathy. *N. Engl. J. Med.* **2019**, *380*, 2295–2306. [CrossRef]
42. Heerspink, H.J.L.; Stefánsson, B.V.; Correa-Rotter, R.; Chertow, G.M.; Greene, T.; Hou, F.F.; Mann, J.F.E.; McMurray, J.J.V.; Lindberg, M.; Rossing, P.; et al. Dapagliflozin in Patients with Chronic Kidney Disease. *N. Engl. J. Med.* **2020**, *383*, 1436–1446. [CrossRef]
43. The EMPA-KIDNEY Collaborative Group; Herrington, W.G.; Staplin, N.; Wanner, C.; Green, J.B.; Hauske, S.J.; Emberson, J.R.; Preiss, D.; Judge, P.; Mayne, K.J.; et al. Empagliflozin in Patients with Chronic Kidney Disease. *N. Engl. J. Med.* **2023**, *388*, 117–127. [CrossRef]
44. Pelletier, R.; Ng, K.; Alkabbani, W.; Labib, Y.; Mourad, N.; Gamble, J.M. Adverse events associated with sodium glucose co-transporter 2 inhibitors: An overview of quantitative systematic reviews. *Ther. Adv. Drug Saf.* **2021**, *12*, 2042098621989134. [CrossRef]
45. Goldenberg, R.M.; Berard, L.D.; Cheng, A.Y.; Gilbert, J.D.; Verma, S.; Woo, V.C.; Yale, J.-F. SGLT2 Inhibitor-associated Diabetic Ketoacidosis: Clinical Review and Recommendations for Prevention and Diagnosis. *Clin. Ther.* **2016**, *38*, 2654–2664.e1. [CrossRef]
46. American Diabetes Association Professional Practice Committee. 16. Diabetes Care in the Hospital: Standards of Care in Diabetes—2024. *Diabetes Care* **2024**, *47* (Suppl. S1), S295–S306. [CrossRef]
47. Bonner, C.; Kerr-Conte, J.J.; Gmyr, V.V.; Queniat, G.G.; Moerman, E.E.; Thévenet, J.J.; Beaucamps, C.C.; Delalleau, N.N.; Popescu, I.I.; Malaisse, W.J.; et al. Inhibition of the glucose transporter SGLT2 with dapagliflozin in pancreatic alpha cells triggers glucagon secretion. *Nat. Med.* **2015**, *21*, 512–517. [CrossRef]
48. Garofalo, C.; Borrelli, S.; Liberti, M.E.; Andreucci, M.; Conte, G.; Minutolo, R. SGLT2 Inhibitors: Nephroprotective Efficacy and Side Effects. *Medicina* **2019**, *55*, 268. [CrossRef] [PubMed]
49. Kamei, J.; Yamamoto, S. Complicated urinary tract infections with diabetes mellitus. J. Infect. *Chemother* **2021**, *27*, 1131–1136.
50. Vasilakou, D.; Karagiannis, T.; Athanasiadou, E.; Mainou, M.; Liakos, A.; Bekiari, E.; Sarigianni, M.; Matthews, D.R.; Tsapas, A. Sodium-glucose cotransporter 2 inhibitors for type 2 diabetes: A systematic review and meta-analysis. *Ann. Intern. Med.* **2013**, *159*, 262–274. [CrossRef] [PubMed]
51. Puckrin, R.; Saltiel, M.P.; Reynier, P.; Azoulay, L.; Yu, O.H.Y.; Filion, K.B. SGLT-2 inhibitors and the risk of infections: A systematic review and meta-analysis of randomized controlled trials. *Acta Diabetol.* **2018**, *55*, 503–514. [CrossRef] [PubMed]
52. Thong, K.Y.; Yadagiri, M.; Barnes, D.J.; Morris, D.S.; Chowdhury, T.A.; Chuah, L.L.; Robinson, A.M.; Bain, S.C.; Adamson, K.A.; Ryder, R.E.J.; et al. Clinical risk factors predicting genital fungal infections with sodium-glucose cotransporter 2 inhibitor treatment: The ABCD nationwide dapagliflozin audit. *Prim. Care Diabetes* **2018**, *12*, 45–50. [CrossRef]
53. Arakaki, R.F. Sodium-glucosecotransporter-2inhibitors and genital and urinary tract infections in type 2 diabetes. *Postgrad. Med.* **2016**, *128*, 409–417. [CrossRef]
54. Nyirjesy, P.; Sobel, J.D.; Fung, A.; Mayer, C.; Capuano, G.; Ways, K.; Usiskin, K. Genital mycotic infections with canagliflozin, a sodium glucose co-transporter 2 inhibitor, in patients with type 2 diabetes mellitus: A pooled analysis of clinical studies. *Curr. Med. Res. Opin.* **2014**, *30*, 1109–1119. [CrossRef]
55. Taylor, S.I.; Blau, J.E.; Rother, K.I. Possible adverse effects of SGLT2 inhibitors on bone. *Lancet Diabetes Endocrinol.* **2015**, *3*, 8–10. [CrossRef] [PubMed]
56. Meier, C.; Schwartz, A.V.; Egger, A.; Lecka-Czernik, B. Effects of diabetes drugs on the skeleton. *Bone* **2016**, *82*, 93–100. [CrossRef] [PubMed]
57. Marso, S.P.; Daniels, G.H.; Brown-Frandsen, K.; Kristensen, P.; Mann, J.F.; Nauck, M.A.; Nissen, S.E.; Pocock, S.; Poulter, N.R.; Ravn, L.S.; et al. Liraglutide and Cardiovascular Outcomes in Type 2 Diabetes. *N. Engl. J. Med.* **2016**, *375*, 311–322. [CrossRef]
58. Marso, S.P.; Bain, S.C.; Consoli, A.; Eliaschewitz, F.G.; Jódar, E.; Leiter, L.A.; Lingvay, I.; Rosenstock, J.; Seufert, J.; Warren, M.L.; et al. Semaglutide and Cardiovascular Outcomes in Patients with Type 2 Diabetes. *N. Engl. J. Med.* **2016**, *375*, 1834–1844. [CrossRef] [PubMed]
59. Gerstein, H.C.; Colhoun, H.M.; Dagenais, G.R.; Diaz, R.; Lakshmanan, M.; Pais, P.; Probstfield, J.; Riesmeyer, J.S.; Riddle, M.C.; Rydén, L.; et al. Dulaglutide and cardiovascular outcomes in type 2 diabetes (REWIND): A double-blind, randomised placebo-controlled trial. *Lancet* **2019**, *394*, 121–130. [CrossRef]
60. Green, J.B.; Hernandez, A.F.; D'Agostino, R.B.; Granger, C.B.; Janmohamed, S.; Jones, N.P.; Leiter, L.A.; Noronha, D.; Russell, R.; Sigmon, K.; et al. Harmony Outcomes: A randomized, double-blind, placebo-controlled trial of the effect of albiglutide on major cardiovascular events in patients with type 2 diabetes mellitus-Rationale, design, and baseline characteristics. *Am. Heart J.* **2018**, *203*, 30–38. [CrossRef]
61. Husain, M.; Birkenfeld, A.L.; Donsmark, M.; Dungan, K.; Eliaschewitz, F.G.; Franco, D.R.; Jeppesen, O.K.; Lingvay, I.; Mosenzon, O.; Pedersen, S.D.; et al. Oral Semaglutide and Cardiovascular Outcomes in Patients with Type 2 Diabetes. *N. Engl. J. Med.* **2019**, *381*, 841–851. [CrossRef]
62. Gerstein, H.C.; Sattar, N.; Rosenstock, J.; Ramasundarahettige, C.; Pratley, R.; Lopes, R.D.; Lam, C.S.P.; Khurmi, N.S.; Heenan, L.; Del Prato, S.; et al. Cardiovascular and Renal Outcomes with Efpeglenatide in Type 2 Diabetes. *N. Engl. J. Med.* **2021**, *385*, 896–907. [CrossRef]
63. Lincoff, A.M.; Brown-Frandsen, K.; Colhoun, H.M.; Deanfield, J.; Emerson, S.S.; Esbjerg, S.; Hardt-Lindberg, S.; Hovingh, G.K.; Kahn, S.E.; Kushner, R.F.; et al. Semaglutide and Cardiovascular Outcomes in Obesity without Diabetes. *N. Engl. J. Med.* **2023**, *389*, 2221–2232. [CrossRef] [PubMed]

64. Perkovic, V.; Tuttle, K.R.; Rossing, P.; Mahaffey, K.W.; Mann, J.F.E.; Bakris, G.; Baeres, F.M.M.; Idorn, T.; Bosch-Traberg, H.; Lausvig, N.L.; et al. Effects of Semaglutide on Chronic Kidney Disease in Patients with Type 2 Diabetes. *N. Engl. J. Med.* **2024**, *391*, 109–121. [CrossRef] [PubMed]
65. Kosiborod, M.N.; Abildstrøm, S.Z.; Borlaug, B.A.; Butler, J.; Rasmussen, S.; Davies, M.; Hovingh, G.K.; Kitzman, D.W.; Lindegaard, M.L.; Møller, D.V.; et al. Semaglutide in Patients with Heart Failure with Preserved Ejection Fraction and Obesity. *N. Engl. J. Med.* **2023**, *389*, 1069–1084. [CrossRef]
66. Hankosky, E.R.; Wang, H.; Neff, L.M.; Kan, H.; Wang, F.; Ahmad, N.N.; Griffin, R.; Stefanski, A.; Garvey, W.T. Tirzepatide Reduces the Predicted Risk of Atherosclerotic Cardiovascular Disease and Improves Cardiometabolic Risk Factors in Adults with Obesity or Overweight: SURMOUNT-1 Post Hoc Analysis. *Diabetes Obes. Metab.* **2024**, *26*, 319–328. [CrossRef]
67. ClinicalTrials.Gov. A Study of Tirzepatide (LY3298176) in Participants with Heart Failure with Preserved Ejection Fraction and Obesity (SUMMIT). ClinicalTrials.Gov Identifier: NCT04847557. Available online: https://clinicaltrials.gov/ct2/show/NCT04847557 (accessed on 1 September 2024).
68. Nicholls, S.J.; Bhatt, D.L.; Buse, J.B.; De Prato, S.; Kahn, S.E.; Lincoff, A.M.; McGuire, D.K.; Nauck, M.A.; Nissen, S.E.; Sattar, N.; et al. Comparison of Tirzepatide and Dulaglutide on Major Adverse Cardiovascular Events in Participants with Type 2 Diabetes Atherosclerotic Cardiovascular Disease: SURPASS-CVOT Design and Baseline Characteristics. *Am. Heart J.* **2024**, *267*, 1–11. [CrossRef]
69. Zhang, Y.; Sun, B.; Feng, D.; Hu, H.; Chu, M.; Qu, Q.; Tarrasch, J.T.; Li, S.; Sun, K.; Kobilka, T.; et al. Cryo-EM structure of the activated GLP-1 receptor in complex with a G protein. *Nature* **2017**, *546*, 248–253. [CrossRef]
70. Richards, P.; Parker, H.E.; Adriaenssens, A.E.; Hodgson, J.M.; Cork, S.C.; Trapp, S.; Gribble, F.M.; Reimann, F. Identification and characterization of GLP-1 receptor-expressing cells using a new transgenic mouse model. *Diabetes* **2014**, *63*, 1224–1233. [CrossRef]
71. Graaf, C.; Donnelly, D.; Wootten, D.; Lau, J.; Sexton, P.; Miller, L.; Ahn, J.; Liao, J.; Fletcher, M.; Yang, D.; et al. Glucagon-Like Peptide-1 and Its Class B G Protein–Coupled Receptors: A Long March to Therapeutic Successes. *Pharmacol. Rev.* **2016**, *68*, 954–1013. [CrossRef] [PubMed]
72. Rajan, S.; Dickson, L.; Mathew, E.; Orr, C.; Ellenbroek, J.; Philipson, L.; Wicksteed, B. Chronic hyperglycemia downregulates GLP-1 receptor signaling in pancreatic β-cells via protein kinase A. *Mol. Metab.* **2015**, *4*, 265–276. [CrossRef]
73. Hemmingsen, B.; Sonne, D.; Metzendorf, M.I.; Richter, B. Dipeptidyl-peptidase (DPP)-4 inhibitors and glucagon-like peptide (GLP)-1 analogues for prevention or delay of type 2 diabetes mellitus and its associated complications in people at increased risk for the development of type 2 diabetes mellitus. *Cochrane Database Syst. Rev.* **2017**, *5*, CD012204. [CrossRef] [PubMed]
74. Kieffer, T.J.; McIntosh, C.H.; Pederson, R.A. Degradation of glucose-dependent insulinotropic polypeptide and truncated glucagon-like peptide 1 in vitro and in vivo by dipeptidyl peptidase IV. *Endocrinology* **1995**, *136*, 3585–3596. [CrossRef]
75. Vinik, A. Advancing therapy in type 2 diabetes mellitus with early, comprehensive progression from oral agents to insulin therapy. *Clin. Ther.* **2007**, *29*, 1236–1253. [CrossRef] [PubMed]
76. Coskun, T.; Sloop, K.W.; Loghin, C.; Alsina-Fernandez, J.; Urva, S.; Bokvist, K.B.; Cui, X.; Briere, D.A.; Cabrera, O.; Roell, W.C.; et al. LY3298176, a novel dual GIP and GLP-1 receptor agonist for the treatment of type 2 diabetes mellitus: From discovery to clinical proof of concept. *Mol. Metab.* **2018**, *18*, 3–14. [CrossRef] [PubMed]
77. Gloerich, M.; Bos, J.L. Epac: Defining a new mechanism for cAMP action. *Annu. Rev. Pharmacol. Toxicol.* **2010**, *50*, 355–375. [CrossRef]
78. Light, P.E.; Manning Fox, J.E.; Riedel, M.J.; Wheeler, M.B. Glucagon-like peptide-1 inhibits pancreatic ATP-sensitive potassium channels via a protein kinase A- and ADP-dependent mechanism. *Mol. Endocrinol.* **2002**, *16*, 2135–2144. [CrossRef]
79. Doyle, M.E.; Egan, J.M. Mechanisms of action of glucagon-like peptide 1 in the pancreas. *Pharmacol. Ther.* **2007**, *113*, 546–593. [CrossRef]
80. Nauck, M.A.; Quast, D.R.; Wefers, J.; Meier, J.J. GLP-1 receptor agonists in the treatment of type 2 diabetes—State-of-the-art. *Mol. Metab.* **2021**, *46*, 101102. [CrossRef]
81. Zhao, X.; Wang, M.; Wen, Z.; Lu, Z.; Cui, L.; Fu, C.; Xue, H.; Liu, Y.; Zhang, Y. GLP-1 Receptor Agonists: Beyond Their Pancreatic Effects. *Front. Endocrinol.* **2021**, *12*, 721135. [CrossRef]
82. Dave, B.P.; Chorawala, M.R.; Shah, I.V.; Shah, N.N.; Bhagat, S.U.; Prajapati, B.G.; Thakkar, P.C. From diabetes to diverse domains: The multifaceted roles of GLP-1 receptor agonists. *Mol. Biol. Rep.* **2024**, *51*, 835. [CrossRef]
83. Bode, B.W. Design, findings and implications of the liraglutide phase III clinical trial program. *Clin. Investig.* **2012**, *2*, 59–72. [CrossRef]
84. Aroda, V.R.; Ahmann, A.; Cariou, B.; Chow, F.; Davies, M.J.; Jódar, E.; Mehta, R.; Woo, V.; Lingvay, I. Comparative efficacy, safety, and cardiovascular outcomes with once-weekly subcutaneous semaglutide in the treatment of type 2 diabetes: Insights from the SUSTAIN 1–7 trials. *Diabetes Metab.* **2019**, *45*, 409–418. [CrossRef] [PubMed]
85. Thethi, T.K.; Pratley, R.; Meier, J.J. Efficacy, safety and cardiovascular outcomes of once-daily oral semaglutide in patients with type 2 diabetes: The PIONEER programme. *Diabetes Obes. Metab.* **2020**, *22*, 1263–1277. [CrossRef]
86. Bersoux, S.; Byun, T.H.; Chaliki, S.S.; Poole, K.G. Pharmacotherapy for obesity: What you need to know. *Cleve. Clin. J. Med.* **2017**, *84*, 951–958. [CrossRef]
87. Baggio, L.L.; Drucker, D.J. Biology of incretins: GLP-1 and GIP. *Gastroenterology* **2007**, *132*, 2131–2157. [CrossRef]
88. van Can, J.; Sloth, B.; Jensen, C.B.; Flint, A.; Blaak, E.E.; Saris, W.H. Effects of the once-daily GLP-1 analog liraglutide on gastric emptying, glycemic parameters, appetite and energy metabolism in obese, non-diabetic adults. *Int. J. Obes.* **2014**, *38*, 784–793. [CrossRef] [PubMed]

89. Blundell, J.; Finlayson, G.; Axelsen, M.; Flint, A.; Gibbons, C.; Kvist, T.; Hjerpsted, J.B. Effects of once-weekly semaglutide on appetite, energy intake, control of eating, food preference and body weight in subjects with obesity. *Diabetes Obes. Metab.* **2017**, *19*, 1242–1251. [CrossRef]
90. McGuire, D.K.; Busui, R.P.; Deanfield, J.; Inzucchi, S.E.; Mann, J.F.E.; Marx, N.; Mulvagh, S.L.; Poulter, N.; Engelmann, M.D.M.; Hovingh, G.K.; et al. Effects of oral semaglutide on cardiovascular outcomes in individuals with type 2 diabetes and established atherosclerotic cardiovascular disease and/or chronic kidney disease: Design and baseline characteristics of SOUL, a randomized trial. *Diabetes Obes. Metab.* **2023**, *25*, 1932–1941. [CrossRef]
91. Caturano, A.; Galiero, R.; Pafundi, P.C.; Cesaro, A.; Vetrano, E.; Palmiero, G.; Rinaldi, L.; Salvatore, T.; Marfella, R.; Sardu, C.; et al. Does a Strict Glycemic Control during Acute Coronary Syndrome Play a Cardioprotective Effect? Pathophysiology and Clinical Evidence. *Diabetes Res. Clin. Pract.* **2021**, *178*, 108959. [CrossRef]
92. Marfella, R.; Sardu, C.; Balestrieri, M.L.; Siniscalchi, M.; Minicucci, F.; Signoriello, G.; Calabrò, P.; Mauro, C.; Pieretti, G.; Coppola, A.; et al. Effects of Incretin Treatment on Cardiovascular Outcomes in Diabetic STEMI-Patients with Culprit Obstructive and Multivessel Non Obstructive-Coronary-Stenosis. *Diabetol. Metab. Syndr.* **2018**, *10*, 1. [CrossRef]
93. Salvatore, T.; Nevola, R.; Pafundi, P.C.; Monaco, L.; Ricozzi, C.; Imbriani, S.; Rinaldi, L.; Sasso, F.C. Incretin Hormones: The Link between Glycemic Index and Cardiometabolic Diseases. *Nutrients* **2019**, *11*, 1878. [CrossRef] [PubMed]
94. Vilsboll, T. No Reactive Hypoglycaemia in Type 2 Diabetic Patients after Subcutaneous Administration of GLP-1 and Intravenous Glucose. *Diabet. Med.* **2001**, *18*, 144–149. [CrossRef]
95. Lyseng-Williamson, K.A. Glucagon-Like Peptide-1 Receptor Analogues in Type 2 Diabetes: Their Use and Differential Features. Clin. *Drug Investig.* **2019**, *39*, 805–819. [CrossRef]
96. Saini, J.; Marino, D.; Badalov, N.; Vugelman, M.; Tenner, S. Drug-Induced Acute Pancreatitis: An Evidence-Based Classification (Revised). *Clin. Transl. Gastroenterol.* **2023**, *14*, e00621. [CrossRef]
97. He, L.; Wang, J.; Ping, F.; Yang, N.; Huang, J.; Li, Y.; Xu, L.; Li, W.; Zhang, H. Association of Glucagon-Like Peptide-1 Receptor Agonist Use with Risk of Gallbladder and Biliary Diseases: A Systematic Review and Meta-analysis of Randomized Clinical Trials. *JAMA Intern. Med.* **2022**, *182*, 513–519. [CrossRef] [PubMed]
98. Zimmermann, T.; Thomas, L.; Baader-Pagler, T.; Haebel, P.; Simon, E.; Reindl, W.; Bajrami, B.; Rist, W.; Uphues, I.; Drucker, D.J.; et al. BI 456906: Discovery and Preclinical Pharmacology of a Novel GCGR/GLP-1R Dual Agonist with Robust Anti-Obesity Efficacy. *Mol. Metab.* **2022**, *66*, 101633. [CrossRef]
99. Thomas, M.K.; Nikooienejad, A.; Bray, R.; Cui, X.; Wilson, J.; Duffin, K.; Milicevic, Z.; Haupt, A.; Robins, D.A. Dual GIP and GLP-1 Receptor Agonist Tirzepatide Improves Beta-cell Function and Insulin Sensitivity in Type 2 Diabetes. *J. Clin. Endocrinol. Metab.* **2021**, *106*, 388–396. [CrossRef]
100. Mori, Y.; Matsui, T.; Hirano, T.; Yamagishi, S.I. GIP as a Potential Therapeutic Target for Atherosclerotic Cardiovascular Disease: A Systematic Review. *Int. J. Mol. Sci.* **2020**, *21*, 1509. [CrossRef]
101. Del Prato, S.; Kahn, S.E.; Pavo, I.; Weerakkody, G.J.; Yang, Z.; Doupis, J.; Aizenberg, D.; Wynne, A.G.; Riesmeyer, J.S.; Heine, R.J.; et al. Tirzepatide versus Insulin Glargine in Type 2 Diabetes and Increased Cardiovascular Risk (SURPASS-4): A Randomised, Open-label, Parallel-Group, Multicentre, Phase 3 Trial. *Lancet* **2021**, *398*, 1811–1824. [CrossRef] [PubMed]
102. Corrao, S.; Pollicino, C.; Maggio, D.; Torres, A.; Argano, C. Tirzepatide against Obesity and Insulin-Resistance: Pathophysiological Aspects and Clinical Evidence. *Front. Endocrinol.* **2024**, *15*, 1402583. [CrossRef]
103. Ludvik, B.; Giorgino, F.; Jódar, E.; Frias, J.P.; Fernández Landó, L.; Brown, K.; Bray, R.; Rodríguez, Á. Once-Weekly Tirzepatide versus Once-Daily Insulin Degludec as Add-On to Metformin with or without SGLT2 Inhibitors in Patients with Type 2 Diabetes (SURPASS-3): A Randomised, Open-Label, Parallel-Group, Phase 3 Trial. *Lancet* **2021**, *398*, 583–598. [CrossRef] [PubMed]
104. Frías, J.P.; Davies, M.J.; Rosenstock, J.; Pérez Manghi, F.C.; Fernández Landó, L.; Bergman, B.K.; Liu, B.; Cui, X.; Brown, K.; SURPASS-2 Investigators. Tirzepatide versus Semaglutide Once Weekly in Patients with Type 2 Diabetes. *N. Engl. J. Med.* **2021**, *385*, 503–515. [CrossRef]
105. Malhotra, A.; Grunstein, R.R.; Fietze, I.; Weaver, T.E.; Redline, S.; Azarbarzin, A.; Sands, S.A.; Schwab, R.J.; Dunn, J.P.; Chakladar, S.; et al. Tirzepatide for the Treatment of Obstructive Sleep Apnea and Obesity. *N. Engl. J. Med.* **2024**, *Epub ahead of print*. [CrossRef] [PubMed]
106. France, N.L.; Syed, Y.Y. Tirzepatide: A Review in Type 2 Diabetes. *Drugs* **2024**, *84*, 227–238. [CrossRef] [PubMed]
107. Mishra, R.; Raj, R.; Elshimy, G.; Zapata, I.; Kannan, L.; Majety, P.; Edem, D.; Correa, R. Adverse Events Related to Tirzepatide. *J. Endocr. Soc.* **2023**, *7*, bvad016. [CrossRef] [PubMed]
108. Loomba, R.; Hartman, M.L.; Lawitz, E.J.; Vuppalanchi, R.; Boursier, J.; Bugianesi, E.; Yoneda, M.; Behling, C.; Cummings, O.W.; Tang, Y.; et al. Tirzepatide for Metabolic Dysfunction-Associated Steatohepatitis with Liver Fibrosis. *N. Engl. J. Med.* **2024**, *391*, 299–310. [CrossRef]
109. Hallakou-Bozec, S.; Vial, G.; Kergoat, M.; Fouqueray, P.; Bolze, S.; Borel, A.L.; Fontaine, E.; Moller, D.E. Mechanism of Action of Imeglimin: A Novel Therapeutic Agent for Type 2 Diabetes. *Diabetes Obes. Metab.* **2021**, *23*, 664–673. [CrossRef]
110. Sanada, J.; Obata, A.; Fushimi, Y.; Kimura, T.; Shimoda, M.; Ikeda, T.; Nogami, Y.; Obata, Y.; Yamasaki, Y.; Nakanishi, S.; et al. Imeglimin Exerts Favorable Effects on Pancreatic β-Cells by Improving Morphology in Mitochondria and Increasing the Number of Insulin Granules. *Sci. Rep.* **2022**, *12*, 13220. [CrossRef]
111. Hozumi, K.; Sugawara, K.; Ishihara, T.; Ishihara, N.; Ogawa, W. Effects of Imeglimin on Mitochondrial Function, AMPK Activity, and Gene Expression in Hepatocytes. *Sci. Rep.* **2023**, *13*, 746. [CrossRef]

112. Detaille, D.; Vial, G.; Borel, A.L.; Cottet-Rouselle, C.; Hallakou-Bozec, S.; Bolze, S.; Fouqueray, P.; Fontaine, E. Imeglimin Prevents Human Endothelial Cell Death by Inhibiting Mitochondrial Permeability Transition without Inhibiting Mitochondrial Respiration. *Cell Death Discov.* **2016**, *2*, 15072. [CrossRef]
113. Dubourg, J.; Fouqueray, P.; Thang, C.; Grouin, J.-M.; Ueki, K. Efficacy and Safety of Imeglimin Monotherapy versus Placebo in Japanese Patients with Type 2 Diabetes (TIMES 1): A Double-Blind, Randomized, Placebo-Controlled, Parallel-Group, Multicenter Phase 3 Trial. *Diabetes Care* **2021**, *44*, 952–959. [CrossRef] [PubMed]
114. Han, H.S.; Kang, G.; Kim, J.S.; Choi, B.H.; Koo, S.H. Regulation of Glucose Metabolism from a Liver-Centric Perspective. *Exp. Mol. Med.* **2016**, *48*, e218. [CrossRef] [PubMed]
115. Matschinsky, F.M. Regulation of pancreatic beta-cell glucokinase: From basics to therapeutics. *Diabetes* **2002**, *51* (Suppl. S3), S394–S404. [CrossRef] [PubMed]
116. Nakamura, A.; Omori, K.; Terauchi, Y. Glucokinase Activation or Inactivation: Which Will Lead to the Treatment of Type 2 Diabetes? *Diabetes Obes. Metab.* **2021**, *23*, 2199–2206. [CrossRef]
117. Agius, L. Hormonal and Metabolite Regulation of Hepatic Glucokinase. *Annu. Rev. Nutr.* **2016**, *36*, 389–415. [CrossRef]
118. Haeusler, R.A.; Camastra, S.; Astiarraga, B.; Nannipieri, M.; Anselmino, M.; Ferrannini, E. Decreased Expression of Hepatic Glucokinase in Type 2 Diabetes. *Mol. Metab.* **2014**, *4*, 222–226. [CrossRef]
119. Haddad, D.; Dsouza, V.S.; Al-Mulla, F.; Al Madhoun, A. New-Generation Glucokinase Activators: Potential Game-Changers in Type 2 Diabetes Treatment. *Int. J. Mol. Sci.* **2024**, *25*, 571. [CrossRef]
120. Wang, P.; Liu, H.; Chen, L.; Duan, Y.; Chen, Q.; Xi, S. Effects of a Novel Glucokinase Activator, HMS5552, on Glucose Metabolism in a Rat Model of Type 2 Diabetes Mellitus. *J. Diabetes Res.* **2017**, *2017*, 5812607. [CrossRef]
121. Vella, A.; Freeman, J.L.R.; Dunn, I.; Keller, K.; Buse, J.B.; Valcarce, C. Targeting Hepatic Glucokinase to Treat Diabetes with TTP399, a Hepatoselective Glucokinase Activator. *Sci. Transl. Med.* **2019**, *11*, eaau3441. [CrossRef]
122. Coskun, T.; Urva, S.; Roell, W.C.; Qu, H.; Loghin, C.; Moyers, J.S.; O'Farrell, L.S.; Briere, D.A.; Sloop, K.W.; Thomas, M.K.; et al. LY3437943, a Novel Triple Glucagon, GIP, and GLP-1 Receptor Agonist for Glycemic Control and Weight Loss: From Discovery to Clinical Proof of Concept. *Cell Metab.* **2022**, *34*, 1234–1247.e9. [CrossRef]
123. Al-Massadi, O.; Fernø, J.; Diéguez, C.; Nogueiras, R.; Quiñones, M. Glucagon Control on Food Intake and Energy Balance. *Int. J. Mol. Sci.* **2019**, *20*, 3905. [CrossRef] [PubMed]
124. Sanyal, A.J.; Kaplan, L.M.; Frias, J.P.; Brouwers, B.; Wu, Q.; Thomas, M.K.; Harris, C.; Schloot, N.C.; Du, Y.; Mather, K.J.; et al. Triple Hormone Receptor Agonist Retatrutide for Metabolic Dysfunction-Associated Steatotic Liver Disease: A Randomized Phase 2a Trial. *Nat. Med.* **2024**, *30*, 2037–2048. [CrossRef] [PubMed]
125. Caturano, A.; Galiero, R.; Loffredo, G.; Vetrano, E.; Medicamento, G.; Acierno, C.; Rinaldi, L.; Marrone, A.; Salvatore, T.; Monda, M.; et al. Effects of a Combination of Empagliflozin Plus Metformin vs. Metformin Monotherapy on NAFLD Progression in Type 2 Diabetes: The IMAGIN Pilot Study. *Biomedicines* **2023**, *11*, 322. [CrossRef]
126. Rawshani, A.; Rawshani, A.; Franzén, S.; Eliasson, B.; Svensson, A.-M.; Miftaraj, M.; McGuire, D.K.; Sattar, N.; Rosengren, A.; Gudbjörnsdottir, S. Mortality and Cardiovascular Disease in Type 1 and Type 2 Diabetes. *N. Engl. J. Med.* **2017**, *376*, 1407–1418. [CrossRef] [PubMed]
127. Fox, C.S.; Matsushita, K.; Woodward, M.; Bilo, H.J.; Chalmers, J.; Heerspink, H.J.L.; Lee, B.J.; Perkins, R.M.; Rossing, P.; Sairenchi, T.; et al. Associations of Kidney Disease Measures with Mortality and End-Stage Renal Disease in Individuals with and without Diabetes: A Meta-Analysis. *Lancet* **2012**, *380*, 1662–1673. [CrossRef]
128. Brownrigg, J.R.; Hughes, C.O.; Burleigh, D.; Karthikesalingam, A.; Patterson, B.O.; Holt, P.J.; Thompson, M.M.; de Lusignan, S.; Ray, K.K.; Hinchliffe, R.J. Microvascular Disease and Risk of Cardiovascular Events among Individuals with Type 2 Diabetes: A Population-Level Cohort Study. *Lancet Diabetes Endocrinol.* **2016**, *4*, 588–597. [CrossRef]
129. Kidney Disease: Improving Global Outcomes (KDIGO) Diabetes Work Group. KDIGO 2022 Clinical Practice Guideline for Diabetes Management in Chronic Kidney Disease. *Kidney Int.* **2022**, *102* (Suppl. S5), S1–S127. [CrossRef]
130. Kengne, A.P.; Patel, A.; Marre, M.; Travert, F.; Lievre, M.; Zoungas, S.; Chalmers, J.; Colagiuri, S.; E Grobbee, D.; Hamet, P.; et al. Contemporary Model for Cardiovascular Risk Prediction in People with Type 2 Diabetes. *Eur. J. Cardiovasc. Prevent. Rehabil.* **2011**, *18*, 393–398. [CrossRef]
131. SCORE2-Diabetes Working Group and the ESC Cardiovascular Risk Collaboration. SCORE2-Diabetes: 10-Year Cardiovascular Risk Estimation in Type 2 Diabetes in Europe. *Eur. Heart J.* **2023**, *44*, 2544–2556. [CrossRef]
132. Visseren, F.L.; Mach, F.; Smulders, Y.M.; Carballo, D.; Koskinas, K.C.; Bäck, M.; Benetos, A.; Biffi, A.; Boavida, J.M.; Capodanno, D.; et al. 2021 ESC Guidelines on Cardiovascular Disease Prevention in Clinical Practice: Developed by the Task Force for Cardiovascular Disease Prevention in Clinical Practice with Representatives of the European Society of Cardiology and 12 Medical Societies with the Special Contribution of the European Association of Preventive Cardiology (EAPC). *Eur. Heart J.* **2021**, *42*, 3227–3337.
133. Wing, R.R.; Bolin, P.; Brancati, F.L.; Bray, G.A.; Clark, J.M.; Coday, M.; Crow, R.S.; Curtis, J.M.; Egan, C.M.; Espeland, M.A.; et al. Cardiovascular Effects of Intensive Lifestyle Intervention in Type 2 Diabetes. *N. Engl. J. Med.* **2013**, *369*, 145–154. [PubMed]
134. Critchley, J.A.; Capewell, S. Mortality Risk Reduction Associated with Smoking Cessation in Patients with Coronary Heart Disease: A Systematic Review. *JAMA* **2003**, *290*, 86–97. [CrossRef] [PubMed]

135. Choi, J.W.; Han, E.; Kim, T.H. Association of Smoking Cessation after New-Onset Type 2 Diabetes with Overall and Cause-Specific Mortality among Korean Men: A Nationwide Population-Based Cohort Study. *BMJ Open Diabetes Res. Care* **2020**, *8*, e001249. [CrossRef]
136. Kim, M.K.; Han, K.; Kim, B.; Kim, J.; Kwon, H.-S. Effects of Exercise Initiation and Smoking Cessation after New-Onset Type 2 Diabetes Mellitus on Risk of Mortality and Cardiovascular Outcomes. *Sci. Rep.* **2022**, *12*, 14603. [CrossRef]
137. Jeong, S.M.; Jeon, K.H.; Shin, D.W.; Han, K.; Kim, D.; Park, S.H.; Cho, M.H.; Lee, C.M.; Nam, K.W.; Lee, S.P. Smoking Cessation, but Not Reduction, Reduces Cardiovascular Disease Incidence. *Eur. Heart J.* **2021**, *42*, 4141–4153. [CrossRef]
138. Joseph, J.J.; Deedwania, P.; Acharya, T.; Aguilar, D.; Bhatt, D.L.; Chyun, D.A.; Di Palo, K.E.; Golden, S.H.; Sperling, L.S.; On behalf of the American Heart Association Diabetes Committee of the Council on Lifestyle and Cardiometabolic Health; et al. Comprehensive Management of Cardiovascular Risk Factors for Adults with Type 2 Diabetes: A Scientific Statement from the American Heart Association. *Circulation* **2022**, *145*, e722–e759. [CrossRef] [PubMed]
139. Diabetes Control and Complications Trial Research Group; Nathan, D.M.; Genuth, S.; Lachin, J.; Cleary, P.; Crofford, O.; Davis, M.; Rand, L.; Siebert, C. The Effect of Intensive Treatment of Diabetes on the Development and Progression of Long-Term Complications in Insulin-Dependent Diabetes Mellitus. *N. Engl. J. Med.* **1993**, *329*, 977–986.
140. UK Prospective Diabetes Study Group. Intensive Blood-Glucose Control with Sulphonylureas or Insulin Compared with Conventional Treatment and Risk of Complications in Patients with Type 2 Diabetes (UKPDS 33). *Lancet* **1998**, *352*, 837–853. [CrossRef]
141. Patel, A.; MacMahon, S.; Chalmers, J.; Neal, B.; Billot, L.; Woodward, M.; Marre, M.; Cooper, M.; Glasziou, P.; Grobbee, D.; et al. Intensive blood glucose control and vascular outcomes in patients with type 2 diabetes. *N. Engl. J. Med.* **2008**, *358*, 2560–2572. [CrossRef]
142. Ismail-Beigi, F.; Craven, T.; Banerji, M.A.; Basile, J.; Calles, J.; Cohen, R.M.; Cuddihy, R.; Cushman, W.C.; Genuth, S.; Grimm, R.H.; et al. Effect of Intensive Treatment of Hyperglycaemia on Microvascular Outcomes in Type 2 Diabetes: An Analysis of the ACCORD Randomised Trial. *Lancet* **2010**, *376*, 419–430. [CrossRef]
143. Nathan, D.M.; DCCT/EDIC Research Group. The Diabetes Control and Complications Trial/Epidemiology of Diabetes Interventions and Complications Study at 30 Years: Overview. *Diabetes Care* **2014**, *37*, 9–16. [CrossRef]
144. Writing Group for the DCCT/EDIC Research Group. Coprogression of Cardiovascular Risk Factors in Type 1 Diabetes during 30 Years of Follow-Up in the DCCT/EDIC Study. *Diabetes Care* **2016**, *39*, 1621–1630. [CrossRef] [PubMed]
145. Holman, R.R.; Paul, S.K.; Bethel, M.A.; Matthews, D.R.; Neil, H.A.W. 10-Year Follow-Up of Intensive Glucose Control in Type 2 Diabetes. *N. Engl. J. Med.* **2008**, *359*, 1577–1589. [CrossRef]
146. Zoungas, S.; Arima, H.; Gerstein, H.C.; Holman, R.R.; Woodward, M.; Reaven, P.; A Hayward, R.; Craven, T.; Coleman, R.L.; Chalmers, J. Effects of Intensive Glucose Control on Microvascular Outcomes in Patients with Type 2 Diabetes: A Meta-Analysis of Individual Participant Data from Randomised Controlled Trials. *Lancet Diabetes Endocrinol.* **2017**, *5*, 431–437. [CrossRef]
147. Turnbull, F.; Abraira, C.; Anderson, R.; Byington, R.; Chalmers, J.; Duckworth, W.; Evans, G.W.; Gerstein, H.C.; Holman, R.R.; Moritz, T.E.; et al. Intensive Glucose Control and Macrovascular Outcomes in Type 2 Diabetes. *Diabetologia* **2009**, *52*, 2288–2298. [CrossRef] [PubMed]
148. Currie, C.J.; Peters, J.R.; Tynan, A.; Evans, M.; Heine, R.J.; Bracco, O.L.; Zagar, T.; Poole, C.D. Survival as a Function of HbA1c in People with Type 2 Diabetes: A Retrospective Cohort Study. *Lancet* **2010**, *375*, 481–489. [CrossRef] [PubMed]
149. Sasso, F.C.; Pafundi, P.C.; Gelso, A.; Bono, V.; Costagliola, C.; Marfella, R.; Sardu, C.; Rinaldi, L.; Galiero, R.; Acierno, C.; et al. High HDL Cholesterol: A Risk Factor for Diabetic Retinopathy? Findings from NO BLIND Study. *Diabetes Res. Clin. Pract.* **2019**, *150*, 236–244. [CrossRef]
150. Zoungas, S.; Chalmers, J.; Ninomiya, T.; Li, Q.; Cooper, M.; Colagiuri, S.; Fulcher, G.; De Galan, B.E.; Harrap, S.; Hamet, P.; et al. Association of HbA1c Levels with Vascular Complications and Death in Patients with Type 2 Diabetes: Evidence of Glycaemic Thresholds. *Diabetologia* **2012**, *55*, 636–643. [CrossRef]
151. International Hypoglycaemia Study Group. Hypoglycaemia, Cardiovascular Disease, and Mortality in Diabetes: Epidemiology, Pathogenesis, and Management. *Lancet Diabetes Endocrinol.* **2019**, *7*, 385–396. [CrossRef]
152. Battelino, T.; Danne, T.; Bergenstal, R.M.; Amiel, S.A.; Beck, R.; Biester, T.; Bosi, E.; Buckingham, B.A.; Cefalu, W.T.; Close, K.L.; et al. Clinical Targets for Continuous Glucose Monitoring Data Interpretation: Recommendations from the International Consensus on Time in Range. *Diabetes Care* **2019**, *42*, 1593–1603. [CrossRef]
153. Dahlén, A.D.; Dashi, G.; Maslov, I.; Attwood, M.M.; Jonsson, J.; Trukhan, V.; Schiöth, H.B. Trends in Antidiabetic Drug Discovery: FDA Approved Drugs, New Drugs in Clinical Trials and Global Sales. *Front. Pharmacol.* **2022**, *12*, 807548. [CrossRef]
154. National Center for Biotechnology Information. PubChem Compound Summary for CID 11949646, Empagliflozin. Available online: https://pubchem.ncbi.nlm.nih.gov/compound/Empagliflozin#section=2D-Structure (accessed on 1 September 2024).
155. National Center for Biotechnology Information. PubChem Compound Summary for CID 9887712, Dapagliflozin. Available online: https://pubchem.ncbi.nlm.nih.gov/compound/Dapagliflozin#section=2D-Structure (accessed on 1 September 2024).
156. National Center for Biotechnology Information. PubChem Compound Summary for CID 24812758, Canagliflozin. Available online: https://pubchem.ncbi.nlm.nih.gov/compound/Canagliflozin#section=2D-Structure (accessed on 1 September 2024).
157. National Center for Biotechnology Information. PubChem Compound Summary for CID 44814423, Ertugliflozin. Available online: https://pubchem.ncbi.nlm.nih.gov/compound/Ertugliflozin#section=2D-Structure (accessed on 1 September 2024).

158. National Center for Biotechnology Information. PubChem Compound Summary for CID 24831714, Sotagliflozin. Available online: https://pubchem.ncbi.nlm.nih.gov/compound/Sotagliflozin#section=2D-Structure (accessed on 1 September 2024).
159. National Center for Biotechnology Information. PubChem Compound Summary for CID 16134956, Liraglutide. Available online: https://pubchem.ncbi.nlm.nih.gov/compound/Liraglutide#section=2D-Structure (accessed on 1 September 2024).
160. National Center for Biotechnology Information. PubChem Compound Summary for CID 171042928, GLP-1 Moiety from Dulaglutide. Available online: https://pubchem.ncbi.nlm.nih.gov/compound/GLP-1-moiety-from-Dulaglutide#section=2D-Structure (accessed on 1 September 2024).
161. National Center for Biotechnology Information. PubChem Compound Summary for CID 56843331, Semaglutide. Available online: https://pubchem.ncbi.nlm.nih.gov/compound/Semaglutide#section=2D-Structure (accessed on 1 September 2024).
162. National Center for Biotechnology Information. PubChem Compound Summary for CID 24812808, Imeglimin. Available online: https://pubchem.ncbi.nlm.nih.gov/compound/Imeglimin#section=2D-Structure (accessed on 1 September 2024).
163. National Center for Biotechnology Information. PubChem Compound Summary for CID 57920094, Dorzagliatin. Available online: https://pubchem.ncbi.nlm.nih.gov/compound/Dorzagliatin#section=2D-Structure (accessed on 1 September 2024).
164. National Center for Biotechnology Information. PubChem Compound Summary for CID 54673176, Cadisegliatin. Available online: https://pubchem.ncbi.nlm.nih.gov/compound/Cadisegliatin#section=2D-Structure (accessed on 1 September 2024).
165. National Center for Biotechnology Information. PubChem Compound Summary for CID 171378578, Retatrutide. Available online: https://pubchem.ncbi.nlm.nih.gov/compound/Retatrutide#section=2D-Structure (accessed on 1 September 2024).
166. National Center for Biotechnology Information. PubChem Compound Summary for CID 166567236, CID 166567236. Available online: https://pubchem.ncbi.nlm.nih.gov/compound/166567236#section=2D-Structure (accessed on 1 September 2024).
167. Sasako, T.; Yamauchi, T.; Ueki, K. Intensified Multifactorial Intervention in Patients with Type 2 Diabetes Mellitus. *Diabetes Metab. J.* **2023**, *47*, 185–197. [CrossRef] [PubMed]
168. Galiero, R.; Caturano, A.; Vetrano, E.; Monda, M.; Marfella, R.; Sardu, C.; Salvatore, T.; Rinaldi, L.; Sasso, F.C. Precision Medicine in Type 2 Diabetes Mellitus: Utility and Limitations. *Diabetes Metab. Syndr. Obes.* **2023**, *16*, 3669–3689. [CrossRef]
169. Sasso, F.C.; Simeon, V.; Galiero, R.; Caturano, A.; De Nicola, L.; Chiodini, P.; Rinaldi, L.; Salvatore, T.; Lettieri, M.; Nevola, R.; et al. The Number of Risk Factors Not at Target Is Associated with Cardiovascular Risk in a Type 2 Diabetic Population with Albuminuria in Primary Cardiovascular Prevention: Post-Hoc Analysis of the NID-2 Trial. *Cardiovasc. Diabetol.* **2022**, *21*, 235. [CrossRef] [PubMed]
170. Sasso, F.C.; Pafundi, P.C.; Simeon, V.; De Nicola, L.; Chiodini, P.; Galiero, R.; Rinaldi, L.; Nevola, R.; Salvatore, T.; Sardu, C.; et al. Efficacy and Durability of Multifactorial Intervention on Mortality and MACEs: A Randomized Clinical Trial in Type-2 Diabetic Kidney Disease. *Cardiovasc. Diabetol.* **2021**, *20*, 145. [CrossRef]
171. Rawshani, A.; Rawshani, A.; Franzén, S.; Sattar, N.; Eliasson, B.; Svensson, A.M.; Zethelius, B.; Miftaraj, M.; McGuire, D.K.; Rosengren, A.; et al. Risk Factors, Mortality, and Cardiovascular Outcomes in Patients with Type 2 Diabetes. *N. Engl. J. Med.* **2018**, *379*, 633–644. [CrossRef] [PubMed]
172. Visseren, F.L.J.; Mach, F.; Smulders, Y.M.; Carballo, D.; Koskinas, K.C.; Bäck, M.; Benetos, A.; Biffi, A.; Boavida, J.M.; Capodanno, D.; et al. 2021 ESC Guidelines on Cardiovascular Disease Prevention in Clinical Practice. *Eur. J. Prev. Cardiol.* **2022**, *29*, 5–115. [CrossRef]
173. Cosentino, F.; Grant, P.J.; Aboyans, V.; Bailey, C.J.; Ceriello, A.; Delgado, V.; Federici, M.; Filippatos, G.; Grobbee, D.E.; Hansen, T.B.; et al. 2019 ESC Guidelines on Diabetes, Pre-Diabetes, and Cardiovascular Diseases Developed in Collaboration with the EASD. *Eur. Heart J.* **2020**, *41*, 255–323. [CrossRef]
174. American Diabetes Association Professional Practice Committee. 9. Pharmacologic Approaches to Glycemic Treatment: Standards of Care in Diabetes—2024. *Diabetes Care* **2024**, *47* (Suppl. S1), S158–S178. [CrossRef]
175. Tsapas, A.; Karagiannis, T.; Avgerinos, I.; Matthews, D.R.; Bekiari, E. Comparative Effectiveness of Glucose-Lowering Drugs for Type 2 Diabetes. *Ann. Intern. Med.* **2021**, *174*, 141. [CrossRef]
176. Salvatore, T.; Galiero, R.; Caturano, A.; Vetrano, E.; Loffredo, G.; Rinaldi, L.; Catalini, C.; Gjeloshi, K.; Albanese, G.; Di Martino, A.; et al. Coronary Microvascular Dysfunction in Diabetes Mellitus: Pathogenetic Mechanisms and Potential Therapeutic Options. *Biomedicines* **2022**, *10*, 2274. [CrossRef]
177. Nevola, R.; Epifani, R.; Imbriani, S.; Tortorella, G.; Aprea, C.; Galiero, R.; Rinaldi, L.; Marfella, R.; Sasso, F.C. GLP-1 Receptor Agonists in Non-Alcoholic Fatty Liver Disease: Current Evidence and Future Perspectives. *Int. J. Mol. Sci.* **2023**, *24*, 1703. [CrossRef]
178. Salvatore, T.; Galiero, R.; Caturano, A.; Rinaldi, L.; Di Martino, A.; Albanese, G.; Di Salvo, J.; Epifani, R.; Marfella, R.; Docimo, G.; et al. An Overview of the Cardiorenal Protective Mechanisms of SGLT2 Inhibitors. *Int. J. Mol. Sci.* **2022**, *23*, 3651. [CrossRef] [PubMed]
179. Caturano, A.; Galiero, R.; Pafundi, P.C. Metformin for Type 2 Diabetes. *JAMA* **2019**, *322*, 1312. [CrossRef] [PubMed]
180. Tonelli, M.; Muntner, P.; Lloyd, A.; Manns, B.J.; Klarenbach, S.; Pannu, N.; James, M.T.; Hemmelgarn, B.R. Risk of coronary events in people with chronic kidney disease compared with those with diabetes: A population-level cohort study. *Lancet* **2012**, *380*, 807–814. [CrossRef] [PubMed]
181. Go, A.S.; Chertow, G.M.; Fan, D.; McCulloch, C.E.; Hsu, C.Y. Chronic kidney disease and the risks of death, cardiovascular events, and hospitalization. *N. Engl. J. Med.* **2004**, *351*, 1296–1305. [CrossRef]

182. Satija, A.; Bhupathiraju, S.N.; Rimm, E.B.; Spiegelman, D.; Chiuve, S.E.; Borgi, L.; Willett, W.C.; Manson, J.E.; Sun, Q.; Hu, F.B. Plant-Based Dietary Patterns and Incidence of Type 2 Diabetes in US Men and Women: Results from Three Prospective Cohort Studies. *PLoS Med.* **2016**, *13*, e1002039. [CrossRef]
183. Alonso-Domínguez, R.; García-Ortiz, L.; Patino-Alonso, M.C.; Sánchez-Aguadero, N.; Gómez-Marcos, M.A.; Recio-Rodríguez, J.I. Effectiveness of A Multifactorial Intervention in Increasing Adherence to the Mediterranean Diet among Patients with Diabetes Mellitus Type 2: A Controlled and Randomized Study (EMID Study). *Nutrients* **2019**, *11*, 162. [CrossRef]
184. Estruch, R.; Ros, E.; Salas-Salvadó, J.; Covas, M.I.; Corella, D.; Arós, F.; Gómez-Gracia, E.; Ruiz-Gutiérrez, V.; Fiol, M.; Lapetra, J.; et al. Primary prevention of cardiovascular disease with a Mediterranean diet supplemented with extravirgin olive oil or nuts. *N. Engl. J. Med.* **2018**, *378*, e34. [CrossRef]
185. Wahid, A.; Manek, N.; Nichols, M.; Kelly, P.; Foster, C.; Webster, P.; Kaur, A.; Smith, C.F.; Wilkins, E.; Rayner, M.; et al. Quantifying the association between physical activity and cardiovascular disease and diabetes: A systematic review and meta-analysis. *J. Am. Heart Assoc.* **2016**, *5*, e002495. [CrossRef]
186. Gardner, C.D.; Landry, M.J.; Perelman, D.; Petlura, C.; Durand, L.R.; Aronica, L.; Crimarco, A.; Cunanan, K.M.; Chang, A.; Dant, C.C.; et al. Effect of a ketogenic diet versus Mediterranean diet on glycated hemoglobin in individuals with prediabetes and type 2 diabetes mellitus: The interventional Keto-Med randomized crossover trial. *Am. J. Clin. Nutr.* **2022**, *116*, 640–652. [CrossRef] [PubMed]
187. Saslow, L.R.; Kim, S.; Daubenmier, J.J.; Moskowitz, J.T.; Phinney, S.D.; Goldman, V.; Murphy, E.J.; Cox, R.M.; Moran, P.; Hecht, F.M. A randomized pilot trial of a moderate carbohydrate diet compared to a very low carbohydrate diet in overweight or obese individuals with type 2 diabetes mellitus or prediabetes. *PLoS ONE.* **2014**, *9*, e91027. [CrossRef]
188. Vetrano, E.; Rinaldi, L.; Mormone, A.; Giorgione, C.; Galiero, R.; Caturano, A.; Nevola, R.; Marfella, R.; Sasso, F.C. Non-alcoholic Fatty Liver Disease (NAFLD), Type 2 Diabetes, and Non-viral Hepatocarcinoma: Pathophysiological Mechanisms and New Therapeutic Strategies. *Biomedicines* **2023**, *11*, 468. [CrossRef] [PubMed]
189. Ibrahim, M.; Barker, M.M.; Ahmad, E.; Ahmed, A.; Annabi, F.A.; Ba-Essa, E.M.; Davies, M.J.; Houeiss, P.; Iraqi, H.; Masood, S.N.; et al. Optimizing Ramadan fasting: A randomised controlled trial for people with type 2 diabetes during Ramadan applying the principles of the ADA/EASD consensus. *Diabetes Metab. Res. Rev.* **2023**, *39*, e3604. [CrossRef]
190. Ueki, K.; Sasako, T.; Okazaki, Y.; Miyake, K.; Nangaku, M.; Ohashi, Y.; Noda, M.; Kadowaki, T.; J-DOIT3 Study Group. Multifactorial intervention has a significant effect on diabetic kidney disease in patients with type 2 diabetes. *Kidney Int.* **2021**, *99*, 256–266. [CrossRef]
191. Gaede, P.; Lund-Andersen, H.; Parving, H.H.; Pedersen, O. Effect of a multifactorial intervention on mortality in type 2 diabetes. *N. Engl. J. Med.* **2008**, *358*, 580–591. [CrossRef] [PubMed]
192. Gaede, P.; Pedersen, O. Intensive integrated therapy of type 2 diabetes: Implications for long-term prognosis. *Diabetes.* **2004**, *53* (Suppl. S3), S39–S47. [CrossRef]
193. Ueki, K.; Sasako, T.; Okazaki, Y.; Kato, M.; Okahata, S.; Katsuyama, H.; Haraguchi, M.; Morita, A.; Ohashi, K.; Hara, K.; et al. Effect of an intensified multifactorial intervention on cardiovascular outcomes and mortality in type 2 diabetes (J-DOIT3): An open-label, randomised controlled trial. *Lancet Diabetes Endocrinol.* **2017**, *5*, 951–964. [CrossRef]
194. Vicente, A.M.; Ballensiefen, W.; Jönsson, J.I. How personalised medicine will transform healthcare by 2030: The ICPerMed vision. *J Transl Med.* **2020**, *18*, 180. [CrossRef]
195. Chong, K.; Chang, J.K.; Chuang, L.M. Recent advances in the treatment of type 2 diabetes mellitus using new drug therapies. *Kaohsiung J. Med. Sci.* **2024**, *40*, 212–220. [CrossRef]
196. Skivington, K.; Matthews, L.; Simpson, S.A.; Craig, P.; Baird, J.; Blazeby, J.M.; Boyd, K.A.; Craig, N.; French, D.P.; McIntosh, E.; et al. A new framework for developing and evaluating complex interventions: Update of Medical Research Council guidance. *BMJ* **2021**, *374*, n2061. [CrossRef] [PubMed]
197. Ma, C.X.; Ma, X.N.; Guan, C.H.; Li, Y.D.; Mauricio, D.; Fu, S.B. Cardiovascular disease in type 2 diabetes mellitus: Progress toward personalized management. *Cardiovasc. Diabetol.* **2022**, *21*, 74. [CrossRef] [PubMed]
198. Galiero, R.; Caturano, A.; Vetrano, E.; Beccia, D.; Brin, C.; Alfano, M.; Di Salvo, J.; Epifani, R.; Piacevole, A.; Tagliaferri, G.; et al. Peripheral Neuropathy in Diabetes Mellitus: Pathogenetic Mechanisms and Diagnostic Options. *Int. J. Mol. Sci.* **2023**, *24*, 3554. [CrossRef] [PubMed]
199. Ghodeshwar, G.K.; Dube, A.; Khobragade, D. Impact of Lifestyle Modifications on Cardiovascular Health: A Narrative Review. *Cureus* **2023**, *15*, e42616. [CrossRef]

biomedicines

MDPI

Review

Stress and the CRH System, Norepinephrine, Depression, and Type 2 Diabetes

Michele Perrelli [1], Pruthvi Goparaju [2], Teodor T. Postolache [3,4,5], Laura del Bosque-Plata [6] and Claudia Gragnoli [2,7,8,9,*]

1 ASL Roma 1, Santo Spirito Hospital, 00193 Rome, Italy; micheleperrelli@hotmail.com
2 Division of Endocrinology, Department of Medicine, Creighton University School of Medicine, Omaha, NE 68124, USA; pruthvigoparaju@creighton.edu
3 Mood and Anxiety Program, Department of Psychiatry, University of Maryland School of Medicine, Baltimore, MD 21201, USA; tpostola@som.umaryland.edu
4 Rocky Mountain Mental Illness Research Education and Clinical Center (MIRECC), Veterans Integrated Service Network (VISN) 19, Military and Veteran Microbiome: Consortium for Research and Education (MVM-CoRE), Aurora, CO 80246, USA
5 Mental Illness Research Education and Clinical Center (MIRECC), Veterans Integrated Service Network (VISN) 5, VA Capitol Health Care Network, Baltimore, MD 21090, USA
6 Nutrigenetics, and Nutrigenomic Laboratory, National Institute of Genomic Medicine, Mexico City 14610, Mexico; ldelbosque@inmegen.gob.mx
7 Department of Public Health Sciences, Penn State College of Medicine, Hershey, PA 17033, USA
8 Klinik für Endokrinologie, Diabetologie und Klinische Ernährung, Universitätsspital Zürich, 8091 Zürich, Switzerland
9 Molecular Biology Laboratory, Bios Biotech Multi-Diagnostic Health Center, 00197 Rome, Italy
* Correspondence: claudia.gragnoli@gmail.com; Tel.: +1-(508)-246-9330

Abstract: Major depressive disorder (MDD) increases the risk of type 2 diabetes (T2D) by 60% in untreated patients, and hypercortisolism is common in MDD as well as in some patients with T2D. Patients with MDD, despite hypercortisolism, show inappropriately normal levels of corticotropin-releasing hormone (CRH) and plasma adrenocorticotropin (ACTH) in the cerebrospinal fluid, which might implicate impaired negative feedback. Also, a positive feedback loop of the CRH–norepinephrine (NE)–CRH system may be involved in the hypercortisolism of MDD and T2D. Dysfunctional CRH receptor 1 (CRHR1) and CRH receptor 2 (CRHR2), both of which are involved in glucose regulation, may explain hypercortisolism in MDD and T2D, at least in a subgroup of patients. CRHR1 increases glucose-stimulated insulin secretion. Dysfunctional *CRHR1* variants can cause hypercortisolism, leading to serotonin dysfunction and depression, which can contribute to hyperglycemia, insulin resistance, and increased visceral fat, all of which are characteristics of T2D. CRHR2 is implicated in glucose homeostasis through the regulation of insulin secretion and gastrointestinal functions, and it stimulates insulin sensitivity at the muscular level. A few studies show a correlation of the *CRHR2* gene with depressive disorders. Based on our own research, we have found a linkage and association (i.e., linkage disequilibrium [LD]) of the genes *CRHR1* and *CRHR2* with MDD and T2D in families with T2D. The correlation of *CRHR1* and *CRHR2* with MDD appears stronger than that with T2D, and per our hypothesis, MDD may precede the onset of T2D. According to the findings of our analysis, *CRHR1* and *CRHR2* variants could modify the response to prolonged chronic stress and contribute to high levels of cortisol, increasing the risk of developing MDD, T2D, and the comorbidity MDD-T2D. We report here the potential links of the CRH system, NE, and their roles in MDD and T2D.

Keywords: CRH; corticotropin releasing hormone receptor; norepinephrine; autonomous sympathetic nervous system; major depressive disorder; depression; type 2 diabetes; HPA axis; stress; cortisol

1. Introduction

1.1. Major Depressive Disorder (MDD) and Type 2 Diabetes (T2D) Prevalence

Both MDD and T2D are widespread global pathologies. Worldwide, about 5% of adults suffer from depression [1], and by 2030, depression is estimated to become the most common disease in the world, according to the World Health Organization [2]. Meanwhile, worldwide, about 10% of adults suffer from T2D [3], with 58% of European Caucasians having impaired fasting glucose (glycemia $\geq$ 100 mg/dL) [4]. This perspective article explores what is known about the role of linkage and association (i.e., linkage disequilibrium [LD]) of the corticotropin-releasing hormone (CRH) *CRHR1* and *CRHR2* genes with MDD and T2D in families with T2D. We searched within PubMed using the keywords "type 2 diabetes, T2D, major depressive disorder, MDD, depression, stress, hypothalamic-pituitary-adrenal axis, HPA, CRH, CRHR, norepinephrine" and included articles reporting valuable concepts on the association of chronic stress, the CRH system, norepinephrine (NE), depression, and T2D, including the genes *CRHR1* and *CRHR2*.

1.2. MDD and T2D Comorbidity

MDD and T2D are often associated, and numerous different genes may underlie their comorbid pathogenesis. As MDD increases the risk of T2D by 60% [5] in patients never previously treated pharmacologically for MDD, genetic predisposition may—at least partially—underlie the MDD-T2D comorbidity, not depending on antidepressant therapy [6]. Conversely, T2D increases the risk for MDD, albeit slightly [5]. Furthermore, depressive symptoms increase both the risk for T2D and, in diabetic patients, the increase in blood sugar levels and the risk of complications and mortality from all causes [7]. While many genes and neuro-endocrine-metabolic pathways are likely implicated in T2D, MDD, and their comorbidity, the hypothalamic–pituitary–adrenal (HPA) axis and the serotonergic system are known to be interconnectedly involved in MDD [8–15] and perhaps also in T2D and associated metabolic alterations [11,15–19]. In fact, the etiology of stress in the pathogenesis of T2D has been reported [20,21]. Also, subjects with depression have higher hair cortisol concentrations than healthy subjects [22]. Similarly, in a cohort of African American adults with and without T2D, elevated hair cortisol, a marker of long-term HPA axis dysregulation, was correlated with increased glycosylated hemoglobin (HbA1c) in the whole group and in the T2D group [19].

Chronic stress acts on the gut–brain axis and has systemic effects, such as the induction of systemic inflammation present in both depression and T2D. Thus, another potential mechanism is represented by the stress-related intestinal microbiota imbalance—also named dysbiosis—which, by impairing the gut–brain–immune axis, can lead to stress-related MDD-T2D comorbidity [23]. In addition, the persistent activation of the sympathetic nervous system (SNS) results in increased levels of proinflammatory cytokines, which *per se* can trigger the HPA axis hyper-response during stress. Furthermore, in the presence of hyperglycemia and/or T2D, the immune system can be dysregulated, thereby augmenting cytokine release, which can increasingly stimulate the HPA axis and can contribute to depression, T2D, and their comorbidity [24].

Furthermore, genetic studies on MDD-T2D comorbidity will disclose mechanisms underlying T2D and MDD and their comorbidity. Finally, confirmation in larger ethnically diverse samples and longitudinal studies will lead to primary prevention targeting individuals at risk for both T2D and MDD and secondary prevention for patients with a confirmed diagnosis of T2D–MDD.

1.3. Hypothalamic–Pituitary–Adrenal (HPA) Axis and Stress

The HPA axis is a neuroendocrine system that regulates the stress response and interacts with the serotonergic, noradrenergic, and dopaminergic brain systems.

In response to prolonged chronic stress, the hypothalamic paraventricular nucleus (PVN) secretes corticotropin-releasing hormone (CRH, aka corticotropin-releasing factor, CRF), which in turn stimulates pituitary corticotropin (ACTH) secretion, resulting in an increased in plasma cortisol produced by the adrenal gland [25]. The PVN also receives circadian signals from the hypothalamic suprachiasmatic nucleus connected to the retina through the retinohypothalamic tract, which also functions as the central circadian clock [26].

Corticotropinergic neurons are present not only in the anterior pituitary gland but also in the hypothalamus, hippocampus, amygdala, and locus coeruleus (LC), located on the floor of the fourth ventricle. CRHR1 and CRHR2 are G-protein-coupled receptors carrying an amino acid sequence homology of 71% [27], binding CRH and stimulating ACTH secretion. CRHR1 and CRHR2 are responsible for the HPA axis response to stress and circadian rhythms. CRHR1 mostly binds CRH, while CRHR2 binds urocortin with an affinity 40 times greater than CRH [28]. *CRHR1* is expressed especially in the hippocampus and generally in the brain, and to a lesser extent in peripheral tissues, such as the adipose tissue and liver. *CRHR2* is mostly expressed in peripheral tissues such as the liver and adipose tissue but is also expressed in the brain [28].

1.4. Resilience, Stress, CRH System, and Depression

Resilience varies among human and non-human primates. Anxious temperament (AT) manifests early in life with physiological and behavioral hyper-reactivity to mildly threatening stimuli. In children, AT predicts psychopathology and risk for anxiety disorders and depression. In monkeys, the function of the anterior hippocampus and the central nucleus amygdala predicts AT, and even if anatomically closely linked, their heritability differs significantly, as the anterior hippocampus metabolic activity is significantly more heritable compared to the central nucleus amygdala metabolic activity, indicating dissimilar influences of genes and environment mediating AT and anxiety and depression risk [29].

Various studies show that the genetic basis of depression may reside, in part, in genes regulating stress-response systems [12,30] such as the HPA axis [31,32]. Various endocrine factors, including CRH and glucocorticoids, have been implicated in the structural and intracellular abnormalities seen in depression [33].

Early life adversity (e.g., early life maternal separation) [34] increases HPA axis activity in rats and humans [31,34] and generates anxious and depressive behaviors in adult mice [35].

In humans, childhood events, like abuse or loss, are closely related to the risk of adult MDD [36]. Early life stress, characterized by altered neural plasticity, leads in subjects with reduced resilience and additional stressors to persistent central nervous system (CNS)–CRH circuit hyperactivity, increased HPA axis sensitization, and sympathetic nervous system (SNS) response. This lasting increased stress sensitization mediates vulnerability to adolescent and adult depression [37]. Furthermore, the CRH system plays a role in psychopathology, anxiety, and depressive disorders triggered by prolonged chronic stress, and various neuro-behavioral-endocrine-sympathetic-immune responses intensely involve the CRH system [31].

1.5. CRH System, Stress, and CRH–Norepinephrine–CRH Circuit

Cortisol secretion accompanying acute stress is a physiological coping response to anxiety triggers. Catecholamine secretion, specifically the major SNS neurotransmitter, norepinephrine (NE), regulated by the catechol-o-methyltransferase (COMT), mediates SNS activation during short-term stress [38]. During induced stress, human bilateral amygdala activity strongly mediates a sympathetic response and attachment insecurity. Thus, under stress, the amygdala activates the central SNS [39]. The brainstem SNS lies in the LC, the main site synthesizing NE, beyond the adrenal medulla. Also, cortical and midbrain areas have noradrenergic neuron projections. To maintain homeostasis, chronic stress usually elicits central nervous system adaptation. Extrahypothalamic CRH and LC-NE systems are the principal components of stress response. In animals, CRH produces various anxiety-, arousal-, and stress-associated behaviors. In the LC, CRH increases the activity of tyrosine hydroxylase (rate-limiting enzyme in the synthesis of catecholamines) and therefore increases the release of NE in the projection areas of the LC. Chronic "unpredictable" stress can maintain CRH neuronal activity and LC-NE system dysregulation, impairing the adaptation system. Further, the NE-CRH interaction may occur in various brain areas, including the hypothalamic PVN and the amygdala central nucleus, where NE stimulates CRH release. The CRH–NE–CRH feed-forward system progressively augments the stress response with repeated exposure. Acute and chronic moderate and "predictable" stresses induce beta-adrenergic receptor down-regulation, which represents stress adaptation. On the contrary, chronic "unpredictable" stress, resembling a model for depression, up-regulates the beta-adrenergic receptor [40]. In rats exposed to 14-day-long chronic "unpredictable" stress, treatment with the selective serotonin-reuptake inhibitor (SSRI) citalopram causes frontal cortex beta-receptor down-regulation; thus, increased 5-hydroxytryptophan (5-HT) availability can preserve beta-receptor down-regulation by NE-potentiating agents. In human depression, CRH–NE hyperactivation of the CRH–NE feed-forward system is implicated in sympathetic activation, hyperarousal, and anxiety. 5-HT reduction is implicated in depression, and an SSRI-mediated 5-HT increase may normalize beta-receptor down-regulation, offering, in prolonged stress, adaptive self-regulation against excessive CRH–NE activity [40]. In cattle, intravenous tryptophan administration attenuates cortisol secretion induced by the intracerebroventricular injection of NE [41].

2. Stress, Depressive Symptoms, T2D, and Our Hypothesis

We hypothesize that a group of depressed patients may have an underlying genetic predisposition to augmented, maladaptive hyperarousal and stress vulnerability activating and self-feeding the CRH–NE–CRH system, characterized by defective CRHR1 and high-normal CRH and NE levels, the latter triggering peripheral cortisol secretion, in the absence of a clear ACTH augmentation. Another theory, depending on the depressed patient subgroups, is that long-lasting chronic stress may be maintained by an enduring imbalance of the HPA axis via CRH and ACTH secretion and hypercortisolism. As the latter can also be triggered by central NE and peripheral adrenal catecholamine secretion, the two hypothesized mechanisms may overlap in some patients presenting with increased ACTH levels beyond increased CRH, NE, and cortisol levels.

Figure 1 illustrates these concepts for how stress and the HPA axis relate to T2D and depression. We hypothesize that receptor resistance of the CRH system can induce hypercortisolism: the CRH system is implicated in the response to depression and prolonged stress [30,32], and *CRH* SNPs are variants of depression risk [32]. Depressed and hypercortisolemic subjects have an attenuated ACTH response to CRH, thus potentially suggesting intact negative feedback. CRH infusion in healthy individuals induces hypercortisolism as in depression but via ACTH [42]. This difference suggests that in depression, hypercortisolism may be due to a defect in the CRHR receptor response with the hypersecretion of CRH and consequently of NE.

A significant cortisol response to a blunted ACTH response may also indicate that the adrenal glands hyper-respond to ACTH due to an ACTH receptor or melanocortin receptor 2 (MC2R) abnormality [43]. The most probable dynamics, however, would be the increase in central NE secretion, triggered by the limbic response to CRH [44]; in turn, NE stimulates the secretion of adrenal cortisol [41,45] and, through positive feedback, also the hypothalamic and limbic secretion of CRH, supporting the central hyperactivation of the HPA system [46,47]. This hypothetical mechanism fully fits with the strong correlation of plasma cortisol with cerebrospinal fluid (CSF) NE in depressed patients [48].

In depressed and control subjects, circadian variations of CSF NE and plasma cortisolemia are superimposable and correlate positively during the day. While healthy individuals have significantly negatively correlated plasma cortisol and CSF-CRH levels, depressed patients have significantly higher circadian CSF NE and plasma cortisol levels, but inappropriately "normal" plasma ACTH and CRH [44]. These studies compellingly suggest that upstream CRH receptor dysfunction may be a cause of depression and that downstream hypercortisolism may further feed into depression by altering the serotonin pathway [14], as well as increasing the risk of T2D and accounting, at least in part, for MDD-T2D comorbidity. The above-mentioned robust correlation of cortisolemia with CSF NE of depressed patients [48] points towards a persistent stress-response dysregulation in depression, independently from any conscious stress, and indicates a bidirectional mutual boosting link between the hyper-noradrenergic state and the hyperfunctioning HPA axis, each triggered and maintained by hypercortisolism through interactions at the central level and the peripheral adrenal level [48].

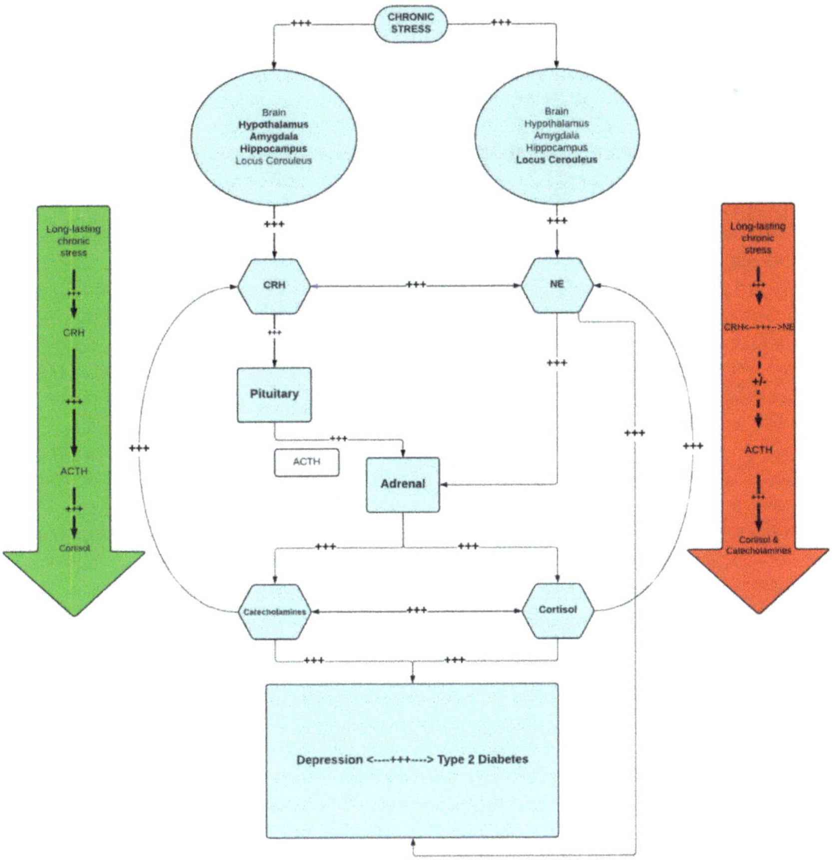

LEGEND:

- *Red Pathway* – Long-lasting chronic stress maintained by high normal CRH and NE levels. NE triggers peripheral cortisol secretion in the absence of a clear ACTH augmentation and peripheral catecholamine secretion.
  Green Pathway – Long-lasting chronic stress maintained by an enduring imbalance of the HPA axis, via CRH, and ACTH and cortisol secretion.
- *Light Blue Overlap* – Both the pathways may overlap in some patients presenting with increased ACTH levels, beyond increased CRH, NE, and cortisol and catecholamine levels.

Figure 1. CRH-NE-CRH Circuit and Hypothalamic-Pituitary-Adrenal Axis Implication in the Comorbidity of Depression and Type 2 Diabetes.

Increased cortisol and reduced HPA axis feedback are alterations present in both depression and T2D [49,50], while T2D, metabolic traits, and MDD are associated with hypercortisolemia [11,15]. The increase in cortisol due to chronic stress, according to our hypothesis, could also lead to T2D. However, anomalies in the feedback and activity of the HPA axis are characteristics found in aging [18].

Also, a potential mechanism may be related to maternal nutritional imbalances, which may permanently affect the offspring by altering the cortisol and sympathetic stress response. Recent studies showed that lower human birth weight—a marker of fetal undernutrition—is correlated in both children and adults to impaired sympathetic nervous system and HPA axis stress responses, which are further linked to depression and T2D [51].

A genetic predisposition to HPA axis hyperactivation and hypercortisolemia could induce glucose intolerance [52], metabolic abnormalities, and depressive symptoms [11]. Various HPA axis receptor genes are related to metabolic alterations [43,53]. Furthermore, hypercortisolemia causes an alteration in serotonergic transmission, which is one of the determinants of depression [12].

To support our hypothesis, studies have shown that CRH injected in rats' brains increases plasmatic epinephrine, NE, and glucagon, leading to hyperglycemia. Of interest, CRH-induced hyperglycemia is present even with hypophysectomy or adrenalectomy; thus, this disease model is not due to the HPA axis but to CRH enhancing both epinephrine and NE secretion [44]. Of note, in congenital adrenal hyperplasia due to 21-hydroxylase deficiency, cortisol precursors are increasingly secreted with ACTH stimulation, indicating impaired cortisol production and compensating increased hypothalamic CRH secretion. In a study, carriers of 21-hydroxylase deficiency (i.e., parents of children with classical congenital adrenal hyperplasia) showed significantly higher state-anxiety scores than healthy subjects, and their mean 24 h urinary free cortisol excretion was significantly associated with psychoticism and paranoid ideation, thereby making them susceptible to anxiety disorders [54].

Of note, the prevalence of subclinical hypercortisolism was found to be significantly higher in hospitalized patients with T2D compared to controls, with 7% of T2D statistically attributable to subclinical hypercortisolism, and subclinical hypercortisolism was significantly related to severe T2D, defined by the presence of insulin treatment, hypertension, and dyslipidemia [55].

A study reported that 30% of T2D patients have significantly elevated basal plasma cortisol levels, higher cortisol levels after a dexamethasone (DEX) suppression test, and a larger response to CRH, without significantly higher ACTH levels. The increased responsiveness to CRH, together with reduced suppression after DEX, may indicate dysfunctional negative HPA axis feedback in T2D. An exaggerated HPA response to the CRH test is also present among depressed patients and the elderly [56,57] and could imply impaired feedback due to a hippocampal glucocorticoid receptor deficit [58]. Of interest, we identified familial linkage to and association with T2D and MDD in the glucocorticoid receptor (*GR* or *NR3C1*) gene [59]. However, the above-mentioned findings could also be due to—at least in some patients—variants in the melanocortin receptor 2 (*MC2R*) gene, which might increase responsiveness to ACTH; in fact, we reported *MC2R* linkage and association to/with T2D; one variant was the opposite allele of the variant causing glucocorticoid deficiency syndrome [60].

However, in T2D, even though cortisol is increased, plasma ACTH values are higher, but not significantly compared to controls without T2D. Even considering the wide variability in ACTH, hypercortisolemia without a significant increase in ACTH suggests a peripheral rather than central alteration, such as hyperactivity of the CRH–NE system.

Among the T2D subjects, cortisol levels during the DEX/CRH test are also significantly positively associated with Hba1c, independent of age, body mass index, hypertension, and dyslipidemia [50].

The diurnal rhythm of cortisol shows a peak 30 min after awakening (cortisol awakening response [CAR]) and a decline during the day with a nadir at midnight [61]. Of note, in healthy subjects, increased fasting cortisolemia at 9 am is associated with glycemia at fasting and 2 h status post oral glucose tolerance test, triglyceride levels, and systolic blood pressure [62], and 24 h urinary free cortisol is associated with insulin resistance, visceral obesity, and lipids [63].

Long-lasting cortisol excess of Cushing's syndrome as well as glucocorticoid treatment cause T2D [64,65]. A flatter diurnal cortisol slope is associated with T2D-related traits (e.g., central adiposity [66], increased cardiovascular disease risk [67]). However, the reported T2D associations with diurnal cortisol patterns are inconsistent. In 3508 adults (50–74 years), inclusive of 238 T2D patients, T2D was associated with a flatter diurnal cortisol slope decline and higher bedtime cortisol, independently from several covariates. However, no association was found between T2D and morning cortisol or CAR [68]. In this study, T2D patients showed a flatter diurnal cortisol slope than healthy subjects, even after adjusting for several potential confounders (e.g., fatigue, BMI, smoking, age, sex, waking time, late saliva collection, employment grade, history of coronary artery disease, cardiovascular medication). A flatter diurnal cortisol slope can be due to low cortisol values on waking or high cortisol values in the evening. T2D patients, compared to control subjects, on average lack significantly higher cortisol waking levels and also have significantly higher bedtime cortisol levels, even after adjusting for covariates [68]. As raised late-night cortisol levels are diagnostic for Cushing's syndrome [69], to exclude Cushing's syndrome patients, subjects with very high cortisol were excluded. Obesity, which is strongly associated with Cushing's syndrome [68], is not driving the results. High late-night salivary cortisol values are reported in T2D without Cushing's syndrome in other studies as well [70]. Also, feelings of tension and anger are associated with flatter diurnal cortisol rhythms, primarily due to their association with higher evening cortisol [71].

Another study showed that T2D patients, compared to healthy subjects, have smaller hippocampal volumes and show a blunted CAR [72]. A study showed that adolescents with insulin resistance have a blunted CAR, smaller hippocampal volumes, and greater frontal lobe atrophy, as compared to control subjects. A smaller CAR is related to higher BMI, associated with higher fasting insulinemia, which is *per se* associated with smaller hippocampal volume and greater frontal lobe atrophy. Thus, HPA impairment may impact brain structures via metabolic abnormalities [73].

Computed tomography (CT) evaluating the adrenal volume in obese patients with and without T2D reports that total adrenal volume is significantly higher in T2D patients versus control subjects and that visceral fat, visceral fat/subcutaneous fat ratio, and total adrenal volume are highly correlated in all subjects tested. These data suggest that visceral obesity, T2D, and enlarged adrenal glands are associated and support that the hypothesized HPA axis hyperactivation in obese subjects may be involved in T2D pathogenesis [74].

A hereditary predisposition to dysfunction of the HPA axis could therefore induce CRH-noradrenergic system abnormalities, causally contributing to depression, T2D, and depression–T2D comorbidity.

3. *CRHR1* Genetic Studies

CRHR1 is an adenylate cyclase-associated membrane receptor and is highly expressed in the neocortex, hippocampus, amygdala, cerebellum, and anterior pituitary gland. *Crhr1* knockout mice show adrenal medullary atrophy, suggesting the peripheral importance of Crhr1 in catecholamine biosynthesis, independent of the central activation of the HPA axis and SNS. Dysfunctional CRHR1 receptors may therefore be responsible for reinforcing the positive feedback of CRH and SNS, peripherally and centrally, with hypersecretion of CRH, bypassing the negative feedback of glucocorticoid receptors. *Crhr1* knockout mice have a depressed HPA axis, low plasma corticosteronemia, and a decreased ACTH and corticosterone response to stress due to marked agenesis of the adrenal glands due to ACTH insufficiency; agenesis is in fact avoided by the administration of ACTH. *CRHR1* variants, therefore, can reduce ACTH release, while catecholamines can positively modulate CRH-dependent ACTH secretion. *Crhr1* knockout mice show, in addition to a reduced stress response, reduced anxious behavior and increased exploratory activity [28,75]. CRHR1 is therefore fundamental in the development of the HPA axis and in the modulation of the anxiety response and behavior, but, in mice, Crhr1 is not essential for the formation of corticotrope cells or for ACTH production in basal conditions [28].

In a study of *Crhr1* knockout mice, Crhr1 appeared to have a bivalent action: its activation in the forebrain glutaminergic system promotes anxious behaviors, whereas in the mesencephalic dopaminergic system, it reduces them. In fact, in mice, while *Crhr1* knockout in prosencephalic glutaminergic neurons leads to reduced anxious behavior and alters neurotransmission in the amygdala and hippocampus, *Crhr1* knockout in mesencephalic dopaminergic neurons leads to the opposite behavior and reduces the release of dopamine by the prefrontal cortex. Thus, CRHR1 may play a bidirectional role in anxiety, as an imbalance between CRHR1-controlled anxiogenic glutamatergic and anxiolytic dopaminergic systems may lead to emotional impairments [76].

Other studies have reported that in young rhesus monkeys, *CRHR1* variants correlate with anxious behavior and brain metabolic activity. Rhesus monkeys' trait anxiety is similar to the childhood risk trait underlying human anxiety and depression. Single nucleotide polymorphisms (SNPs) of *CRHR1* modulate metabolic activity in the intraparietal sulcus, precuneus, amygdala, and anterior hippocampus, thereby influencing key neural structures of anxious behavior and contributing to psychopathology triggered by childhood trauma [77].

Further work has confirmed that the *CRHR1* gene is associated with depression, increasing the risk of depression after childhood trauma [37,78] and the risk of suicide in males [79]. Three main haplotypes depend on the *CRHR1* SNPs rs7209436, rs4792887, and rs110402 (i.e., CCG, 35.3%, CTG, 32.9%, TCA, 30.4%). The *CRHR1*-rs110402 or TCA haplotype contributes to MDD in child abuse cases [80]. MDD significantly associates with the allelic and genotypic rs242939 SNP and the GGT haplotype formed by the rs1876828, rs242939, and rs242941 alleles [81]. Very anxious subjects suffering from MDD who are homozygous carriers of the GAG haplotype are more sensitive to the antidepressant fluoxetine or desipramine; even highly anxious MDD patients and carriers of the rs242941 G/G genotype associated with the homozygous GAG haplotype have a high response to fluoxetine [82,83].

We previously found no studies on human *CRHR1* and T2D. We were the first to report the role of *CRHR1* in familial T2D, familial MDD, and T2D–MDD [84]. Of note, the *CRHR1* 17q12 locus is associated with T2D [85] and metabolic syndrome [86]. Pancreatic beta cells express CRHR1 on their surface, which stimulates cell proliferation and insulin secretion in a glucose-dependent manner [87]. An alteration in the CRHR1 receptor could therefore be a cause of hyperglycemia and T2D.

4. *CRHR2* Genetic Studies

The *CRHR2* gene is expressed in the brain; *Crhr2* knockout mice show reduced stress response [88], hypersensitivity to stress, and anxiety behavior [89,90]. The CRHR2 receptor has urocortins 1, 2, and 3 as ligands [91]. Studies with urocortin analogues have highlighted a strategic role of CRHR2 in glucose homeostasis: it reduces insulin secretion and inhibits gastric emptying and glucose absorption [92] both directly and indirectly through the strengthening of mechano-sensitive gastric vagal afferents [93]; furthermore, the CRHR2 receptor is abundantly expressed at the muscle level and increases insulin sensitivity in this tissue [94,95]. Male *Crhr2* knockout mice develop hepatic steatosis and metabolic syndrome [96]. A few studies have investigated the potential involvement of *CRHR2* in depressive disorders, finding a positive correlation of some alleles with MDD [97] or its mediated resistance to pharmacological treatment [98]. The *CRHR2* 7p21-p15 locus is, however, related to T2D [99,100]; blood glucose, high-density lipoprotein, and triglyceride values [101]; MDD [102]; and bipolar disorder [103,104]. Indeed, bipolar disorder and depression share various genes [105]. *Crhr2* knockout mice have arterial hypertension and reduced sustained hypophagia [88]; thus, *CRHR2* variants might contribute to hypertension and obesity. A recent study showed an association between *CRHR2* SNPs and T2D in a body of pooled genotypic data from 32 genome-wide association studies of European ancestry (GWAS) [106]. We were the first to report the *CRHR2* linkage and association with familial T2D, MDD, and T2D–MDD comorbidity [107].

5. Conclusions

HPA axis dysregulation may contribute to T2D and MDD, alone or in combination, due to dysfunctional CRHR1 and CRHR2 receptors. According to our hypothesis, an impaired function of CRHR1 would fuel the CRH–NE–CRH circuit, supporting the hyperactivation of the HPA axis with increased secretion of NE and cortisol, the latter especially implicated in metabolic and depressive disorders. The CRHR2 receptor also appears to be related to metabolic and depressive disorders. Reduced functioning of CRHR2 could contribute to the pathogenesis of T2D and MDD. Future studies to investigate our hypothesis are warranted, including genetic studies of the *CRHR1* and *CRHR2* genes in various ethnicities.

Author Contributions: C.G. conceived, drafted, and supervised the manuscript. M.P. co-drafted and critically revised the manuscript. T.T.P., L.d.B.-P. and P.G. critically revised the manuscript and implemented manuscript sections. All authors have read and agreed to the published version of the manuscript.

Funding: This publication was supported in part with the funds received under Nebraska Laws 2021, LB 380, Section 109 awarded to C.G. (PI), Creighton University School of Medicine, through the Nebraska Department of Health & Human Services (DHHS). Its contents represent the views of the authors and do not necessarily represent the official views of the State of Nebraska or DHHS.

Conflicts of Interest: The authors declare no conflicts of interest.

References

1. World Health Organization. Depressive Disorder (Depression). 2023. Available online: https://www.who.int/news-room/fact-sheets/detail/depression (accessed on 3 March 2024).
2. Malhi, G.S.; Mann, J.J. Depression. *Lancet* **2018**, *392*, 2299–2312. [CrossRef] [PubMed]
3. IDF Diabetes Atlas. Diabetes around the World in 2021. Available online: https://diabetesatlas.org/#:~:text=Diabetes%20around%20the%20world%20in%202021:,-%20and%20middle-income%20countries (accessed on 22 May 2024).
4. Yip, W.C.Y.; Sequeira, I.R.; Plank, L.D.; Poppitt, S.D. Prevalence of Pre-Diabetes across Ethnicities: A Review of Impaired Fasting Glucose (IFG) and Impaired Glucose Tolerance (IGT) for Classification of Dysglycaemia. *Nutrients* **2017**, *9*, 1273. [CrossRef] [PubMed]
5. Mezuk, B.; Eaton, W.W.; Albrecht, S.; Golden, S.H. Depression and type 2 diabetes over the lifespan: A meta-analysis. *Diabetes Care* **2008**, *31*, 2383–2390. [CrossRef] [PubMed]
6. Demakakos, P.; Pierce, M.B.; Hardy, R. Depressive symptoms and risk of type 2 diabetes in a national sample of middle-aged and older adults: The English longitudinal study of aging. *Diabetes Care* **2010**, *33*, 792–797. [CrossRef] [PubMed]
7. Rustad, J.K.; Musselman, D.L.; Nemeroff, C.B. The relationship of depression and diabetes: Pathophysiological and treatment implications. *Psychoneuroendocrinology* **2011**, *36*, 1276–1286. [CrossRef] [PubMed]
8. Messaoud, A.; Mensi, R.; Douki, W.; Neffati, F.; Najjar, M.F.; Gobbi, G.; Valtorta, F.; Gaha, L.; Comai, S. Reduced peripheral availability of tryptophan and increased activation of the kynurenine pathway and cortisol correlate with major depression and suicide. *World J. Biol. Psychiatry* **2018**, *20*, 1–9. [CrossRef]
9. Fakhoury, M. Revisiting the Serotonin Hypothesis: Implications for Major Depressive Disorders. *Mol. Neurobiol.* **2016**, *53*, 2778–2786. [CrossRef] [PubMed]
10. Mangold, D.; Marino, E.; Javors, M. The cortisol awakening response predicts subclinical depressive symptomatology in Mexican American adults. *J. Psychiatr. Res.* **2011**, *45*, 902–909. [CrossRef] [PubMed]
11. Vogelzangs, N.; Suthers, K.; Ferrucci, L.; Simonsick, E.M.; Ble, A.; Schrager, M.; Bandinelli, S.; Lauretani, F.; Giannelli, S.V.; Penninx, B.W. Hypercortisolemic depression is associated with the metabolic syndrome in late-life. *Psychoneuroendocrinology* **2007**, *32*, 151–159. [CrossRef]
12. Pompili, M.; Serafini, G.; Innamorati, M.; Moller-Leimkuhler, A.M.; Giupponi, G.; Girardi, P.; Tatarelli, R.; Lester, D. The hypothalamic-pituitary-adrenal axis and serotonin abnormalities: A selective overview for the implications of suicide prevention. *Eur. Arch. Psychiatry Clin. Neurosci.* **2010**, *260*, 583–600. [CrossRef]
13. Yokoyama, K.; Yamada, T.; Mitani, H.; Yamada, S.; Pu, S.; Yamanashi, T.; Matsumura, H.; Nakagome, K.; Kaneko, K. Relationship between hypothalamic-pituitary-adrenal axis dysregulation and insulin resistance in elderly patients with depression. *Psychiatry Res.* **2015**, *226*, 494–498. [CrossRef] [PubMed]

14. Feng, G.; Kang, C.; Yuan, J.; Zhang, Y.; Wei, Y.; Xu, L.; Zhou, F.; Fan, X.; Yang, J. Neuroendocrine abnormalities associated with untreated first episode patients with major depressive disorder and bipolar disorder. *Psychoneuroendocrinology* **2019**, *107*, 119–123. [CrossRef] [PubMed]
15. Joseph, J.J.; Golden, S.H. Cortisol dysregulation: The bidirectional link between stress, depression, and type 2 diabetes mellitus. *Ann. N. Y. Acad. Sci.* **2017**, *1391*, 20–34. [CrossRef] [PubMed]
16. Cataldo Bascunan, L.R.; Lyons, C.; Bennet, H.; Artner, I.; Fex, M. Serotonergic regulation of insulin secretion. *Acta Physiol.* **2019**, *225*, e13101. [CrossRef] [PubMed]
17. Bennet, H.; Balhuizen, A.; Medina, A.; Dekker Nitert, M.; Ottosson Laakso, E.; Essen, S.; Spegel, P.; Storm, P.; Krus, U.; Wierup, N.; et al. Altered serotonin (5-HT) 1D and 2A receptor expression may contribute to defective insulin and glucagon secretion in human type 2 diabetes. *Peptides* **2015**, *71*, 113–120. [CrossRef]
18. Bjorntorp, P. Alterations in the ageing corticotropic stress-response axis. *Novartis Found. Symp.* **2002**, *242*, 46–58; discussion 58–65.
19. Lehrer, H.M.; Dubois, S.K.; Maslowsky, J.; Laudenslager, M.L.; Steinhardt, M.A. Hair cortisol concentration and glycated hemoglobin in African American adults. *Psychoneuroendocrinology* **2016**, *72*, 212–218. [CrossRef] [PubMed]
20. Sunena; Mishra, D.N. Stress Etiology of Type 2 Diabetes. *Curr. Diabetes Rev.* **2022**, *18*, e240222201413. [CrossRef] [PubMed]
21. Sharma, K.; Akre, S.; Chakole, S.; Wanjari, M.B. Stress-Induced Diabetes: A Review. *Cureus* **2022**, *14*, e29142. [CrossRef]
22. Koumantarou Malisiova, E.; Mourikis, I.; Darviri, C.; Nicolaides, N.C.; Zervas, I.M.; Papageorgiou, C.; Chrousos, G.P. Hair cortisol concentrations in mental disorders: A systematic review. *Physiol. Behav.* **2021**, *229*, 113244. [CrossRef]
23. Lisco, G.; Giagulli, V.A.; De Pergola, G.; Guastamacchia, E.; Jirillo, E.; Vitale, E.; Triggiani, V. Chronic Stress as a Risk Factor for Type 2 Diabetes: Endocrine, Metabolic, and Immune Implications. *Endocr. Metab. Immune Disord. Drug Targets* **2024**, *24*, 321–332. [CrossRef] [PubMed]
24. Mosili, P.; Mkhize, B.C.; Sibiya, N.H.; Ngubane, P.S.; Khathi, A. Review of the direct and indirect effects of hyperglycemia on the HPA axis in T2DM and the co-occurrence of depression. *BMJ Open Diabetes Res. Care* **2024**, *12*, e003218. [CrossRef] [PubMed]
25. Herman, J.P.; McKlveen, J.M.; Ghosal, S.; Kopp, B.; Wulsin, A.; Makinson, R.; Scheimann, J.; Myers, B. Regulation of the Hypothalamic-Pituitary-Adrenocortical Stress Response. *Compr. Physiol.* **2016**, *6*, 603–621. [CrossRef] [PubMed]
26. Bedont, J.L.; Blackshaw, S. Constructing the suprachiasmatic nucleus: A watchmaker's perspective on the central clockworks. *Front. Syst. Neurosci.* **2015**, *9*, 74. [CrossRef] [PubMed]
27. Vale, W.; Vaughan, J.; Perrin, M. Corticotropin-Releasing Factor (CRF) Family of Ligands and Their Receptors. *Endocrinol.* **1997**, *7*, 3S–9S. [CrossRef]
28. Smith, G.W.; Aubry, J.M.; Dellu, F.; Contarino, A.; Bilezikjian, L.M.; Gold, L.H.; Chen, R.; Marchuk, Y.; Hauser, C.; Bentley, C.A.; et al. Corticotropin releasing factor receptor 1-deficient mice display decreased anxiety, impaired stress response, and aberrant neuroendocrine development. *Neuron* **1998**, *20*, 1093–1102. [CrossRef]
29. Oler, J.A.; Fox, A.S.; Shelton, S.E.; Rogers, J.; Dyer, T.D.; Davidson, R.J.; Shelledy, W.; Oakes, T.R.; Blangero, J.; Kalin, N.H. Amygdalar and hippocampal substrates of anxious temperament differ in their heritability. *Nature* **2010**, *466*, 864–868. [CrossRef]
30. Keck, M.E. Corticotropin-releasing factor, vasopressin and receptor systems in depression and anxiety. *Amino Acids* **2006**, *31*, 241–250. [CrossRef]
31. Naert, G.; Ixart, G.; Maurice, T.; Tapia-Arancibia, L.; Givalois, L. Brain-derived neurotrophic factor and hypothalamic-pituitary-adrenal axis adaptation processes in a depressive-like state induced by chronic restraint stress. *Mol. Cell Neurosci.* **2011**, *46*, 55–66. [CrossRef]
32. Bao, A.M.; Swaab, D.F. Corticotropin-releasing hormone and arginine vasopressin in depression focus on the human postmortem hypothalamus. *Vitam. Horm.* **2010**, *82*, 339–365. [CrossRef]
33. Gold, P.W. Endocrine Factors in Key Structural and Intracellular Changes in Depression. *Trends Endocrinol. Metab.* **2021**, *32*, 212–223. [CrossRef] [PubMed]
34. Brand, S.; Wilhelm, F.H.; Kossowsky, J.; Holsboer-Trachsler, E.; Schneider, S. Children suffering from separation anxiety disorder (SAD) show increased HPA axis activity compared to healthy controls. *J. Psychiatr. Res.* **2010**, *45*, 452–459. [CrossRef] [PubMed]
35. Kolber, B.J.; Boyle, M.P.; Wieczorek, L.; Kelley, C.L.; Onwuzurike, C.C.; Nettles, S.A.; Vogt, S.K.; Muglia, L.J. Transient early-life forebrain corticotropin-releasing hormone elevation causes long-lasting anxiogenic and despair-like changes in mice. *J. Neurosci.* **2010**, *30*, 2571–2581. [CrossRef] [PubMed]
36. Chapman, D.P.; Whitfield, C.L.; Felitti, V.J.; Dube, S.R.; Edwards, V.J.; Anda, R.F. Adverse childhood experiences and the risk of depressive disorders in adulthood. *J. Affect. Disord.* **2004**, *82*, 217–225. [CrossRef] [PubMed]
37. Heim, C.; Newport, D.J.; Mletzko, T.; Miller, A.H.; Nemeroff, C.B. The link between childhood trauma and depression: Insights from HPA axis studies in humans. *Psychoneuroendocrinology* **2008**, *33*, 693–710. [CrossRef] [PubMed]
38. Kopin, I.J.; Lake, R.C.; Ziegler, M. Plasma levels of norepinephrine. *Ann. Intern. Med.* **1978**, *88*, 671–680. [CrossRef] [PubMed]
39. Lemche, E.; Giampietro, V.P.; Surguladze, S.A.; Amaro, E.J.; Andrew, C.M.; Williams, S.C.; Brammer, M.J.; Lawrence, N.; Maier, M.A.; Russell, T.A.; et al. Human attachment security is mediated by the amygdala: Evidence from combined fMRI and psychophysiological measures. *Hum. Brain Mapp.* **2006**, *27*, 623–635. [CrossRef] [PubMed]
40. Asakura, M.; Nagashima, H.; Fujii, S.; Sasuga, Y.; Misonoh, A.; Hasegawa, H.; Osada, K. Influences of chronic stress on central nervous systems. *Nihon Shinkei Seishin Yakurigaku Zasshi* **2000**, *20*, 97–105. [PubMed]
41. Sutoh, M.; Kasuya, E.; Yayou, K.; Ohtani, F.; Kobayashi, Y. Intravenous tryptophan administration attenuates cortisol secretion induced by intracerebroventricular injection of noradrenaline. *Anim. Sci. J.* **2016**, *87*, 266–270. [CrossRef]

42. Gold, P.W.; Kling, M.A.; Khan, I.; Calabrese, J.R.; Kalogeras, K.; Post, R.M.; Avgerinos, P.C.; Loriaux, D.L.; Chrousos, G.P. Corticotropin releasing hormone: Relevance to normal physiology and to the pathophysiology and differential diagnosis of hypercortisolism and adrenal insufficiency. *Adv. Biochem. Psychopharmacol.* **1987**, *43*, 183–200.
43. Clark, A.J.; Metherell, L.A. Mechanisms of disease: The adrenocorticotropin receptor and disease. *Nat. Clin. Pract. Endocrinol. Metab.* **2006**, *2*, 282–290. [CrossRef] [PubMed]
44. Brown, M.R.; Fisher, L.A.; Spiess, J.; Rivier, C.; Rivier, J.; Vale, W. Corticotropin-releasing factor: Actions on the sympathetic nervous system and metabolism. *Endocrinology* **1982**, *111*, 928–931. [CrossRef] [PubMed]
45. Walker, S.W.; Lightly, E.R.; Milner, S.W.; Williams, B.C. Catecholamine stimulation of cortisol secretion by 3-day primary cultures of purified zona fasciculata/reticularis cells isolated from bovine adrenal cortex. *Mol. Cell Endocrinol.* **1988**, *57*, 139–147. [CrossRef] [PubMed]
46. Calogero, A.E.; Gallucci, W.T.; Chrousos, G.P.; Gold, P.W. Catecholamine effects upon rat hypothalamic corticotropin-releasing hormone secretion in vitro. *J. Clin. Investig.* **1988**, *82*, 839–846. [CrossRef]
47. Al-Damluji, S.; Perry, L.; Tomlin, S.; Bouloux, P.; Grossman, A.; Rees, L.H.; Besser, G.M. Alpha-adrenergic stimulation of corticotropin secretion by a specific central mechanism in man. *Neuroendocrinology* **1987**, *45*, 68–76. [CrossRef] [PubMed]
48. Wong, M.L.; Kling, M.A.; Munson, P.J.; Listwak, S.; Licinio, J.; Prolo, P.; Karp, B.; McCutcheon, I.E.; Geracioti, T.D., Jr.; DeBellis, M.D.; et al. Pronounced and sustained central hypernoradrenergic function in major depression with melancholic features: Relation to hypercortisolism and corticotropin-releasing hormone. *Proc. Natl. Acad. Sci. USA* **2000**, *97*, 325–330. [CrossRef] [PubMed]
49. Zunszain, P.A.; Anacker, C.; Cattaneo, A.; Carvalho, L.A.; Pariante, C.M. Glucocorticoids, cytokines and brain abnormalities in depression. *Prog. Neuropsychopharmacol. Biol. Psychiatry* **2010**, *35*, 722–729. [CrossRef]
50. Bruehl, H.; Rueger, M.; Dziobek, I.; Sweat, V.; Tirsi, A.; Javier, E.; Arentoft, A.; Wolf, O.T.; Convit, A. Hypothalamic-pituitary-adrenal axis dysregulation and memory impairments in type 2 diabetes. *J. Clin. Endocrinol. Metab.* **2007**, *92*, 2439–2445. [CrossRef]
51. Krishnaveni, G.V.; Srinivasan, K. Maternal Nutrition and Offspring Stress Response-Implications for Future Development of Non-Communicable Disease: A Perspective from India. *Front. Psychiatry* **2019**, *10*, 795. [CrossRef]
52. Pivonello, R.; De Leo, M.; Vitale, P.; Cozzolino, A.; Simeoli, C.; De Martino, M.C.; Lombardi, G.; Colao, A. Pathophysiology of diabetes mellitus in Cushing's syndrome. *Neuroendocrinology* **2010**, *92* (Suppl. S1), S77–S81. [CrossRef]
53. Qi, L.; Kraft, P.; Hunter, D.J.; Hu, F.B. The common obesity variant near MC4R gene is associated with higher intakes of total energy and dietary fat, weight change and diabetes risk in women. *Hum. Mol. Genet.* **2008**, *17*, 3502–3508. [CrossRef] [PubMed]
54. Kyritsi, E.M.; Koltsida, G.; Farakla, I.; Papanikolaou, A.; Critselis, E.; Mantzou, E.; Zoumakis, E.; Kolaitis, G.; Chrousos, G.P.; Charmandari, E. Psychological vulnerability to stress in carriers of congenital adrenal hyperplasia due to 21-hydroxylase deficiency. *Hormones* **2017**, *16*, 42–53. [CrossRef] [PubMed]
55. Chiodini, I.; Torlontano, M.; Scillitani, A.; Arosio, M.; Bacci, S.; Di Lembo, S.; Epaminonda, P.; Augello, G.; Enrini, R.; Ambrosi, B.; et al. Association of subclinical hypercortisolism with type 2 diabetes mellitus: A case-control study in hospitalized patients. *Eur. J. Endocrinol.* **2005**, *153*, 837–844. [CrossRef]
56. Heuser, I.; Yassouridis, A.; Holsboer, F. The combined dexamethasone/CRH test: A refined laboratory test for psychiatric disorders. *J. Psychiatr. Res.* **1994**, *28*, 341–356. [CrossRef]
57. Heuser, I.J.; Gotthardt, U.; Schweiger, U.; Schmider, J.; Lammers, C.H.; Dettling, M.; Holsboer, F. Age-associated changes of pituitary-adrenocortical hormone regulation in humans: Importance of gender. *Neurobiol. Aging* **1994**, *15*, 227–231. [CrossRef]
58. Heuser, I.; Lammers, C.H. Stress and the brain. *Neurobiol. Aging* **2003**, *24* (Suppl. S1), S69–S76; discussion S81–S62. [CrossRef]
59. Amin, M.; Syed, S.; Wu, R.; Postolache, T.T.; Gragnoli, C. Familial Linkage and Association of the NR3C1 Gene with Type 2 Diabetes and Depression Comorbidity. *Int. J. Mol. Sci.* **2022**, *23*, 11951. [CrossRef] [PubMed]
60. Amin, M.; Ott, J.; Wu, R.; Postolache, T.T.; Gragnoli, C. Implication of Melanocortin Receptor Genes in the Familial Comorbidity of Type 2 Diabetes and Depression. *Int. J. Mol. Sci.* **2022**, *23*, 8350. [CrossRef]
61. Adam, E.K.; Kumari, M. Assessing salivary cortisol in large-scale, epidemiological research. *Psychoneuroendocrinology* **2009**, *34*, 1423–1436. [CrossRef]
62. Phillips, D.I.; Barker, D.J.; Fall, C.H.; Seckl, J.R.; Whorwood, C.B.; Wood, P.J.; Walker, B.R. Elevated plasma cortisol concentrations: A link between low birth weight and the insulin resistance syndrome? *J. Clin. Endocrinol. Metab.* **1998**, *83*, 757–760. [CrossRef]
63. Misra, M.; Bredella, M.A.; Tsai, P.; Mendes, N.; Miller, K.K.; Klibanski, A. Lower growth hormone and higher cortisol are associated with greater visceral adiposity, intramyocellular lipids, and insulin resistance in overweight girls. *Am. J. Physiol. Endocrinol. Metab.* **2008**, *295*, E385–E392. [CrossRef]
64. Newell-Price, J.; Bertagna, X.; Grossman, A.B.; Nieman, L.K. Cushing's syndrome. *Lancet* **2006**, *367*, 1605–1617. [CrossRef]
65. Clore, J.N.; Thurby-Hay, L. Glucocorticoid-induced hyperglycemia. *Endocr. Pract.* **2009**, *15*, 469–474. [CrossRef]
66. Kumari, M.; Chandola, T.; Brunner, E.; Kivimaki, M. A nonlinear relationship of generalized and central obesity with diurnal cortisol secretion in the Whitehall II study. *J. Clin. Endocrinol. Metab.* **2010**, *95*, 4415–4423. [CrossRef]
67. Kumari, M.; Shipley, M.; Stafford, M.; Kivimaki, M. Association of diurnal patterns in salivary cortisol with all-cause and cardiovascular mortality: Findings from the Whitehall II study. *J. Clin. Endocrinol. Metab.* **2011**, *96*, 1478–1485. [CrossRef]
68. Hackett, R.A.; Steptoe, A.; Kumari, M. Association of diurnal patterns in salivary cortisol with type 2 diabetes in the Whitehall II study. *J. Clin. Endocrinol. Metab.* **2014**, *99*, 4625–4631. [CrossRef]

69. Carroll, T.; Raff, H.; Findling, J.W. Late-night salivary cortisol for the diagnosis of Cushing syndrome: A meta-analysis. *Endocr. Pract.* **2009**, *15*, 335–342. [CrossRef]
70. Liu, H.; Bravata, D.M.; Cabaccan, J.; Raff, H.; Ryzen, E. Elevated late-night salivary cortisol levels in elderly male type 2 diabetic veterans. *Clin. Endocrinol.* **2005**, *63*, 642–649. [CrossRef]
71. Adam, E.K.; Hawkley, L.C.; Kudielka, B.M.; Cacioppo, J.T. Day-to-day dynamics of experience--cortisol associations in a population-based sample of older adults. *Proc. Natl. Acad. Sci. USA* **2006**, *103*, 17058–17063. [CrossRef]
72. Bruehl, H.; Wolf, O.T.; Convit, A. A blunted cortisol awakening response and hippocampal atrophy in type 2 diabetes mellitus. *Psychoneuroendocrinology* **2009**, *34*, 815–821. [CrossRef]
73. Ursache, A.; Wedin, W.; Tirsi, A.; Convit, A. Preliminary evidence for obesity and elevations in fasting insulin mediating associations between cortisol awakening response and hippocampal volumes and frontal atrophy. *Psychoneuroendocrinology* **2012**, *37*, 1270–1276. [CrossRef]
74. Godoy-Matos, A.F.; Vieira, A.R.; Moreira, R.O.; Coutinho, W.F.; Carraro, L.M.; Moreira, D.M.; Pasquali, R.; Meirelles, R.M. The potential role of increased adrenal volume in the pathophysiology of obesity-related type 2 diabetes. *J. Endocrinol. Investig.* **2006**, *29*, 159–163. [CrossRef]
75. Timpl, P.; Spanagel, R.; Sillaber, I.; Kresse, A.; Reul, J.M.; Stalla, G.K.; Blanquet, V.; Steckler, T.; Holsboer, F.; Wurst, W. Impaired stress response and reduced anxiety in mice lacking a functional corticotropin-releasing hormone receptor 1. *Nat. Genet.* **1998**, *19*, 162–166. [CrossRef]
76. Refojo, D.; Schweizer, M.; Kuehne, C.; Ehrenberg, S.; Thoeringer, C.; Vogl, A.M.; Dedic, N.; Schumacher, M.; von Wolff, G.; Avrabos, C.; et al. Glutamatergic and dopaminergic neurons mediate anxiogenic and anxiolytic effects of CRHR1. *Science* **2011**, *333*, 1903–1907. [CrossRef]
77. Rogers, J.; Raveendran, M.; Fawcett, G.L.; Fox, A.S.; Shelton, S.E.; Oler, J.A.; Cheverud, J.; Muzny, D.M.; Gibbs, R.A.; Davidson, R.J.; et al. CRHR1 genotypes, neural circuits and the diathesis for anxiety and depression. *Mol. Psychiatry* **2013**, *18*, 700–707. [CrossRef]
78. Heim, C.; Bradley, B.; Mletzko, T.C.; Deveau, T.C.; Musselman, D.L.; Nemeroff, C.B.; Ressler, K.J.; Binder, E.B. Effect of Childhood Trauma on Adult Depression and Neuroendocrine Function: Sex-Specific Moderation by CRH Receptor 1 Gene. *Front. Behav. Neurosci.* **2009**, *3*, 41. [CrossRef]
79. Wasserman, D.; Wasserman, J.; Rozanov, V.; Sokolowski, M. Depression in suicidal males: Genetic risk variants in the CRHR1 gene. *Genes. Brain Behav.* **2009**, *8*, 72–79. [CrossRef]
80. Ressler, K.J.; Bradley, B.; Mercer, K.B.; Deveau, T.C.; Smith, A.K.; Gillespie, C.F.; Nemeroff, C.B.; Cubells, J.F.; Binder, E.B. Polymorphisms in CRHR1 and the serotonin transporter loci: Gene x gene x environment interactions on depressive symptoms. *Am. J. Med. Genet. B Neuropsychiatr. Genet.* **2010**, *153B*, 812–824. [CrossRef]
81. Liu, Z.; Zhu, F.; Wang, G.; Xiao, Z.; Wang, H.; Tang, J.; Wang, X.; Qiu, D.; Liu, W.; Cao, Z.; et al. Association of corticotropin-releasing hormone receptor1 gene SNP and haplotype with major depression. *Neurosci. Lett.* **2006**, *404*, 358–362. [CrossRef]
82. Licinio, J.; O'Kirwan, F.; Irizarry, K.; Merriman, B.; Thakur, S.; Jepson, R.; Lake, S.; Tantisira, K.G.; Weiss, S.T.; Wong, M.L. Association of a corticotropin-releasing hormone receptor 1 haplotype and antidepressant treatment response in Mexican-Americans. *Mol. Psychiatry* **2004**, *9*, 1075–1082. [CrossRef]
83. Liu, Z.; Zhu, F.; Wang, G.; Xiao, Z.; Tang, J.; Liu, W.; Wang, H.; Liu, H.; Wang, X.; Wu, Y.; et al. Association study of corticotropin-releasing hormone receptor1 gene polymorphisms and antidepressant response in major depressive disorders. *Neurosci. Lett.* **2007**, *414*, 155–158. [CrossRef]
84. Del Bosque-Plata, L.; Amin, M.; Gonzalez-Ramirez, R.; Wu, R.; Postolache, T.T.; Vergare, M.; Gordon, D.; Gragnoli, C. LD block disorder-specific pleiotropic roles of novel CRHR1 in type 2 diabetes and depression disorder comorbidity. *Eur. Arch. Psychiatry Clin. Neurosci.* **2023**. [CrossRef]
85. Spurdle, A.B.; Thompson, D.J.; Ahmed, S.; Ferguson, K.; Healey, C.S.; O'Mara, T.; Walker, L.C.; Montgomery, S.B.; Dermitzakis, E.T.; Fahey, P.; et al. Genome-wide association study identifies a common variant associated with risk of endometrial cancer. *Nat. Genet.* **2011**, *43*, 451–454. [CrossRef]
86. Cheng, C.Y.; Lee, K.E.; Duggal, P.; Moore, E.L.; Wilson, A.F.; Klein, R.; Bailey-Wilson, J.E.; Klein, B.E. Genome-wide linkage analysis of multiple metabolic factors: Evidence of genetic heterogeneity. *Obesity* **2009**, *18*, 146–152. [CrossRef] [PubMed]
87. Huising, M.O.; van der Meulen, T.; Vaughan, J.M.; Matsumoto, M.; Donaldson, C.J.; Park, H.; Billestrup, N.; Vale, W.W. CRFR1 is expressed on pancreatic beta cells, promotes beta cell proliferation, and potentiates insulin secretion in a glucose-dependent manner. *Proc. Natl. Acad. Sci. USA* **2010**, *107*, 912–917. [CrossRef] [PubMed]
88. Coste, S.C.; Kesterson, R.A.; Heldwein, K.A.; Stevens, S.L.; Heard, A.D.; Hollis, J.H.; Murray, S.E.; Hill, J.K.; Pantely, G.A.; Hohimer, A.R.; et al. Abnormal adaptations to stress and impaired cardiovascular function in mice lacking corticotropin-releasing hormone receptor-2. *Nat. Genet.* **2000**, *24*, 403–409. [CrossRef]
89. Bale, T.L.; Contarino, A.; Smith, G.W.; Chan, R.; Gold, L.H.; Sawchenko, P.E.; Koob, G.F.; Vale, W.W.; Lee, K.F. Mice deficient for corticotropin-releasing hormone receptor-2 display anxiety-like behaviour and are hypersensitive to stress. *Nat. Genet.* **2000**, *24*, 410–414. [CrossRef]
90. Kishimoto, T.; Radulovic, J.; Radulovic, M.; Lin, C.R.; Schrick, C.; Hooshmand, F.; Hermanson, O.; Rosenfeld, M.G.; Spiess, J. Deletion of crhr2 reveals an anxiolytic role for corticotropin-releasing hormone receptor-2. *Nat. Genet.* **2000**, *24*, 415–419. [CrossRef] [PubMed]

91. Kuperman, Y.; Chen, A. Urocortins: Emerging metabolic and energy homeostasis perspectives. *Trends Endocrinol. Metab.* **2008**, *19*, 122–129. [CrossRef]
92. Grunddal, K.V.; Trammell, S.A.J.; Baech-Laursen, C.; Andersen, D.B.; Xu, S.F.S.; Andersen, H.; Gillum, M.P.; Ghiasi, S.M.; Novak, I.; Tyrberg, B.; et al. Opposing roles of the entero-pancreatic hormone urocortin-3 in glucose metabolism in rats. *Diabetologia* **2022**, *65*, 1018–1031. [CrossRef]
93. Li, H.; Page, A.J. Activation of CRF2 receptor increases gastric vagal afferent mechanosensitivity. *J. Neurophysiol.* **2019**, *122*, 2636–2642. [CrossRef] [PubMed]
94. Borg, M.L.; Massart, J.; Schonke, M.; De Castro Barbosa, T.; Guo, L.; Wade, M.; Alsina-Fernandez, J.; Miles, R.; Ryan, A.; Bauer, S.; et al. Modified UCN2 Peptide Acts as an Insulin Sensitizer in Skeletal Muscle of Obese Mice. *Diabetes* **2019**, *68*, 1403–1414. [CrossRef] [PubMed]
95. Jamieson, P.M.; Cleasby, M.E.; Kuperman, Y.; Morton, N.M.; Kelly, P.A.; Brownstein, D.G.; Mustard, K.J.; Vaughan, J.M.; Carter, R.N.; Hahn, C.N.; et al. Urocortin 3 transgenic mice exhibit a metabolically favourable phenotype resisting obesity and hyperglycaemia on a high-fat diet. *Diabetologia* **2011**, *54*, 2392–2403. [CrossRef] [PubMed]
96. Paruthiyil, S.; Hagiwara, S.I.; Kundassery, K.; Bhargava, A. Sexually dimorphic metabolic responses mediated by CRF(2) receptor during nutritional stress in mice. *Biol. Sex. Differ.* **2018**, *9*, 49. [CrossRef]
97. Ishitobi, Y.; Nakayama, S.; Yamaguchi, K.; Kanehisa, M.; Higuma, H.; Maruyama, Y.; Ninomiya, T.; Okamoto, S.; Tanaka, Y.; Tsuru, J.; et al. Association of CRHR1 and CRHR2 with major depressive disorder and panic disorder in a Japanese population. *Am. J. Med. Genet. B Neuropsychiatr. Genet.* **2012**, *159B*, 429–436. [CrossRef] [PubMed]
98. Papiol, S.; Arias, B.; Gasto, C.; Gutierrez, B.; Catalan, R.; Fananas, L. Genetic variability at HPA axis in major depression and clinical response to antidepressant treatment. *J. Affect. Disord.* **2007**, *104*, 83–90. [CrossRef] [PubMed]
99. Wiltshire, S.; Hattersley, A.T.; Hitman, G.A.; Walker, M.; Levy, J.C.; Sampson, M.; O'rahilly, S.; Frayling, T.M.; Bell, J.I.; Lathrop, G.M.; et al. A genomewide scan for loci predisposing to type 2 diabetes in a U.K. population (The Diabetes UK Warren 2 Repository): Analysis of 573 pedigrees provides independent replication of a susceptibility locus on chromosome 1q. *Am. J. Hum. Genet.* **2001**, *69*, 553–569. [CrossRef] [PubMed]
100. Leak, T.S.; Langefeld, C.D.; Keene, K.L.; Gallagher, C.J.; Lu, L.; Mychaleckyj, J.C.; Rich, S.S.; Freedman, B.I.; Bowden, D.W.; Sale, M.M. Chromosome 7p linkage and association study for diabetes related traits and type 2 diabetes in an African-American population enriched for nephropathy. *BMC Med. Genet.* **2010**, *11*, 22. [CrossRef] [PubMed]
101. Tam, C.H.; Lam, V.K.; So, W.Y.; Ma, R.C.; Chan, J.C.; Ng, M.C. Genome-wide linkage scan for factors of metabolic syndrome in a Chinese population. *BMC Genet.* **2010**, *11*, 14. [CrossRef]
102. Camp, N.J.; Lowry, M.R.; Richards, R.L.; Plenk, A.M.; Carter, C.; Hensel, C.H.; Abkevich, V.; Skolnick, M.H.; Shattuck, D.; Rowe, K.G.; et al. Genome-wide linkage analyses of extended Utah pedigrees identifies loci that influence recurrent, early-onset major depression and anxiety disorders. *Am. J. Med. Genet. B Neuropsychiatr. Genet.* **2005**, *135B*, 85–93. [CrossRef]
103. Kremeyer, B.; Garcia, J.; Muller, H.; Burley, M.W.; Herzberg, I.; Parra, M.V.; Duque, C.; Vega, J.; Montoya, P.; Lopez, M.C.; et al. Genome-wide linkage scan of bipolar disorder in a colombian population isolate replicates Loci on chromosomes 7p21-22, 1p31, 16p12 and 21q21-22 and identifies a novel locus on chromosome 12q. *Hum. Hered.* **2010**, *70*, 255–268. [CrossRef] [PubMed]
104. Hamshere, M.L.; Schulze, T.G.; Schumacher, J.; Corvin, A.; Owen, M.J.; Jamra, R.A.; Propping, P.; Maier, W.; Orozco y Diaz, G.; Mayoral, F.; et al. Mood-incongruent psychosis in bipolar disorder: Conditional linkage analysis shows genome-wide suggestive linkage at 1q32.3, 7p13 and 20q13.31. *Bipolar Disord.* **2009**, *11*, 610–620. [CrossRef] [PubMed]
105. Pregelj, P. Psychosis and depression—A neurobiological view. *Psychiatr. Danub.* **2009**, *21* (Suppl. S1), S102–S105.
106. Mahajan, A.; Taliun, D.; Thurner, M.; Robertson, N.R.; Torres, J.M.; Rayner, N.W.; Payne, A.J.; Steinthorsdottir, V.; Scott, R.A.; Grarup, N.; et al. Fine-mapping type 2 diabetes loci to single-variant resolution using high-density imputation and islet-specific epigenome maps. *Nat. Genet.* **2018**, *50*, 1505–1513. [CrossRef]
107. Amin, M.; Ott, J.; Gordon, D.; Wu, R.; Postolache, T.T.; Vergare, M.; Gragnoli, C. Comorbidity of Novel CRHR2 Gene Variants in Type 2 Diabetes and Depression. *Int. J. Mol. Sci.* **2022**, *23*, 9819. [CrossRef]

biomedicines

MDPI

Review

Role of Oxidative Stress in Tuberculosis Meningitis Infection in Diabetics

Inesa Navasardyan [1], Stephanie Yeganyan [1], Helena Nguyen [1], Payal Vaghashia [1], Selvakumar Subbian [2] and Vishwanath Venketaraman [1,*]

1 College of Osteopathic Medicine of the Pacific, Western University of Health Sciences, Pomona, CA 91766, USA; inesa.navasardyan@westernu.edu (I.N.); stephanie.yeganyan@westernu.edu (S.Y.); helena.nguyen@westernu.edu (H.N.); payal.vaghashia@westernu.edu (P.V.)

2 Public Health Research Center, New Jersey Medical School, Rutgers University, Newark, NJ 07103, USA; subbiase@njms.rutgers.edu

* Correspondence: vvenketaraman@westernu.edu; Tel.: +1-909-706-3736

Abstract: Tuberculosis meningitis (TBM) is a result of the invasion of the meninges with the bacilli of *Mycobacterium tuberculosis* (Mtb), leading to inflammation of the meninges around the brain or spinal cord. Oxidative stress occurs when the body's cells become overwhelmed with free radicals, particularly reactive oxygen species (ROS). ROS plays a significant role in the pathogenesis of TBM due to their toxic nature, resulting in impairment of the body's ability to fight off infection. ROS damages the endothelial cells and impairs the defense mechanisms of the blood–brain barrier (BBB), which contributes to CNS susceptibility to the bacteria causing TBM. Diabetes mellitus (DM) is a common condition that is characterized by the impairment of the hormone insulin, which is responsible for modulating blood glucose levels. The increased availability of glucose in individuals with diabetes results in increased cellular activity and metabolism, leading to heightened ROS production and, in turn, increased susceptibility to TBM. In this review, we summarize our current understanding of oxidative stress and its role in both TBM and DM. We further discuss how increased oxidative stress in DM can contribute to the likelihood of developing TBM and potential therapeutic approaches that may be of therapeutic value.

Keywords: *Mycobacterium tuberculosis*; tuberculosis meningitis; diabetes; oxidative stress

1. Introduction

Tuberculous meningitis (TBM) is an extrapulmonary manifestation of *Mycobacterium tuberculosis* (Mtb) infection of the central nervous system (CNS), resulting in non-suppurative inflammation of the meninges of the brain or spinal cord [1,2]. In humans, TBM is thought to be secondary to pulmonary tuberculosis (TB), the most predominant form of TB that begins with inhalation of Mtb into the lungs, where it infects alveolar macrophages, neutrophils, and dendritic cells, and continues to replicate [3]. Impaired anti-mycobacterial immune responses can lead to a severe form of cavitary TB that can further result in the dissemination of Mtb to the CNS [4]. Experimental models have proposed several mechanisms that promote entry of Mtb across the blood–brain barrier (BBB), allowing access to the CNS. Research shows that invasion of the BBB by Mtb results in cytoskeletal actin rearrangements of brain cells [5]. Furthermore, specific genes were found to be upregulated during Mtb invasion of the BBB, suggesting the role of possible Mtb virulence factors in transmission [5]. In addition, Mtb-infected macrophages can penetrate the BBB, with simultaneous elevation in the levels of vascular endothelial growth factor (VEGF), suggesting VEGF's possible role in Mtb invasion [6]. Although it is difficult to quantify the true global burden of TBM due to poor diagnostics and surveillance, research suggests that TBM contributes to about 5–10% of all extrapulmonary tuberculosis (TB) cases, and approximately 1–10% of TB patients develop TBM, strongly depending on the local prevalence [7]. Among the major factors that affect TBM diagnosis and prognosis are age and HIV prevalence. Over 80% of individuals with TBM were HIV-infected in a high HIV prevalence setting [8]. In children, a higher rate of TBM can be due to a weakened or immature immune system. Researchers found that 30% of children with TBM were in contact with an individual with pulmonary Mtb, in contrast to only 13% of adults with TBM [9]. Nevertheless, TBM remains the most fatal manifestation among all forms of tuberculosis, with a significant frequency of mortality and morbidity, reaching approximately 40% [10,11].

Diabetes mellitus (DM) is a chronic condition in which the body fails to produce and respond to insulin, resulting in elevated glucose levels [12]. Common characteristics of individuals living with DM include thirst, frequent urination, and weight loss. Type 1 diabetes (T1D) is characterized by cell-mediated auto-immune destruction of the pancreatic β-cells responsible for producing insulin. Conversely, type 2 diabetes (T2D) is attributed to insulin resistance and reduced insulin secretion [13]. Currently, there are 29.1 million individuals living with DM in the United States, with T2D being more prevalent than T1D [14]. Both T1D and T2D are associated with genetic predispositions and lifestyle factors [15]. Current treatment strategies for DM include lifestyle changes and insulin therapy, which works to mimic the body's innate insulin secretion. Depending on the stage of the disease, exogenous insulin can be used for both T1D and T2D and has been shown to reduce complications associated with DM, such as neuropathy, retinopathy, and kidney disease [16]. For patients suffering from T2D, lifestyle intervention and metformin, a medication that increases insulin sensitivity, were shown to decrease the incidence of diabetes by 58% and 31%, respectively [17]. More targeted approaches, such as exosome therapy, are being considered as future treatments for DM [18].

Oxidative stress occurs when there exists an imbalance between the production of reactive oxygen species (ROS) and the capacity of antioxidants to remove such toxic substances from the body [19]. ROS are natural byproducts of physiological processes in the body important for cell signaling; however, it is when the production of ROS exceeds the ability of the body to effectively remove such substances that the body experiences a state of oxidative stress, leading to cell tissue damage [19]. The increase in cellular activity and metabolism observed in individuals with diabetes renders them particularly susceptible to increased oxidative stress [20]. The role of oxidative stress in the pathogenesis of TBM has been studied. The aim of this review is to provide several mechanisms in which increased oxidative stress in diabetic patients may increase one's likelihood of developing TBM.

2. TB and Diabetes

Diabetes can have a significant impact on Mtb infection, including increased susceptibility to active TB infection, altered immune responses, and poor treatment outcomes. Multiple studies have shown that asymptomatic infection with Mtb, termed latent TB infection (LTBI), is found in higher numbers among individuals with pre-diabetes and T2D compared to those without [21,22]. Diabetes is also a well-studied risk factor for the progression from LTBI to active TB disease [23,24]. T2D predisposes individuals to develop active TB and, thus, as the prevalence of T2D increases, the global burden of TB is also thought to increase. Recent evidence suggests that, in addition to hyperglycemia, hypercholesterolemia, and elevated triglyceride levels associated with DM, diabetes is also a main contributor to the increased susceptibility to TB [24].

Chronic inflammation and altered immune defense mechanisms in diabetics may compromise the ability of the host immune system to combat Mtb infection [25]. Furthermore, the ability of immune cells to recognize and destroy Mtb may be impaired, allowing the bacteria to replicate and manifest elsewhere, such as in the meninges in the case of TBM. For instance, there exists an inverse relationship between the activity of natural killer (NK) cells and hyperglycemia, wherein an increase in blood sugar levels is associated with an observed decrease in NK cell function in the innate and adaptive immune response against infection [26]. Moreover, another study demonstrated that endoplasmic reticulum (ER) stress as a result of uncontrolled hyperglycemia led to the downregulation of natural-killer receptor group 2, member D (NKG2D), a well-studied NK cell-activating receptor [27]. Induced hyperglycemia was found to impair neutrophil degranulation, a mechanism of pathogen clearance involving extracellular destruction [28]. Moreover, long-term high-glucose concentrations sensitize macrophages to cytokine stimulation while reducing the phagocytic and bactericidal function of macrophages essential in fighting pathogens [29]. Lastly, the role of cytokines in the increased susceptibility of diabetics to infection has been studied. Upregulation of pro-inflammatory IL-6 and TNF-α has been observed in diabetics, whereas there is a reduction in the circulating levels of anti-inflammatory IL-10 [30,31]. Thus, cytokine dysregulation in diabetic individuals, involving an increase in pro-inflammatory cytokines along with a decrease in anti-inflammatory cytokines, results in a chronic inflammatory cellular state, increasing one's susceptibility to infection (Figure 1).

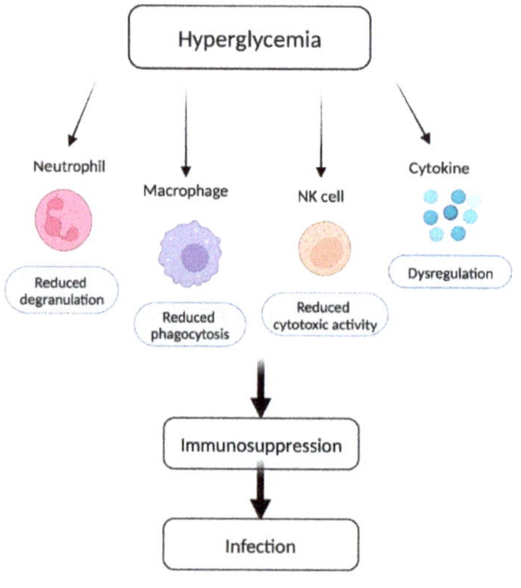

Figure 1. As blood sugar levels rise, the immune system operates with less efficiency, leading to increased vulnerability to infections, such as *Mycobacterium tuberculosis* (Mtb). Neutrophils and macrophages, crucial for combating infections, exhibit restricted degranulation and phagocytic activity in individuals with diabetes. Hyperglycemia contributes to a decline in natural killer (NK) cell functionality, resulting in diminished cytotoxic activity. Additionally, diabetic individuals experience cytokine dysregulation, which gives rise to a state of chronic inflammation.

Multidrug-resistant TB (MDR-TB) is characterized by the resistance to at least isoniazid and rifampin, two potent drugs used in the treatment of TB. Diabetes, in particular T2D, is associated with a two-fold increased risk of MDR-TB [32]. Whole-genome sequencing of clinical isolates of Mtb revealed several mutations in individuals with T2D conferring resistance to isoniazid, ethionamide, fluoroquinolone, and rifampicin [33]. Interestingly, the serum concentrations of isoniazid and pyrazinamide were reduced in TB patients with T2D compared to those without T2D, which may be attributed to the generally higher BMI observed in T2D patients and/or the increased metabolic rate of anti-TB drugs in diabetics [34,35].

The relationship between DM and TB infection has been well studied. In this review, however, we provide novel insight into the potential mechanisms that predispose diabetic individuals to the extrapulmonary manifestation of TB infection into TBM.

3. Pathogenesis of TBM in Humans

Following Mtb infection of the cells of the CNS, slow-progressive meningitis develops with clinical symptoms such as headaches, vomiting, fever, and neck stiffness, indistinguishable from other meningitis types [36]. If untreated, TBM progresses to severe clinical conditions, including unconsciousness, focal neurological deficits, cranial nerve palsies, seizures, raised intracranial pressure, and hemiparesis. These symptoms are driven by the exacerbated inflammation caused by Mtb infection [36]. Elevated levels of pro-inflammatory cytokines, including tumor necrosis factor-alpha (TNF-α) released by infected immune cells into the CNS, contribute to the local and systemic inflammation in TBM, with the fifth and third cranial nerves being involved in approximately 50% of patients [37]. In advanced TBM, about 10% of patients report either hemiplegia or paraplegia, and death is almost inevitable at this stage, without proper therapeutic interventions [38]. Pleocytosis with lymphocyte predominance (150–1000 leukocytes/μL), enriched with neutrophils and lymphocytes, low glucose levels with the cerebrospinal fluid (CSF) to plasma glucose ratios of <0.5, and high protein content (0.8–2.0 g/dL) are some of the essential laboratory findings in the CSF of patients with TBM [10]. Furthermore, in patients with human immunodeficiency virus (HIV) co-infection, TBM is characterized by the absence of mononuclear leukocytes and the prominent presence of neutrophils (>1000 cells/μL) in the CSF, mimicking acute pyogenic bacterial meningitis [10]. Elevated levels of inflammatory cytokines are commonly noted in the plasma and CSF of patients with TBM. Radiographically, patients with TBM show basal meningeal exudates, infarction, tuberculomas, and hydrocephalus [10].

4. Oxidative Stress in the Pathogenesis of TBM

Increased production of reactive oxygen species (ROS) has been found to be intimately involved in the pathogenesis of TB and TBM [4,39]. Upon exposure to Mtb infection, the host immune system activates several defense mechanisms to control the infection, one of which includes the generation of ROS. Although ROS is initially produced to protect against infection, its overproduction leads to host tissue damage, including brain tissue, contributing to the pathogenesis of TBM. Increased ROS levels have been shown to impair the host immune response against Mtb infection and, in turn, allow infection to ensue in other parts of the body, including the brain [40]. Biomarkers identified from cerebrospinal fluid (CSF) samples from individuals with TBM demonstrated increased inflammation, disruption of the BBB, and impairment of amyloid-β (Aβ) metabolism [41].

Cellular damage and inflammation play a significant role in the pathogenesis of TBM. Both pro- and anti-inflammatory cytokines have been shown to be induced in individuals with TBM; however, it is the imbalance between the two that is responsible for the pathogenesis and prognosis of TBM [4]. Damage to cellular structures including lipids, proteins, and nucleic acids induced by excessive ROS production may lead to chronic inflammation and, in turn, increases the likelihood of TBM [42].

ROS may also have a significant impact on the integrity of the BBB. The lining of the BBB acts to protect the CNS by regulating the passage of molecules between the bloodstream and the brain. The BBB consists of tightly connected cells, including endothelial cells, astrocytes and pericytes. Increased ROS production and the resulting oxidative stress have been shown to damage endothelial cells crucial for the integrity of the BBB, resulting in increased permeability of the BBB to infection, including Mtb [43]. Subsequent impairment of tight junctions between endothelial cells also contributes to the dysregulation of the BBB. Moreover, ROS-induced production of pro-inflammatory stimuli, such as the redox-sensitive transcription factor NF-kB, can further impair the BBB by promoting leukocyte adhesion and extravasation, leading to increased neuroinflammation [43]. Furthermore, the BBB employs antioxidant defense mechanisms, such as superoxide dismutase (SOD) and glutathione peroxidase (GPx), to neutralize ROS and maintain redox homeostasis; however, in conditions of ROS overproduction, these antioxidants become overwhelmed and lead to subsequent damage of the BBB [44]. Lastly, increased ROS production may result in the upregulation of matrix metalloproteinases (MMPs), which are enzymes found to degrade components of the extracellular matrix, including those in the BBB, further disrupting the integrity of tight junctions and basal lamina of the BBB [43]. In summary, the accumulation of ROS leads to increased permeability of the BBB, allowing the infiltration of harmful and infectious agents such as Mtb, leading to the culmination of Mtb infection in the meninges. Thus, the increase in ROS production seen in diabetics may significantly increase an individual's susceptibility to TBM.

Impaired metabolism of Aβ peptide metabolism and its resulting aggregation is a well-known pathological hallmark of Alzheimer's disease. However, emerging evidence suggests that Aβ aggregation and deposition may also be implicated in the pathogenesis of diabetes and related neurodegenerative and neurovascular changes [45]. Hyperglycemia is associated with increased amyloid precursor protein (APP), leading to an increase in Aβ peptide production and increased permeability through endothelial tight junctions [46]. Furthermore, insulin resistance, a hallmark of T2DM, has been shown to impair Aβ clearance through the BBB, resulting in Aβ accumulation in the brain [46]. Oxidative stress, such as that seen in diabetic patients, further promotes Aβ aggregation [47]. Thus, one may argue that the increase in Aβ peptides observed in CSF samples of diabetic individuals suffering from TBM may be partly attributed to oxidative stress.

5. Oxidative Stress in Diabetes

Oxidative stress is implicated in the onset of insulin resistance due to the impairment of insulin signaling pathways, as well as in β-cell dysfunction and apoptosis, reducing the number of functional pancreatic β-cells [48]. Persistent hyperglycemia makes those with diabetes particularly susceptible to oxidative stress due to enhanced ROS production as well as impaired antioxidant defense mechanisms [49]. Thus, therapeutic interventions targeting oxidative stress in diabetes management through modulating ROS production or antioxidant supplementation have gained attention (Figure 2).

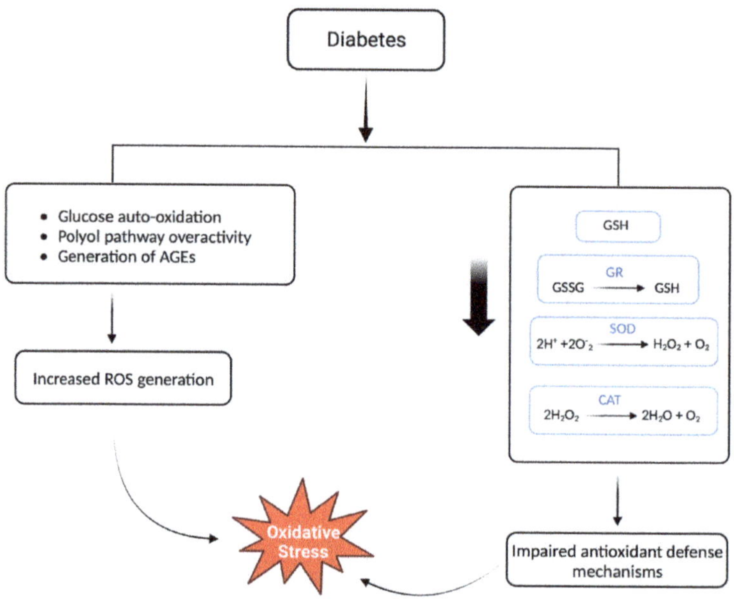

Figure 2. Hyperglycemia in individuals with diabetes leads to an elevation in glucose auto-oxidation, the activation of the polyol pathway, and the formation of advanced glycation end products (AGEs). These processes collectively contribute to an increased generation of reactive oxygen species (ROS), which subsequently results in increased oxidative stress. Furthermore, diabetes is associated with reduced levels of antioxidants such as glutathione, as well as diminished activity of antioxidant enzymes such as glutathione reductase (GR), superoxide dismutase (SOD), and catalase (CAT). The compromised functioning of the antioxidant defense system in diabetic individuals results in the accumulation of ROS, ultimately leading to increased oxidative stress and subsequent damage.

5.1. Increased ROS Production in Diabetics

Diabetes may lead to an overproduction of ROS primarily through increased glucose auto-oxidation, activation of the polyol pathway, and the generation of advanced glycation end products (AGEs) [50]. Hyperglycemia is considered a significant source of ROS in the body since the increased availability of glucose contributes to an elevated rate of cellular processes involving glucose and, thus, an increase in ROS generation [50]. Glucose auto-oxidation is described as the spontaneous oxidation of glucose in the presence of oxygen or other electron acceptors. Under normal conditions, glucose exists in equilibrium with its enediol; however, under conditions of glucose auto-oxidation, an enediol radical is formed [51]. Glucose auto-oxidation is a significant source of free radical formation, such as hydrogen peroxide (H_2O_2) and superoxide anion [50]. The polyol pathway, also termed the sorbitol pathway, involves the conversion of glucose to sorbitol and then to fructose, using the enzyme aldose reductase (AR). This pathway is another mechanism through which hyperglycemia can lead to ROS generation [52]. Overactivity of AR under hyperglycemia conditions subjects' diabetics to increased activity of the polyol pathway and, thus, increased ROS generation [52]. The conversion of glucose to sorbitol involves the consumption and depletion of NADPH, a necessary component of the host antioxidant defense system against ROS [52]. Lastly, the increased formation of AGEs in diabetes has been shown to increase ROS [53]. AGEs are modified proteins or lipids that have been non-enzymatically glycated and oxidized in response to glucose exposure. AGEs may interact with receptors for advanced glycation end products (RAGE) to increase ROS production via NADPH oxidases within the mitochondria, resulting in increased inflammation and tissue damage [54].

5.2. Impaired Antioxidant Defense Mechanisms in Diabetics

Antioxidants play a crucial role in the response against the production of ROS by effectively counteracting the detrimental effects of free radicals and mitigating the onset of oxidative stress. Consequently, impaired functionality of the antioxidant defense mechanism results in the accumulation of harmful species and, in turn, increased oxidative stress and damage. Due to the high metabolic activity in the brain, it relies on antioxidant defense mechanisms to exert neuroprotective effects by scavenging ROS and defending against oxidative damage, yet their efficiency is compromised in diabetics [55]. Diabetes is associated with reduced levels of antioxidants, such as glutathione, and antioxidant enzymes, such as glutathione reductase (GR), superoxide dismutase (SOD), and catalase (CAT) [56]. Another study revealed a positive correlation between GR, CAT, and SOD with malondialdehyde (MDA), a marker of oxidative stress [57].

Levels of glutathione have been reported to be decreased in individuals with diabetes compared to non-diabetic individuals [58,59]. The active and reduced form of glutathione (GSH) plays a crucial role in ROS scavenging, whereas the oxidized form of glutathione (GSSG) is often increased in conditions of oxidative stress. Thus, a reduced plasma GSH/GSSG ratio, such as that seen in diabetic individuals, may be used as an indicator of oxidative stress [60]. One study attributed GSH deficiency in patients with T2DM to the limited availability of glutathione precursors and, upon dietary administration of the GSH precursor amino acids cysteine and glycine, GSH levels were restored, and levels of oxidative stress and oxidative damage were reduced [58]. Another study using a diabetic mouse model demonstrated that liposomal glutathione (L-GSH) supplementation used in combination with rifampicin improved the treatment response against Mtb infection [61]. Moreover, GR is the enzyme responsible for maintaining glutathione in its reduced and active form by catalyzing the reduction of GSSG with the use of an NADPH electron donor. The decrease in GR activity in diabetics results in increased levels of GSSG and, thus, a diminishment in the levels of GSH and its ability to combat oxidative damage [62].

SODs are a group of enzymes that defend against ROS via the dismutation of superoxide radicals (O2-) to molecular oxygen and H_2O_2. Superoxide radicals produced in excess amounts lead to cell damage and, therefore, must be regulated by the action of

SOD [63]. The expression and activity of the several isoforms of SOD varies in diabetes. Cytosolic CuZn-SOD (SOD1) and extracellular CuZn-SOD (SOD3) were downregulated in KK/Ta-Akita diabetic mouse models susceptible to diabetic nephropathy, whereas no significant change in mitochondrial Mn-SOD was observed [64]. Another study found reduced serum levels of extracellular SOD to be associated with polyneuropathy in individuals with recent-onset diabetes [65].

CAT is an antioxidant enzyme that catalyzes the reduction of H_2O_2 into water and molecular oxygen, protecting the body from oxidative damage. Although CAT activity in the brain is lower compared to other tissues and organs, such as the liver and kidney, it is still regarded as an important antioxidant necessary for proper brain function [66]. Inhibition of CAT activity is associated with enhanced cytotoxicity and increased levels of ROS, namely the accumulation of hydrogen peroxide that is responsible for compromised neurological function [66]. Low levels of catalase activity and the subsequent accumulation of H_2O_2 contribute to the pathogenesis of T2DM and related diabetic complications [67].

5.3. Role of Inflammation in Oxidative Stress and Diabetes

There also exists an intricate relationship between inflammation and oxidative stress in the context of diabetes, wherein diabetes-mediated inflammation triggers the production of pro-inflammatory molecules as well as the production of ROS by immune cells, aimed at combating pathogens [68]. Although these events are initially protective, chronic inflammation in diabetes leads to sustained ROS production, causing cellular damage and depletion of antioxidant defenses [69]. Moreover, the presence of excess adipose tissue in patients with T2D leads to the release of pro-inflammatory molecules, such as IL-6 and TNF-α, intensifying oxidative stress [70]. Additionally, the hexosamine pathway demonstrates the effects of hyperglycemia in the alteration of gene expression and contribution to diabetic complications, including tissue-type plasminogen activator inhibitor-1 (PAI-1) and transforming growth factor-β1 (TGF-β1) [68]. PAI-1 and TGF-β1 play a crucial role in the production of ROS and promotion of oxidative stress in diabetic nephropathy and neuropathy, respectively [68]. Finally, oxidative stress resulting from a pro-inflammatory state has been shown to impair insulin secretion and beta-cell function, ultimately worsening hyperglycemia [71]. Inflammation clearly plays a pivotal role in the advancement of oxidative stress, making it a potential therapeutic target in diabetic individuals, as observed using metformin.

6. Effects of Anti-Diabetic Agents on Oxidative Stress

DM is commonly managed through lifestyle modifications and medications. Metformin is the currently recommended first-line treatment of T2DM and exerts its effects by inhibiting hepatic gluconeogenesis and increasing insulin sensitivity, resulting in enhanced glucose uptake and reduced blood glucose levels [72,73]. One study demonstrated that rats treated with metformin exhibited an associated decrease in oxidative stress markers, such as conjugated dienes and thiobarbituric acid-reactive substances (TBARS), when compared to control groups [74].

Metformin has been proposed to lower oxidative stress through its inhibition of the mitochondrial electron transport chain (ETC) [72]. The ETC comprises four complexes that work together to generate an electrochemical gradient that ultimately results in the generation of ATP. However, the ETC can work in reverse, a process that has been proposed to be inhibited by metformin [72]. By inhibiting complex, I (NADH: ubiquinone oxidoreductase), metformin directly lowers mitochondrial-induced production of ROS, decreasing oxidative stress [72] (Figure 3).

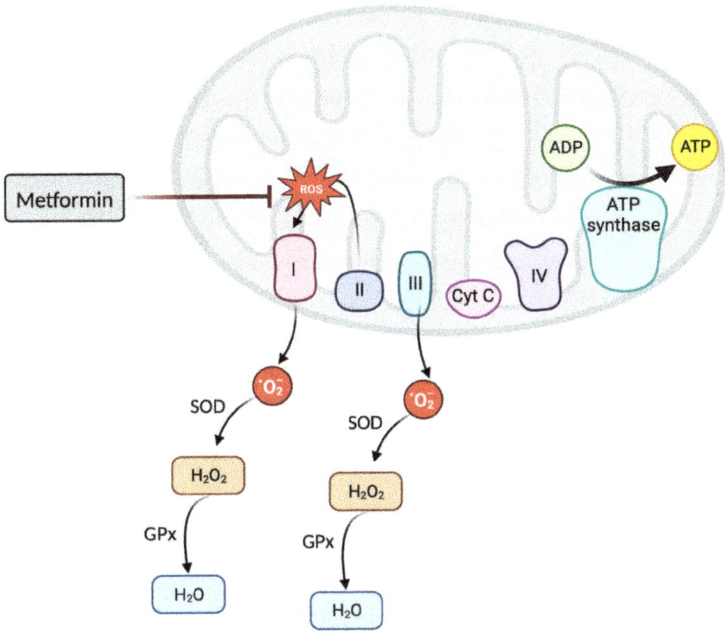

Figure 3. The electron transport chain (ETC) is composed of four complexes that collaborate to generate energy within the mitochondria. Typically, mitochondria produce reactive oxygen species (ROS) through complexes I and III during respiration. Nonetheless, the ETC may also function in reverse, allowing electrons that enter complex II to circulate back to complex I. This reversal leads to the generation of ROS. Metformin has been suggested as a potential inhibitor of this phenomenon, thereby potentially decreasing ROS production and aiding in the regulation of oxidative stress.

As previously mentioned, increased AGEs in diabetic patients can lead to increased ROS production. Metformin also plays a protective role against AGEs. In a three-month study of T2DM patients treated with metformin, there was a significant reduction in levels of RAGE isoforms, β-amyloid, and inflammatory cytokines, indicating a decrease in oxidative stress and tissue inflammation [75].

Anti-diabetic treatments have also been shown to affect antioxidant function and levels. For example, paraoxonase 1 (PON 1) is an enzyme that primarily functions in the liver as an antioxidant against lipid oxidation [76]. In a study conducted using a rat model, metformin was associated with increased PON 1 activity in diabetic rats, increasing its protection against ROS [77]. However, previous studies regarding metformin and antioxidant capacity were unable to quite confirm its direct effects. While the previous study showed an increase in antioxidant activity, metformin has been shown to instead prevent antioxidant levels from increasing. The study theorized that this could be due to metformin limiting the production of ROS in the first place, eliminating the need for increased antioxidant activity [78].

It is evident that metformin plays a protective role in protecting diabetic patients against oxidative stress by decreasing the production of harmful species and/or increasing antioxidant activity within cells. Nevertheless, further studies involving the direct effects of metformin as well as its specific mechanism of action are warranted.

7. Potential Therapeutic Strategies

The current antibiotics-based regimen for TBM treatment is the same used to treat pulmonary TB. This standard TB therapy regimen consists of a combination of isoniazid (INH), rifampin (RIF), pyrazinamide (PZA), and ethambutol (ETH) administered for

2 months, followed by INH plus RIF for another 4–10 months [37,79]. For these antibiotics to be effective against TBM, they must cross the BBB and reach the therapeutic concentration at the site of infection in the brain [10,38]. It was reported that RIF and ETH poorly cross the BBB, and limited studies are available on the anti-TB drug distribution in various compartments of the brain [10,37,38,80]. Additionally, the pharmacokinetic characterization of the anti-TBM drug to understand the efficient therapeutic concentration in the brain is yet to be determined [81]. Anti-inflammatory agents, such as corticosteroids, are often used in conjunction with anti-TB drugs to improve TBM treatment. However, the immunosuppressive nature of corticosteroids poses the risk of acquiring new infections and reactivation of latent TB. Therefore, new and improved therapeutic strategies are urgently needed for the efficient management of TBM [82,83].

Metformin is associated with reduced intracellular growth of Mtb in infected mice and enhanced efficacy of anti-TB drugs [84]. In Mtb-infected mice treated with both metformin and traditional anti-TB medications, including isoniazid (INH) or ethionamide (ETH), mice treated with metformin and INH were reported to have a lower bacterial load in their lungs compared to mice treated with INH alone [84]. Based on the discussion above, metformin used in combination with additional therapies to combat oxidative stress may have additional therapeutic value in the prevention and treatment of diabetic patients with TBM. Supplementing metformin with oral vitamin D, a nonenzymatic antioxidant, has been shown to further reduce advanced oxidation protein products [85]. However, it is important to note that metformin has been associated with respiratory side effects such as hypoxia secondary to lactic acidosis caused by metformin [86]. In T2DM patients with pulmonary conditions, such as chronic obstructive pulmonary disease (COPD), metformin was associated with increased bacterial pneumonia infections and usage of ventilators [87]. Therefore, when treating TBM, especially when symptoms of respiratory insufficiency are present, the risks should be carefully evaluated before treating with metformin.

Though metformin is the first-line treatment for T2DM, other medications, such as sulfonylureas, a-glucosidase inhibitors, and meglitinides, are also approved to act as glucose-lowering agents [88]. Pharmaceutical therapies that are specifically associated with decreased biomarkers of oxidative stress in animal models include, but are not limited to, thiazolidinediones, pioglitazone, and statins [89]. Statins are commonly prescribed to T2DM patients as preventative care since diabetes is a risk factor for the development of cardiovascular pathologies. In addition to managing lipid levels within the body, statins also possess anti-inflammatory properties. They have been reported to decrease inflammation via reduced C-reactive proteins [90]. In human endothelial cells exposed to hyperglycemic environments, atorvastatin and simvastatin have been shown to decrease production of ROS through the inhibition of HMG-CoA reductase in cholesterol synthesis [91]. Sodium-glucose cotransporter-2 (SGLT2) inhibitors can also be used to lower blood glucose levels by inhibiting glucose reabsorption within the kidneys. Similar to statins, they interrupt oxidative stress production pathways, leading to lowered ROS generation as well as reduced inflammatory biomarkers, such as AGEs [92]. Lower blood glucose and reduced oxidative stress markers have also been reported after vitamin C supplementation [93]. Overall, these pharmaceutical therapies have pleiotropic benefits that extend beyond their intended use. Statins and SGLT2 inhibitors were intended for lipid and glucose control and meant to reduce T2DM complications. However, patients can also benefit from their anti-inflammatory effects, leading to improved overall clinical outcomes.

High levels of H_2O_2 may stimulate further production of ROS; hence, there is a need to limit the levels of H_2O_2. GSH, in the presence of GPx, may be used to manage mitochondrial ROS production by reducing H_2O_2 to water [94]. Oral administration of the GSH precursors cysteine and glycine resulted in individuals with T2DM having restored rates of GSH synthesis and, in turn, reduced oxidative stress and oxidant damage plasma markers [58,95]. Considering that individuals with T2DM exhibit an associated reduction in levels of GSH, GSH supplementation may be an option to help combat oxidative stress and prevent TBM in these patients (Figure 4).

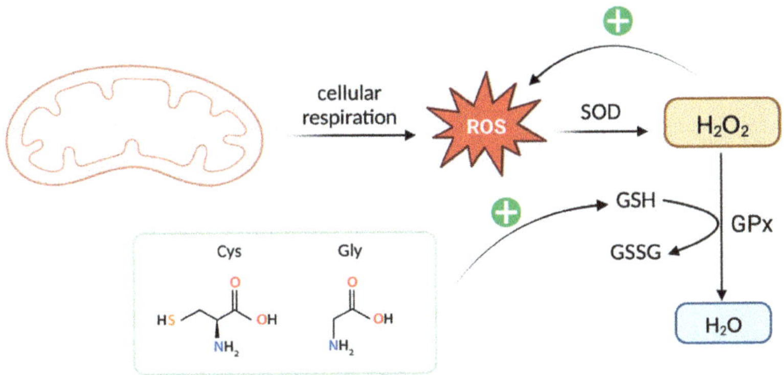

Figure 4. Reactive oxygen species (ROS) are generated by the mitochondria as a consequence of cellular respiration. In the presence of superoxide dismutase (SOD), ROS undergoes catalysis to form hydrogen peroxide (H_2O_2). Glutathione (GSH), aided by the presence of glutathione peroxidase (GPx), functions to counteract H_2O_2 by converting it into water, thereby assisting in the regulation of oxidative stress. Nevertheless, when the levels of H_2O_2 become elevated, they can trigger the production of additional ROS, thereby intensifying oxidative stress within the cellular environment. Administering precursors of GSH, such as cysteine and glycine, aids in the restoration of GSH levels. As a result, this helps to manage H_2O_2 levels and subsequently control oxidative stress.

Moreover, supplementation of metformin with oral vitamin D, a non-enzymatic antioxidant, has been shown to further reduce advanced oxidation protein products [85]. A spectrum of pharmacologic therapies has been associated with decreased biomarkers of oxidative stress in animal models, including thiazolidinediones, pioglitazone, and statins [89]. A reduction in blood glucose levels and oxidative stress biomarkers has also been reported following vitamin C supplementation [93]. Though fruits can increase glucose levels within the body, various studies have shown that sweet limes, oranges, apples, cranberries, grapes, pomegranate, and blueberries have been identified as harboring antioxidant properties and, thus, reduce oxidative stress levels among diabetic patients [93]. Furthermore, regular exercise can both reduce ROS production and enhance antioxidant capabilities, while also increasing insulin sensitivity, resulting in better glucose uptake into cells and lowering blood glucose levels [93]. Such exercises that have been shown to counteract the effects of oxidative stress are Tai chi, Pilates, and moderate-intensity aerobic exercises.

Hence, since oxidative stress is highly implicated in the pathogenesis of TBM, we propose that the aforementioned therapeutic strategies may offer protective benefits beyond Mtb lung infections and can prevent TBM, specifically in diabetic patients.

8. Discussion

We have discussed the association of TBM with DM in terms of oxidative stress and susceptibility to infection. Individuals with diabetes, particularly T2D, exhibit heightened levels of oxidative stress, leading to cellular damage and inflammation. This condition may compromise the ability of the immune system to fight Mtb infection, particularly in the CNS.

Whereas the host immune system generates ROS in the defense against exposure to Mtb, the overproduction of ROS in diabetics leads to tissue damage, including brain tissue, contributing to the development of TBM. ROS may also impact the integrity of the BBB—the major defense mechanism of the CNS. Damage to the endothelial cells lining the BBB increases permeability to pathogens and contributes to the development of TBM. Oxidative stress may also play a role in the accumulation and aggregation of Aβ peptides in the brain, an identified biomarker of TBM. Diabetes leads to an overproduction of ROS in addition to impaired antioxidant defense mechanisms, further contributing to a state of oxidative stress. Several factors, such as glucose auto-oxidation, glucose metabolism, and AGEs, contribute to the increased generation of ROS in individuals with diabetes. Moreover, the impairment of antioxidants, such as GSH, and antioxidant enzymes, such as GR, CAT, and SOD, worsen the effects of ROS and oxidative stress. The combination of increased ROS production and reduced antioxidant defense mechanisms creates a state of oxidative stress, leading to cellular damage and inflammation.

Considering the role of oxidative stress in the pathogenesis of TBM and the increased levels of oxidative stress in diabetes, we propose the use of antioxidants and other therapies targeting oxidative stress in the treatment of TBM. This article also highlights the role of metformin, a common diabetes medication, in reducing oxidative stress in diabetic patients. Thus, combining metformin with additional therapies, such as vitamin D or GSH supplementation, is a novel therapeutic strategy that may have significant value in combatting oxidative stress and improving treatment outcomes in diabetic patients and preventing the development of TBM. Overall, this review sheds light on the complex relationship between TBM and diabetes co-infection, with emphasis on the role of oxidative stress, suggesting that targeting oxidative stress through various therapeutic approaches could have beneficial effects in preventing TBM in diabetics.

Nevertheless, the limitations inherent in this review involve the fundamental nature of literature reviews, which inherently rely upon previously published studies and their accessibility. Specifically, we encountered a lack of comprehensive data pertaining to the direct relationship between TBM and DM. One anticipated challenge within the potential therapies proposed in this review is the establishment of a non-human model for the purpose of investigating the coexistence of DM and TBM to study the effect of various therapies. Moreover, the prospective therapeutic interventions suggested for mitigating oxidative stress, notably the employment of metformin, predominantly draw upon evidence derived from animal models, and a paucity of human-related data persists. These gaps in the current knowledge, pervasive within the available literature, inevitably constrain the capacity to offer efficacious and pragmatic potential therapeutic strategies. Thus, there exists a need for additional research in this field to build upon the existing findings and contribute to the expanding body of evidence that supports the connection between oxidative stress and the co-occurrence of TBM in individuals with diabetes.

Author Contributions: Conceptualization, I.N. and V.V.; software, I.N.; validation, V.V.; writing—original draft preparation, I.N., S.Y., H.N., S.S. and P.V.; writing—review and editing, I.N., S.S. and V.V.; supervision, V.V. All authors have read and agreed to the published version of the manuscript.

Funding: This research received no external funding.

Institutional Review Board Statement: Not applicable.

Informed Consent Statement: Not applicable.

Conflicts of Interest: The authors declare no conflict of interest.

References

1. Donald, P.R.; Donald, P.R.; Schaaf, H.S.; Schoeman, J.F. Tuberculous meningitis and miliary tuberculosis: The Rich focus revisited. *J. Infect.* **2005**, *50*, 193–195. [CrossRef] [PubMed]
2. Sharma, P.; Garg, R.K.; Verma, R.; Singh, M.K.; Shukla, R. Incidence, predictors and prognostic value of cranial nerve involvement in patients with tuberculous meningitis: A retrospective evaluation. *Eur. J. Intern. Med.* **2011**, *22*, 289–295. [CrossRef] [PubMed]
3. Manyelo, C.M.; Solomons, R.S.; Walzl, G.; Chegou, N.N. Tuberculous Meningitis: Pathogenesis, Immune Responses, Diagnostic Challenges, and the Potential of Biomarker-Based Approaches. *J. Clin. Microbiol.* **2021**, *59*, e01771-20. [CrossRef]
4. Davis, A.G.; Rohlwink, U.K.; Proust, A.; Figaji, A.A.; Wilkinson, R.J. The pathogenesis of tuberculous meningitis. *J. Leukoc. Biol.* **2019**, *105*, 267–280. [CrossRef] [PubMed]
5. Jain, S.K.; Paul-Satyaseela, M.; Lamichhane, G.; Kim, K.S.; Bishai, W.R. *Mycobacterium tuberculosis* invasion and traversal across an in vitro human blood-brain barrier as a pathogenic mechanism for central nervous system tuberculosis. *J. Infect. Dis.* **2006**, *193*, 1287–1295. [CrossRef] [PubMed]

6. van Leeuwen, L.M.; Boot, M.; Kuijl, C.; Picavet, D.I.; van Stempvoort, G.; van der Pol, S.M.A.; de Vries, H.E.; van der Wel, N.N.; van der Kuip, M.; van Furth, A.M.; et al. Mycobacteria employ two different mechanisms to cross the blood-brain barrier. *Cell Microbiol.* **2018**, *20*, e12858. [CrossRef]
7. Dodd, P.J.; Osman, M.; Cresswell, F.V.; Stadelman, A.M.; Lan, N.H.; Thuong, N.T.T.; Muzyamba, M.; Glaser, L.; Dlamini, S.S.; Seddon, J.A. The global burden of tuberculous meningitis in adults: A modelling study. *PLoS Glob. Public Health.* **2021**, *1*, e0000069. [CrossRef]
8. Marais, S.; Pepper, D.J.; Schutz, C.; Wilkinson, R.J.; Meintjes, G. Presentation and outcome of tuberculous meningitis in a high HIV prevalence setting. *PLoS ONE* **2011**, *6*, e20077. [CrossRef]
9. Miftode, E.G.; Dorneanu, O.S.; Leca, D.A.; Juganariu, G.; Teodor, A.; Hurmuzache, M.; Nastase, E.V.; Anton-Paduraru, D.T. Tuberculous Meningitis in Children and Adults: A 10-Year Retrospective Comparative Analysis. *PLoS ONE* **2015**, *10*, e0133477. [CrossRef]
10. Török, M.E. Tuberculous meningitis: Advances in diagnosis and treatment. *Br. Med. Bull.* **2015**, *113*, 117–131. [CrossRef]
11. Navarro-Flores, A.; Fernandez-Chinguel, J.E.; Pacheco-Barrios, N.; Soriano-Moreno, D.R.; Pacheco-Barrios, K. Global morbidity and mortality of central nervous system tuberculosis: A systematic review and meta-analysis. *J. Neurol.* **2022**, *269*, 3482–3494. [CrossRef] [PubMed]
12. Genuth, S.M.; Palmer, J.P.; Nathan, D.M. Classification and Diagnosis of Diabetes. In *Diabetes in America*, 3rd ed.; Cowie, C.C., Casagrande, S.S., Menke, A., Cissell, M.A., Eberhardt, M.S., Meigs, J.B., Gregg, E.W., Knowler, W.C., Barrett-Connor, E., Becker, D.J., et al., Eds.; National Institute of Diabetes and Digestive and Kidney Diseases: Bethesda, MD, USA, 2018; Chapter 1.
13. Permutt, M.A.; Wasson, J.; Cox, N. Genetic epidemiology of diabetes. *J. Clin. Investig.* **2005**, *115*, 1431–1439. [CrossRef] [PubMed]
14. Centers for Disease Control and Prevention. National Diabetes Statistics Report Website. Available online: https://www.cdc.gov/diabetes/data/statistics-report/index.html (accessed on 26 July 2023).
15. Tuomi, T. Type 1 and type 2 diabetes: What do they have in common? *Diabetes* **2005**, *54* (Suppl. 2), S40–S45. [CrossRef] [PubMed]
16. Diabetes Control and Complications Trial Research Group; Nathan, D.M.; Genuth, S.; Lachin, J.; Cleary, P.; Crofford, O.; Davis, M.; Rand, L.; Siebert, C. The effect of intensive treatment of diabetes on the development and progression of long-term complications in insulin-dependent diabetes mellitus. *N. Engl. J. Med.* **1993**, *329*, 977–986. [CrossRef] [PubMed]
17. Diabetes Prevention Program Research Group; Knowler, W.C.; Fowler, S.E.; Hamman, R.F.; Christophi, C.A.; Hoffman, H.J.; Brenneman, A.T.; Brown-Friday, J.O.; Goldberg, R.; Venditti, E.; et al. 10-year follow-up of diabetes incidence and weight loss in the Diabetes Prevention Program Outcomes Study. *Lancet* **2009**, *374*, 1677–1686. [CrossRef]
18. Zhu, M.; Wu, J.; Gao, J. Exosomes for diabetes syndrome: Ongoing applications and perspective. *Biomater. Sci.* **2022**, *10*, 2154–2171. [CrossRef]
19. Burton, G.J.; Jauniaux, E. Oxidative stress. *Best. Pr. Res. Clin. Obs. Gynaecol.* **2011**, *25*, 287–299. [CrossRef]
20. Giacco, F.; Brownlee, M. Oxidative stress and diabetic complications. *Circ. Res.* **2010**, *107*, 1058–1070. [CrossRef]
21. Hensel, R.L.; Kempker, R.R.; Tapia, J.; Oladele, A.; Blumberg, H.M.; Magee, M.J. Increased risk of latent tuberculous infection among persons with pre-diabetes and diabetes mellitus. *Int. J. Tuberc. Lung Dis.* **2016**, *20*, 71–78. [CrossRef]
22. Salindri, A.D.; Haw, J.S.; Amere, G.A.; Alese, J.T.; Umpierrez, G.E.; Magee, M.J. Latent tuberculosis infection among patients with and without type-2 diabetes mellitus: Results from a hospital case-control study in Atlanta. *BMC Res. Notes.* **2021**, *14*, 252. [CrossRef]
23. Workneh, M.H.; Bjune, G.A.; Yimer, S.A. Prevalence and associated factors of tuberculosis and diabetes mellitus comorbidity: A systematic review. *PLoS ONE* **2017**, *12*, e0175925. [CrossRef] [PubMed]
24. Ngo, M.D.; Bartlett, S.; Ronacher, K. Diabetes-Associated Susceptibility to Tuberculosis: Contribution of Hyperglycemia vs. *Dyslipidemia. Microorganisms* **2021**, *9*, 2282. [CrossRef] [PubMed]
25. Abbas, U.; Masood, K.I.; Khan, A.; Irfan, M.; Saifullah, N.; Jamil, B.; Hasan, Z. Tuberculosis and diabetes mellitus: Relating immune impact of co-morbidity with challenges in disease management in high burden countries. *J. Clin. Tuberc. Other Mycobact. Dis.* **2022**, *29*, 100343. [CrossRef] [PubMed]
26. Kim, J.H.; Park, K.; Lee, S.B.; Kang, S.; Park, J.S.; Ahn, C.W.; Nam, J.S. Relationship between natural killer cell activity and glucose control in patients with type 2 diabetes and prediabetes. *J. Diabetes Investig.* **2019**, *10*, 1223–1228. [CrossRef]
27. Berrou, J.; Fougeray, S.; Venot, M.; Chardiny, V.; Gautier, J.F.; Dulphy, N.; Toubert, A.; Peraldi, M.N. Natural killer cell function, an important target for infection and tumor protection, is impaired in type 2 diabetes. *PLoS ONE* **2013**, *8*, e62418. [CrossRef] [PubMed]
28. Stegenga, M.E.; van der Crabben, S.N.; Blümer, R.M.; Levi, M.; Meijers, J.C.; Serlie, M.J.; Tanck, M.W.; Sauerwein, H.P.; van der Poll, T. Hyperglycemia enhances coagulation and reduces neutrophil degranulation, whereas hyperinsulinemia inhibits fibrinolysis during human endotoxemia. *Blood* **2008**, *112*, 82–89. [CrossRef]
29. Pavlou, S.; Lindsay, J.; Ingram, R.; Xu, H.; Chen, M. Sustained high glucose exposure sensitizes macrophage responses to cytokine stimuli but reduces their phagocytic activity. *BMC Immunol.* **2018**, *19*, 24. [CrossRef]
30. Goyal, R.; Faizy, A.F.; Siddiqui, S.S.; Singhai, M. Evaluation of TNF-α and IL-6 Levels in Obese and Non-obese Diabetics: Pre- and Postinsulin Effects. *N. Am. J. Med. Sci.* **2012**, *4*, 180–184. [CrossRef]
31. Naz, S.; Shafique, N.; Sharif, S.; Manzoor, F.; Saifi, S.Z.; Firasat, S.; Kaul, H. Association of Interleukin 10 (IL-10) Gene with Type 2 Diabetes Mellitus by Single Nucleotide Polymorphism of Its Promotor Region G/A 1082. *Crit. Rev. Eukaryot. Gene. Expr.* **2020**, *30*, 285–289. [CrossRef]

32. Huangfu, P.; Ugarte-Gil, C.; Golub, J.; Pearson, F.; Critchley, J. The effects of diabetes on tuberculosis treatment outcomes: An updated systematic review and meta-analysis. *Int. J. Tuberc. Lung Dis.* **2019**, *23*, 783–796. [CrossRef]
33. Ruesen, C.; Chaidir, L.; Ugarte-Gil, C.; van Ingen, J.; Critchley, J.A.; Hill, P.C.; Ruslami, R.; Santoso, P.; Huynen, M.A.; Dockrell, H.M.; et al. Diabetes is associated with genotypically drug-resistant tuberculosis. *Eur. Respir. J.* **2020**, *55*, 1901891. [CrossRef] [PubMed]
34. Kumar, A.K.; Chandrasekaran, V.; Kannan, T.; Murali, A.L.; Lavanya, J.; Sudha, V.; Swaminathan, S.; Ramachandran, G. Anti-tuberculosis drug concentrations in tuberculosis patients with and without diabetes mellitus. *Eur. J. Clin. Pharmacol.* **2017**, *73*, 65–70. [CrossRef] [PubMed]
35. Alfarisi, O.; Mave, V.; Gaikwad, S.; Sahasrabudhe, T.; Ramachandran, G.; Kumar, H.; Gupte, N.; Kulkarni, V.; Deshmukh, S.; Atre, S.; et al. Effect of Diabetes Mellitus on the Pharmacokinetics and Pharmacodynamics of Tuberculosis Treatment. *Antimicrob. Agents Chemother.* **2018**, *62*, e01383-18. [CrossRef] [PubMed]
36. Gupta, M.; Munakomi, S. CNS Tuberculosis. In *StatPearls*; StatPearls Publishing: Treasure Island, FL, USA, 2023.
37. Davis, A.; Meintjes, G.; Wilkinson, R.J. Treatment of Tuberculous Meningitis and Its Complications in Adults. *Curr. Treat. Options Neurol.* **2018**, *20*, 5. [CrossRef] [PubMed]
38. Thwaites, G.E.; van Toorn, R.; Schoeman, J. Tuberculous meningitis: More questions, still too few answers. *Lancet Neurol.* **2013**, *12*, 999–1010. [CrossRef]
39. Shastri, M.D.; Shukla, S.D.; Chong, W.C.; Dua, K.; Peterson, G.M.; Patel, R.P.; Hansbro, P.M.; Eri, R.; O'Toole, R.F. Role of Oxidative Stress in the Pathology and Management of Human Tuberculosis. *Oxid. Med. Cell Longev.* **2018**, *2018*, 7695364. [CrossRef]
40. de Martino, M.; Lodi, L.; Galli, L.; Chiappini, E. Immune Response to *Mycobacterium tuberculosis*: A Narrative Review. *Front. Pediatr.* **2019**, *7*, 350. [CrossRef]
41. Stroffolini, G.; Guastamacchia, G.; Audagnotto, S.; Atzori, C.; Trunfio, M.; Nigra, M.; Di Stefano, A.; Di Perri, G.; Calcagno, A. Low cerebrospinal fluid Amyloid-βeta 1-42 in patients with tuberculous meningitis. *BMC Neurol.* **2021**, *21*, 449. [CrossRef]
42. Pizzino, G.; Irrera, N.; Cucinotta, M.; Pallio, G.; Mannino, F.; Arcoraci, V.; Squadrito, F.; Altavilla, D.; Bitto, A. Oxidative Stress: Harms and Benefits for Human Health. *Oxid. Med. Cell Longev.* **2017**, *2017*, 8416763. [CrossRef]
43. Lehner, C.; Gehwolf, R.; Tempfer, H.; Krizbai, I.; Hennig, B.; Bauer, H.C.; Bauer, H. Oxidative stress and blood-brain barrier dysfunction under particular consideration of matrix metalloproteinases. *Antioxid. Redox Signal.* **2011**, *15*, 1305–1323. [CrossRef]
44. Lee, K.H.; Cha, M.; Lee, B.H. Neuroprotective Effect of Antioxidants in the Brain. *Int. J. Mol. Sci.* **2020**, *21*, 7152. [CrossRef] [PubMed]
45. Stanciu, G.D.; Bild, V.; Ababei, D.C.; Rusu, R.N.; Cobzaru, A.; Paduraru, L.; Bulea, D. Link Between Diabetes and Alzheimer's Disease due to the Shared Amyloid Aggregation and Deposition Involving both Neurodegenerative Changes and Neurovascular Damages. *J. Clin. Med.* **2020**, *9*, 1713. [CrossRef]
46. Chao, A.C.; Lee, T.C.; Juo, S.H.; Yang, D.I. Hyperglycemia Increases the Production of Amyloid Beta-Peptide Leading to Decreased Endothelial Tight Junction. *CNS Neurosci. Ther.* **2016**, *22*, 291–297. [CrossRef] [PubMed]
47. Jurcău, M.C.; Andronie-Cioara, F.L.; Jurcău, A.; Marcu, F.; Ţiţ, D.M.; Paşcalău, N.; Nistor-Cseppentö, D.C. The Link between Oxidative Stress, Mitochondrial Dysfunction and Neuroinflammation in the Pathophysiology of Alzheimer's Disease: Therapeutic Implications and Future Perspectives. *Antioxidants* **2022**, *11*, 2167. [CrossRef] [PubMed]
48. Rains, J.L.; Jain, S.K. Oxidative stress, insulin signaling, and diabetes. *Free Radic. Biol. Med.* **2011**, *50*, 567–575. [CrossRef]
49. Asmat, U.; Abad, K.; Ismail, K. Diabetes mellitus and oxidative stress-A concise review. *Saudi Pharm. J.* **2016**, *24*, 547–553. [CrossRef]
50. Tangvarasittichai, S. Oxidative stress, insulin resistance, dyslipidemia and type 2 diabetes mellitus. *World J. Diabetes* **2015**, *6*, 456–480. [CrossRef]
51. González, P.; Lozano, P.; Ros, G.; Solano, F. Hyperglycemia and Oxidative Stress: An Integral, Updated and Critical Overview of Their Metabolic Interconnections. *Int. J. Mol. Sci.* **2023**, *24*, 9352. [CrossRef]
52. Yan, L.J. Redox imbalance stress in diabetes mellitus: Role of the polyol pathway. *Anim. Model. Exp. Med.* **2018**, *1*, 7–13. [CrossRef]
53. Nowotny, K.; Jung, T.; Höhn, A.; Weber, D.; Grune, T. Advanced glycation end products and oxidative stress in type 2 diabetes mellitus. *Biomolecules* **2015**, *5*, 194–222. [CrossRef]
54. Cepas, V.; Collino, M.; Mayo, J.C.; Sainz, R.M. Redox Signaling and Advanced Glycation Endproducts (AGEs) in Diet-Related Diseases. *Antioxidants* **2020**, *9*, 142. [CrossRef] [PubMed]
55. Kurutas, E.B. The importance of antioxidants which play the role in cellular response against oxidative/nitrosative stress: Current state. *Nutr. J.* **2016**, *15*, 71. [CrossRef] [PubMed]
56. Tiwari, B.K.; Pandey, K.B.; Abidi, A.B.; Rizvi, S.I. Markers of Oxidative Stress during Diabetes Mellitus. *J. Biomark.* **2013**, *2013*, 378790. [CrossRef] [PubMed]
57. Kumawat, M.; Sharma, T.K.; Singh, I.; Singh, N.; Ghalaut, V.S.; Vardey, S.K.; Shankar, V. Antioxidant Enzymes and Lipid Peroxidation in Type 2 Diabetes Mellitus Patients with and without Nephropathy. *N. Am. J. Med. Sci.* **2013**, *5*, 213–219. [CrossRef]
58. Sekhar, R.V.; McKay, S.V.; Patel, S.G.; Guthikonda, A.P.; Reddy, V.T.; Balasubramanyam, A.; Jahoor, F. Glutathione synthesis is diminished in patients with uncontrolled diabetes and restored by dietary supplementation with cysteine and glycine. *Diabetes Care* **2011**, *34*, 162–167. [CrossRef]

59. Lagman, M.; Ly, J.; Saing, T.; Kaur Singh, M.; Vera Tudela, E.; Morris, D.; Chi, P.T.; Ochoa, C.; Sathananthan, A.; Venketaraman, V. Investigating the causes for decreased levels of glutathione in individuals with type II diabetes. *PLoS ONE* **2015**, *10*, e0118436. [CrossRef]
60. Calabrese, V.; Cornelius, C.; Leso, V.; Trovato-Salinaro, A.; Ventimiglia, B.; Cavallaro, M.; Scuto, M.; Rizza, S.; Zanoli, L.; Neri, S.; et al. Oxidative stress, glutathione status, sirtuin and cellular stress response in type 2 diabetes. *Biochim. Biophys. Acta* **2012**, *1822*, 729–736. [CrossRef]
61. Beever, A.; Kachour, N.; Owens, J.; Sasaninia, K.; Kolloli, A.; Kumar, R.; Ramasamy, S.; Sisliyan, C.; Khamas, W.; Subbian, S.; et al. L-GSH Supplementation in Conjunction with Rifampicin Augments the Treatment Response to *Mycobacterium tuberculosis* in a Diabetic Mouse Model. *Front. Pharmacol.* **2022**, *13*, 879729. [CrossRef]
62. Ferlita, S.; Yegiazaryan, A.; Noori, N.; Lal, G.; Nguyen, T.; To, K.; Venketaraman, V. Type 2 Diabetes Mellitus and Altered Immune System Leading to Susceptibility to Pathogens, Especially *Mycobacterium tuberculosis*. *J. Clin. Med.* **2019**, *8*, 2219. [CrossRef]
63. Wang, Y.; Branicky, R.; Noë, A.; Hekimi, S. Superoxide dismutases: Dual roles in controlling ROS damage and regulating ROS signaling. *J. Cell Biol.* **2018**, *217*, 1915–1928. [CrossRef]
64. Fujita, H.; Fujishima, H.; Chida, S.; Takahashi, K.; Qi, Z.; Kanetsuna, Y.; Breyer, M.D.; Harris, R.C.; Yamada, Y.; Takahashi, T. Reduction of renal superoxide dismutase in progressive diabetic nephropathy. *J. Am. Soc. Nephrol.* **2009**, *20*, 1303–1313. [CrossRef] [PubMed]
65. Strom, A.; Kaul, K.; Brüggemann, J.; Ziegler, I.; Rokitta, I.; Püttgen, S.; Szendroedi, J.; Müssig, K.; Roden, M.; Ziegler, D. Lower serum extracellular superoxide dismutase levels are associated with polyneuropathy in recent-onset diabetes. *Exp. Mol. Med.* **2017**, *49*, e394. [CrossRef] [PubMed]
66. Azami, S.; Forouzanfar, F. Therapeutic potentialities of green tea (*Camellia sinensis*) in ischemic stroke: Biochemical and molecular evidence. *Metab. Brain Dis.* 2023; *Online ahead of print*. [CrossRef]
67. Góth, L. Catalase deficiency and type 2 diabetes. *Diabetes Care* **2008**, *31*, e93. [CrossRef] [PubMed]
68. Caturano, A.; D'Angelo, M.; Mormone, A.; Russo, V.; Mollica, M.P.; Salvatore, T.; Galiero, R.; Rinaldi, L.; Vetrano, E.; Marfella, R.; et al. Oxidative Stress in Type 2 Diabetes: Impacts from Pathogenesis to Lifestyle Modifications. *Curr. Issues Mol. Biol.* **2023**, *45*, 6651–6666. [CrossRef] [PubMed]
69. Luc, K.; Schramm-Luc, A.; Guzik, T.J.; Mikolajczyk, T.P. Oxidative stress and inflammatory markers in prediabetes and diabetes. *J. Physiol. Pharmacol.* **2019**, *70*. [CrossRef]
70. Oguntibeju, O.O. Type 2 diabetes mellitus, oxidative stress and inflammation: Examining the links. *Int. J. Physiol. Pathophysiol. Pharmacol.* **2019**, *11*, 45–63.
71. Sreedhar, A.; Zhao, Y. Uncoupling protein 2 and metabolic diseases. *Mitochondrion* **2017**, *34*, 135–140. [CrossRef]
72. Kelly, B.; Tannahill, G.M.; Murphy, M.P.; O'Neill, L.A. Metformin Inhibits the Production of Reactive Oxygen Species from NADH:Ubiquinone Oxidoreductase to Limit Induction of Interleukin-1β (IL-1β) and Boosts Interleukin-10 (IL-10) in Lipopolysaccharide (LPS)-activated Macrophages. *J. Biol. Chem.* **2015**, *290*, 20348–20359. [CrossRef]
73. Tseng, C.H. Metformin Decreases Risk of Tuberculosis Infection in Type 2 Diabetes Patients. *J. Clin. Med.* **2018**, *7*, 264. [CrossRef]
74. Malínská, H.; Oliyarnyk, O.; Škop, V.; Šilhavý, J.; Landa, V.; Zídek, V.; Mlejnek, P.; Šimáková, M.; Strnad, H.; Kazdová, L.; et al. Effects of Metformin on Tissue Oxidative and Dicarbonyl Stress in Transgenic Spontaneously Hypertensive Rats Expressing Human C-Reactive Protein. *PLoS ONE* **2016**, *11*, e0150924. [CrossRef]
75. Adeshara, K.A.; Bangar, N.S.; Doshi, P.R.; Diwan, A.; Tupe, R.S. Action of metformin therapy against advanced glycation, oxidative stress and inflammation in type 2 diabetes patients: 3 months follow-up study. *Diabetes Metab. Syndr.* **2020**, *14*, 1449–1458. [CrossRef]
76. Litvinov, D.; Mahini, H.; Garelnabi, M. Antioxidant and anti-inflammatory role of paraoxonase 1: Implication in arteriosclerosis diseases. *N. Am. J. Med. Sci.* **2012**, *4*, 523–532. [CrossRef] [PubMed]
77. Roxo, D.F.; Arcaro, C.A.; Gutierres, V.O.; Costa, M.C.; Oliveira, J.O.; Lima, T.F.O.; Assis, R.P.; Brunetti, I.L.; Baviera, A.M. Curcumin combined with metformin decreases glycemia and dyslipidemia, and increases paraoxonase activity in diabetic rats. *Diabetol. Metab. Syndr.* **2019**, *11*, 33. [CrossRef] [PubMed]
78. Diniz Vilela, D.; Gomes Peixoto, L.; Teixeira, R.R.; Belele Baptista, N.; Carvalho Caixeta, D.; Vieira de Souza, A.; Machado, H.L.; Pereira, M.N.; Sabino-Silva, R.; Espindola, F.S. The Role of Metformin in Controlling Oxidative Stress in Muscle of Diabetic Rats. *Oxid. Med. Cell Longev.* **2016**, *2016*, 6978625. [CrossRef] [PubMed]
79. Nahid, P.; Dorman, S.E.; Alipanah, N.; Barry, P.M.; Brozek, J.L.; Cattamanchi, A.; Chaisson, L.H.; Chaisson, R.E.; Daley, C.L.; Grzemska, M.; et al. Official American Thoracic Society/Centers for Disease Control and Prevention/Infectious Diseases Society of America Clinical Practice Guidelines: Treatment of Drug-Susceptible Tuberculosis. *Clin. Infect. Dis.* **2016**, *63*, e147–e195. [CrossRef]
80. Mehta, K.; Narayanan, N.; Heysell, S.K.; Bisson, G.P.; Subbian, S.; Kurepina, N.; Kreiswirth, B.N.; Vinnard, C. Pharmacogenetic variability and the probability of site of action target attainment during tuberculosis meningitis treatment: A physiologically based pharmacokinetic modeling and simulations study. *Tuberculosis* **2022**, *137*, 102271. [CrossRef]
81. Te Brake, L.H.M.; de Knegt, G.J.; de Steenwinkel, J.E.; van Dam, T.J.P.; Burger, D.M.; Russel, F.G.M.; van Crevel, R.; Koenderink, J.B.; Aarnoutse, R.E. The Role of Efflux Pumps in Tuberculosis Treatment and Their Promise as a Target in Drug Development: Unraveling the Black Box. *Annu. Rev. Pharmacol. Toxicol.* **2018**, *58*, 271–291. [CrossRef]

82. Kumar, R.; Kolloli, A.; Singh, P.; Vinnard, C.; Kaplan, G.; Subbian, S. Thalidomide and Phosphodiesterase 4 Inhibitors as Host Directed Therapeutics for Tuberculous Meningitis: Insights from the Rabbit Model. *Front. Cell Infect. Microbiol.* **2020**, *9*, 450. [CrossRef]
83. Davis, A.G.; Donovan, J.; Bremer, M.; Van Toorn, R.; Schoeman, J.; Dadabhoy, A.; Lai, R.P.J.; Cresswell, F.V.; Boulware, D.R.; Wilkinson, R.J.; et al. Host Directed Therapies for Tuberculous Meningitis. *Wellcome Open Res.* **2021**, *5*, 292. [CrossRef]
84. Singhal, A.; Jie, L.; Kumar, P.; Hong, G.S.; Leow, M.K.; Paleja, B.; Tsenova, L.; Kurepina, N.; Chen, J.; Zolezzi, F.; et al. Metformin as adjunct antituberculosis therapy. *Sci. Transl. Med.* **2014**, *6*, 263ra159. [CrossRef]
85. Cojic, M.; Kocic, R.; Klisic, A.; Kocic, G. The Effects of Vitamin D Supplementation on Metabolic and Oxidative Stress Markers in Patients with Type 2 Diabetes: A 6-Month Follow Up Randomized Controlled Study. *Front. Endocrinol.* **2021**, *12*, 610893. [CrossRef] [PubMed]
86. Zhu, A.; Teng, Y.; Ge, D.; Zhang, X.; Hu, M.; Yao, X. Role of metformin in treatment of patients with chronic obstructive pulmonary disease: A systematic review. *J. Thorac. Dis.* **2019**, *11*, 4371–4378. [CrossRef] [PubMed]
87. Yen, F.S.; Wei, J.C.; Yang, Y.C.; Hsu, C.C.; Hwu, C.M. Respiratory outcomes of metformin use in patients with type 2 diabetes and chronic obstructive pulmonary disease. *Sci. Rep.* **2020**, *10*, 10298. [CrossRef]
88. American Diabetes Association. 9. Pharmacologic Approaches to Glycemic Treatment: Standards of Medical Care in Diabetes-2020. *Diabetes Care* **2020**, *43* (Suppl. 1), S98–S110, Erratum in: *Diabetes Care* **2020**, *43*, 1979. [CrossRef] [PubMed]
89. Johansen, J.S.; Harris, A.K.; Rychly, D.J.; Ergul, A. Oxidative stress and the use of antioxidants in diabetes: Linking basic science to clinical practice. *Cardiovasc. Diabetol.* **2005**, *4*, 5. [CrossRef]
90. Eldor, R.; Raz, I. American Diabetes Association indications for statins in diabetes: Is there evidence? *Diabetes Care* **2009**, *32* (Suppl. 2), S384–S391. [CrossRef]
91. Choi, S.W.; Ho, C.K. Antioxidant properties of drugs used in Type 2 diabetes management: Could they contribute to, confound or conceal effects of antioxidant therapy? *Redox Rep.* **2018**, *23*, 1–24. [CrossRef]
92. Klen, J.; Dolžan, V. SGLT2 Inhibitors in the Treatment of Diabetic Kidney Disease: More than Just Glucose Regulation. *Pharmaceutics* **2023**, *15*, 1995. [CrossRef]
93. Wronka, M.; Krzemińska, J.; Młynarska, E.; Rysz, J.; Franczyk, B. The Influence of Lifestyle and Treatment on Oxidative Stress and Inflammation in Diabetes. *Int. J. Mol. Sci.* **2022**, *23*, 15743. [CrossRef]
94. Nuhu, F.; Gordon, A.; Sturmey, R.; Seymour, A.M.; Bhandari, S. Measurement of Glutathione as a Tool for Oxidative Stress Studies by High Performance Liquid Chromatography. *Molecules* **2020**, *25*, 4196. [CrossRef]
95. To, K.; Cao, R.; Yegiazaryan, A.; Owens, J.; Nguyen, T.; Sasaninia, K.; Vaughn, C.; Singh, M.; Truong, E.; Medina, A.; et al. Effects of Oral Liposomal Glutathione in Altering the Immune Responses Against *Mycobacterium tuberculosis* and the *Mycobacterium bovis* BCG Strain in Individuals with Type 2 Diabetes. *Front. Cell Infect. Microbiol.* **2021**, *11*, 657775. [CrossRef] [PubMed]

biomedicines

MDPI

Systematic Review

Comparative Efficacy and Safety of Weekly GLP-1/GIP Agonists vs. Weekly Insulin in Type 2 Diabetes: A Network Meta-Analysis of Randomized Controlled Trials

Hazem Ayesh [1,*], Sajida Suhail [2], Suhail Ayesh [2] and Kevin Niswender [3]

1 Deaconess Health System, Evansville, IN 47708, USA
2 Gene Medical Labs, Gaza 00972, Palestine; sajidasuhail91@gmail.com (S.S.); profayesh@gmail.com (S.A.)
3 Department of Medicine, Division of Diabetes, Endocrinology, and Metabolism, Vanderbilt University Medical Center, Nashville, TN 37232, USA; kevin.niswender@vumc.org
* Correspondence: hazimayesh@gmail.com

Abstract: Background: Diabetes mellitus (DM) significantly impacts global health due to its complications and the economic burden it places on healthcare systems. The rise of novel once-weekly diabetes medications with different mechanisms of action necessitates an evaluation of their relative efficacy and safety. Objectives: This study compares the efficacy and tolerability of once-weekly insulin analogs (icodec and BIF) with once-weekly GLP-1/GIP agonists (semaglutide, exenatide, tirzepatide, dulaglutide) in managing type 2 diabetes mellitus (T2DM). Methods: We conducted a network meta-analysis (NMA) using data from randomized controlled trials (RCTs) that compared these treatments with a baseline of daily basal insulin. Primary outcomes included changes in HbA1c, body weight, and tolerability. Results: The analysis integrated data from 25 RCTs, involving 18,257 patients. Tirzepatide significantly outperformed other treatments in reducing HbA1c and promoting weight loss. Weekly insulins, compared to GLP-1/GIP agonists, showed a more tolerable profile and were beneficial for certain patient demographics emphasizing weight stability. Conclusion: Our findings suggest that while once-weekly GLP-1/GIP agonists provide superior glycemic control and weight management, weekly insulins offer viable options for patients prioritizing fewer side effects and weight stability. This comprehensive comparison aids in refining personalized treatment strategies for T2DM management.

Keywords: diabetes management; once-weekly insulin; GLP-1/GIP receptor agonists; HbA1c reduction; treatment tolerability

1. Introduction

Diabetes mellitus (DM) imposes a substantial global burden, contributing significantly to morbidity and mortality rates, particularly due to associated complications such as cardiovascular disease, renal dysfunction, and neurological impairments [1,2]. Moreover, the economic impact of diabetes on healthcare systems is considerable [2]. Hence, optimizing diabetes management is imperative, especially given the escalating prevalence of this metabolic disorder.

There are remarkable advancements in the practice of diabetes, particularly in the realm of once-weekly agents designed to enhance treatment adherence and simplify patient management [3,4]. However, the proliferation of these agents has created a complex decision-making landscape for healthcare providers, necessitating evidence-based strategies for personalized treatment plans [4].

Among the recent advancements are glucagon-like peptide-1 (GLP-1) agonists and glucose-dependent insulinotropic peptide (GIP) dual agonists and once-weekly insulin, which offer promising avenues for diabetes management [5,6]. These novel agents offer intriguing alternatives to traditional therapies, potentially revolutionizing the treatment paradigm. Nonetheless, the challenge lies in personalizing therapy in order to optimize treatment outcomes while minimizing adverse effects and the risk of polypharmacy.

Our study aims to address this challenge by comparing the efficacy, safety, and tolerability profiles of once-weekly insulin formulations, such as icodec and BIF, against once-weekly GLP-1/GIP agonists, including semaglutide, exenatide, tirzepatide, and dulaglutide. Specifically, we will evaluate their impact on glycated hemoglobin (HbA1c) levels, body weight, and tolerability, providing valuable insights into their relative efficacy and safety profiles.

Conducting a comprehensive comparison through network meta-analysis (NMA) represents a significant endeavor with far-reaching implications. NMA enables the integration of data from diverse randomized controlled trials (RCTs), offering a robust framework for assessing the comparative efficacy and safety of different treatment modalities. By elucidating the relative merits of once-weekly GLP-1/GIP agonists and insulin formulations, our analysis aims to inform clinical decision-making, guide guideline development, and inform healthcare policies. Ultimately, this endeavor seeks to enhance the delivery of personalized and effective care for individuals living with type 2 diabetes mellitus (T2DM).

2. Methods

The protocol for this network meta-analysis was registered in OSF registries (https://osf.io/p7szu, accessed on 30 May 2024) [7]. Results were reported according to preferred reporting items for systematic reviews and meta-analyses (PRISMA) guidelines [8].

2.1. Data Sources

We conducted a comprehensive search in the databases Scopus, PubMed, Cochrane, and Web of Science from inception to 5 April 2024 (search strategy detailed in Supplement S1).

2.2. Study Selection

We included randomized controlled trials (RCTs) involving individuals diagnosed with type 2 diabetes mellitus that evaluated weekly GLP-1/GIP agonists and weekly insulin in comparison to daily insulin. The primary outcome measures evaluated were glycemic control (HbA1c levels and fasting plasma glucose), weight change, and safety parameters (incidence of hypoglycemia and adverse events). We excluded non-randomized studies, observational studies, extension studies, exploratory analyses, post hoc analyses, and animal studies. Additionally, we excluded studies involving individuals without type 2 diabetes mellitus, pediatric populations, studies that did not have daily insulin as a comparator, and studies not reporting relevant outcomes related to efficacy and safety.

2.3. Data Extraction

The primary efficacy outcome extracted from each RCT was the mean change from baseline in hemoglobin A1c (HbA1c). Secondary efficacy outcomes included mean changes from baseline in fasting plasma glucose (FPG) and body weight (BW). Safety outcomes encompassed the incidence of hypoglycemia, treatment-emergent adverse events (TEAE), and rates of treatment discontinuation due to adverse events.

In our analysis, we calculated the standard error (SE) of the mean with the equation: SE = (CI_width)/(2 × z_value), where CI_width denotes the breadth of the confidence interval and z_value is the z-score corresponding to the targeted confidence level [9]. This approach enabled us to estimate the SE when only the confidence interval (CI) and the mean of the data were provided [9]. We selected data for analysis that represented the longest follow-up periods and included comparisons with daily basal insulin since there is no direct comparison between GLP-1/GIP and weekly insulin. In cases where the original studies reported data as medians and ranges, we converted these to means and standard deviations to ensure uniformity in our analysis [10].

2.4. Risk of Bias Assessment

The risk of bias was assessed using the RoB2 tool [11]. This evaluation covered several domains, deviations from intended interventions, randomization process, missing outcome data, outcome measurement, and selection of the reported results.

2.5. Statistical Analysis

We performed frequentist random effects network meta-analysis that compared multiple treatments by analyzing data from various studies, allowing for both direct and indirect comparisons. This method synthesizes evidence to determine the relative efficacy of each treatment, even if some treatments were not directly compared in any individual study [12].

For continuous outcomes (HbA1c, FPG, BW), we calculated mean differences (MDs) with 95% confidence intervals (CIs). For binary outcomes (TEAE, hypoglycemic events, incidence of serious adverse events, and treatment discontinuation due to adverse events), we calculated risk ratios (RRs) with 95% CIs.

Pairwise comparisons were conducted for direct comparisons [13]. We validated the transitivity assumption by utilizing node splitting to compare direct and indirect outcomes, ensuring their consistency [14]. Heterogeneity was evaluated by comparing the magnitude of the common between-study variance ($\tau 2$) for each outcome with empirical distributions of heterogeneity variances [15]. We also created surface under the cumulative ranking curve (SUCRA) graphs for efficacy outcomes and conducted meta-regression analyses for age, BMI, and diabetes duration [16]. SUCRA provides a hierarchical ranking of treatments facilitating comparison across studies [16]. We conducted a sensitivity analysis to ensure the robustness of our results by applying a Bayesian network meta-analysis model with meta-regression (accounting for age, BMI, and duration) for efficacy outcomes, thereby confirming the findings of our network meta-analysis.

We performed the analysis using RStudio version number 4.3.2 (31 October 2023) and R packages: netmeta version number 2.9-0, gemtc version number 1.0-2, and rjags version number 4.15 [17–20]. The certainty of evidence was evaluated using the confidence in network meta-analysis (CINeMA) framework and online application (https://cinema.ispm.unibe.ch/, accessed on 30 May 2024) [21].

3. Results

3.1. Study Characteristics

A total of 25 trials [22–46] were included in the analysis (Figure 1). The network of trials comparing HbA1c is shown in Figure 2. The characteristics of studies and patients' baseline features are presented in Supplement S2.

The mean age of participants in the included studies was 57.8 years (standard deviation [SD]: 11.2), with 57.8% being male. The mean body mass index (BMI) was 31.2 kg/m^2 (SD: 5.6). The mean HbA1c level was 8.3% (SD: 0.8), and the mean duration of diabetes was 11.0 years (SD: 7.7).

There was substantial heterogeneity in HbA1c, fasting plasma glucose (FPG), body weight (BW), risk of adverse events, and risk of hypoglycemia. Overall, global inconsistency was minimal. The primary outcome's risk of bias was low in 20 trials, with 5 trials presenting some concerns. Comparison-adjusted funnel plots indicated no publication bias for HbA1c, hypoglycemia, FPG, and body weight, but there was some indication of publication bias for the incidence of adverse events. (Supplement S4). The certainty of evidence was generally moderate to high for each of the main comparisons, with some comparisons having low certainty. All data from certainty analysis are included in (Supplement S6).

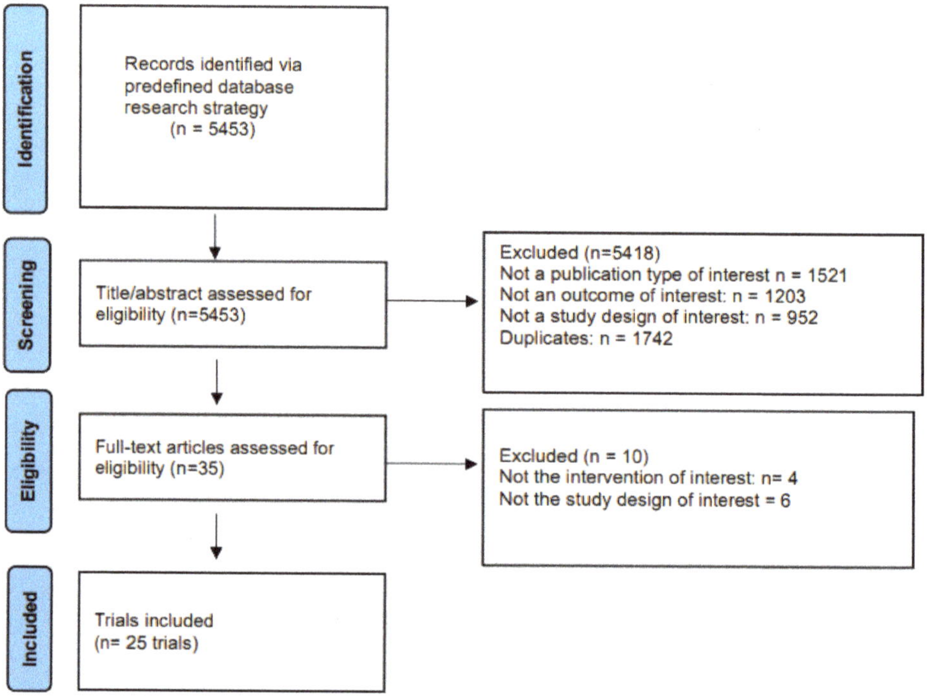

Figure 1. PRISMA flowchart for study selection.

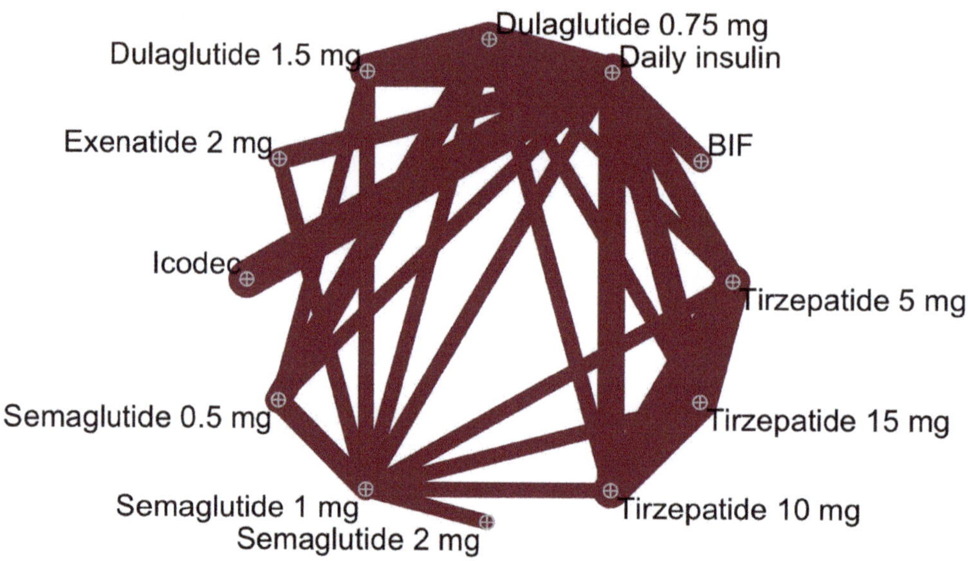

Figure 2. Meta-analysis networks for change in HbA1c level. Each circle indicates a treatment node. Lines connecting two nodes represent direct comparisons between two treatments; the thickness of the lines is proportional to the number of trials directly comparing the two connected treatments.

3.2. *HbA1c*

We evaluated the effects of GLP-1/GIP receptor agonists and weekly insulin analogs on HbA1c reduction, using daily insulin as the active comparator. The analysis encompassed 25 studies involving 18,257 patients. Tirzepatide showed the highest efficacy with the 15 mg dose achieving a mean difference (MD) in HbA1c reduction of −1.29 (95% CI: −1.44 to −1.14), followed by the 10 mg dose with an MD of −1.16 (95% CI: −1.31 to −1.02), and the 5 mg dose with an MD of −0.94 (95% CI: −1.09 to −0.79). Semaglutide showed substantial HbA1c reductions across dosages: the 2 mg dose had an MD of −1.00 (95% CI: −1.34 to −0.65), the 1 mg dose at −0.82 (95% CI: −0.98 to −0.65), and the 0.5 mg dose at −0.47 (95% CI: −0.65 to −0.29). Exenatide 2 mg also contributed with an MD of −0.27 (95% CI: −0.46 to −0.08). Among the weekly insulin analogs, icodec demonstrated a modest but significant reduction in HbA1c compared to daily insulin, with an MD of −0.16 (95% CI: −0.30 to −0.02). BIF, however, did not demonstrate a statistically significant change, with an MD of 0.08 (95% CI: −0.17 to 0.33). Detailed results of pairwise comparisons can be found in Supplement S5, and network meta-analysis results are presented in Figure 3. The SUCRA ranking is depicted in Figure 4, and confirms tirzepatide 15 mg as the top-ranked treatment for HbA1c reduction, unaffected by patient age, BMI, or diabetes duration according to our meta-regression analyses. Meta-regression results are depicted in Supplement S7.

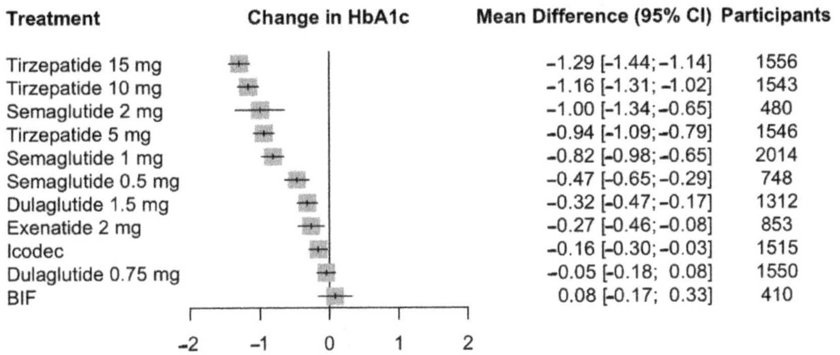

Figure 3. Network meta-analysis results for change from baseline. HbA1c compared with daily insulin. Effect sizes are presented as mean difference (MD) and 95% confidence intervals (CI). Treatments are presented according to their effect estimate compared with glargine. Abbreviations: HbA1c: hemoglobin A1c, BIF: basal insulin Fc.

3.3. *FPG*

Our analysis focused on the impact of GLP-1/GIP receptor agonists and weekly insulin analogs on fasting plasma glucose (FPG) levels, using daily insulin as the baseline for comparison. The pooled data from 18,257 patients reveal that tirzepatide at 15 mg had the most substantial effect on reducing FPG, with a mean difference (MD) of −0.70 mmol/L (95% CI: −1.00 to −0.41), and the 10 mg dose showed a significant decrease with an MD of −0.55 mmol/L (95% CI: −0.84 to −0.25). The 5 mg dose of tirzepatide also suggested a reduction in FPG levels, with an MD of −0.21 mmol/L (95% CI: −0.50 to 0.09), although this was not statistically significant. Semaglutide displayed varied effects across dosages: the 2 mg dose led to a reduction with an MD of −0.45 mmol/L (95% CI: −1.19 to 0.28), the 1 mg dose had a non-significant impact with an MD of −0.12 mmol/L (95% CI: −0.47 to 0.22), and the 0.5 mg dose increased FPG levels slightly with an MD of 0.47 mmol/L (95% CI: 0.09 to 0.85). Exenatide 2 mg had an MD of 0.34 mmol/L (95% CI: −0.08 to 0.76), indicating a possible, but not statistically significant, increase. BIF and icodec had MDs of 0.60 mmol/L (95% CI: 0.15 to 1.05) and −0.06 mmol/L (95% CI: −0.35 to 0.22), respectively, reflecting a significant increase for BIF and a non-significant difference for icodec. Detailed results of pairwise comparisons can be found in Supplement S5. Network meta-analysis results are presented in Figure 5. Meta-regression results are depicted in Supplement S7.

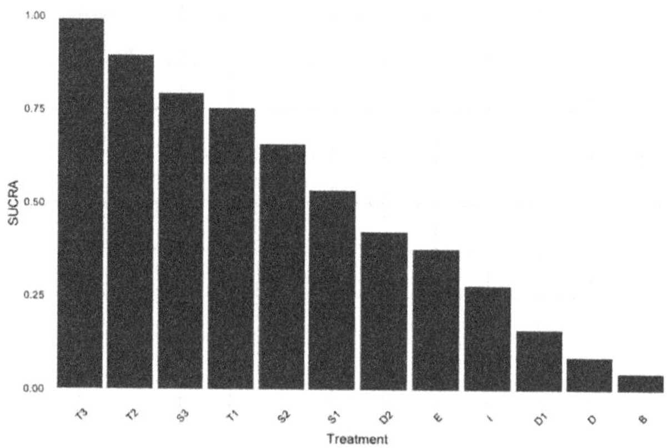

Figure 4. The surface under the cumulative ranking (SUCRA) plot displays the ranking probabilities of treatments in reducing hemoglobin A1c (HbA1c). Higher SUCRA scores indicate a greater likelihood of lowering HbA1c. Abbreviations: T3: tirzepatide 15 mg, T2: tirzepatide 10 mg, T1: tirzepatide 5 mg, S3: semaglutide 2 mg, S2: semaglutide 1 mg, S1: semaglutide 0.5 mg, D2: dulaglutide 1.5 mg, E: exenatide 2 mg, I: icodec, D: daily insulin, B: BIF, D1: dulaglutide 0.75 mg.

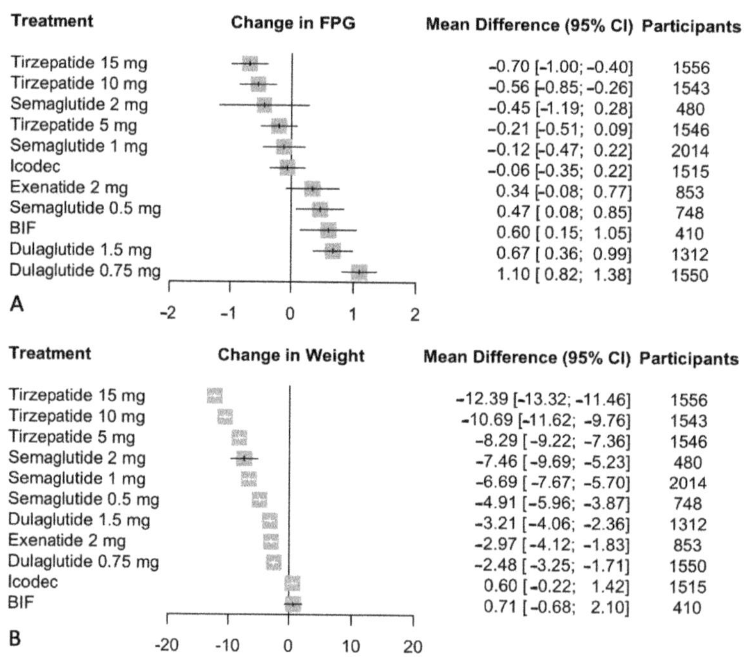

Figure 5. (**A**) Network meta-analysis results for change from baseline in FPG compared with daily insulin. (**B**). Network meta-analysis results for change from baseline in weight compared with daily insulin. Effect sizes are presented as mean difference (MD) and 95% confidence intervals (CI). Treatments are presented according to their effect estimate compared with daily insulin. Abbreviations: FPG: fasting plasma glucose, BIF: basal insulin Fc.

3.4. BW

We evaluated the effects of GLP-1/GIP receptor agonists and weekly insulin analogs on weight loss, using daily insulin as the active comparator. We pooled data from 25 studies encompassing 18,257 patients. Tirzepatide showed the most notable weight loss, with the 15 mg dose achieving a mean difference (MD) of −12.39 kg (95% CI: −13.32 to −11.46), and the 10 mg and 5 mg doses showing MDs of −10.69 kg (95% CI: −11.62 to −9.76) and −8.29 kg (95% CI: −9.22 to −7.36), respectively. Significant reductions in weight were also seen with semaglutide, with the 2 mg dose resulting in an MD of −7.46 kg (95% CI: −9.69 to −5.23), the 1 mg dose at −6.69 kg (95% CI: −7.67 to −5.70), and the 0.5 mg dose at −4.91 kg (95% CI: −5.96 to −3.87). Dulaglutide at 1.5 mg and 0.75 mg also showed substantial weight reductions, with MDs of −3.21 kg (95% CI: −4.06 to −2.36) and −2.48 kg (95% CI: −3.25 to −1.71), respectively. Exenatide 2 mg contributed to weight loss with an MD of −2.97 kg (95% CI: −4.12 to −1.83). In contrast, icodec showed a non-significant trend toward weight gain with an MD of 0.60 kg (95% CI: −0.22 to 1.42). BIF suggested a potential increase in weight, with an MD of 0.71 kg (95% CI: −0.68 to 2.10), although this was not statistically significant. Detailed results of pairwise comparisons can be found in Supplement S5. Network meta-analysis results are presented in Figure 5. Meta-regression results are depicted in Supplement S7.

3.5. Hypoglycemia

We conducted a comprehensive analysis to assess the risk of hypoglycemia associated with GLP-1/GIP receptor agonists and weekly insulin analogs, using daily insulin as the baseline comparator. The analysis pooled results from multiple studies that reported level 1 (≤70 mg/dL) and level 2 (≤55 mg/dL) hypoglycemia. It indicated that tirzepatide has a low risk of hypoglycemia, particularly with the 5 mg dose (RR 0.26, 95% CI: 0.17 to 0.40), followed by the 10 mg dose (RR 0.32, 95% CI: 0.21 to 0.49), and the 15 mg dose (RR 0.42, 95% CI: 0.27 to 0.64). Semaglutide also presents a low risk of hypoglycemia across its dosages, with the 2 mg dose showing the most significant effect (RR 0.30, 95% CI: 0.11 to 0.80). Exenatide 2 mg showed a low risk of hypoglycemia as well (RR 0.35, 95% CI: 0.20 to 0.60). In contrast, icodec (RR 1.31, 95% CI: 0.94 to 1.84) and BIF (RR 1.41, 95% CI: 0.74 to 2.70) did not demonstrate a significant reduction in hypoglycemia risk compared to daily insulin. Dulaglutide doses also showed a reduction in hypoglycemia risk, with RRs of 0.56 (95% CI: 0.39 to 0.83) for the 1.5 mg dose and 0.51 (95% CI: 0.35 to 0.75) for the 0.75 mg dose. The network meta-analysis results are presented in Figure 6.

Regarding the subgroup analysis for level 2 hypoglycemia, tirzepatide demonstrated a significant reduction in the risk of severe hypoglycemic episodes across all doses: the 10 mg dose achieved a risk ratio (RR) of 0.50 (95% CI: 0.36 to 0.71), the 5 mg dose an RR of 0.52 (95% CI: 0.37 to 0.74), and the 15 mg dose an RR of 0.65 (95% CI: 0.46 to 0.91), all indicating statistically significant decreases. Similarly, semaglutide showed substantial reductions, with the 2 mg dose showing an RR of 0.22 (95% CI: 0.09 to 0.52), the 1 mg dose an RR of 0.44 (95% CI: 0.28 to 0.68), and the 0.5 mg dose an RR of 0.36 (95% CI: 0.20 to 0.65). Exenatide 2 mg also notably decreased the risk with an RR of 0.40 (95% CI: 0.28 to 0.59). In contrast, dulaglutide, icodec, and BIF did not demonstrate statistically significant effects: dulaglutide's 1.5 mg and 0.75 mg doses had RRs of 0.55 (95% CI: 0.16 to 1.86) and 0.33 (95% CI: 0.09 to 1.22), respectively; icodec had an RR of 1.19 (95% CI: 0.84 to 1.70); and BIF showed an RR of 0.97 (95% CI: 0.62 to 1.51). The network meta-analysis results are presented in Figure 6.

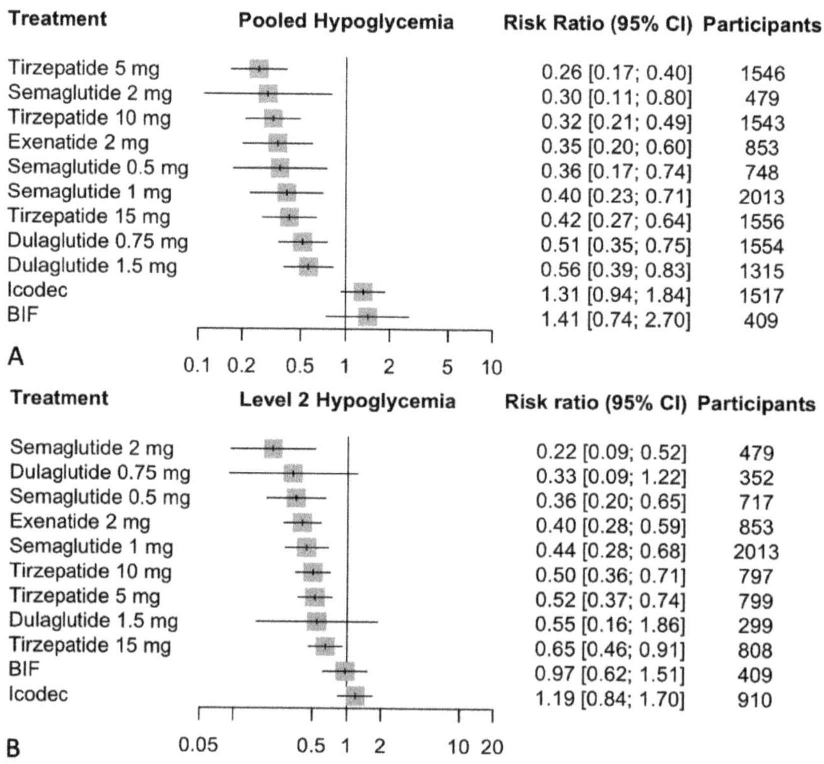

Figure 6. (**A**) Network meta-analysis results for change from baseline in pooled hypoglycemia. (**B**) Network meta-analysis results for change from baseline in level 2 (≤55 mg/dL) hypoglycemia. Effect sizes are presented as risk ratio (RR) and 95% confidence intervals (CI). Treatments are presented according to their effect estimate compared with daily insulin. Abbreviations: BIF: basal insulin Fc.

3.6. Incidence of Any Adverse Events

Our comprehensive analysis assessed the incidence of adverse events associated with GLP-1/GIP receptor agonists and weekly insulin analogs, using daily insulin as the baseline comparator. The results indicated that tirzepatide had the highest incidence of adverse events, with the 15 mg dose showing a risk ratio (RR) of 1.22 (95% CI: 1.04 to 1.43), followed by the 10 mg dose at an RR of 1.18 (95% CI: 1.01 to 1.38). The 5 mg dose also showed an increased risk of adverse events with an RR of 1.10 (95% CI: 0.95 to 1.29). Semaglutide demonstrated an increased incidence as well, particularly the 1 mg dose with an RR of 1.13 (95% CI: 0.96 to 1.33), and the 2 mg dose with an RR of 1.23 (95% CI: 0.91 to 1.66). Exenatide 2 mg reported a notable increase in adverse events with an RR of 1.20 (95% CI: 0.95 to 1.51). Dulaglutide doses showed an elevated risk with RRs of 1.08 (95% CI: 0.92 to 1.27) for the 0.75 mg dose and 1.14 (95% CI: 0.96 to 1.35) for the 1.5 mg dose. In contrast, icodec and BIF did not demonstrate a statistically significant increase in adverse events compared to daily insulin, with RRs of 1.07 (95% CI: 0.92 to 1.25) and 1.11 (95% CI: 0.81 to 1.52), respectively. The network meta-analysis results are presented in Figure 7.

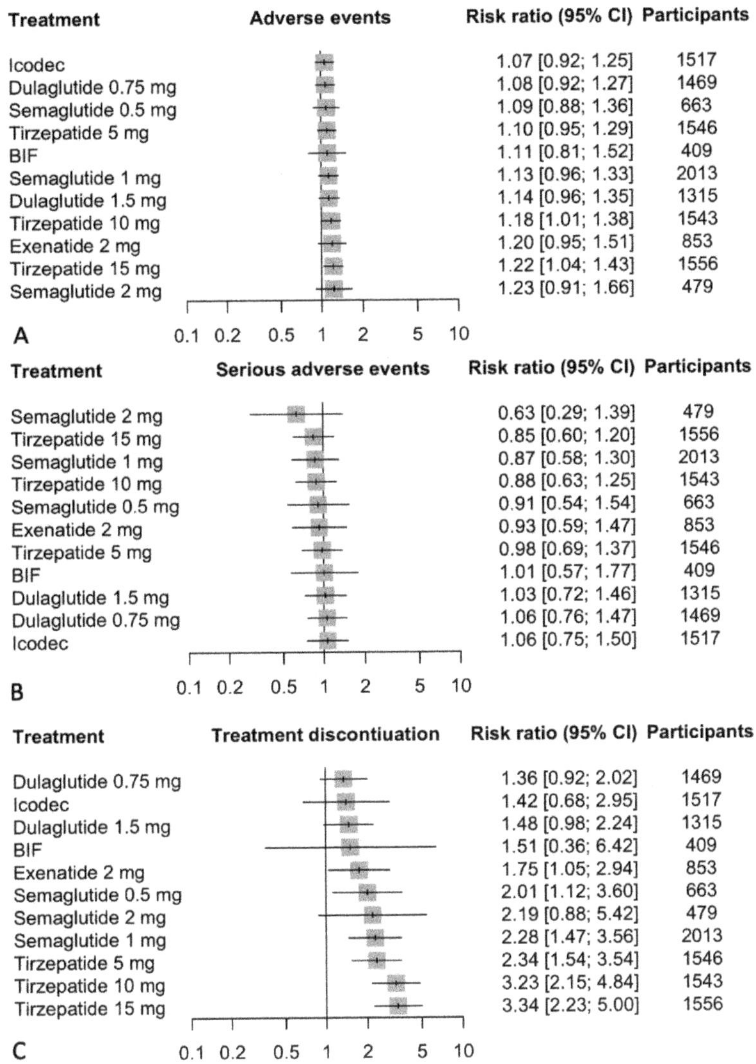

Figure 7. Network meta-analysis results for (**A**) incidence in adverse events. (**B**) incidence in serious adverse events. (**C**) treatment discontinuation due to adverse events compared with daily insulin. Treatments are presented according to their effect estimate compared with daily insulin. Effect sizes are presented as risk ratio (RR) and 95% confidence intervals (CI). Abbreviations: BIF: basal insulin Fc.

3.7. Incidence of Any Serious Events

Our analysis evaluated the incidence of serious adverse events associated with GLP-1/GIP receptor agonists and weekly insulin analogs, with daily insulin serving as the comparator. The results indicate that the majority of treatments did not demonstrate a statistically significant increase in the risk of serious adverse events compared to daily insulin. Specifically, tirzepatide showed non-significant differences across its doses, with the 15 mg dose having a risk ratio (RR) of 0.85 (95% CI: 0.60 to 1.20), the 10 mg dose an RR of 0.88 (95% CI: 0.63 to 1.25), and the 5 mg dose an RR of 0.98 (95% CI: 0.69 to 1.37). Similarly, semaglutide's doses all presented non-significant risks, with the 2 mg dose at an RR of 0.63 (95% CI: 0.29 to 1.39), the 1 mg dose at an RR of 0.87 (95% CI: 0.58 to 1.30), and the 0.5 mg dose at an RR of 0.91 (95% CI: 0.54 to 1.54). Exenatide 2 mg and icodec also showed no significant increase in risk with RRs of 0.93 (95% CI: 0.59 to 1.47) and 1.06 (95% CI: 0.75 to 1.50), respectively. The same trend was observed with dulaglutide, where both the 1.5 mg and 0.75 mg doses had non-significant RRs of 1.03 (95% CI: 0.72 to 1.46) and 1.06 (95% CI: 0.76 to 1.47). Additionally, BIF exhibited a reduced risk, though not statistically significant, with an RR of 1.01 (95% CI: 0.57 to 1.77). The network meta-analysis results are presented in Figure 7.

3.8. Treatment Discontinuation Due to Adverse Events

Our analysis examined treatment discontinuation due to adverse events among GLP-1/GIP receptor agonists and weekly insulin analogs, using daily insulin as the baseline comparator. The findings reveal that tirzepatide had the highest rates of discontinuation due to adverse events, with the 15 mg dose showing a risk ratio (RR) of 3.34 (95% CI: 2.23 to 5.00), followed closely by the 10 mg dose at an RR of 3.23 (95% CI: 2.15 to 4.84). The 5 mg dose also exhibited a significantly increased risk with an RR of 2.34 (95% CI: 1.54 to 3.54). Semaglutide similarly led to higher discontinuation rates, particularly the 1 mg dose with an RR of 2.28 (95% CI: 1.47 to 3.56), the 2 mg dose at an RR of 2.19 (95% CI: 0.88 to 5.42), and the 0.5 mg dose at an RR of 2.01 (95% CI: 1.12 to 3.60). Exenatide 2 mg also showed a notably high rate of discontinuation due to adverse events with an RR of 1.75 (95% CI: 1.05 to 2.94). In contrast, dulaglutide and icodec had less pronounced effects, with dulaglutide's 1.5 mg dose showing a borderline significant increase in discontinuation rates (RR 1.48, 95% CI: 0.98 to 2.24), while its 0.75 mg dose and icodec did not show statistically significant increases. BIF also did not demonstrate a significant difference in discontinuation rates compared to daily insulin (RR 1.51, 95% CI: 0.36 to 6.42). The network meta-analysis results are presented in Figure 7. Table 1 below summarizes the results of the study.

Table 1. Summary of the results of the network meta-analysis. Abbreviations: HbA1c: hemoglobin A1c, MD: mean difference, CI: confidence interval, BIF: basal insulin Fc, BW: body weight, FPG: fasting plasma glucose, RR: risk ratio, mg: milligrams, kg: kilograms, mmol/L: millimoles per liter.

Outcome	Most Favorable Intervention	Treatment Effect	Least Favorable Intervention	Treatment Effect
Change in HbA1c	Tirzepatide 15 mg	MD: −1.29% (95% CI: −1.44 to −1.14)	BIF	MD: 0.08 (95% CI: −0.17 to 0.33)
Change in FPG	Tirzepatide 15 mg	MD: −0.70 mmol/L (95% CI: −1.00 to −0.41)	Dulaglutide 0.75 mg	MD: 1.10 (95% CI: 0.82 to 1.38)
Change in BW	Tirzepatide 15 mg	MD: −12.39 kg (95% CI: −13.32 to −11.46)	BIF	MD: 0.71 (95% CI: −0.68 to 2.10)
Pooled hypoglycemia	Tirzepatide 5 mg	RR: 0.26 (95% CI: 0.17 to 0.40)	BIF	RR: 1.41 (95% CI: 0.74 to 2.70)
Level 2 hypoglycemia	Semaglutide 2 mg	RR: 0.22 (95% CI: 0.09 to 0.52)	Icodec	RR: 1.19 (95% CI: 0.84 to 1.70)
Incidence of any adverse events	Icodec	RR: 1.07 (95% CI: 0.92 to 1.25)	Semaglutide 2 mg	RR: 1.23 (95% CI: 0.91 to 1.66)
Serious adverse events	Semaglutide 2 mg	RR: 0.63 (95% CI: 0.29 to 1.39)	Icodec	RR: 1.06 (95% CI: 0.75 to 1.50)
Treatment discontinuation due to adverse events	Dulaglutide 0.75 mg	RR: 1.36 (95% CI: 0.92 to 2.02)	Tirzepatide 15 mg	RR: 3.34 (95% CI: 2.23 to 5.00)

4. Discussion

This systematic review and network meta-analysis incorporated data from 23 trials to evaluate the efficacy and safety of GLP-1/GIP receptor agonists and weekly insulin analogs, focusing on their effects on HbA1c reduction, fasting plasma glucose (FPG), body weight (BW), incidence of hypoglycemia, and adverse events. Our analysis not only underscores the variability in efficacy across different treatment modalities but also highlights important safety and tolerability concerns associated with these therapies.

Tirzepatide emerged as the standout treatment, significantly reducing HbA1c levels and body weight across all its dosages when compared to insulin glargine, the active comparator. The superior efficacy of tirzepatide, particularly at the 15 mg dose, is consistent with its dual mechanism of action as both a GLP-1 and GIP receptor agonist, which may offer enhanced metabolic control over single-mechanism treatments. In contrast, weekly insulin analogs like icodec showed modest HbA1c reductions but showed lower efficacy in controlling body weight, sometimes even leading to weight gain. However, these insulins could be a viable option for individuals in low to moderate weight categories where significant weight loss is not a primary treatment goal. This suggests a potential niche for weekly insulins in personalized diabetes management, particularly for patients where weight stability is preferred or where GLP-1/GIP receptor agonists' effects on weight are contraindicated. These results are consistent with works in the literature that showed 3 to 9 kg weight gain in the first year after starting insulin therapy [47].

The analysis reveals that while higher doses of GLP-1/GIP receptor agonists such as tirzepatide showed higher efficacy, they are also associated with an increased incidence of adverse events and treatment discontinuations. The most common adverse events include gastrointestinal side effects such as nausea, vomiting, and abdominal pain, in addition to hypoglycemia. Gastrointestinal adverse events were more common at higher doses of GLP-1/GIP. On the other hand, hypoglycemia and injection sit reaction were more common with weekly insulin. These findings are consistent with the current literature [48].

Lower doses of these agents, while slightly less efficacious in reducing HbA1c and body weight, demonstrate better tolerability, making them suitable for patients who may be sensitive to the side effects of higher doses. Considering the convenience of weekly insulin, our data suggest that a combination therapy involving low doses of GLP-1/GIP agonists with weekly insulin might be a viable strategy for achieving good glycemic control with reduced side effects. This approach would leverage the benefits of both treatments: the metabolic efficacy of GLP-1/GIP agonists and the convenience and tolerability profile of weekly insulin but would increase expense.

The substantial heterogeneity detected in the incidence of adverse events and hypoglycemia across studies suggests that individual patient factors and underlying health conditions play a significant role in the safety profiles of these therapies. The presence of some publication bias for adverse events calls for cautious interpretation of the safety data.

The findings of this meta-analysis have significant implications for clinical practice. The high efficacy of GLP-1/GIP receptor agonists in reducing both HbA1c and body weight makes them attractive options for patients struggling with weight management in addition to glycemic control. However, for patients where weight loss is not necessary or desired, weekly insulins offer an effective alternative that maintains weight stability while still providing good glycemic control. Combining lower doses of GLP-1/GIP agonists with weekly insulin may enhance patient adherence and satisfaction by reducing the frequency of injections and side effects while maintaining efficacy.

Further research is needed to explore the long-term outcomes of these treatments, particularly regarding cardiovascular health, renal function, and mortality. Additionally, studies should aim to identify patient characteristics that predict better tolerance and response to these therapies, which could enable more personalized treatment approaches.

This investigation has yielded insights into the comparative efficacy, safety, and patient reception of once-weekly GLP-1/GIP agonist treatments and basal insulin in the context of type 2 diabetes mellitus (T2DM). There are, however, several limitations to our study. The novelty of the examined therapies has resulted in a limited selection of studies for inclusion, which, in turn, has introduced a notable degree of heterogeneity to our findings. Moreover, the analysis predominantly reflects short-term effects, underscoring the need for extended longitudinal research to comprehensively discern the long-term impacts of these treatments on the progression of T2DM, associated complications, and the quality of life of the patients. Variations in the duration of studies, as well as the demographic and baseline health characteristics of participants, inject a level of variability that may limit the broad applicability of our findings. The methodology of network meta-analysis, dependent on indirect treatment comparisons, is inherently complex and operates under assumptions like transitivity and consistency that are critical to the integrity of our conclusions. Inconsistencies in defining and documenting adverse events in clinical trials further complicate the precision of our adverse event data. Finally, the very nature of meta-analysis, contingent on the quality and inclusiveness of existing research, carries an omnipresent risk of publication bias that cannot be completely negated.

5. Conclusions

In conclusion, this network meta-analysis provides comprehensive insights into the comparative efficacy and safety of GLP-1/GIP receptor agonists and weekly insulin analogs. It highlights the need for balancing efficacy with safety in diabetes management, and the importance of individualizing treatment plans based on patient-specific factors and preferences. Our findings underscore the superior efficacy of GLP-1/GIP agonists in both glycemic control and weight management. However, weekly insulins remain a crucial part of the therapeutic arsenal, especially for individuals where significant weight loss is not desired or patients who cannot tolerate GLP-1/GIP agonists. The integration of these agents into clinical practice should consider patient-specific factors such as baseline body weight, potential side effects, and individual health goals to optimize outcomes in diabetes care.

Supplementary Materials: The following supporting information can be downloaded at: https://www.mdpi.com/article/10.3390/biomedicines12091943/s1. Supplement S1: Search strategy. Supplement S2: Baseline characteristics of included studies. Supplement S3: Risk of bias assessment of included trials for each outcome. Supplement S4: Comparison-adjusted funnel plots. Supplement S5: Pairwise meta-analysis results. Supplement S6: Certainty of the effect estimates. Supplement S7: Meta-regression results. Supplement S8: Summary of the excluded studies. Supplement S9: Evaluation of heterogeneity and inconsistency under full design-by-treatment interaction random effects model. References [22–46,49–58] are cited in the supplementary materials.

Author Contributions: H.A.: writing—review and editing, writing—original draft, visualization, validation, supervision, software, resources, project administration, methodology, investigation, formal analysis, data curation, and conceptualization; S.S.: data curation, formal analysis, software, and review of the final draft; S.A.: conceptualization, writing—original draft, validation, and review of final draft; K.N.: writing—review and editing, conceptualization, project administration, and funding acquisition. All authors have read and agreed to the published version of the manuscript.

Funding: This research received no external funding.

Institutional Review Board Statement: Not applicable.

Informed Consent Statement: Not applicable.

Data Availability Statement: The original contributions presented in the study are included in the article/Supplementary Materials, further inquiries can be directed to the corresponding author.

Conflicts of Interest: The authors declare no conflicts of interest.

Abbreviations

DM	Diabetes mellitus
GLP-1	Glucagon-like peptide-1
GIP	Glucose-dependent insulinotropic peptide
NMA	Network meta-analysis
RCT	Randomized controlled trial
HbA1c	Hemoglobin A1c
BW	Body weight
FPG	Fasting plasma glucose
TEAE	Treatment-emergent adverse events
SE	Standard error
CI	Confidence interval
RR	Risk ratio
T2DM	Type 2 diabetes mellitus
SUCRA	Surface under the cumulative ranking curve
PRISMA	Preferred reporting items for systematic reviews and meta-analyses

References

1. Leon, B.M.; Maddox, T.M. Diabetes and cardiovascular disease: Epidemiology, biological mechanisms, treatment recommendations and future research. *World J. Diabetes* **2015**, *6*, 1246–1258. [CrossRef] [PubMed]
2. Fan, W. Epidemiology in diabetes mellitus and cardiovascular disease. *Cardiovasc. Endocrinol.* **2017**, *6*, 8–16. [CrossRef] [PubMed]
3. Kerr, D.; Rajpura, J.R.; Namvar, T. Evaluating Patient and Provider Preferences for a Once-Weekly Basal Insulin in Adults with Type 2 Diabetes. *Patient Prefer. Adherence* **2024**, *18*, 411–424. [CrossRef] [PubMed]
4. Cornell, S. A review of GLP-1 receptor agonists in type 2 diabetes: A focus on the mechanism of action of once-weekly agents. *J. Clin. Pharm. Ther.* **2020**, *45* (Suppl. S1), 17–27. [CrossRef]
5. Rizvi, A.A.; Rizzo, M. The Emerging Role of Dual GLP-1 and GIP Receptor Agonists in Glycemic Management and Cardiovascular Risk Reduction. *Diabetes Metab. Syndr. Obes.* **2022**, *15*, 1023–1030. [CrossRef]
6. Scheen, A.J. Dual GIP/GLP-1 receptor agonists: New advances for treating type-2 diabetes. *Ann. D'endocrinologie* **2023**, *84*, 316–321. [CrossRef]
7. Ayesh, H. Comparative Efficacy and Safety of Weekly GLP-1/GIP Agonists versus Weekly Insulin in Type 2 Diabetes: A Network Meta-Analysis of Randomized Controlled Trials. 2024. Available online: https://osf.io/p7szu (accessed on 30 May 2024).
8. Page, M.J.; McKenzie, J.E.; Bossuyt, P.M.; Boutron, I.; Hoffmann, T.C.; Mulrow, C.D.; Shamseer, L.; Tetzlaff, J.M.; Akl, E.A.; Brennan, S.E.; et al. The PRISMA 2020 statement: An updated guideline for reporting systematic reviews. *BMJ* **2021**, *372*, n71. [CrossRef]
9. Altman, D.G.; Bland, J.M. Standard deviations and standard errors. *BMJ* **2005**, *331*, 903. [CrossRef]
10. Wan, X.; Wang, W.; Liu, J.; Tong, T. Estimating the sample mean and standard deviation from the sample size, median, range and/or interquartile range. *BMC Med. Res. Methodol.* **2014**, *14*, 135. [CrossRef]
11. Sterne, J.A.C.; Savović, J.; Page, M.J.; Elbers, R.G.; Blencowe, N.S.; Boutron, I.; Cates, C.J.; Cheng, H.-Y.; Corbett, M.S.; Eldridge, S.M.; et al. RoB 2: A revised tool for assessing risk of bias in randomised trials. *BMJ* **2019**, *366*, l4898. [CrossRef]
12. Shim, S.R.; Kim, S.J.; Lee, J.; Rücker, G. Network meta-analysis: Application and practice using R software. *Epidemiol. Health* **2019**, *41*, e2019013. [CrossRef] [PubMed]
13. Dias, S.; Caldwell, D.M. Network meta-analysis explained. *Arch. Dis. Child. Fetal Neonatal Ed.* **2019**, *104*, F8–F12. [CrossRef] [PubMed]
14. Jansen, J.P.; Fleurence, R.; Devine, B.; Itzler, R.; Barrett, A.; Hawkins, N.; Lee, K.; Boersma, C.; Annemans, L.; Cappelleri, J.C. Interpreting indirect treatment comparisons and network meta-analysis for health-care decision making: Report of the ISPOR Task Force on Indirect Treatment Comparisons Good Research Practices: Part 1. *Value Health* **2011**, *14*, 417–428. [CrossRef] [PubMed]
15. Rhodes, K.M.; Turner, R.M.; Higgins, J.P. Predictive distributions were developed for the extent of heterogeneity in meta-analyses of continuous outcome data. *J. Clin. Epidemiol.* **2015**, *68*, 52–60. [CrossRef]
16. Mbuagbaw, L.; Rochwerg, B.; Jaeschke, R.; Heels-Andsell, D.; Alhazzani, W.; Thabane, L.; Guyatt, G.H. Approaches to interpreting and choosing the best treatments in network meta-analyses. *Syst. Rev.* **2017**, *6*, 79. [CrossRef]
17. RStudio Team. *RStudio: Integrated Development Environment for R*; RStudio, PBC: Boston, MA, USA, 2020. Available online: http://www.rstudio.com/ (accessed on 30 May 2024).
18. Balduzzi, S.; Rücker, G.; Nikolakopoulou, A.; Papakonstantinou, T.; Salanti, G.; Efthimiou, O.; Schwarzer, G. netmeta: An R Package for Network Meta-Analysis Using Frequentist Methods. *J. Stat. Softw.* **2023**, *106*, 1–40. [CrossRef]

19. van Valkenhoef, G.; Kuiper, J. gemtc: Network Meta-Analysis Using Bayesian Methods. 2023. Available online: https://cran.r-project.org/web/packages/gemtc/gemtc.pdf (accessed on 30 May 2024).
20. Plummer, M. rjags: Bayesian Graphical Models Using MCMC. 2024. Available online: https://cran.r-project.org/web//packages/rjags/rjags.pdf (accessed on 19 August 2024).
21. Nikolakopoulou, A.; Higgins, J.P.T.; Papakonstantinou, T.; Chaimani, A.; Del Giovane, C.; Egger, M.; Salanti, G. CINeMA: An approach for assessing confidence in the results of a network meta-analysis. *PLoS Med.* **2020**, *17*, e1003082. [CrossRef]
22. Ahmann, A.J.; Capehorn, M.; Charpentier, G.; Dotta, F.; Henkel, E.; Lingvay, I.; Holst, A.G.; Annett, M.P.; Aroda, V.R. Efficacy and Safety of Once-Weekly Semaglutide Versus Exenatide ER in Subjects With Type 2 Diabetes (SUSTAIN 3): A 56-Week, Open-Label, Randomized Clinical Trial. *Diabetes Care* **2018**, *41*, 258–266. [CrossRef]
23. Aroda, V.R.; Bain, S.C.; Cariou, B.; Piletic, M.; Rose, L.; Axelsen, M.; Rowe, E.; DeVries, J.H. Efficacy and safety of once-weekly semaglutide versus once-daily insulin glargine as add-on to metformin (with or without sulfonylureas) in insulin-naive patients with type 2 diabetes (SUSTAIN 4): A randomised, open-label, parallel-group, multicentre, multinational, phase 3a trial. *Lancet Diabetes Endocrinol.* **2017**, *5*, 355–366. [CrossRef]
24. Bajaj, H.S.; Bergenstal, R.M.; Christoffersen, A.; Davies, M.J.; Gowda, A.; Isendahl, J.; Lingvay, I.; Senior, P.A.; Silver, R.J.; Trevisan, R.; et al. Switching to Once-Weekly Insulin Icodec Versus Once-Daily Insulin Glargine U100 in Type 2 Diabetes Inadequately Controlled on Daily Basal Insulin: A Phase 2 Randomized Controlled Trial. *Diabetes Care* **2021**, *44*, 1586–1594. [CrossRef]
25. Blonde, L.; Jendle, J.; Gross, J.; Woo, V.; Jiang, H.; Fahrbach, J.L.; Milicevic, Z. Once-weekly dulaglutide versus bedtime insulin glargine, both in combination with prandial insulin lispro, in patients with type 2 diabetes (AWARD-4): A randomised, open-label, phase 3, non-inferiority study. *Lancet* **2015**, *385*, 2057–2066. [CrossRef]
26. Diamant, M.; Van Gaal, L.; Stranks, S.; Northrup, J.; Cao, D.; Taylor, K.; Trautmann, M. Once weekly exenatide compared with insulin glargine titrated to target in patients with type 2 diabetes (DURATION-3): An open-label randomised trial. *Lancet* **2010**, *375*, 2234–2243. [CrossRef] [PubMed]
27. Frias, J.; Chien, J.; Zhang, Q.; Chigutsa, E.; Landschulz, W.; Syring, K.; Wullenweber, P.; Haupt, A.; Kazda, C. Safety and efficacy of once-weekly basal insulin Fc in people with type 2 diabetes previously treated with basal insulin: A multicentre, open-label, randomised, phase 2 study. *Lancet Diabetes Endocrinol.* **2023**, *11*, 158–168. [CrossRef]
28. Frías, J.P.; Auerbach, P.; Bajaj, H.S.; Fukushima, Y.; Lingvay, I.; Macura, S.; Søndergaard, A.L.; Tankova, T.I.; Tentolouris, N.; Buse, J.B. Efficacy and safety of once-weekly semaglutide 2·0 mg versus 1·0 mg in patients with type 2 diabetes (SUSTAIN FORTE): A double-blind, randomised, phase 3B trial. *Lancet Diabetes Endocrinol.* **2021**, *9*, 563–574. [CrossRef]
29. Frías, J.P.; Davies, M.J.; Rosenstock, J.; Pérez Manghi, F.C.; Fernández Landó, L.; Bergman, B.K.; Liu, B.; Cui, X.; Brown, K. Tirzepatide versus Semaglutide Once Weekly in Patients with Type 2 Diabetes. *N. Engl. J. Med.* **2021**, *385*, 503–515. [CrossRef] [PubMed]
30. Gao, L.; Lee, B.W.; Chawla, M.; Kim, J.; Huo, L.; Du, L.; Huang, Y.; Ji, L. Tirzepatide versus insulin glargine as second-line or third-line therapy in type 2 diabetes in the Asia-Pacific region: The SURPASS-AP-Combo trial. *Nat. Med.* **2023**, *29*, 1500–1510. [CrossRef]
31. Giorgino, F.; Benroubi, M.; Sun, J.H.; Zimmermann, A.G.; Pechtner, V. Efficacy and Safety of Once-Weekly Dulaglutide Versus Insulin Glargine in Patients With Type 2 Diabetes on Metformin and Glimepiride (AWARD-2). *Diabetes Care* **2015**, *38*, 2241–2249. [CrossRef]
32. Inagaki, N.; Atsumi, Y.; Oura, T.; Saito, H.; Imaoka, T. Efficacy and safety profile of exenatide once weekly compared with insulin once daily in Japanese patients with type 2 diabetes treated with oral antidiabetes drug(s): Results from a 26-week, randomized, open-label, parallel-group, multicenter, noninferiority study. *Clin. Ther.* **2012**, *34*, 1892–1908.e1891. [CrossRef]
33. Inagaki, N.; Takeuchi, M.; Oura, T.; Imaoka, T.; Seino, Y. Efficacy and safety of tirzepatide monotherapy compared with dulaglutide in Japanese patients with type 2 diabetes (SURPASS J-mono): A double-blind, multicentre, randomised, phase 3 trial. *Lancet Diabetes Endocrinol.* **2022**, *10*, 623–633. [CrossRef] [PubMed]
34. Kimura, T.; Katakura, Y.; Shimoda, M.; Kawasaki, F.; Yamabe, M.; Tatsumi, F.; Matsuki, M.; Iwamoto, Y.; Anno, T.; Fushimi, Y.; et al. Comparison of clinical efficacy and safety of weekly glucagon-like peptide-1 receptor agonists dulaglutide and semaglutide in Japanese patients with type 2 diabetes: Randomized, parallel-group, multicentre, open-label trial (COMING study). *Diabetes Obes. Metab.* **2023**, *25*, 3632–3647. [CrossRef]
35. Lingvay, I.; Asong, M.; Desouza, C.; Gourdy, P.; Kar, S.; Vianna, A.; Vilsboll, T.; Vinther, S.; Mu, Y. Once-Weekly Insulin Icodec vs Once-Daily Insulin Degludec in Adults With Insulin-Naive Type 2 Diabetes: The ONWARDS 3 Randomized Clinical Trial. *JAMA* **2023**, *330*, 228–237. [CrossRef] [PubMed]
36. Ludvik, B.; Giorgino, F.; Jodar, E.; Frias, J.P.; Fernandez Lando, L.; Brown, K.; Bray, R.; Rodriguez, A. Once-weekly tirzepatide versus once-daily insulin degludec as add-on to metformin with or without SGLT2 inhibitors in patients with type 2 diabetes (SURPASS-3): A randomised, open-label, parallel-group, phase 3 trial. *Lancet* **2021**, *398*, 583–598. [CrossRef] [PubMed]
37. Mathieu, C.; Ásbjörnsdóttir, B.; Bajaj, H.S.; Lane, W.; Matos, A.; Murthy, S.; Stachlewska, K.; Rosenstock, J. Switching to once-weekly insulin icodec versus once-daily insulin glargine U100 in individuals with basal-bolus insulin-treated type 2 diabetes (ONWARDS 4): A phase 3a, randomised, open-label, multicentre, treat-to-target, non-inferiority trial. *Lancet* **2023**, *401*, 1929–1940. [CrossRef] [PubMed]

38. Philis-Tsimikas, A.; Asong, M.; Franek, E.; Jia, T.; Rosenstock, J.; Stachlewska, K.; Watada, H.; Kellerer, M. Switching to once-weekly insulin icodec versus once-daily insulin degludec in individuals with basal insulin-treated type 2 diabetes (ONWARDS 2): A phase 3a, randomised, open label, multicentre, treat-to-target trial. *Lancet Diabetes Endocrinol.* **2023**, *11*, 414–425. [CrossRef]
39. Pratley, R.E.; Aroda, V.R.; Lingvay, I.; Lüdemann, J.; Andreassen, C.; Navarria, A.; Viljoen, A. Semaglutide versus dulaglutide once weekly in patients with type 2 diabetes (SUSTAIN 7): A randomised, open-label, phase 3b trial. *Lancet Diabetes Endocrinol.* **2018**, *6*, 275–286. [CrossRef]
40. Del Prato, S.; Kahn, S.E.; Pavo, I.; Weerakkody, G.J.; Yang, Z.; Doupis, J.; Aizenberg, D.; Wynne, A.G.; Riesmeyer, J.S.; Heine, R.J.; et al. Tirzepatide versus insulin glargine in type 2 diabetes and increased cardiovascular risk (SURPASS-4): A randomised, open-label, parallel-group, multicentre, phase 3 trial. *Lancet* **2021**, *398*, 1811–1824. [CrossRef]
41. Rosenstock, J.; Bain, S.C.; Gowda, A.; Jodar, E.; Liang, B.; Lingvay, I.; Nishida, T.; Trevisan, R.; Mosenzon, O.; Investigators, O.T. Weekly Icodec versus Daily Glargine U100 in Type 2 Diabetes without Previous Insulin. *N. Engl. J. Med.* **2023**, *389*, 297–308. [CrossRef]
42. Rosenstock, J.; Bajaj, H.S.; Janež, A.; Silver, R.; Begtrup, K.; Hansen, M.V.; Jia, T.; Goldenberg, R. Once-weekly insulin for type 2 diabetes without previous insulin treatment. *N. Engl. J. Med.* **2020**, *383*, 2107–2116. [CrossRef]
43. Takahashi, Y.; Nomoto, H.; Yokoyama, H.; Takano, Y.; Nagai, S.; Tsuzuki, A.; Cho, K.Y.; Miya, A.; Kameda, H.; Takeuchi, J.; et al. Improvement of glycaemic control and treatment satisfaction by switching from liraglutide or dulaglutide to subcutaneous semaglutide in patients with type 2 diabetes: A multicentre, prospective, randomized, open-label, parallel-group comparison study (SWITCH-SEMA 1 study). *Diabetes Obes. Metab.* **2023**, *25*, 1503–1511. [CrossRef]
44. Tuttle, K.R.; Lakshmanan, M.C.; Rayner, B.; Busch, R.S.; Zimmermann, A.G.; Woodward, D.B.; Botros, F.T. Dulaglutide versus insulin glargine in patients with type 2 diabetes and moderate-to-severe chronic kidney disease (AWARD-7): A multicentre, open-label, randomised trial. *Lancet Diabetes Endocrinol.* **2018**, *6*, 605–617. [CrossRef]
45. Wang, J.; Li, H.-Q.; Xu, X.-H.; Kong, X.-C.; Sun, R.; Jing, T.; Ye, L.; Su, X.-F.; Ma, J.-H. The Effects of Once-Weekly Dulaglutide and Insulin Glargine on Glucose Fluctuation in Poorly Oral-Antidiabetic Controlled Patients with Type 2 Diabetes Mellitus. *BioMed Res. Int.* **2019**, *2019*, 2682657. [CrossRef] [PubMed]
46. Bue-Valleskey, J.M.; Kazda, C.M.; Ma, C.; Chien, J.; Zhang, Q.; Chigutsa, E.; Landschulz, W.; Haupt, A.; Frias, J.P. Once-Weekly Basal Insulin Fc Demonstrated Similar Glycemic Control to Once-Daily Insulin Degludec in Insulin-Naive Patients with Type 2 Diabetes: A Phase 2 Randomized Control Trial. *Diabetes Care* **2023**, *46*, 1060–1067. [CrossRef] [PubMed]
47. Brown, A.; Guess, N.; Dornhorst, A.; Taheri, S.; Frost, G. Insulin-associated weight gain in obese type 2 diabetes mellitus patients: What can be done? *Diabetes Obes. Metab.* **2017**, *19*, 1655–1668. [CrossRef] [PubMed]
48. Hayes, M.R.; Borner, T.; De Jonghe, B.C. The Role of GIP in the Regulation of GLP-1 Satiety and Nausea. *Diabetes* **2021**, *70*, 1956–1961. [CrossRef]
49. Umpierrez, G.; Tofé Povedano, S.; Pérez Manghi, F.; Shurzinske, L.; Pechtner, V. Efficacy and safety of dulaglutide monotherapy versus metformin in type 2 diabetes in a randomized controlled trial (AWARD-3). *Diabetes Care* **2014**, *37*, 2168–2176. [CrossRef]
50. Wysham, C.; Blevins, T.; Arakaki, R.; Colon, G.; Garcia, P.; Atisso, C.; Kuhstoss, D.; Lakshmanan, M. Efficacy and safety of dulaglutide added onto pioglitazone and metformin versus exenatide in type 2 diabetes in a randomized controlled trial (AWARD-1). *Diabetes Care* **2014**, *37*, 2159–2167. [CrossRef]
51. Weinstock, R.S.; Guerci, B.; Umpierrez, G.; Nauck, M.A.; Skrivanek, Z.; Milicevic, Z. Safety and efficacy of once-weekly dulaglutide versus sitagliptin after 2 years in metformin-treated patients with type 2 diabetes (AWARD-5): A randomized, phase III study. *Diabetes Obes. Metab.* **2015**, *17*, 849–858. [CrossRef]
52. Dungan, K.M.; Povedano, S.T.; Forst, T.; Gonzalez, J.G.G.; Atisso, C.; Sealls, W.; Fahrbach, J.L. Once-weekly dulaglutide versus once-daily liraglutide in metformin-treated patients with type 2 diabetes (AWARD-6): A randomised, open-label, phase 3, non-inferiority trial. *Lancet* **2014**, *384*, 1349–1357. [CrossRef]
53. Dungan, K.M.; Weitgasser, R.; Perez Manghi, F.; Pintilei, E.; Fahrbach, J.L.; Jiang, H.H.; Shell, J.; Robertson, K.E. A 24-week study to evaluate the efficacy and safety of once-weekly dulaglutide added on to glimepiride in type 2 diabetes (AWARD-8). *Diabetes Obes. Metab.* **2016**, *18*, 475–482. [CrossRef]
54. Pozzilli, P.; Norwood, P.; Jodar, E.; Davies, M.J.; Ivanyi, T.; Jiang, H.; Woodward, D.B.; Milicevic, Z. Placebo-controlled, randomized trial of the addition of once-weekly glucagon-like peptide-1 receptor agonist dulaglutide to titrated daily insulin glargine in patients with type 2 diabetes (AWARD-9). *Diabetes Obes. Metab.* **2017**, *19*, 1024–1031. [CrossRef]
55. Chen, Y.H.; Huang, C.-N.; Cho, Y.M.; Li, P.; Gu, L.; Wang, F.; Yang, J.; Wang, W.Q. Efficacy and safety of dulaglutide monotherapy compared with glimepiride in East-Asian patients with type 2 diabetes in a multicentre, double-blind, randomized, parallel-arm, active comparator, phase III trial. *Diabetes Obes. Metab.* **2018**, *20*, 2121–2130. [CrossRef] [PubMed]
56. Battelino, T.; Bergenstal, R.M.; Rodriguez, A.; Fernandez Lando, L.; Bray, R.; Tong, Z.; Brown, K. Efficacy of once-weekly tirzepatide versus once-daily insulin degludec on glycaemic control measured by continuous glucose monitoring in adults with type 2 diabetes (SURPASS-3 CGM): A substudy of the randomised, open-label, parallel-group, phase 3 SURPASS-3 trial. *Lancet Diabetes Endocrinol.* **2022**, *10*, 407–417. [CrossRef] [PubMed]

57. Gastaldelli, A.; Cusi, K.; Fernández Landó, L.; Bray, R.; Brouwers, B.; Rodríguez, Á. Effect of tirzepatide versus insulin degludec on liver fat content and abdominal adipose tissue in people with type 2 diabetes (SURPASS-3 MRI): A substudy of the randomised, open-label, parallel-group, phase 3 SURPASS-3 trial. *Lancet Diabetes Endocrinol.* **2022**, *10*, 393–406. [CrossRef] [PubMed]
58. Wilson, J.M.; Nikooienejad, A.; Robins, D.A.; Roell, W.C.; Riesmeyer, J.S.; Haupt, A.; Duffin, K.L.; Taskinen, M.R.; Ruotolo, G. The dual glucose-dependent insulinotropic peptide and glucagon-like peptide-1 receptor agonist, tirzepatide, improves lipoprotein biomarkers associated with insulin resistance and cardiovascular risk in patients with type 2 diabetes. *Diabetes Obes. Metab.* **2020**, *22*, 2451–2459. [CrossRef]

MDPI AG
Grosspeteranlage 5
4052 Basel
Switzerland
Tel.: +41 61 683 77 34

Biomedicines Editorial Office
E-mail: biomedicines@mdpi.com
www.mdpi.com/journal/biomedicines

www.ingramcontent.com/pod-product-compliance
Lightning Source LLC
Chambersburg PA
CBHW061841210926
51850CB00006B/942
* 9 7 8 3 7 2 5 8 5 5 5 7 5 *